# THE HERBAL RESURRECTION

*A Foundational Framework for Modern Western Herbal Practice*

Featuring 282 Fully Explained Herbs · The Fifteen Core Herbal Categories · The Foundational 52

**Fred V. Jenkins**

*Author · Herbal Researcher · System Developer*

Herbal Resurrection Publishing · ISBN 979-8-9953605-1-6

**The Herbal Resurrection**
*A Foundational Framework for Modern Western Herbal Practice*


Published by
**Herbal Resurrection Publishing**

For updates, educational materials, and instructor resources related to this work, visit:
**www.herbalresurrection.com**

This work is intended for educational and informational purposes and is designed to support the study and understanding of herbal medicine.

Cataloging information for this title is available from the publisher.

ISBN: 979-8-9953605-1-6

Printed and distributed by **IngramSpark**

# Dedication

This work is dedicated to the memory and legacy of Dr. Sebi, and to the never-ending mission of today's remarkable herbalists and healers – Rosemary Gladstar, David Winston, Stephen Buhner, Dr. Yahki Rapha Eloh, and countless others whose wisdom and tireless devotion to healing continue to uplift, encourage, and inspire me everyday.

Within these pages lies my humble contribution to the enduring work of these masterful herbal practitioners.

To my beloved daughter Shanise – your light and constant encouragement have carried me through the most worrisome times.

To my big sister Peggy — thank you for always being there with honest advice and love. I miss you, Sis.

And to my dear mother Ruth, who has gone on to her reward – your nurturing and loving spirit continues to guide me still all the time — to this day.

Much love to you all my family.

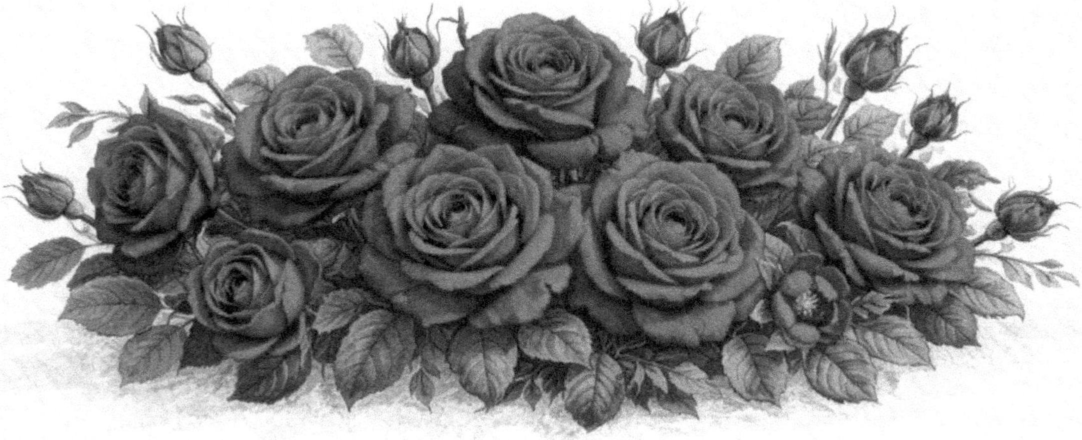

# Preface

In every generation, people have looked to the earth for answers, for relief, and for renewal. The plants recorded in this book are not just remedies of old — they are living reminders that healing has always been within reach. Nature has preserved these herbs with a purpose: to restore balance to our bodies, clarity to your minds, and peace to your spirits.

This book is not simply a listing of plants and their uses. It is a *resurrection* — a return to truths that modern life has tried to bury, but which remain as vital as the very breath itself. My hope is that you, the reader, will see in these pages not only practical remedies but also a reflection of divine order: that nothing has been created without a cure, and no ailment is without some answer in nature's design.

As you read, you join a long line of *seekers* who trusted in the *Creator's* provision and in the quiet power of Mother earth. May this work guide you, steady you, and remind you that you are never far from the healing you need.

— *Fred Vincent Jenkins*

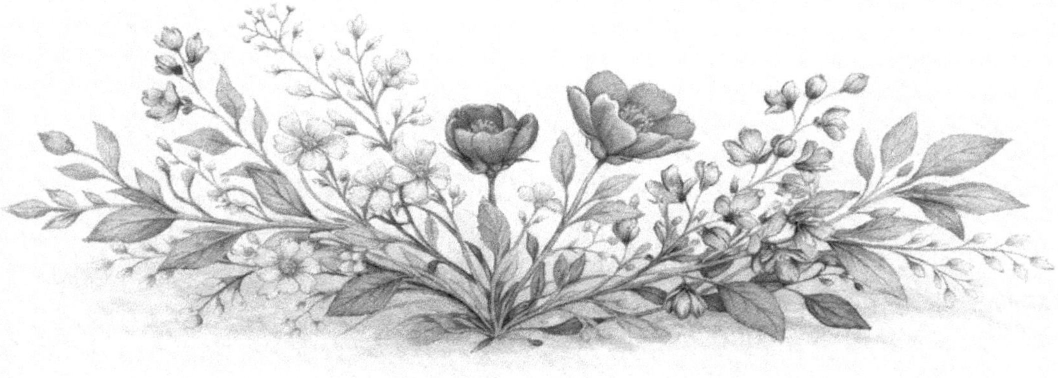

## What is The Foundation of Modern Herbal Practice?

**The foundation of modern herbal practice is the integration of traditional herbal wisdom, system-based energetics, disciplined materia medica knowledge, ethical safety standards, and evidence-informed application—used to support the whole person rather than suppress isolated symptoms.**

Modern herbal practice today draws upon long-established traditions while applying structured understanding and responsible use. Herbs are studied individually according to their actions, energetics, preparation methods, and safety considerations, and are applied within the context of human physiology rather than isolated conditions. This book teaches recognition, understanding, and responsible use—not diagnosis or medical treatment.

Rather than focusing solely on symptom relief, modern herbalism emphasizes system-based balance and pattern recognition across areas such as digestion, circulation, immunity, inflammation, and nervous system function. Ethical use, informed dosage, and safety awareness are central to this approach, which respects herbs as whole, synergistic agents that support long-term balance and resilience.

# Safety Notes & Responsible Use

Herbs can be effective allies. You should 'always' use them with care, common sense, and respect for your body.

**Quick Principles**

• **Start low and go slow**. Try one new herb at a time first.
• **Choose quality**: use reputable, identity-tested sources.
• **Match the herb to the person** (age, medications, health goals).

**Who Should obtain Medical advice before herbal intervention**

• **Pregnant or nursing individuals**; infants and young children.
• **People with chronic conditions** (heart, liver, kidney, autoimmune, psychiatric).
• **Anyone taking prescription meds** (anticoagulants, heart meds, antidepressants, diabetes, anti-seizure, immunosuppressants).
• **Those scheduled for surgery** (pause non-essential herbs ~2 weeks prior unless advised otherwise).

**Common Interactions & Cautions (examples)**

• **Anticoagulants**: ginkgo, garlic, ginseng, ginger, turmeric may increase bleeding risk.
• **St. John's wort:** can reduce levels of many meds (e.g., antidepressants, birth control).
• **Blood pressure/heart meds:** whole-root licorice may raise Blood pressure; Hawthorn can potentiate cardiac effects.
• **Sedatives/CNS depressants:** go slowly with valerian, kava, hops.
• **Liver health:** avoid internal comfrey; use caution with high-dose or prolonged kava.

**Topical & Preparations**

• **Patch test salves/essential-oil blends;** dilute essential oils properly (many are not for internal use).
• **Tinctures contain alcohol;** choose glycerites if sensitive.
• **Allergies:** if sensitive to a plant family (e.g., ragweed for chamomile), proceed cautiously.

**Sourcing & Storage**

• Prefer identity-tested herbs from reputable suppliers; avoid endangered species and questionable wildcrafting.
• Store dried herbs in airtight jars away from heat/light; typical shelf life ~6–12 months (aromatics fade sooner).

**When to Seek Medical Care (Do Not Delay)**

• Trouble breathing, chest pain, severe allergic reaction (swelling, hives).
• Fainting, severe abdominal pain, blood in stool/vomit.
• Sudden neurological symptoms (weakness, slurred speech) or high fever that persists.

The information presented in this book is for educational purposes only and is not intended as a substitute for professional medical advice, diagnosis, or treatment. Always consult a qualified healthcare professional before making any health-related decisions.

The "Scientific Backing" summaries throughout this book are educational overviews based on published botanical, pharmacological, and clinical literature. They are intended to introduce the current state of scientific evidence relating to traditional and modern herbal use rather than to provide exhaustive literature reviews for each individual herb. Readers wishing to explore the primary scientific literature are encouraged to consult Appendix A — *Selected Scientific Literature for Further Study* — where representative peer-reviewed studies, authoritative monographs, and additional scientific resources are organized according to the Fifteen Core Herbal Categories used throughout this book.

# TABLE OF CONTENTS

*The Herbal Resurrection — Fred V. Jenkins*


**FRONT MATTER**

| | |
|---|---|
| Title Page | i |
| Copyright Page | ii |
| Dedication | iii |
| Preface | vi |
| What is the Foundation of Modern Herbal Practice? | vii |
| Safety Notes & Responsible Use | viii |
| Disclaimer | ix |
| About the Scientific Backing Sections | ix |
| Table of Contents | x |
| The Herbal Resurrection — Opening Declaration | xi |
| Message to the Reader | xii–xiv |
| Heads Up Message | xv |
| The 15 Core Herbal Categories | xv–xvii |
| The Foundational 52 | xviii–xxi |
| How to Use This Book | xxii–xxvi |
| How the Book Is Rated & Rating Chart | xxvii–xxxii |
| Welcome to the Garden of Herbs | xxxiii |
| The Herb Garden (Illustration) | xxxiv |

**MAIN HERBAL SECTION**

| | |
|---|---|
| **Herb Pages (Aloe Vera to Zedoary)** | 1–903 |

**REFERENCE & STUDY SECTIONS**

| | |
|---|---|
| **Medical Herbal Support Charts I–XXXIII** | 905–982 |
| Symptoms Index | 983–988 |
| Glossary | 989–992 |
| Herb Index (Alphabetized) | 993–998 |
| Core Herbal Category Index | 999–1006 |
| Bonus Pages | 1007–1013 |

**BACK MATTER**

| | |
|---|---|
| Obtaining Herbs Safely and Responsibly | 1014–1016 |

| | |
|---|---|
| Thank You Page | 1018 |
| Appendix A: Selected Scientific Literature for Further Study | 1022–1066 |
| Additional Resources & Continuing Study | 1067–1068 |
| Herbal Resurrection Student Workbook | 1069–1070 |
| Herbal Resurrection Teacher's Manual | 1071–1072 |
| Selected Sources & Supporting Context | 1073–1074 |
| Architecture of the 15 Core Herbal Categories | 1075–1077 |
| Author Biography | 1078 |
| Review This Book | 1079 |
| For Those Who Wish to Study Herbalism Further | 1080–1082 |
| A Final Word, Closing Reflection & Disclaimer | 1083 |
| *Moon Over the Garden (Illustration)* | 1084 |
| Your Final Notes Page | 1085 |

# *THE HERBAL RESURRECTION'S OPENING DECLARATION*

***The Herbal Resurrection*** is more than a traditional herbal textbook—it is a carefully structured reference designed to serve as a reliable guide and long-term companion for those seeking a clearer and more organized approach to herbal study. It was created to bring together depth, clarity, structure, simplicity, and completeness into a single, unified, and practical resource.

This book was created to serve as both an anchor and a launch point—a foundational work for readers who wish to study and understand herbs with greater clarity and confidence. Rather than requiring readers to piece together information from multiple sources, *The Herbal Resurrection* brings herbal knowledge into a single, cohesive, and structured framework.

This volume presents a highly organized herbal reference designed to bring clarity to a complex field. In addition to serving as a detailed materia medica, it introduces a practical system for understanding, organizing, and applying herbal knowledge. This system is designed not only to present herbal information, but to develop the ability to distinguish between similar herbs based on real-world application and pattern recognition. **It is designed to support both independent study and structured learning.**

Within these pages, you will be introduced to two central pillars of this system:
- **The 15 Core Herbal Categories** — a functional classification system designed to organize the major therapeutic roles of medicinal herbs within modern Western practice.
- **The Foundational 52** — a curated body of cornerstone herbs representing essential plant knowledge that every developing herbal practitioner can benefit from understanding early in their study.

Together, these components establish a clear and efficient entry point into herbal study. They demonstrate how a focused group of foundational herbs can provide a strong working base for understanding and addressing many of the most common conditions encountered in everyday practice.

By combining breadth of content with a consistent structural approach, *The Herbal Resurrection* presents each herb in deliberate detail while organizing a wide-ranging materia medica within a single, unified system.
Rather than requiring readers to navigate multiple texts written from differing perspectives, *The Herbal Resurrection* offers a more consistent, structured, and accessible pathway into the study of herbal medicine.

## A Message to the Reader

### *Understanding the Heart of Herbal Mastery*

For thousands of years, healers across cultures—monks, midwives, shamans, physicians, and wise elders—have worked with plants not merely by memorizing endless lists, but by recognizing the patterns that unite herbs within coherent systems of healing. Through careful observation, tradition, and generations of practical application, a consistent understanding emerges:

**Herbal mastery does not begin with knowing hundreds of herbs.**
**It begins with understanding the patterns that connect them.**

Across global herbal traditions, a relatively small group of plants appears again and again. These herbs—or close botanical equivalents—have been relied upon for generations to address many of the most common conditions encountered in everyday life. In this book, these herbs are referred to as **The Foundational 52**.

In addition, when viewed through a functional lens, the vast majority of medicinal herbs commonly used in modern Western herbal practice can be meaningfully organized into one or more **15 Core Herbal Categories.** These 'categories' will be introduced to you in the following section.

These categories help clarify:

- **why an herb works**
- **how it supports the body**
- **when it may be most appropriate**
- **how to approach its use with safety**
- **and how herbs can be combined thoughtfully**

As these patterns become familiar, confusion begins to fade.
Clarity replaces guesswork and confidence replaces uncertainty.
This structure forms the foundation of *The Herbal Resurrection*.

---

### Why This Matters for You

Whether you are new to herbal study or continuing your learning, this book is designed to provide:

- a clear point of entry
- a consistent structure
- and a reliable way to understand how herbs function

Within these pages, you will learn:

• the 15 Core Herbal Categories
• how each herb expresses its functional role
• how to evaluate herbs with greater clarity
• how to approach their use with safety and awareness
• and how a focused group of foundational herbs can support a wide range of everyday concerns

## This is more than a reference book.

As you explore this work, you will begin to recognize what experienced healers throughout history have long understood:
**Herbal mastery is not about knowing many herbs—**
**but knowing the right ones, and knowing them well.**

Over time, patterns begin to emerge. Therapeutic tendencies become clearer, and herbs are seen not merely as individual remedies, but as part of a larger, more coherent system of understanding.

Through this perspective, the relationship between the **Foundational 52** and the **15 Core Herbal Categories** comes into clearer focus—revealing a practical and structured way to organize and approach Western herbal knowledge with greater consistency and confidence.

Welcome to *The Herbal Resurrection*—a work designed to bring clarity, structure, and a more coherent approach to the study of herbal medicine.

## One Moment Please.

Before you explore the unique and wonderful herb pages within this book, let me first show you the deeper logic behind its structure. To understand why the Foundational 52 are so useful, it is helpful to first understand the 15 Core Herbal Categories—how they function, how they interrelate, and how they simplify the vast world of herbal medicine into a form that is easier to understand.
What follows is the underlying framework that supports *The Herbal Resurrection*.

---

## The Architecture Behind the Herbs
## Understanding the 15 Core Herbal Categories and the Foundational 52

Before any herb can be fully understood, it must be placed within a larger structure. One of the greatest challenges in herbal study has never been a lack of information—but a lack of organization. Across cultures and traditions, thousands of herbs have been documented, each described through different languages, philosophies, and medical perspectives. For many learners, this abundance can lead not to clarity, but to confusion.

The structure presented in *The Herbal Resurrection* is designed to address that challenge.

Rather than organizing herbs solely by culture, geography, or botanical family, this work introduces a functional framework—a way of understanding what herbs do, how they behave in the body, and why certain plants appear consistently across healing traditions.

From this perspective emerge two central pillars that form the backbone of this framework:

---

# The Missing Map in Herbal Learning

The **15 Core Herbal Categories** did not originate from theory alone. They emerged through long-term pattern recognition—by observing how herbs behave across systems, cultures, and clinical traditions. When stripped of language differences and philosophical overlays, nearly all medicinal herbs naturally fall into functional roles that repeat consistently.

These roles form a unifying framework that simplifies the vast world of herbal medicine into a structure the human mind can actually work with.

In this book, **every herb is organized using the Universal 15 Core Herbal Categories**. Each herb in this book is assigned **one Primary Core**, reflecting its dominant role in the body, along with **Secondary Cores** that show additional areas of support that the herb also offers.

Here are the '15' Core herbal Categories that nearly all medicinal herbs fall under:

### The 15 Core Herbal Categories

---

#### 1. Adaptogens

Support stress resilience, recovery, and systemic balance across multiple body systems.
*(e.g., Ashwagandha, Rhodiola, Eleuthero)*

---

#### 2. Nervous System Support (Nervines)

Support nerve function, emotional balance, stress response, and sleep regulation.
*(e.g., Skullcap, Chamomile, St. John's Wort)*

---

#### 3. Digestive System Support

Support digestion, absorption, motility, and overall gut function.
*(e.g., Ginger, Peppermint, Fennel)*

---

#### 4. Immune System Support

Support, strengthen, and help regulate the body's immune response.
*(e.g., Echinacea, Astragalus, Reishi)*

---

#### 5. Respiratory System Support

Support lung function, airway clarity, mucus balance, and respiratory health.
*(e.g., Mullein, Thyme, Elecampane)*

---

#### 6. Cardiovascular System Support

Support heart function, circulation, blood flow, and vascular integrity.
*(e.g., Hawthorn, Cayenne, Ginkgo Biloba)*

---

#### 7. Anti-Inflammatory & Pain Support

Help reduce inflammation and support the body's natural pain response without suppressing healing.
*(e.g., Turmeric, Willow Bark, Boswellia)*

---

#### 8. Liver & Detoxification Support

Support liver function, bile flow, and the body's natural detoxification pathways.
*(e.g., Milk Thistle, Dandelion Root, Burdock Root)*

---

#### 9. Kidney & Urinary Support

Support fluid balance, filtration, mineral regulation, and urinary tract health.

*(e.g., Nettle, Corn Silk, Uva Ursi)*

---

**10. Endocrine & Hormonal Support**
Support hormonal balance and communication across endocrine glands.
*(e.g., Vitex, Maca, Licorice Root)*

---

**11. Lymphatic & Skin Support**
Support lymphatic movement, fluid drainage, and healthy skin expression.
*(e.g., Cleavers, Red Clover, Calendula)*

---

**12. Antimicrobial Support**
Provide natural defense against bacterial, viral, fungal, and parasitic challenges.
*(e.g., Garlic, Oregano, Olive Leaf)*

---

**13. Reproductive & Women's Health Support**
Support reproductive function, menstrual balance, uterine tone, and menopausal transition.
*(e.g., Red Raspberry Leaf, Dong Quai, Black Cohosh)*

---

**14. Nutritional & Tonic Support**
Provide nourishment, rebuild vitality, and support long-term tissue strength and resilience.
*(e.g., Nettle, Reishi, Astragalus)*

---

**15. Foundational / Systemic Support**
Support overall physiological balance by acting across multiple systems and improving the body's responsiveness.
*(e.g., Chamomile, Licorice Root, Yarrow)*

These categories act as a **map, not a method**. Their purpose is not to tell you *how* to use herbs, but to show you *where* each herb belongs within the larger landscape of medicinal healing. By understanding the Core Category an herb falls into, patterns begin to emerge—why different cultures may choose different plants to address the same condition, and why some herbs can substitute for one another while others cannot.

This shift—from memorizing long lists of individual herbs, as was common in the past, to understanding the **roles** herbs play and how they relate to one another—is what is believed will fuel the transformation of beginning herbal study 'today' from simple accumulation into true orderly comprehension.

## The Foundational 52 Under the Microscope
### *Why Mastery Does Not Require Hundreds of Herbs*

As the Core Categories become clear, another important pattern begins to emerge: not all herbs carry the same foundational importance.

Across medical systems worldwide, a relatively small group of herbs appears again and again. These plants are not prominent by accident. They are versatile, reliable, time-tested, and capable of addressing a wide range of common human conditions when properly understood.

In this book, this group of herbs is referred to as **The Foundational 52**.

The Foundational 52 represents a carefully selected collection of 52 essential herbs which, when understood and applied skillfully, provide a practical working foundation for supporting many of the most common health concerns encountered in everyday life by people.

These herbs form a functional core—capable of addressing a wide range of conditions—while also preparing the reader to understand and integrate additional herbs with greater clarity and confidence.

They have been selected not because other herbs lack value, but because these particular plants consistently demonstrate a combination of versatility, adaptability, and foundational usefulness across a broad range of applications.

Together, they provide a focused and efficient starting point for building herbal understanding without unnecessary complexity or overlap.

---

**Without further introduction, the following pages present this selected group of 52 foundational herbs:**

# THE FOUNDATIONAL 52

*The Universal Herbal Cabinet — 52 Cornerstone Herbs for Foundational Herbal Mastery*

---

| | |
|---|---|
| 1. *Ashwagandha* | 27. *Echinacea* |
| 2. *Astragalus* | 28. *Ginkgo Biloba* |
| 3. *Reishi* | 29. *Boswellia* |
| 4. *Ginger* | 30. *Willow Bark* |
| 5. *Turmeric* | 31. *Mullein* |
| 6. *Garlic* | 32. *Thyme* |
| 7. *Cayenne* | 33. *Oregano (Oil & Leaf)* |
| 8. *Hawthorn* | 34. *Olive Leaf* |
| 9. *Yarrow* | 35. *Fennel* |
| 10. *Slippery Elm* | 36. *Chamomile (Roman & German)* |
| 11. *Milk Thistle* | 37. *Marshmallow Root* |
| 12. *Agrimony* | 38. *Dandelion (Root & Leaf)* |
| 13. *Peppermint* | 39. *Plantain Leaf* |
| 14. *Licorice Root* | 40. *Corn Silk* |
| 15. *Cleavers* | 41. *Nettle (Leaf & Seed)* |
| 16. *Burdock Root* | 42. *Uva Ursi* |
| 17. *Red Clover* | 43. *Vitex (Chaste Tree Berry)* |
| 18. *Calendula* | 44. *Red Raspberry Leaf* |

| | |
|---|---|
| 19. *Skullcap* | 45. *Black Cohosh* |
| 20. *Lemon Balm* | 46. *Cramp Bark* |
| 21. *Passionflower* | 47. *Boneset* |
| 22. *St. John's Wort* | 48. *Motherwort* |
| 23. *Eleuthero* | 49. *Catnip* |
| 24. *Rhodiola* | 50. *Gentian* |
| 25. *Schisandra* | 51. *Horsetail* |
| 26. *Elderberry* | 52. *Cranesbill* |

## The Foundational 52 — The Universal Herbal Cabinet

These 52 cornerstone herbs, referred to throughout this book as the **Foundational 52**, represent far more than a simple list of plants. Together, they form a practical herbal cabinet—a focused collection capable of addressing many of the most common functional imbalances experienced across everyday life.

These include, but are not limited to, concerns related to inflammation, infection, digestion, pain, stress, bleeding, immune weakness, and circulatory imbalance. When understood by their functional roles rather than by isolated names alone, the herbs within the Foundational 52 provide a broad and useful working foundation for herbal understanding.

They have earned this designation not through novelty, but through consistency, reliability, versatility, and enduring usefulness across traditions and time.
For this reason, familiarity with both the **15 Core Herbal Categories** and the **Foundational 52** can provide readers with a strong foundation for deeper herbal study.

Together, they offer a clear structural starting point—one that helps replace confusion with clarity, and scattered information with a more organized understanding.
What has been presented here is the underlying framework that gives *The Herbal Resurrection* its structure and coherence. Its purpose is to orient the reader and to introduce a more organized way of approaching herbal knowledge.

At this time I invite you to set the framework aside for a moment and simply enjoy the book itself.
***The Herbal Resurrection: A Foundational Framework for Modern Western Herbal Practice*** was created to stand alone as a complete and unified reference—one that brings together depth, clarity, structure, and breadth in a single volume for study, reflection, and daily reference.
This is a book meant to remain with you over time—a companion to return to again and again as your understanding deepens.
Take your time.
Explore freely.
And above all—
**Enjoy.**

# HOW TO USE THIS BOOK

**A Gentle On-Ramp for Learning the Herbs**

---

## Before You Begin

If you are new to herbalism—or returning after time away—it's normal to feel a little unsure at first. Many people open a large herbal book and quietly wonder, *"Is this going to be too much for me?"*

Let's set that worry aside right now.

This book was written to be **learned slowly**, **used flexibly**, and **returned to often**. You are not expected to understand everything at once. You are not expected to memorize. And you are certainly not expected to be perfect.

Think of this book as a **guide**, not a test.

You can move through it at your own pace, pause when needed, and come back as often as you like. The herbs will still be here, and so will the learning.

---

## What This Book Is Meant to Do

Many beginner books focus on quick answers—*this herb for that symptom*. That can be helpful, but it often leaves people unsure **why** something works or **when** it might not.

This book takes a gentler, deeper approach.

Instead of rushing to outcomes, it helps you understand:

- what different herbs *do* in the body
- how they support systems rather than chase symptoms
- and how to choose herbs thoughtfully, not reactively

You don't need prior training to use this book. Curiosity and patience are enough to begin.

---

## How the Book Is Organized (In Simple Terms)

Every herb in this book is presented in the same basic way. Once you understand one page, the rest will feel familiar.

You may use this book like a **Table of Contents for healing**—finding a topic, system, or concern—and then reading more deeply where it feels relevant.

There are also charts and indexes to help you look things up quickly. You don't need to read from beginning to end. Most people don't.

---

# How to Read an Herb Page (Without Feeling Overwhelmed)

Let's walk through a page together.

### 🌿 Core Herbal Category

This section tells you the *type* of herb it is — which of the **15 Core Herbal Categories** it belongs to and what *function* it serves in the human body.
You can think of it like a **job description**.
For example, some herbs:

- nourish and rebuild
- calm and soothe
- stimulate movement or clearing

The **Primary Core** shows which of the 15 categories the herb falls under and the *main healing function* it performs best in the body.
The **Secondary Cores** explain the other *supporting functions* the herb also performs, but on a smaller scale than its primary role.
You don't need to memorize these — just notice the patterns as you read.

---

### 🌿 How It Works

This section explains, in plain language, **the manner in which the herb operates in the human body.**
If that sounds abstract, think of it this way:

- Some herbs help the body to *slow down*
- Some help it to *warm up*
- Some help it to *clear congestion*
- Some help it to *rebuild strength*

That's all this section is trying to show you.

---

### 🌱 Primary Uses

These are just the common, traditional ways that the herb has normally been used by people.

---

## 🔄 Same / Similar Foundation

This section highlights other herbs that share the **same or a closely related foundational role** in the body as the herb you are currently reviewing.
This does **not** mean the herbs are identical—no two herbs are ever truly the same. Each plant has its own chemistry, strengths, and safety profile. However, two or more herbs **can perform the same or a similar functional role** when supporting a particular system or condition.
This section is especially useful in three situations:

1. **Safety or contraindication:**
 When an herb cannot be used because a person has a medical condition, sensitivity, or medication conflict that could be adversely affected. In these cases, a different herb may be chosen that performs the same function **without posing the same risk**.

2. **Multiple conditions:**
 When a person has more than one condition to address, and an herb is needed that supports the primary concern **while also assisting a secondary condition**.

3. **Suitability and strength:**
 When an herb is too strong or not strong enough for the individual. This commonly applies to infants, older adults, pregnant or nursing individuals, or those who require a gentler or more targeted option.

Think of this section like a set of tools: a screwdriver and a wrench may both help complete a task, but they are not interchangeable. Each has a best use depending on the situation. This section helps readers make **appropriate, informed substitutions** while maintaining functional intent.

---

## ⭐ Herbal Confidence Index

This rating reflects how **reliable, safe, and consistent** an herb has been over time.
A lower rating does not mean an herb is weak or bad. Often, it means the herb is **strong and needs respect**, timing, or supervision.

---

# Where to Start If You're New

You do not need to start with the most powerful herbs.
Most beginners do best by first getting to know **gentle, supportive plants**—the ones that nourish, steady, and teach you how your body responds.
Good starting places include:

- Nutritive herbs

- Gentle immune supporters

- Digestive tonics
- Mild nervines (calming herbs that are not sedating)

These herbs allow learning through experience, not risk.
As confidence grows, understanding grows naturally with it.

---

## A Few Important Safety Notes

This book includes herbs of many strengths.
You will see:

- ● herbs that are broadly safe when used thoughtfully
- ● herbs that require moderation and awareness
- ● herbs that require professional supervision

If a page clearly says **"Supervision Required,"** please take that seriously. Those herbs are included for knowledge, not experimentation.
Learning herbalism is not about pushing limits. It's about **knowing where the edges are**.

---

## How to Study Without Stress

You don't need a schedule or a plan.
Many readers simply:

- read one herb at a time
- notice which ideas repeat
- compare similar herbs
- and slowly build familiarity

If something doesn't make sense right away, that's okay. Understanding often arrives *after* repetition.
Herbal learning is more like learning a language than memorizing facts. Over time, it begins to feel natural.

## A Final Reassurance

You don't have to rush.
You don't have to know everything.
You don't have to get it "right."
This book is meant to grow with you.
If you approach it with patience and respect, it will quietly teach you how to think, observe, and choose wisely—one herb at a time.
So don't worry about it. You'll get it. Just take your time. And if ever you don't understand something, simply read it again.

The 'next' page explains to you how 'each' of the herbs which appear in this book has received it's 'rating' by the author.

## Herbal Confidence Index — Explanation Page

Each herb featured in ***The Herbal Resurrection*** has been carefully evaluated and assigned a **Herbal Confidence Index** by this author to give readers a quick, trustworthy sense of an herb's overall reliability, safety, and effectiveness in everyday use.
Please keep in mind, however, that these are my *own* personal ratings, and they may or may not necessarily reflect the evaluations or conclusions of other knowledgeable herbalists, practitioners, researchers, or medical professionals. They are offered not as a replacement for established expertise, but as a carefully considered guide based on my own study, experience, and observations over time.

These ratings, however, reflect a balanced combination of scientific support, historical use, consistency of results, and safety profile, rather than popularity or marketing. They are based on long-term observation of how well each herb performs when used correctly and responsibly.

### Understanding the Star Levels

★★★★★ – **Cornerstone Herb**

Represents herbs of outstanding reputation and reliability — highly effective, safe for most users, and supported by both tradition and research. These are the "foundation herbs" of natural healing.

★★★★ – **Strong Herb**

Highly effective and dependable but may carry minor cautions, narrower dosage ranges, or have slightly stronger alternatives. Still a very good choice for regular use.

### ⭐⭐⭐ – **Moderate Herb**

Helpful and useful, yet requiring more attention to dosage, duration, or individual sensitivity. Often effective but less universal than the top tiers.

### ⭐⭐ – **Occasional Herb**

Herbs that show benefits only in certain situations, or where risk, toxicity, or limited data reduce confidence. May still serve a purpose with expert guidance.

### ⭐ – **Minimal or Experimental Herb**

Herbs with little proven reliability, normally are particularly 'dangerous' and are best avoided except under professional supervision. Included primarily for historical or educational completeness.

### 🌿 **Author's Choice Philosophy**

The Herbal Confidence Index is not a popularity scale. It is the author's personal measure of how trustworthy an herb truly is for ordinary people seeking safe, natural results.

Each rating balances the *power of the plant* with its *margin of safety* — giving more weight to herbs that can heal without harm, and less to those that require caution or complex preparation.

This page is meant to help you interpret the ratings found at the end of every herb's Herbal Reflections section. Use it as your guide for understanding the author's standards of quality and safety throughout this book.

# 🌿 Herbal Confidence Index — Reference Chart

(A Complement to the Author's Explanation)

| Star Rating | Title / Tier Name | Meaning & Reader Guidance | Example Herbs |
|---|---|---|---|
| ⭐⭐⭐⭐⭐ | **Cornerstone Herb** | Highly effective, safe for daily use, well-researched, globally trusted. Suitable for most adults when used moderately. | Chamomile · Nettle Leaf · Ginger · Milk Thistle · Fenugreek |
| ⭐⭐⭐⭐ | **Strong Herb** | Very effective and dependable but with mild cautions (e.g., dosage awareness or narrow range). | Oregano Oil · Hops · Sage · Valerian · Cinnamon |
| ⭐⭐⭐½ | **Balanced / Conditional Herb** | Useful for specific needs; safe for most users but requires attention to timing, combination, or user type. | Lady's Mantle · Nettle Seed · Lemon Balm · Maca Root |
| ⭐⭐⭐ | **Specialized Herb** | Potent and effective under certain conditions but not for routine or unsupervised use. | Tribulus · Black Cohosh · Bitter Melon · Ginkgo |
| ⭐⭐ | **High-Risk / Expert Herb** | May cause adverse effects or interact with medications; should be used with professional guidance only. | Goat's Rue · Calaguala · European Mistletoe |

| | | | |
|---|---|---|---|
| ⭐ | **Danger / Obsolete Herb** | Historically valuable but no longer recommended due to safety risks or toxicity; for external/educational reference only. | Pennyroyal · Tansy (internal use) |

---

**Color Code Reference:**

🟢 Green = Generally safe for self-use (Cornerstone & Strong Herbs)

🟡 Yellow = Caution; dose or duration awareness advised

🔴 Red = Use only under trained supervision or avoid entirely

## ⚠ Caution-Level Key

| Symbol | Color (digital) | Text Label | Meaning |
|---|---|---|---|
| ● | Green | **Safe (General Use)** | Broadly safe for self-care and daily use. |
| ● | Yellow | **Caution (Moderate Use)** | Use with dosage awareness or limited duration. |
| ● | Red | **Supervision Required** | Restricted; professional guidance or avoidance advised. |

**In black-and-white editions, read the **text label** instead of the color.
Each caution line throughout the book follows this same hybrid format which reads either: '**SAFE**', '**CAUTION**' or **'SUPERVISION REQUIRED'.**

---

## Author's Note

The Herbal Confidence Index reflects some several years of research, combining safety, consistency, and traditional respect for the plant world.
It helps readers instantly gauge whether a herb is:

- **Everyday-safe**,
- **Occasional or monitored**, or
- **Specialized for expert use.**

Read this chart together with the "🌿 **Herbal Confidence Index — Explanation Page"** for a complete understanding of how ratings are chosen.

*Ultrà iacet scientia quae tē līberābit.*

## Welcome to the Garden of Healing Herbs!

From the ancient temples of Egypt to the mountain valleys of China, from the rainforests of South America to the quiet meadows of Europe, *herbs have always been humankind's oldest companions in healing.* Long before modern medicine, communities around the globe relied on the wisdom of plants to restore balance, comfort pain, and bring wellness to both body and spirit.

The herbs you are about to explore in this book are drawn from *every corner of the world. Some have been revered for centuries as sacred tonics, while others were humble remedies passed down in family traditions. Together, they represent a living tapestry of natural medicine that continues to inspire and heal.*

In the pages that follow, you will discover:

- *The histories behind many herbs and how they were treasured by different cultures.*
- *Their primary uses, backed by traditional knowledge and modern insights.*
- *Guidance on forms and preparations, from teas to tinctures to oils.*
- *Practical notes on cautions, safe use, and expected results.*

This is not just a catalog of plants, but an invitation into a *tradition as old as* humanity itself – *a tradition where nature holds the key to vitality,* and *you're about to enter through that door.*

— *Perge* —

# le jardin des herbes

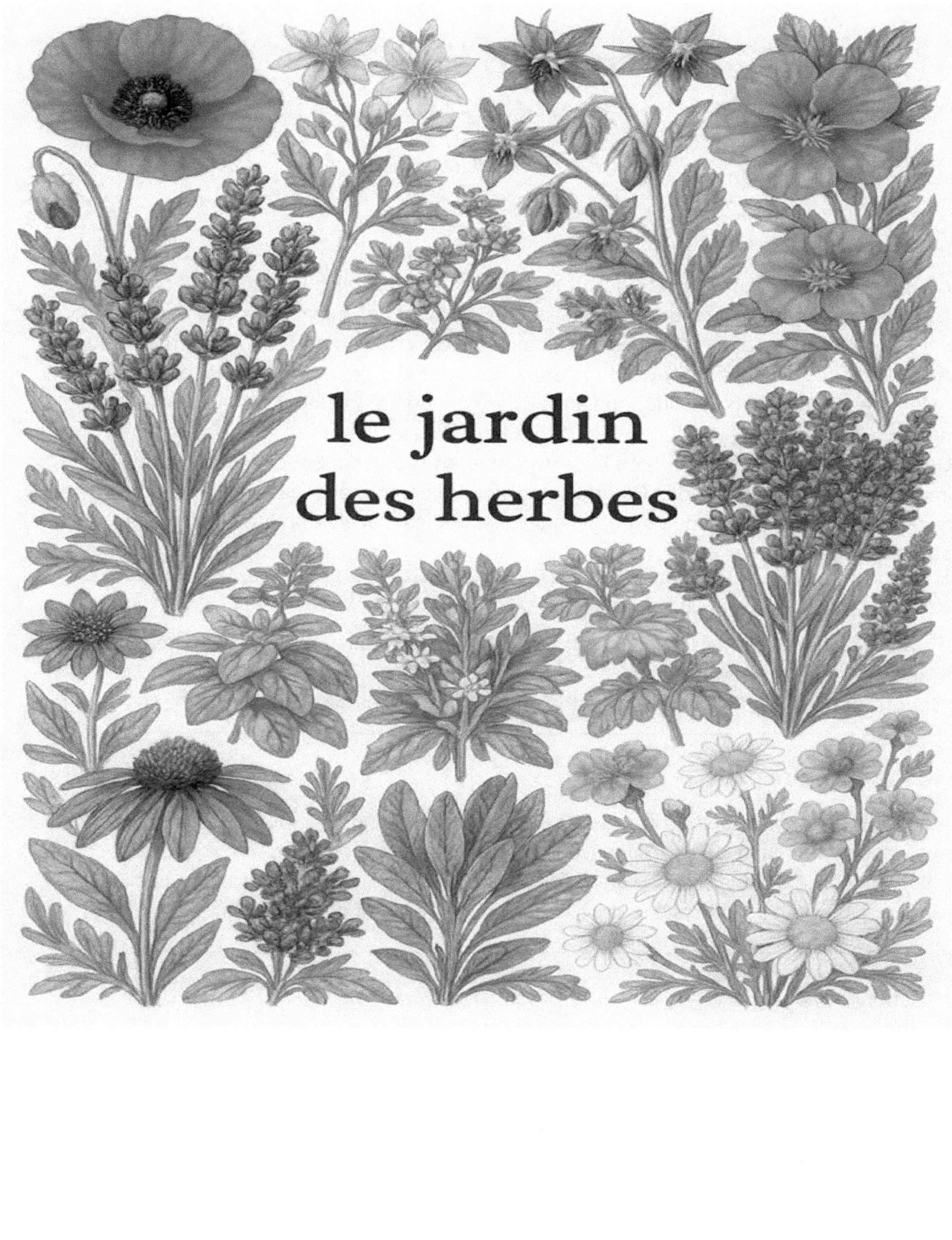

# ALOE VERA

★★★★★

*Aloe barbadensis*

**Aloe Vera** is a cooling, soothing herb widely used for burns, skin irritation, and digestive discomfort such as acid reflux and constipation. Its inner gel supports wound healing, hydrates dry tissue, reduces inflammation, and calms irritated mucous membranes. Internally, purified Aloe gel or juice is commonly used to gently cleanse the digestive tract, support immune response, and assist blood sugar balance, making it one of the most versatile household healing herbs.

Used for thousands of years, Aloe Vera was revered in ancient Egypt as the "plant of immortality" and recognized in Chinese medicine, Ayurveda, and classical Greek medicine. Its thick, succulent leaves and cooling gel have secured its place as both a medicinal and cosmetic staple across cultures.

---

🌿 **Core Herbal Category — Aloe Vera**

**Primary Core: Digestive System Support** with (cooling principles that calm heat and irritated tissues)

**Secondary Cores:** Digestive Support · Skin Support · Immune Support

---

## How It Works

Aloe Vera coats and soothes irritated tissues with mucilaginous compounds that reduce friction, heat, and inflammation. This protective layer supports tissue repair in the digestive tract and helps normalize bowel function. On the skin, Aloe hydrates, cools, and supports cellular regeneration, with its effects most noticeable in conditions of dryness, heat, or irritation.

---

## Primary Use

Soothes burns, wounds, eczema, and irritation
Heals digestive lining (ulcers, IBS, reflux)
Supports hydration and skin regeneration
Aids liver and colon detox
Supports nutrient absorption and gut flora balance

---

## Scientific Backing

Contains over 75 bioactive compounds, including vitamins A, C, E, B12, enzymes, and amino acids. Clinical studies demonstrate accelerated burn and wound healing, along with improvement in peptic ulcers due to anti-inflammatory and mucosal-protective effects.

---

## Forms Available

Fresh inner gel (from leaf)
Bottled gel or juice (inner fillet preferred)
Capsules or softgels
Topical creams and ointments
Freeze-dried powder

---

## How to Use (Dosage & Methods)

• **Internal (Juice/Gel):** 1–2 oz inner-leaf gel or juice once daily for digestive support. *(Avoid latex.)*
• **Capsules:** 300–500 mg freeze-dried inner leaf, 1–2× daily.
• **Topical Gel:** Apply thinly to irritated or burned skin 2–3× daily.
• **Smoothies:** Blend 1–2 tbsp fresh gel once daily.

---

## Caution Level ▨ Caution

Generally safe when used properly. The yellow latex beneath the leaf skin is a strong laxative and may irritate the intestines; avoid internal use of latex. Use purified inner fillet only.

---

## 🚹 🚺 Gender-Specific Safety

● **Men:** Supports digestive, skin, and immune balance without hormonal effects. Safe for topical use and short internal courses when sourced pure.

● **Women:** Helpful for digestive sluggishness, skin irritation, and heat-related imbalance. External use is safe; internal use should be moderate and periodic.

● **Pregnancy / Nursing:** Avoid internal use of latex or high-dose juice due to laxative and uterine-stimulating potential. External gel use is generally safe.

---

## ⌛ Expected Results

Topical relief: Immediate–24 hrs
Digestive support: 2–5 days
Skin healing: 7–14 days
Systemic benefits: 14–21 days

---

## DIY Recipe — Aloe Gut-Healing Juice

Blend 2 tbsp fresh inner Aloe gel with ½ cup cucumber, juice of ½ lemon, and 1 cup water. Drink once daily on an empty stomach.

---

## Same/Similar Results

● Slippery Elm, ● Marshmallow Root, ● Licorice Root, ● Chamomile, ● Plantain Leaf

---

## Shelf Life / Potency After Preparation

Fresh gel: 24–48 hrs refrigerated (strongest in first 24 hrs).
Bottled inner fillet juice: 1–2 months after opening (refrigerated).
Powder/freeze-dried: 12–24 months airtight.
Topical products: 12–18 months after opening.
Fresh blends: Best within 24 hrs refrigerated.

---

## Herbal Reflections of Aloe Vera

Aloe Vera reflects nature's cooling intelligence — a gentle balancer that soothes both surface and internal tissues. Beyond burns, it quietly nourishes cells, calms gut irritation, and supports renewal without forcing detox, making it a foundational herb for restoration and balance.

⭐ **Herbal Confidence Index:** 🌿 🌿 🌿 🌿 🌿 (5/5 green stars — a time-honored cornerstone herb revered for exceptional healing of skin, burns, and internal tissues; safe, versatile, and widely accessible.)

---

# AGRIMONY

★★★★

*Agrimonia eupatoria*

**Agrimony** is a gentle astringent herb used to relieve diarrhea, soothe indigestion, and reduce inflammation of the digestive tract. Its toning action supports the throat, gut, and urinary system while also assisting liver and gallbladder function. Traditionally, it has been valued for strengthening tissues, calming irritation, and supporting balanced digestion and metabolism. With deep roots in European folk medicine, Agrimony was historically associated with protection and healing. Its name derives from the Greek *argemone*, meaning "plant that heals the eye." Known for its small yellow flowers and mild fragrance, it has remained a dependable remedy since medieval times.

---

🌿 **Core Herbal Category — Agrimony**
**Primary Core: Digestive System Support** with (toning principles that gently tighten and restore tissue integrity)
**Secondary Cores:** Digestive · Liver & Gallbladder · Urinary · Nervous System · Foundational / Systemic Support

---

## How It Works

Agrimony works through gentle astringent compounds that tone and strengthen irritated or weakened tissues without excessive dryness. This action restores integrity to the digestive and urinary linings. Mild bitter compounds stimulate liver and gallbladder function, while subtle nervine effects help ease internal tension that can aggravate digestive imbalance.

---

## Primary Uses

Relieves diarrhea and gastrointestinal inflammation
Soothes sore throat and mouth ulcers (gargle)
Supports liver and gallbladder detox
Promotes healing of minor cuts and wounds
Strengthens bladder and urinary tract tone

---

## Scientific Backing

Contains tannins, flavonoids, and coumarins with mild antimicrobial, antioxidant, and anti-inflammatory effects. Small studies support traditional use for soothing mucous membranes and improving tissue tone in the digestive and urinary systems.

---

## Forms Available

Dried herb (tea)
Tincture or liquid extract
Capsules or tablets
Topical compress or poultice

---

## How to Use (Dosage & Methods)

- **Tea:** 1–2 tsp dried herb per cup hot water; steep 10–15 min. Drink 1–2× daily.
- **Tincture:** 2–4 mL, up to 3× daily.
- **Gargle:** Strong tea used warm for sore throat or mouth irritation.
- **Topical:** Apply cooled tea or diluted tincture to minor skin issues.

---

## Shelf Life / Potency After Preparation

Dried herb: 1–2 years airtight.
Prepared tea: 12–24 hrs refrigerated.
Tinctures: 3–5 years.
Tea and gargles are most potent within the first 6–12 hrs; topical preparations work best when freshly made.

---

## Caution Level ▨ Caution

Generally well tolerated. Excess use may reduce iron absorption due to tannins. Consult a practitioner if using blood-pressure or diabetes medications.

---

## 🚹 🚺 Gender-Specific Safety

● **Men:** Supports liver, digestion, and urinary comfort. Useful for mild hemorrhoids or digestive sluggishness. Avoid prolonged heavy use.
● **Women:** Traditionally used to tone tissues, ease menstrual discomfort, and reduce digestive bloating. Safe as tea or mild extract.
● **Pregnancy / Nursing:** Use cautiously due to mild uterine-toning effects. Occasional weak tea is generally tolerated; avoid concentrated tinctures without guidance.

---

## ⌛ Expected Results

Digestive relief: 1–2 days
Throat comfort: Immediate–1–2 uses
Liver/bladder support: 14–21 days

---

## DIY Recipe — Soothing Agrimony Gargle

Steep 1 tbsp dried Agrimony in 1 cup boiling water for 10 minutes. Cool, strain, and gargle 3–4× daily for throat or mouth irritation.

---

## Same/Similar Results

● Marshmallow Root, ● Slippery Elm, ● Plantain Leaf, ● Sage, ● Chamomile, ● Yarrow, ● Blackberry Leaf, ● Goldenseal

---

## Herbal Reflections of Agrimony

Agrimony is a quiet restorer that strengthens tissues while soothing irritation. Milder than stronger astringents like Goldenseal, it is well suited for steady, daily support — demonstrating how gentle remedies often produce the most lasting results.

★ **Herbal Confidence Index:** 🌿 🌿 🌿 🌿 (4/5 green stars — a dependable, balanced astringent that tones and soothes without harshness; especially effective for digestive and throat comfort.)

# ALFALFA

★★★★★

*Medicago sativa*

**Alfalfa** is a deeply nutritive herb used to support heart health, lower cholesterol, and restore vitality through mineral and vitamin replenishment. It supports digestion, reduces inflammation, aids gentle detoxification, and helps balance hormones, making it especially valuable during menopause or recovery from depletion. Rich in protein, trace minerals, and phytonutrients, Alfalfa functions as a long-term restorative tonic rather than a fast-acting stimulant.
Cultivated for over 2,000 years, Alfalfa originated in ancient Persia and spread through Greece and Rome as a prized food and medicine. Its name, meaning "father of all foods," reflects its exceptional nutritional density. Today, Alfalfa leaves and sprouts are widely used as both nourishment and medicine in natural health traditions worldwide.

---

**Core Herbal Category — Alfalfa**
**Primary Core: Nutritional & Tonic Support** (rich in restorative principles that rebuild tissues and mineral reserves)
**Secondary Cores:** Digestive · Hormonal · Blood

---

## How It Works

Alfalfa supplies a broad spectrum of vitamins, minerals, amino acids, and phytonutrients that support cellular repair and metabolic resilience. Its nutritive action rebuilds depleted tissues and strengthens overall vitality over time. Mild phytoestrogens assist hormonal balance, while chlorophyll and antioxidants support gentle detoxification and blood quality. Consistent use restores strength gradually and sustainably.

---

## Primary Uses

Nutritional tonic and recovery support
Menopausal and hormonal balance
Supports lactation in nursing mothers
Aids detoxification and pH balance
Mild diuretic and digestive tonic

---

## Scientific Backing

Rich in phytoestrogens, saponins, amino acids, and antioxidants. Studies show support for cholesterol and blood-sugar regulation, immune modulation, and easing menopausal symptoms, with laboratory research confirming antioxidant activity.

## Forms Available

Dried leaf (tea or capsules)
Fresh sprouts (food use)
Liquid extract or tincture
Powder for smoothies or green drinks

## How to Use (Dosage & Methods)

- **Tea:** 1–2 tsp dried leaf per cup hot water; steep 10 min. Drink 1–2× daily.
- **Capsules / Powder:** 1–2 g daily with meals.
- **Tincture:** 2–4 mL, up to 3× daily.
- **Food Use:** Add fresh sprouts to salads or sandwiches.

## Caution Level — ● Caution

Avoid use with lupus or autoimmune disorders due to immune stimulation. Use modestly in pregnancy. High vitamin K content may interact with anticoagulants; consult a clinician if on blood thinners.

## Gender-Specific Safety

● **Men:** Supports stamina, joint comfort, and cholesterol balance. Safe for daily use as tea, powder, or capsules; avoid high-dose sprout extracts if using anticoagulants.

● **Women:** Nourishes reproductive health, hair, nails, and hormonal balance. Helpful during menopause or post-menstrual fatigue. Use moderate food-like amounts; avoid concentrated extracts during hormonal therapy.

● **Pregnancy / Nursing:** Generally safe in dietary forms (tea or food). Avoid potent extracts or sprout concentrates due to hormonal activity.

## ⌛ Expected Results

Nutrient renewal: 5–7 days
Hormonal balance: 14–21 days
Detox / pH support: 21–28 days

## Same / Similar Results

● Nettle Leaf, ● Red Raspberry Leaf, ● Dandelion Leaf, ● Dong Quai, ● Spirulina

## Shelf Life / Potency After Preparation

**Shelf Life:**
Dried leaves: 1–2 years · Powder: 6–12 months · Tinctures: 3–5 years · Fresh sprouts: 3–5 days refrigerated
**Potency:**
Tea retains full nutritive value 12–24 hrs refrigerated; powders ~24 hrs once mixed; tinctures retain long-term potency.

---

## DIY Recipe — Alfalfa Vitality Tea Blend

Combine 1 tsp dried Alfalfa leaf, 1 tsp Nettle, and 1 tsp Red Raspberry Leaf. Steep in 2 cups hot water for 10 minutes. Drink daily to restore minerals and support hormonal balance.

---

## Herbal Reflections of Alfalfa

Alfalfa is a quiet builder of strength — nourishing rather than forcing change. True to its title as the Father of All Foods, it restores balance through steady mineral-rich nourishment. Its benefits accumulate gently, making it ideal for long-term vitality, menopausal steadiness, and recovery from depletion.

🌟 **Herbal Confidence Index:** 🌿 🌿 🌿 🌿 🌿
*(5/5 green stars — steady, nourishing, and remarkably safe for long-term vitality.)*

# ANGELICA ROOT

★★★★

*Angelica archangelica*

**Angelica Root** is a warming, aromatic herb used to support digestion, ease bloating and gas, and stimulate appetite. It is traditionally valued for relieving menstrual discomfort, promoting circulation, and supporting respiratory strength. Its gentle nervine action helps calm tension associated with cold, stagnation, or fatigue, making it a balancing remedy for both physical and emotional states.

Angelica has a long history in European and Asian herbal traditions and was once called the "holy spirit root" for its protective reputation. In Chinese medicine it is closely associated with women's reproductive health, while its fragrant roots have also been used in liqueurs and culinary preparations, reflecting its dual medicinal and cultural importance.

---

🌿 **Core Herbal Category — Angelica Root**

**Primary Core: Cardiovascular System Support** with (warming principles that promote movement)

**Secondary Cores:** Digestive · Women's Reproductive · Nervine · Respiratory · Foundational / Systemic Support

---

## How It Works

Angelica Root gently warms the body and stimulates circulation, helping move stagnant blood and energy. Its aromatic compounds relax smooth muscle tissue, easing cramping and improving blood flow to the pelvis and digestive organs. Carminative actions reduce gas and support appetite, while mild nervine effects help calm tension linked to cold or stagnation. Together, these actions restore warmth, movement, and rhythmic balance.

---

## Primary Uses

Relieves menstrual cramps and supports cycle regularity
Supports menopausal comfort
Stimulates circulation and warmth
Aids digestion (bloating, poor appetite)
Restores vitality after illness or fatigue

---

## Scientific Backing

Contains ligustilide, ferulic acid, and coumarins with antispasmodic, vasodilatory, and mild estrogenic activity. Traditional and clinical evidence supports its use for menstrual regulation, menopausal balance, and circulatory enhancement through smooth-muscle relaxation and improved blood flow.

---

## Forms Available

Dried root (tea or decoction)
Capsules or powdered root
Traditional women's formulas (Chinese and European)

---

## How to Use (Dosage & Methods)

- **Tea / Decoction:** Simmer 1 tsp dried root in 1 cup water for 10 min; drink 1–2× daily.
- **Tincture:** 1–3 mL, up to 3× daily for digestion, circulation, or menstrual sluggishness.
- **Capsules:** 300–600 mg powdered root, 1–2× daily.
- **Topical:** Diluted essential oil (never neat) for tight muscles or cold extremities.
- **Timing:** Best taken before meals to stimulate appetite and digestive flow.

---

## Caution Level — ◍ Caution

Avoid during pregnancy due to uterine-stimulating potential. Use care with blood-thinning medications or hormone-sensitive conditions. May increase photosensitivity; avoid excessive sun exposure immediately after use.

---

## 🚹 🚺 Gender-Specific Safety

● **Men:** Supports circulation, digestion, and respiratory ease. Helpful for cold limbs or sluggish metabolism. Safe in moderate doses; avoid high amounts if using blood thinners.

● **Women:** Traditionally used as a uterine and menstrual balancer. Eases cramps and supports menopausal steadiness. Avoid during pregnancy or heavy bleeding.

● **Pregnancy / Nursing:** Avoid entirely in pregnancy. Nursing women should use only under professional supervision due to active coumarins.

---

## ⌛ Expected Results

Digestive comfort: 3–5 days
Menstrual relief: 7–14 days or within 1–2 cycles
Circulatory support: 14–21 days
Post-illness recovery: 21–28 days

---

## Same / Similar Results

Dong Quai, Red Clover, Black Cohosh, Vitex, Wild Yam

---

## Shelf Life / Potency After Preparation

Dried root: 1–2 years airtight in a cool, dark place.
Powders: 6–12 months.
Tinctures: 3–5 years.
Teas/decoctions are strongest within 12–24 hrs refrigerated; powdered blends ~24 hrs; tinctures retain long-term potency.

---

## DIY Recipe — Angelica Root Menstrual Support Tea

Simmer 1 tsp dried Angelica root with 1 tsp Ginger and 1 tsp Cinnamon in 2 cups water for 15 minutes. Strain and sip warm before and during the menstrual cycle.

---

## Herbal Reflections of Angelica Root

Angelica Root is warming and centering, restoring movement where stagnation exists. Long regarded as a "holy spirit root," it supports circulation, menstrual harmony, and renewed vitality without force when used with respect and care.

**Herbal Confidence Index:**

*(4/5 green stars — a deeply restorative circulatory and women's balancing tonic with broad, time-tested effectiveness when used wisely.)*

# TONGKAT ALI

★★★★

Eurycoma longifolia

**Tongkat Ali** is a traditional Southeast Asian medicinal root valued for supporting male vitality, physical endurance, and stress-related hormonal balance. Long used in Malaysian, Indonesian, and Thai herbal systems, it is most often applied for fatigue, reduced drive, and age-related decline in strength rather than acute performance enhancement.

Rather than acting as a direct stimulant, Tongkat Ali works by supporting healthy stress adaptation and hormonal signaling, particularly through moderating excess cortisol and encouraging balanced testosterone expression. Its benefits develop gradually with consistent use, making it best suited for short-to-moderate cycles instead of continuous daily intake.

---

🌿 **Core Herbal Category — Tongkat Ali**
**Primary Core: Adaptogens** with (restorative principles that support hormonal balance)
**Secondary Cores:** Endocrine · Vitality · Energy

---

## How It Works

Tongkat Ali helps regulate stress hormones, particularly by lowering excess cortisol that can suppress vitality and testosterone function. Bitter tonic compounds support endocrine signaling, allowing natural testosterone expression without forced stimulation. Over time, this rebalancing improves energy, strength, and resilience, which is why structured cycling is recommended.

---

## Primary Uses

Supports healthy testosterone balance
Enhances male vitality and stamina
Assists stress adaptation and cortisol regulation
Supports libido and reproductive energy
Promotes physical strength and endurance

---

## Scientific Backing

Contains quassinoids (including eurycomanone), alkaloids, and bioactive peptides linked to adaptogenic and hormone-modulating activity. Research in *Journal of the International Society of Sports Nutrition*, *Phytotherapy Research*, and *Andrologia* suggests support for healthy testosterone levels, reduced cortisol, improved performance, fatigue resistance, and libido—consistent with traditional restorative use.

## Forms Available

Dried root powder
Capsules (whole-root preparations preferred)
Decoction (traditional use)
Standardized extracts (use with caution)

---

## How to Use (Dosage & Methods)

**Root Powder / Capsules:** 200–400 mg once daily, preferably in the morning.
**Traditional Decoction:** Simmer 1–2 tsp chopped root in water for 20–30 min; consume once daily for limited cycles.
**Cycling Guidance:** Use 4–8 weeks, then break 2–4 weeks.

---

## Caution Level — ● Supervision Recommended

Not for long-term continuous use. Avoid during pregnancy or breastfeeding. Use caution with heart conditions or hypertension. High doses may cause restlessness or irritability. Avoid combining with stimulant medications.

---

## Gender-Specific Safety

● **Men:** Effective for restoring vitality, stress resilience, and hormonal balance when used responsibly and cycled.
● **Women:** Not typically recommended due to androgenic activity unless under professional guidance.
● **Pregnancy / Nursing:** Avoid use.

---

## ⌛ Expected Results

Energy and stamina: 1–2 weeks
Libido support: 2–4 weeks
Hormonal balance: 3–6 weeks
Full adaptogenic benefit: 4–8 weeks (cycled)

---

## DIY Recipe — Tongkat Ali Vitality Decoction

Simmer 1 tsp chopped root in 2 cups water for 25 minutes. Strain and drink once daily. Use no longer than 8 weeks continuously.

---

## Same / Similar Results

Maca Root · Tribulus · Pumpkin Seed · Horny Goat Weed

---

## Shelf Life / Potency After Preparation

Dried root: 2–3 years · Capsules: 1–2 years · Decoction: 24 hrs refrigerated

---

## Herbal Reflections of Tongkat Ali

Tongkat Ali restores strength through recalibration, not stimulation. Its discipline-based action rebuilds vitality where stress and depletion have eroded it. Used wisely and cycled, it supports renewed balance; used recklessly, it teaches restraint.

**Herbal Confidence Index:**

*(4/5 green stars — highly effective men's vitality and adaptogenic herb when used responsibly; powerful and best cycled.)*

---

# ARNICA

★★★★

*Arnica montana*

**Arnica** is a trusted topical herb for reducing pain, easing swelling, and speeding recovery from bruises, sprains, and muscle soreness. Applied externally, it relieves inflammation, calms joint pain, and supports healing after minor injuries. While some traditions reference diluted internal forms, Arnica must be handled with care and is primarily used topically.

A cornerstone of European folk medicine, Arnica—often called the "mountain daisy"—has been relied upon by healers, athletes, and laborers for fast-acting injury relief. Its long record of use makes it a mainstay of natural first-aid care.

---

🌿 **Core Herbal Category — Arnica**

**Primary Core: Anti-Inflammatory & Pain Support** with (resolving principles that reduce swelling and tissue trauma)

**Secondary Cores:** Pain · Circulatory · Tissue

---

## How It Works

Arnica interrupts inflammatory signaling at injury sites, reducing swelling, pain, and tissue congestion. Its active compounds stimulate local circulation to clear pooled blood and inflammatory byproducts responsible for bruising. This focused, topical action accelerates visible recovery without systemic penetration.

---

## Primary Uses

Bruises and swelling
Muscle soreness and joint pain
Sprains and blunt injuries
Post-surgical recovery (topical)
Inflammatory skin conditions (diluted)

---

## Scientific Backing

Contains sesquiterpene lactones (notably helenalin) that inhibit inflammatory pathways. Evidence supports reduced bruising, swelling, and pain with external use, often comparable to OTC creams for mild-to-moderate cases.

---

## Forms Available

Topical creams, gels, and salves
Infused herbal oils
Homeopathic tablets or pellets (diluted only)
Tinctures for external use (heavily diluted)

---

## How to Use (Dosage & Methods)

- **Topical Cream/Gel:** Apply thinly to affected areas 2–3× daily.
- **Homeopathic (Internal):** Only homeopathic potencies (e.g., 6X, 30C); follow label directions.
- **Compress:** 1–2 tsp dried flowers per cup warm water; apply 10–15 min.
- **Massage Oil:** Use pre-diluted oil on unbroken skin only.

**Important:** Never apply to broken skin or ingest whole-plant extracts.

---

## Caution Level — ▨ Caution

Toxic if ingested in raw form. External use on unbroken skin only. Avoid open wounds unless product specifies safety. Patch-test if sensitive to Asteraceae plants.

---

## Gender-Specific Safety

● **Men:** Excellent for bruises, soreness, and joint inflammation; safe externally after activity or injury.
● **Women:** Helpful for backache, postpartum bruising, and general soreness; topical use only.
● **Pregnancy / Nursing:** Avoid internal use completely; external use only with guidance and short duration.

---

## ⌛ Expected Results

Bruising & swelling: 24–48 hrs
Muscle soreness: 2–6 hrs
Joint inflammation: 3–5 days with regular use

---

## Same / Similar Results

● Comfrey · ● Turmeric · ● Ginger · ● St. John's Wort · ● Witch Hazel

---

## Shelf Life / Potency After Preparation

Dried flowers: 1–2 years airtight.
Infused oils: 12–18 months.
Commercial creams/gels: 1–3 years (per expiration).

Infused oils are strongest in the first 6–12 months.

---

## DIY Recipe — Arnica Muscle Recovery Salve

Infuse dried flowers in olive or jojoba oil for 2 weeks. Strain and combine with melted beeswax (1:4 wax-to-oil). Apply thinly to sore areas. **Never use on open wounds.**

---

## Herbal Reflections of Arnica

Arnica is the herbal first responder—precise, fast, and focused. It reduces inflammation and speeds visible recovery rather than rebuilding tissue, earning its place as a trusted ally for swift, respectful healing.

**Herbal Confidence Index:**

*(4/5 green stars — exceptional topical anti-inflammatory and pain reliever; powerful and external use only.)*

# ARTICHOKE LEAF

★★★★

*Cynara scolymus*

**Artichoke Leaf** is a classic liver and digestive herb used to stimulate bile flow, support hepatic function, and improve fat metabolism. It eases indigestion, bloating, and post-meal discomfort while contributing to healthier cholesterol balance and blood sugar regulation. Its steady bitter action makes it one of the most reliable herbs for long-term metabolic and digestive vitality. Valued since ancient Rome and Greece, Artichoke Leaf was used both as food and medicine throughout Mediterranean cultures. Its continued use reflects centuries of consistent success in supporting digestion and liver efficiency through gentle, non-forcing means.

---

**Core Herbal Category — Artichoke Leaf**
**Primary Core: Liver & Detoxification Support** with (bile-stimulating principles that support hepatic function)
**Secondary Cores:** Digestive · Cholesterol

---

## How It Works

Artichoke Leaf stimulates bile production and improves bile flow from the liver and gallbladder, enhancing fat digestion and waste elimination. Improved bile activity reduces digestive sluggishness, bloating, and nausea while supporting cholesterol processing. Over time, this tonic action strengthens liver efficiency without aggressive detox effects.

---

## Primary Uses

Liver support and protection
Lowering LDL ("bad") cholesterol
Supporting bile production and flow
Indigestion, bloating, and nausea
Gallbladder support

---

## Scientific Backing

Rich in cynarin and chlorogenic acid. Clinical studies demonstrate hepatoprotective effects, improved liver enzyme balance, and measurable reductions in LDL cholesterol with consistent use.

---

## Forms Available

Capsules or tablets
Tinctures or liquid extracts
Dried leaf (tea or decoction)

---

## How to Use (Dosage & Methods)

- **Capsules/Tablets:** 300–600 mg standardized extract (2.5–5% cynarin), 1–2× daily
- **Tincture:** 2–4 mL up to 3× daily before meals
- **Tea/Decoction:** 1–2 tsp dried leaf steeped 10–15 min (very bitter)
- **Timing:** Best taken before meals to stimulate bile flow

---

## ⚠ Caution Level — ● Caution

Avoid with bile duct obstruction or Asteraceae allergy. Use cautiously with gallstones or bile disorders. Consult a provider if pregnant or nursing.

---

## Gender-Specific Safety

● **Men:** Supports cholesterol balance, liver detox, and digestion.
● **Women:** Supports hormone-related digestion and skin clarity via liver balance.
● **Pregnancy / Nursing:** Use cautiously; avoid concentrated extracts unless supervised.

---

## ⌛ Expected Results

Digestive relief: 1–2 hours
Liver support: 14–28 days
Cholesterol balance: 28–42 days

---

## Same / Similar Results

● Dandelion Root · ● Milk Thistle · ● Gentian · ● Turmeric · ● Burdock Root

---

## Shelf Life / Potency After Preparation

Dried leaf: 1–2 years airtight
Powders: 6–12 months
Tinctures: 3–5 years
Teas/decoctions: best within 12–24 hrs refrigerated

---

## DIY Recipe — Artichoke Digestive Decoction

Simmer 1 tbsp dried Artichoke Leaf in 2 cups water for 10 minutes. Strain and sip before meals.

---

## Herbal Reflections of Artichoke Leaf

Artichoke Leaf is a steady liver guardian. Less dramatic than Milk Thistle, it excels at regulating bile flow, digestion, and metabolic balance. Its bitterness awakens digestive intelligence, making it a subtle but deeply reliable ally in modern dietary excess.

🌟 **Herbal Confidence Index:** 🌿 🌿 🌿 🌿

*(4/5 green stars — dependable liver and digestive tonic valued for bile flow and cholesterol regulation.)*

---

# ASHWAGANDHA

★★★★★

*Withania somnifera*

**Ashwagandha** is a classic adaptogenic root used to support stress regulation, nervous system stability, and long-term energy resilience. It is commonly applied for fatigue, disrupted sleep, mental strain, and recovery from prolonged stress, with effects that build gradually rather than through immediate stimulation.

Traditionally central to Ayurvedic medicine, Ashwagandha supports balanced adrenal and immune function by helping moderate stress responses and promote physiological equilibrium. Its actions are cumulative and restorative, making it well suited for sustained use during periods of depletion, overwork, or emotional strain.

---

🌿 **Core Herbal Category — Ashwagandha**

**Primary Core: Adaptogens** with (adaptogenic principles that build stress resilience and support adrenal and nervous-system equilibrium)

**Secondary Cores:** Nervous System · Endocrine · Sleep · Immune · Vitality

---

## How It Works

Ashwagandha helps regulate the stress response by supporting healthy cortisol rhythms rather than forcing stimulation or sedation. This allows the nervous and endocrine systems to recover from chronic stress, gradually improving sleep, mental clarity, energy stability, and immune resilience. Its benefits build steadily with consistent use.

---

## Primary Uses

Reduces stress and anxiety
Supports adrenal and nervous system health
Enhances memory and cognitive focus
Balances thyroid and hormonal function
Improves sleep quality and deep rest
Supports reproductive vitality

---

## Scientific Backing

Research shows Ashwagandha lowers cortisol, improves sleep quality, enhances cognition, and increases stress resilience. Studies also support benefits for thyroid balance, male fertility, anxiety regulation, and stress-related exhaustion, aligning with its Ayurvedic classification as a *rasayana* tonic.

## Forms Available

Powder (often mixed with warm milk)
Capsules or tablets
Liquid extract / tincture
Included in tonics and adaptogenic blends

## How to Use (Dosage & Methods)

- **Capsules:** 300–600 mg standardized extract (1.5–5% withanolides), 1–2× daily
- **Powder:** ½–1 tsp in warm milk or plant milk once daily
- **Tincture:** 2–4 mL up to 2× daily
- **Timing:** Morning for stress resilience; evening for sleep support

## ⚠ Caution Level — ◍ Caution

Avoid during pregnancy unless supervised. May interact with sedatives, thyroid medications, or immunosuppressants. Start low if sensitive; may cause drowsiness or excess warmth in some individuals.

## Gender-Specific Safety

● **Men:** Supports stamina, testosterone balance, strength recovery, and mental focus.
● **Women:** Supports thyroid balance, sleep quality, anxiety relief, and hormonal steadiness.
● **Pregnancy / Nursing:** Traditionally nourishing postpartum; avoid high internal doses during pregnancy unless guided.

## ⌛ Expected Results

Stress reduction: 7–14 days
Sleep improvement: 3–7 days
Hormone/adrenal recovery: 14–28 days
Cognitive clarity & stamina: 21–35 days

## Same / Similar Results

● Rhodiola · ● Maca · ● Holy Basil · ● Lemon Balm · ● Eleuthero

## Shelf Life / Potency After Preparation

Powder: 1–2 years airtight

Capsules: 2–3 years
Tinctures: 3–5 years
Prepared tonics: best fresh; 12–24 hrs refrigerated
Teas: retain potency ~12 hrs

---

## DIY Recipe — Ashwagandha Sleep Tonic

Mix ½ tsp Ashwagandha powder into 1 cup warm milk (or plant milk). Add cinnamon and honey. Drink 30 minutes before bed.

---

## Herbal Reflections of Ashwagandha

Ashwagandha rebuilds what stress erodes. It restores rather than pushes, teaching the nervous system how to exhale again. With steady use, it demonstrates that calm strength is the most enduring form of power.

🌟 **Herbal Confidence Index:** 🌿 🌿 🌿 🌿 🌿

*(5/5 green stars — cornerstone adaptogen offering deep restoration, nervous-system nourishment, and exceptional long-term safety.)*

# ASTRAGALUS

★★★★★

*Astragalus membranaceus*

**Astragalus Root** is a cornerstone tonic used to strengthen immune resistance, boost baseline energy, and support recovery from fatigue. It also supports cardiovascular tone and circulation and is valued for building long-term resilience during seasonal changes and periods of stress. Rather than acting like a quick "immune booster," Astragalus is used to steadily fortify the body over time.

Used in Chinese medicine for over 2,000 years, Astragalus is known as **Huang Qi** ("yellow leader") and was prized for its golden roots and restorative qualities. Today it remains a respected daily-tonic herb bridging traditional practice and modern herbal wellness.

---

🌿 **Core Herbal Category — Astragalus**

**Primary Core: Adaptogens** with (strengthening principles that build resilience)

**Secondary Cores:** Immune · Energy · Longevity

---

## How It Works

Astragalus strengthens immune tone rather than overstimulating immune response. It supports defensive barrier function, promotes healthy white-blood-cell activity, and improves recovery after illness. With consistent use, it increases resistance to stress, fatigue, and seasonal challenges. Its benefits are cumulative, making it ideal for long-term use (not as an acute-fever remedy).

---

## Primary Uses

Strengthens immune system resistance

Enhances stamina and baseline energy

Supports cardiovascular and circulatory tone

Helps resist stress, fatigue, and seasonal illness

Promotes tissue repair and healthy aging

---

## Scientific Backing

Contains polysaccharides, saponins, and flavonoids with immunomodulatory and antioxidant activity. Research supports antiviral effects, reduced inflammation, improved immune signaling, and tissue-repair support. Human studies show benefits for immune tone, recovery, and cardiovascular support with consistent use.

---

## Forms Available

Dried root slices (tea, broths, soups)
Powder (capsules or smoothies)
Tablets and tinctures

---

## How to Use (Dosage & Methods)

- **Tea/Decoction:** Simmer 1–2 tbsp sliced root in 3 cups water for 20–30 min; drink 1–2× daily.
- **Tincture:** 2–4 mL, 2–3× daily for long-term vitality and immune tone.
- **Capsules/Powder:** 1,000–2,000 mg daily in divided doses.
- **Food Use:** Add 2–4 root slices to soups/stews; remove before eating.
- **Timing:** Best used consistently; avoid during acute fever.

---

## ⚠ Caution Level — ● Caution

Avoid during active fever or acute infection unless professionally guided. May interact with immunosuppressive medications. Use cautiously in autoimmune conditions.

---

## Gender-Specific Safety

● **Men:** Supports immune defense, stamina, and cardiovascular tone without hormonal stimulation. Safe long term; pause during acute fever.

● **Women:** Supports energy, immune recovery, and circulation; helpful after illness or adrenal depletion. Avoid during active infections/fever.

● **Pregnancy / Nursing:** Generally safe in food/tea amounts. Avoid high-dose extracts early in pregnancy; may support energy and immunity during nursing.

---

## ⌛ Expected Results

Immune tone improvement: 7–14 days
Energy and stamina: 1–2 weeks
Recovery & longevity effects: cumulative with steady use

---

## Same / Similar Results

● Ginseng · ● Eleuthero · ● Cat's Claw · ● Echinacea · ● Reishi

---

## Shelf Life / Potency After Preparation

**Shelf Life:** Dried root 2–3 years airtight · Powder ~1 year · Tinctures 4–6 years

**Potency:** Decoctions strongest within 24–36 hrs refrigerated · Soups retain support ~24 hrs · Tinctures maintain long-term potency

---

## DIY Recipe — Astragalus Immunity Tea

Simmer 1 tbsp root slices in 3 cups water for 30–45 minutes. Strain and drink 1 cup daily. Optional: ginger or cinnamon.

---

## Herbal Reflections of Astragalus

Astragalus is the quiet guardian—building protection before weakness appears. Where Echinacea rallies short-term defense and Ginseng stimulates, Astragalus strengthens the foundation that helps illness not take hold. Its medicine is consistency: resilience built long before it is tested.

🌟 **Herbal Confidence Index:** 🌿 🌿 🌿 🌿 🌿

*(5/5 green stars — cornerstone immune and vitality tonic; exceptionally safe and effective for long-term daily use.)*

---

# *BLESSED THISTLE*

★★★★

*Cnicus benedictus*

Blessed Thistle is a strong bitter herb used to stimulate digestion, increase appetite, and promote bile flow. It is also traditionally used to support lactation, relieve indigestion, and strengthen the body during depletion. Herbalists value it for restoring digestive drive and functional tone—especially when appetite and digestion feel weak.
Used since medieval times, Blessed Thistle was regarded as a protective herb and was cultivated in monastery gardens. Its name reflects the reverence given to its role in strengthening the body, and it remains a respected traditional remedy today.

---

🌿 **Core Herbal Category — Blessed Thistle**
**Primary Core: Digestive System Support** with (bitter tonic principles that stimulate digestion, bile flow, and appetite)
**Secondary Cores:** Liver Support · Lactation Support · Circulatory Support

---

## How It Works

Blessed Thistle activates bitter taste receptors, increasing saliva, stomach acid, and bile release. This sharpens appetite signaling and improves digestive efficiency before and during meals. Enhanced bile flow supports fat breakdown and internal clearance. Its benefits come through strong bitter stimulation rather than nourishment, restoring digestive tone and momentum.

---

## Primary Uses

Stimulates digestion and bile production
Supports liver detoxification
Aids hormonal balance
Promotes lactation
May reduce inflammation

---

## Scientific Backing

Contains sesquiterpene lactones (especially **cnicin**) that stimulate digestive secretions. Research notes galactagogue potential and mild antimicrobial effects.

---

## Forms Available

Dried leaves and stems (tea)
Powdered herb (very bitter; use sparingly)
Tincture or liquid extract

---

## How to Use (Dosage & Methods)

- **Tea:** 1 tsp dried herb per cup hot water; steep 5–10 min. Drink 1–2× daily.
- **Tincture:** 1–2 mL up to 3× daily for sluggish digestion, gas, or liver support.
- **Capsules:** 300–500 mg, 1–2× daily as a bitter tonic.
- **Bitters Use:** Take before meals for appetite, stomach acid, and bile flow.
- **Note:** Works best taken prior to eating and used steadily for several days.

---

## ⚠ Caution Level — ◍ Caution

Avoid during pregnancy. Use caution with ulcers or acid reflux. May trigger allergy in those sensitive to Asteraceae plants.

---

## 🚹 🚺 Gender-Specific Safety

● **Men:** Supports appetite, digestion, and liver tone; helpful for dietary heaviness. Avoid excessive dosing.

● **Women:** Traditionally valued for postpartum recovery and milk flow; may support PMS-related bloating and digestion. Stop if nausea occurs.

● **Pregnancy / Nursing:** Avoid during pregnancy. Traditionally used for lactation under guidance.

---

## ⌛ Expected Results

Digestive stimulation: 1–3 days
Lactation support: 5–10 days
Liver support: builds with ongoing use

---

## Same / Similar Results

● Milk Thistle · ● Dandelion Root · ● Burdock Root · ● Dong Quai · ● Fenugreek

---

## Shelf Life / Potency After Preparation

Dried herb: 1–2 years airtight · Powder: 9–12 months · Tinctures: 3–5 years · Teas: strongest within 12 hrs refrigerated

---

### DIY Recipe — Blessed Liver Tonic Tea

Steep 1 tsp dried Blessed Thistle in 1 cup hot water for 5–7 minutes. Drink 1–2× daily.

---

### Herbal Reflections of Blessed Thistle

Blessed Thistle works like a clear bell for digestion—bracing, bitter, and direct. It awakens appetite, rallies digestive secretions, and helps the body process what has grown heavy or stagnant. Its medicine is not comfort, but clarity and renewed momentum.

⭐ **Herbal Confidence Index:** 🌿🌿🌿🌿

*(4/5 green stars — reliable digestive and liver bitter with historical depth and dependable effectiveness.)*

# MILK THISTLE

★★★★★

*Silybum marianum*

**Milk Thistle** is a premier liver-protective herb used to support detoxification and help regenerate damaged liver tissue. It supports digestion, reduces inflammation, and may assist cholesterol balance, blood sugar stability, and skin clarity through improved liver function. Herbalists rely on Milk Thistle for shielding the body from toxin burden and restoring vitality, making it a cornerstone detox and repair herb.
Used since classical times by Greek and Roman physicians and later European healers, Milk Thistle is now one of the most studied herbs in modern herbal medicine. Its key compound, **silymarin**, is strongly associated with liver-cell protection and repair, and its long history supports its reputation for reliable, safe use.

---

🌿 **Core Herbal Category — Milk Thistle**
**Primary Core: Liver & Detoxification Support** with (silymarin-rich principles that promote hepatic repair and regeneration)
**Secondary Cores:** Detoxification Support · Skin Support · Gallbladder Support · Antioxidant

---

## How It Works

Milk Thistle stabilizes liver cell membranes and supports protein synthesis within hepatic cells. Its active compounds help protect liver tissue from oxidative injury while promoting regeneration of damaged cells. By improving bile processing, it supports detoxification and waste clearance, strengthening liver resilience and functional capacity over time.

---

## Primary Uses

Supports liver detoxification and repair
Improves gallbladder flow
Aids recovery from medication or alcohol strain
Promotes clearer skin through liver balance
Provides antioxidant protection

---

## Scientific Backing

Contains **silymarin**, widely studied for liver protection, membrane stabilization, reduced inflammation, and tissue regeneration. Milk Thistle remains one of the most researched liver-support herbs in modern herbal practice.

## Forms Available

Standardized extract capsules (70–80% silymarin)
Tincture or liquid extract
Crushed seeds for tea
Ground seeds / powder blends

## How to Use (Dosage & Methods)

- **Capsules/Tablets:** 150–300 mg standardized extract (70–80% silymarin), 1–2× daily
- **Tincture:** 2–4 mL, 2× daily
- **Powder (Seeds):** ½–1 tsp freshly ground seeds daily
- **Tea:** Steep crushed seeds 10–15 min; drink 1–2× daily
- **Consistency Note:** Best taken **4+ weeks** for skin clarity, detox support, and liver repair

## ⚠ Caution Level — ● Caution

Generally well tolerated; may cause mild stomach upset. Avoid if allergic to Asteraceae. May interact with medications processed through the liver.

## Gender-Specific Safety

● **Men:** Supports detox, cholesterol balance, hormone metabolism, and metabolic recovery.
● **Women:** Supports skin clarity, PMS-related sluggishness, and liver-related mood shifts.
● **Pregnancy / Nursing:** Generally safe in food or tea amounts; avoid high-dose extracts unless guided.

## ⌛ Expected Results

Skin and digestive clarity: 14–28 days
Liver repair and regeneration: 6–12 weeks

## Same / Similar Results

● Dandelion Root · ● Schisandra · ● Yellow Dock · ● Artichoke Leaf · ● Burdock Root

## Shelf Life / Potency After Preparation

Whole seeds: 2–3 years airtight · Ground powder: 9–12 months · Extracts: 2–4 years · Tinctures: 4–6 years · Tea: strongest within 12–24 hrs refrigerated

## DIY Recipe — Liver Restoration Tea

Simmer 1 tsp crushed Milk Thistle seeds with ½ tsp Dandelion Root and a pinch of Ginger in 1½ cups water for 15 minutes. Drink 1–2× daily.

---

## Herbal Reflections of Milk Thistle

Milk Thistle restores what life wears down. Where bitters clear and tonics strengthen, Milk Thistle encourages the liver to rebuild and rise again—reminding us that true healing is not only detoxification, but regeneration.

---

🌟 **Herbal Confidence Index:** 🌿 🌿 🌿 🌿 🌿
*(5/5 green stars — cornerstone liver-regenerating herb; exceptionally safe, deeply restorative, and strongly evidence-supported.)*

---

# BLUE VERVAIN

★★★★

*Verbena hastata*

**Blue Vervain** is a classic nervine that releases stored tension, eases anxiety, and supports emotional steadiness without heavy sedation. It is used for stress headaches, tight neck/shoulders, mild low mood, and stress-related digestive spasms. Its bitter-nervine action helps the body shift out of fight-or-flight, often improving digestion and sleep while calming the mind.

Honored in many traditions—including European ritual use and Native American herbal practice—Blue Vervain has long been associated with purification, protection, and peace. Its delicate purple flowers reflect its gentle but meaningful role in mind–body harmony.

---

🌿 **Core Herbal Category — Blue Vervain**

**Primary Core: Nervous System Support (Nervines)** with (relaxing principles that release stored tension)

**Secondary Cores:** Digestive · Liver · Antispasmodic

---

## How It Works

Blue Vervain relaxes an over-contracted nervous system, easing tight muscles and calming stress-driven nerve signaling. Its bitter-nervine effect helps reduce headaches, digestive tension, and emotional overload, allowing the body to settle into a more balanced state. This "release" often improves sleep and digestion while supporting steadier mood.

---

## Primary Uses

Relieves anxiety and nervous tension
Supports restful sleep and clearer thinking
Loosens neck/shoulder stress and muscle tightness
Aids stress-related digestive discomfort (spasm, cramping)
Supports liver processing linked to mood and irritability
Helps tension headaches and emotional overload patterns

---

## Scientific Backing

Contains iridoid glycosides (verbenalin, hastatoside) and flavonoids associated with mild sedative/anxiolytic effects, antispasmodic activity, and anti-inflammatory, liver-supportive action. Preclinical research supports nervous-system calming and tension reduction.

## Forms Available

Dried aerial parts (tea)
Tincture / liquid extract
Capsules
Powder (less common)

## How to Use (Dosage & Methods)

- **Tea:** 1–2 tsp dried herb; steep 10–15 min; 1–2× daily
- **Tincture:** 1–2 mL up to 3× daily for tension, anxiety, or PMS stress
- **Capsules:** 300–500 mg, 1–2× daily
- **Topical Compress:** Apply cooled tea to neck/shoulders for muscle ease

**Tip:** Often best in the evening or during overwhelm. Avoid very high doses (naturally strong bitterness).

## ⚠ Caution Level — Caution

Avoid during pregnancy due to traditional uterine-stimulating effects. Use care with sedatives or antidepressants. Large doses may cause nausea or excessive relaxation/drowsiness.

## Gender-Specific Safety

**Men:** Helpful for irritability, neck tension, and emotional buildup. Safe in moderate doses; large doses may cause drowsiness.

**Women:** Supports PMS tension, stress headaches, and emotional overwhelm. Often best in short 1–2 week cycles if needed. Use moderately if prone to heavy menstrual bleeding.

**Pregnancy / Nursing:** Avoid entirely during pregnancy. During nursing, mild tea may be acceptable only with professional guidance; stronger preparations may affect infant digestion and may reduce milk flow.

## ⌛ Expected Results

Nervous-system calm: 30–60 minutes
Improved sleep & emotional steadiness: 3–5 days
Reduced neck/shoulder tension: 3–7 days
Liver & hormonal balance support: 1–2 weeks

## Same / Similar Results

Passionflower · Lemon Balm · Chamomile · Skullcap · Valerian Root

## Shelf Life / Potency After Preparation

Dried herb: 1–2 years airtight/dark · Tincture: 3–5 years · Powder: 6–12 months · Prepared tea: best within 24 hrs refrigerated

## DIY Recipe — Vervain Nervous System Tea

1 tsp Blue Vervain + 1 tsp Lemon Balm. Steep 8–10 minutes. Sip before bed or during stress for grounding and relaxation.

## Herbal Reflections of Blue Vervain

Blue Vervain teaches release—unclenching the body and softening the mind when stress has tightened everything. It clears the fog of emotional overload and supports calm strength through gentle unwinding, reminding us that softness can be powerful.

🌟 **Herbal Confidence Index:** 🌿 🌿 🌿 🌿 🌿 (5/5 green stars — a foundational nervine for emotional, muscular, and digestive calming; safe, reliable, and deeply restorative for stress-tension patterns.)

# BONESET

★★★★

*Eupatorium perfoliatum*

**Boneset** is a herb that **reduces fever, relieves flu symptoms, and eases body aches and chills**. It is also used to **stimulate the immune system, clear congestion, and support recovery from colds and respiratory infections**. Herbalists often recommend Boneset to **shorten the duration of seasonal illness, relieve stubborn coughs, and promote sweating to break fevers**, making it a powerful ally during times of sickness.

Boneset has a long history in Native American and early American herbal traditions, valued for its ability to help with "breakbone fever" caused by influenza. Its bitter taste and strong action made it a trusted household remedy in colonial times. With its tall stems and clusters of white flowers, Boneset remains one of the most respected herbs for fighting seasonal infections and supporting overall resilience.

---

## 🌿 Core Herbal Category — Boneset

**Primary Core: Immune System Support** with (febrile principles that guide effective immune response)

**Secondary Cores:** Fever · Respiratory · Musculoskeletal

---

## How It Works

Boneset works by supporting the immune system's natural fever response, helping the body mount a coordinated defense rather than suppressing symptoms prematurely. Its bitter and diaphoretic compounds encourage sweating, which assists toxin release and temperature regulation during acute illness. By easing deep body aches and tension often associated with flu-like conditions, Boneset helps the body move through infection more efficiently. Its action is short-term and targeted, making it most appropriate during acute immune challenges rather than daily tonic use.

---

## Primary Uses

• Eases flu, colds, and fevers • Promotes sweating and detoxification • Relieves deep muscle and joint aches • Supports immune response • Helps clear viral congestion • Mild laxative for occasional constipation

## Scientific Backing

Boneset contains **sesquiterpene lactones, polysaccharides, and flavonoids** shown to exhibit antiviral, anti-inflammatory, and immunomodulatory actions. Early studies support its historical role in fever management and viral infection recovery through increased immune activation and diaphoretic effects.

---

## Forms Available

• Dried leaves and flowering tops (tea/infusion) • Tincture or liquid extract • Capsules (less common)

---

## How to Use (Dosage & Methods)

• **Tea / Hot Infusion** Steep 1–2 tsp dried Boneset in hot water for 10–15 minutes. Drink 1 cup, up to 2× daily for fever, chills, or flu-like body aches. (*Extremely bitter — combine with Peppermint or Ginger if needed.*)
• **Tincture**
1–2 mL, up to 3× daily during acute symptoms.
Reduce to 1–2× daily as symptoms ease.
• **Short-Term Only**
Use for **3–7 days** during active illness. Not for long-term use due to pyrrolizidine alkaloid content.
• **Timing**
For fevers and chills, take warm before rest to encourage sweating and natural temperature regulation.

---

## Caution Level: Caution

• High doses may cause nausea/vomiting. • Avoid during pregnancy and nursing. • Contains **pyrrolizidine alkaloids** — restrict to **short-term** use. • Avoid long-term or excessive dosing. • Use under guidance if you have liver conditions or take hepatotoxic medications.

---

## Gender-Specific Safety

**Men:** Effective for fevers, chills, deep aches, viral fatigue, and supporting immune strength. Safe for **short-term 3–7 day use**. Avoid high doses; potential liver irritation if overused.

**Women:**
Supportive for feverish exhaustion, chills, and flu-related aches. Diaphoretic action helps regulate temperature and speed recovery. Safe for short-term tea/tincture use; discontinue when symptoms improve.

● **Pregnancy / Nursing:**
Avoid completely. Not considered safe due to PA content and potential uterine-stimulating effects.

---

## Expected Results

• Sweating and fever softening: **6–12 hours** • Relief of deep aches and chills: **24–48 hours** • Immune strengthening and appetite return: **3–5 days**

---

## Same / Similar Results

● Elderflower • ● Yarrow • ● Echinacea • ● Goldenrod • ● Catnip

---

## Shelf Life / Potency After Preparation

**Shelf Life:** • Dried herb: 1–2 years • Tincture: 3–5 years • Capsules: shelf-life stable per manufacturer
**Potency After Preparation:**
• Hot infusions strongest within **12 hours** (keep warm or gently reheat).
• Refrigerated teas: use within **24 hours**.
• Tinctures maintain long-term consistency and offer the most stable potency.

---

## DIY Recipe — Flu-Busting Boneset Tea

Steep 1 tsp dried Boneset in 1 cup hot water for 10 minutes. Drink hot, 2–3× daily at the first sign of flu or chills. Combine with **Elderflower + Yarrow** to enhance fever relief and immune activation.

---

## Herbal Reflections of Boneset

Boneset is the herb of endurance and renewal — guiding the body through the full fever process rather than suppressing it. It brings warmth to the surface, loosens tension deep in the bones, and supports the body's natural intelligence to recover. Where Yarrow cools and Elderflower softens, Boneset steadies — the quiet strength in the middle of a storm.

---

## ⭐ Herbal Confidence Index: 🌿 🌿 🌿 🌿 🌿

(5/5 green stars — a time-honored immune and fever specialist, powerful yet dependable when used short-term during acute illness.)

# BORAGE

★★★★

*Borago officinalis*

**Borage** is a herb that **reduces inflammation, supports adrenal health, and improves skin conditions such as eczema and rashes**. It is also used to **ease stress, lift mood, and strengthen the heart and lungs**, making it valuable for both emotional and physical well-being. Herbalists often turn to Borage to **restore courage, balance hormones, and promote overall vitality**, giving rise to its reputation as the "herb of gladness."
Borage has been cultivated since the Middle Ages, praised for its edible flowers and leaves as well as its healing power. Its star-shaped blue blossoms were used in wines and tonics to cheer the spirit, while ancient texts mention its use for courage before battle. Today, Borage remains popular as both a medicinal herb and a culinary delight, treasured for its beauty and health benefits alike.

---

### Core Herbal Category — Borage

**Primary Core: Nutritional & Tonic Support** with (restorative principles that nourish stressed tissues)
**Secondary Cores:** Nervous · Skin · Hormonal · Anti-Inflammatory

---

### How It Works

Borage works by supplying the body with nourishing fatty acids, minerals, and plant compounds that help restore tissues stressed by fatigue or chronic strain. Its rich gamma-linolenic acid (GLA) content supports healthy inflammatory balance and skin integrity while gently buffering the stress response. This nutritive action calms and strengthens rather than stimulates, making Borage especially useful for dry, depleted, or overheated systems. With consistent use, it promotes steady restoration of resilience and tissue health.

---

## Primary Uses

• Supports mood and emotional resilience • Aids adrenal fatigue and stress recovery • Reduces inflammation and joint discomfort • Soothes coughs and mild lung congestion • Promotes skin hydration and tissue repair

---

## Scientific Backing

Borage seed oil is rich in **gamma-linolenic acid (GLA)** — clinically studied for reducing inflammation, improving eczema, easing PMS and menopausal symptoms, and supporting joint health. The leaves and flowers provide mild nervine action, trace minerals, and anti-inflammatory benefits, while GLA aids hormonal and cellular repair, making Borage a versatile herb for systemic resilience.

---

## Forms Available

• Borage seed oil (capsules or liquid) • Fresh/dried leaves and flowers (tea) • Topical creams, infused oils • Edible flowers and leaves (culinary use)

---

## How to Use (Dosage & Methods)

• **Tea** Steep 1–2 tsp dried Borage leaf or flower in 1 cup hot water for 10 minutes. Drink 1–2× daily for mood support, adrenal nourishment, or respiratory soothing.
• **Capsules (Seed Oil)**
500–1,000 mg Borage seed oil (standardized for GLA), 1× daily for skin hydration, PMS balancing, or inflammatory support.
*(Take with food.)*
• **Tincture**
2–4 mL, 1–2× daily for adrenal stress, nervous tension, or mild mood lifting.
• **Topical Use**
Apply Borage-infused oil or cream to inflamed, dry, or irritated skin 1–2× daily.
• **Timing**
Tea is best for stress and lung support.
Seed oil is best for skin, inflammation, and hormonal balance.

---

## Caution Level: Caution

• Avoid large internal doses of leaves due to trace **pyrrolizidine alkaloids (PAs)**. • Prefer **PA-free seed oil** for long-term use. • Avoid internal use during pregnancy. • Use caution with liver conditions. • Discontinue if digestive or skin irritation occurs.

---

## Gender-Specific Safety

**Men:** Supports adrenal recovery, stamina, emotional resilience, and joint comfort. Helpful during periods of stress, fatigue, or inflammation. Internal use should be moderate and preferably PA-free. Tea or capsule use is generally safe short-term.

**Women:**
Commonly used to ease PMS, menopausal discomfort, mood swings, and stress-related fatigue. Borage oil is especially supportive for skin health and hormonal regulation. Avoid concentrated extracts during pregnancy or with liver disorders.

**Pregnancy / Nursing:**

Avoid internal use unless advised by a clinician.
Topical use of PA-free oils/creams is generally safe.

---

## Expected Results

**Short-Term (7–14 days):** • Softer, better-hydrated skin • Reduced inflammatory flare-ups
**Mid-Term (21–28 days):**
- Relief from PMS symptoms
- Improved joint comfort and emotional steadiness
- Noticeable reduction in adrenal fatigue

**Long-Term (30–60 days):**
- Stronger resilience to stress
- Clearer skin and improved hormonal balance
- More stable mood and vitality

---

### Same / Similar Results

Lemon Balm • Evening Primrose • Chamomile • Ashwagandha • Dong Quai

---

### Shelf Life / Potency After Preparation

**Shelf Life:** • Borage seed oil: 6–12 months (refrigerated, light-protected) • Dried leaves: 1 year • Topical oils/creams: 6–12 months
**Potency After Preparation:**
- Seed oil delivers strongest GLA benefits when used daily within active shelf life.
- Teas are most effective within **12–24 hours** refrigerated.
- Topicals maintain potency until natural rancidity or separation occurs.

---

### DIY Recipe — Nourishing Borage Tea

Steep 1 tsp dried Borage leaf in 1 cup hot water for 8 minutes. Add mint or lemon for flavor. Drink 1–2× daily for adrenal and mood support.

---

### Herbal Reflections of Borage

Borage brings calm where the spirit feels heavy — moistening dryness, softening inflammation, and restoring confidence gently. Its minerals nourish depleted nerves, while its cooling oils soothe irritation and help the heart lighten. Unlike strong stimulants, Borage rebuilds by replenishing, inviting a quiet strength that feels like peace returning to the body.

---

### Herbal Confidence Index:

(4/5 green stars — uplifting adrenal and skin tonic; rich in GLA, reliable for stress relief, hormonal balance, and skin restoration with steady use.)

# BURDOCK ROOT

★★★★★

*Arctium lappa*

**Burdock Root** is a classic cleansing herb used to support blood and lymph purification, promote liver and kidney function, and improve chronic skin conditions such as acne and eczema. It also supports digestion, reduces inflammation, and is often used to aid joint comfort and blood sugar balance—especially during seasonal shifts or long-standing imbalance.
Used in both Western and Asian traditions for centuries, Burdock is also a valued food in Japan ("gobo"). Its deep root reflects its reputation for steady endurance and long-term internal clearing.

---

**Core Herbal Category — Burdock Root**
**Primary Core: Liver & Detoxification Support** with (deep-cleansing principles that support elimination and blood purification)
**Secondary Cores:** Lymphatic · Digestive · Skin · Inflammatory

---

## How It Works

Burdock supports gradual elimination by strengthening liver, kidneys, and lymphatic flow, helping remove metabolic waste and inflammatory byproducts. Bitter/alterative compounds improve clearance through digestion, urine, and skin, reducing internal congestion. By supporting nutrient assimilation and steady detox pathways, it improves "blood quality" and calms inflammatory responses. Best for long-term rebalancing rather than aggressive detox.

---

## Primary Uses

Detoxifies blood and lymphatic system
Supports liver and kidney function
Clears skin issues (eczema, acne, boils)
Aids digestion and elimination
Provides antioxidant and anti-inflammatory support
Supports blood sugar balance

---

## Scientific Backing

Contains phenolic acids, quercetin, chlorogenic acid, and other antioxidants associated with liver support and inflammation reduction. Inulin acts as a prebiotic to support gut flora, digestion, and immune balance. Studies highlight potential benefits for metabolic support, skin clarity, and detoxification pathways.

---

## Forms Available

Dried root (tea/decoction)
Capsules or powders
Tincture or liquid extract
Fresh root as food ("gobo")

---

## How to Use (Dosage & Methods)

- **Decoction (Tea):** Simmer 1–2 tbsp chopped root in 2 cups water for 20 min; drink 1–2× daily.
- **Tincture:** 2–4 mL up to 3× daily.
- **Capsules/Powder:** 500–1,000 mg, 1–2× daily.
- **Food Use:** Add fresh root to soups, stews, or stir-fries.
- **Timing:** Works best with consistent use for several weeks for skin/lymph/liver improvement.

---

## Caution Level — ▨ Caution

Avoid during pregnancy or breastfeeding unless supervised. May lower blood sugar—monitor carefully if diabetic. Source from clean soil (deep roots can absorb contaminants/heavy metals). Discontinue if rash, nausea, or digestive upset occurs.

---

## Gender-Specific Safety

● **Men:** Strong daily detoxifier for clarity, energy, and skin support; supports healthy liver metabolism. Safe long term in moderate use.
● **Women:** Helpful for PMS-related acne, hormonal shifts, lymph stagnation, chronic skin issues, and bloating; safe in moderate ongoing use.
● **Pregnancy / Nursing:** Avoid internal use unless professionally supervised. Topical compresses for irritated skin are generally safe.

---

## ⌛ Expected Results

Skin clarity: 7–14 days
Digestive regularity: 3–5 days
Deeper detoxification/vitality: 14–28 days, with continued gains over long-term use

---

## Same / Similar Results

● Dandelion Root • ● Red Clover • ● Yellow Dock • ● Milk Thistle • ● Nettle Leaf

---

## Shelf Life / Potency After Preparation

**Shelf Life:** Dried root 1–2 years · Powder 9–12 months · Fresh root 1–2 weeks refrigerated · Tincture 3–5 years
**Potency:** Decoctions strongest within 24–36 hrs refrigerated · Teas ~24 hrs · Tinctures preserve detox/prebiotic support long term

---

## DIY Recipe — Burdock Liver Detox Tea

Simmer 1 tbsp dried Burdock Root in 2 cups water for 15 minutes. Strain and drink 1 cup morning and evening for up to 14 days to support liver and lymph cleansing.

---

## Herbal Reflections of Burdock Root

Burdock cleanses with patience, supporting liver, lymph, and gut like a steady current washing debris from within. It softens inflammation, clears pathways, and restores vitality one day at a time—gentle enough for consistency, strong enough for real change.

🌟 **Herbal Confidence Index:** 🌿 🌿 🌿 🌿 🌿

*(5/5 green stars — dependable long-term detoxifier; gentle yet powerful for restoring skin, liver, lymph, and digestive vitality.)*

# CALENDULA

★★★★★

Calendula officinalis

**Calendula** is a premier tissue-healing herb that soothes irritation, reduces inflammation, and supports wound repair. It is widely used in natural first aid for cuts, rashes, burns, and infections, and is also used internally to calm digestive upset, support lymphatic flow, and ease menstrual cramping. Its versatility and gentleness make it a staple for both external and internal healing.
Often called "marigold," Calendula has been revered across European, Ayurvedic, and Native American traditions and associated with warmth and renewal for centuries.

---

🌿 **Core Herbal Category — Calendula**
**Primary Core: Lymphatic & Skin Support** with (gentle regenerative principles that protect and restore tissues)
**Secondary Cores:** Lymphatic · Anti-Inflammatory · Digestive

---

## How It Works

Calendula supports steady tissue regeneration while calming inflammation and protecting sensitive skin and mucosal surfaces. Flavonoids/resins support local circulation and healthy wound repair. Internally, these soothing actions calm irritated digestive linings and promote lymphatic movement, reducing stagnation and low-grade inflammation. Mild but persistent, it is ideal for sensitive tissues and longer healing timelines.

---

## Primary Uses

Accelerates wound and skin healing
Reduces inflammation in tissues
Soothes eczema, diaper rash, sunburn
Supports defense against fungal/bacterial imbalance
Supports oral and gum repair
Eases digestive irritation

---

## Scientific Backing

Contains flavonoids, triterpenoids, carotenoids, and volatile oils with anti-inflammatory, antimicrobial, and tissue-regenerating actions. Research supports improved wound closure, reduced microbial load, increased collagen activity, and faster epithelial repair.

## Forms Available

Dried flowers (tea, compress, rinse)
Salves, oils, creams
Tinctures and liquid extracts
Mouthwash or throat-rinse preparations

## How to Use (Dosage & Methods)

- **Tea:** 1–2 tsp dried flowers per cup; steep 10–15 min; drink 1–2× daily.
- **Tincture:** 2–4 mL up to 2× daily.
- **Topical:** Apply infused oil/salve/cream 1–3× daily to cuts, rashes, burns, inflamed skin.
- **Gargle/Rinse:** Use cooled tea for mouth ulcers, gum irritation, sore throat.

## Caution Level — ● Safe

Gentle and safe for regular use. If allergic to ragweed/daisies/marigold-family plants, test cautiously. Avoid internal use in early pregnancy due to mild uterine-stimulating potential. Discontinue if rash or digestive upset occurs.

## Gender-Specific Safety

● **Men:** Supports skin repair, oral/gum healing, and mild liver/lymph support; safe topically and in short internal use as tea.

● **Women:** Supports menstrual comfort, postpartum healing, and skin clarity; safe in moderate internal or topical use.

● **Pregnancy / Nursing:** Safe externally throughout pregnancy/lactation. Internally, keep to mild tea and avoid concentrated doses in early pregnancy.

## ⌛ Expected Results

Skin soothing: 24–48 hours
Wound closure: 2–4 days
Oral/gum improvement: 3–5 days
Digestive inflammation reduction: 3–7 days

## Same / Similar Results

● Chamomile • ● Plantain Leaf • ● Comfrey • ● Goldenseal • ● Lavender

## Shelf Life / Potency After Preparation

**Shelf Life:** Dried petals 1–2 years · Oils/salves/creams 6–12 months · Tinctures 3–5 years
**Potency:** Teas/rinses best within 24 hrs refrigerated · Oils/salves stay active through shelf life if sealed/cool · Tinctures remain stable long term

---

## DIY Recipe — Calendula Skin-Healing Salve

Infuse 1 cup dried petals in 1 cup olive oil over low heat for 2–3 hours. Strain, stir in ¼ cup melted beeswax, pour into jars, and cool. Apply to cuts, burns, or rashes.

---

## Herbal Reflections of Calendula

Calendula is sunlight in plant form—calming what is inflamed and guiding recovery with gentle order. Where Plantain draws and Comfrey knits, Calendula refines: easing irritation, supporting clean closure, and encouraging steady repair in skin and deeper tissues.

⭐ **Herbal Confidence Index:** 🌿 🌿 🌿 🌿 🌿
*(5/5 green stars — cornerstone skin and tissue healer; clinically supported, extremely safe, and indispensable in home and clinical herbal care.)*

# CALIFORNIA POPPY

★★★★

Eschscholzia californica

**California Poppy** is a gentle nervine used to reduce anxiety, calm restlessness, and improve sleep quality. It can also ease nervous tension and mild pain (including tension headaches), offering non-addictive support for stress and insomnia in both adults and sensitive nervous systems. It is often favored when a calmer transition into sleep is needed without heavy sedation.

Traditionally used in Native American medicine (and at times as food), California Poppy later became a respected Western herbal calming remedy. Known for its bright orange flowers and symbolic association with peace and rest, it remains valued for dependable nervous-system soothing.

---

🌿 **Core Herbal Category — California Poppy**

**Primary Core: Nervous System Support (Nervines)** with (calming principles that ease nervous-system tension)

**Secondary Cores:** Sleep · Pain Relief · Mood

---

## How It Works

California Poppy gently relaxes the nervous system without creating dependency. Its calming alkaloids reduce neural excitability, quiet mental restlessness, ease muscle tension, and soften pain perception. This helps the body shift into rest and sleep while usually maintaining clarity during waking hours. Supportive rather than forceful, it is often suitable for sensitive systems.

---

## Primary Uses

Insomnia and disturbed sleep
Anxiety and nervousness
Restlessness and agitation
Mild pain and tension headaches
Hyperactivity or nighttime wakefulness in children

---

## Scientific Backing

Contains californidine, eschscholtzine, protopine, and related alkaloids studied for sedative, anxiolytic, and analgesic properties. Research supports gentle relaxation without dependency, positioning it as a calmer alternative to stronger sleep aids for some users.

## Forms Available

Tincture or liquid extract
Dried aerial parts (tea)
Capsules or standardized extracts
Glycerite (for children)
Homeopathic preparations

## How to Use (Dosage & Methods)

- **Tea:** 1–2 tsp dried herb per cup; steep 10–15 min; drink 1–2× daily for anxiety/restlessness/sleep.
- **Tincture:** 1–2 mL up to 3× daily; take 30–60 min before bed for sleep support.
- **Capsules:** 300–500 mg extract, 1–2× daily.
- **Children's Use:** Mild tea or glycerite only—strictly under professional guidance.
- **Timing:** For anxiety, space doses; for sleep, take in the evening/before bed.

## Caution Level — ● Caution

May cause drowsiness—avoid driving, alcohol, or sedatives. Not recommended during pregnancy except under guidance. Use smaller amounts for children. Avoid combining with prescription sleep aids or strong anxiolytics.

## Gender-Specific Safety

● **Men:** Helps reduce anxiety, muscle tension, and overthinking; supports deeper sleep. Safe in tea/tincture/capsule form; avoid combining with sedatives or alcohol.

● **Women:** Helpful for PMS irritability, emotional stress, menopausal restlessness, and nighttime tension; safe in moderate use.

● **Pregnancy / Nursing:** Use cautiously and only with professional supervision. Mild tea for occasional relaxation is typically tolerated; consistent internal use is discouraged.

## Expected Results

Calming effect: 30–60 minutes
Improved sleep: 5–7 nights of consistent use
Mood steadiness: 1–2 weeks of regular intake

## Same / Similar Results

● Chamomile • ● Passionflower • ● Lemon Balm • ● Valerian • ● Kava * ● Lavender

### Shelf Life / Potency After Preparation

**Shelf Life:** Dried aerial parts 1–2 years · Alcohol tincture 3–5 years · Capsules ~2 years (cool/airtight)
**Potency:** Tea best within 12–24 hrs refrigerated · Tinctures remain stable for years and are reliable for bedtime dosing

---

### DIY Recipe — California Poppy Bedtime Tea

Combine 1 tsp California Poppy + 1 tsp Chamomile + a pinch of Lemon Balm. Steep 10 minutes. Drink 30 minutes before bed.

---

### Herbal Reflections of California Poppy

California Poppy is a soft sunset for the nervous system—quieting tension and encouraging natural rest without heaviness. Where Valerian can feel abrupt, California Poppy is subtle: the steady exhale at day's end, inviting the mind and body to release.
🌟 **Herbal Confidence Index:** 🌿🌿🌿🌿½
*(4.5/5 green stars — gentle yet effective nervine for sleep, anxiety, restlessness, and emotional balance without dependency.)*

---

# CAYENNE PEPPER

★★★★★

Capsicum annuum

**Cayenne Pepper** is a fast-acting circulatory stimulant that increases warmth, boosts metabolism, supports digestion, and can relieve pain—especially when used topically. Herbalists also use Cayenne as a "catalyst herb," meaning small amounts can enhance absorption and drive companion herbs deeper into the body. Its active compound **capsaicin** works quickly, making Cayenne valuable for cold extremities, sluggish circulation, and topical pain support.

Used for thousands of years in Native American medicine and cuisine and later spread worldwide, Cayenne has been used to restore warmth, support the heart, and revive energy. It remains both a kitchen staple and an herbal cornerstone.

---

**Core Herbal Category — Cayenne Pepper**

**Primary Core: Cardiovascular System Support** with (rapid warming principles that activate blood movement)

**Secondary Cores:** Digestive · Pain Relief (Topical) · Metabolic · Catalyst

---

## How It Works

Cayenne stimulates circulation by increasing blood flow through capsaicin-driven vascular and nerve signaling. This warming action improves oxygen delivery and nutrient transport and helps disperse stagnation. Internally it increases digestive secretions and metabolic activity; externally it reduces pain by desensitizing local nerve endings. Because it amplifies response, it is often used in small amounts to activate other herbs rather than as a stand-alone daily tonic.

---

## Primary Uses

Improves circulation and vascular tone
Enhances metabolism and thermogenesis
Boosts digestion and nutrient absorption
Supports mild high or low blood pressure (context dependent)
Reduces joint, muscle, and nerve pain (topical use)
Helps clear sinus and chest congestion

---

## Scientific Backing

Capsaicin is well studied for analgesic, anti-inflammatory, vasodilatory, and thermogenic effects.

Research supports increased peripheral circulation, metabolic heat/fat oxidation, and topical pain relief for neuropathy and arthritic discomfort. Topical capsaicin is FDA-recognized for pain relief in certain conditions.

---

## Forms Available

Dried powder or flakes
Capsules (standardized capsaicin content)
Tincture or liquid extract
Infused oils and salves
Creams/ointments/patches (0.025–0.1% capsaicin)

---

## How to Use (Dosage & Methods)

- **Capsules:** 300–500 mg with food, 1–2× daily.
- **Tincture:** 5–10 drops up to 2× daily for warmth/sinus clearing/sluggish digestion.
- **Tea/Tonic:** A small pinch in hot water with lemon or ginger for congestion/coldness.
- **Topical:** Apply capsaicin cream (0.025–0.1%) to sore areas 2× daily (patch test first).
- **Catalyst Use:** Add small amounts to blends/tinctures to enhance absorption and penetration.

---

## Caution Level — ▨ Caution

May irritate stomach lining—avoid with ulcers, reflux, or gastritis. Avoid contact with eyes, mucous membranes, or open wounds. Use caution with blood thinners, hypertension meds, or heart meds. Avoid during gallbladder inflammation or active liver irritation. Discontinue if significant burning or GI distress occurs. Avoid concentrated forms during pregnancy unless supervised.

---

## Gender-Specific Safety

● **Men:** Supports circulation, stamina, and metabolic vigor; use moderate food-level or diluted doses to avoid GI irritation/burning.

● **Women:** Helpful for sluggish circulation and as a warming digestive aid; moderate culinary use is generally safe. Avoid heavy daily dosing during pregnancy.

● **Pregnancy / Nursing:** Safe in food amounts. Avoid concentrated capsules/tinctures (may increase heat or GI irritation). Nursing individuals should keep doses small to avoid possible infant digestive effects.

---

## ⌛ Expected Results

Circulatory warmth: 30–60 minutes
Topical pain relief: 15–30 minutes (best with consistent use)

Metabolic support: gradual with regular use
Cardiovascular support: cumulative over time

---

## Same / Similar Results

Ginger • Turmeric • Black Pepper • Garlic • Mustard Seed • Ginkgo

---

## Shelf Life / Potency After Preparation

**Shelf Life:** Powder/flakes 2–3 years · Oils/salves/creams 6–12 months · Tinctures 3–5 years
**Potency:** Internal tonics best fresh within hours · Topicals hold potency through shelf life if stored cool · Tinctures remain stable long term

---

## DIY Recipe — Cayenne Pain-Relief Oil

Combine 1 tbsp Cayenne powder with ½ cup olive oil. Warm gently 10 minutes, strain, and cool. Apply sparingly to sore joints/muscles (patch test first). Never apply to open wounds.

---

## DIY Recipe — Cayenne Circulation Tonic

Mix ¼ tsp Cayenne powder with warm water and lemon. Drink once daily to support circulation and digestive fire (reduce amount if sensitive).

---

## Herbal Reflections of Cayenne Pepper

Cayenne is the herbal spark—quick, catalytic, and unmistakably warming. It awakens circulation, ignites digestion, and helps move what feels cold or stuck. Used with respect, it becomes a synergist, amplifying other herbs and reminding us that sometimes healing begins with a single spark.

**Herbal Confidence Index:**

*(5/5 green stars — powerhouse circulatory stimulant; boosts metabolism, relieves pain, and enhances herbal effectiveness with speed and strong safety when used properly.)*

# ROMAN CHAMOMILE

★★★★

Chamaemelum nobile

**Roman Chamomile** is a gentle but effective calming herb prized for relaxing the mind, easing tension, and soothing the skin. Native to Western Europe and the Mediterranean, it differs from German Chamomile by being lower-growing, sweeter in aroma, and often favored for topical use and children's remedies. Its golden blossoms carry an apple-like scent and a long history as a comfort herb for emotional and physical distress.

Internally, it calms nerves, eases digestive upset, and supports sleep. Externally, it cools inflamed skin, helps minor wound repair, and soothes sunburns or rashes—offering steady comfort for body and mind.

---

**Core Herbal Category — Roman Chamomile**

**Primary Core: Nervous System Support (Nervines)** with (gentle calming principles that soothe the nervous system)

**Secondary Cores:** Digestive · Anti-Inflammatory · Sleep · Pediatric

---

## How It Works

Roman Chamomile gently reduces nervous-system overactivity, easing irritability, tension, and restlessness without heavy sedation. Aromatic compounds relax smooth muscle, reducing stress-linked digestive cramping and discomfort. Mild anti-inflammatory action soothes irritated tissues internally and externally. Its soft, non-forceful nature makes it well suited for children, sensitive individuals, and long-term calming support.

---

## Primary Uses

Calms nervousness, anxiety, and insomnia
Soothes upset stomach, gas, and mild nausea
Relieves cramps and digestive tension
Reduces skin inflammation and irritation
Supports children's sleep and emotional balance

---

## Scientific Backing

Contains esters (notably isobutyl angelate), flavonoids, and sesquiterpenes linked to antispasmodic, calming, anti-inflammatory, and skin-soothing effects. Research supports benefits for anxiety reduction, sleep support, digestive relaxation, and topical soothing in irritated or inflamed skin. Its milder profile suits sensitive users.

---

## Forms Available

Dried flowers (tea/infusion)
Tincture / glycerite
Essential oil (aromatherapy; topical use only when diluted)
Creams, infused oils, compresses

---

## How to Use (Dosage & Methods)

- **Tea:** Steep 1–2 tsp flowers in 1 cup hot water for 10 min; drink 1–2× daily.
- **Tincture:** 1–2 mL up to 3× daily for anxiety, cramping, or restlessness.
- **Topical:** Apply cooled tea or use a diluted essential-oil compress for irritated skin or puffiness.
- **Aromatherapy:** Diffuse 3–5 drops essential oil to promote calm and sleep.

---

## Shelf Life / Potency After Preparation

**Shelf Life:** Dried flowers 1–2 years (airtight/dark) · Tincture 3–5 years · Essential oil 2–3 years (cool/sealed)
**Potency:** Tea strongest within 12–24 hrs refrigerated · Compresses best made fresh daily · Essential-oil blends retain strength for months if protected from heat/light

---

## Caution Level — ● Safe

Well tolerated for most adults and children. Possible cross-sensitivity in those allergic to ragweed/marigold/daisy family plants. Avoid excessive essential-oil use near eyes. Internal tincture use during pregnancy should be supervised.

---

## Gender-Specific Safety (GS)

● **Men:** Supports calm, digestion, and sleep without hormonal effects; suitable for daily tea use.
● **Women:** Soothes PMS irritability, digestive tension, and emotional restlessness; gentle enough for regular use and skin support.
● **Pregnancy / Nursing:** Safe as a mild tea. Avoid concentrated tinctures or essential oils unless guided; mild topical or inhaled use is typically well tolerated.

---

## ⌛ Expected Results

Digestive ease: 30–60 minutes
Nervous relaxation & sleep improvement: 1–3 days of consistent use

Skin relief: within 1–3 applications

## DIY Recipe — Roman Chamomile Comfort Tea

Steep 1–2 tsp dried flowers in 1 cup hot water for 10 minutes. Add honey or lemon if desired.

## DIY Recipe — Skin-Calming Compress

Brew strong chamomile tea, cool slightly, soak a cloth, and apply to irritated or sunburned skin for 10–15 minutes.

## Same / Similar Results

German Chamomile • Lavender • Lemon Balm • Calendula Lavender

## Herbal Reflections of Roman Chamomile

Roman Chamomile whispers peace where tension gathers. It softens the stomach, loosens the breath, and invites the nervous system back toward ease. Where stronger nervines push or sedate, Roman Chamomile comforts—steady, patient, and restorative.

**Herbal Confidence Index:**

*(4/5 green stars — gentle but remarkably effective nervine; exceptionally safe, soothing for digestion and skin, and ideal for children and sensitive individuals.)*

# CHICKWEED

★★★★

*Stellaria media*

**Chickweed** is a cooling, soothing herb used for itchy rashes, eczema, and inflamed skin, and it is also taken internally to calm heat, support gentle detoxification, and ease constipation. Herbalists often use it to support lymphatic flow, reduce congestion, and bring balance when the body feels overheated, irritated, or "stuck."

Long valued in European and Native American traditions, Chickweed has also been eaten as a tender spring green. Its delicate star-shaped flowers mirror its quiet strength: nourishing, cooling, and steady.

---

🌿 **Core Herbal Category — Chickweed**

**Primary Core: Lymphatic & Skin Support** with (cooling moistening principles that calm heat and irritation)

**Secondary Cores:** Lymphatic Support · Digestive Support · Nutritive Support

---

## How It Works

Chickweed cools and coats irritated tissues, helping ease heat, dryness, and inflammation internally and externally. Demulcent action soothes mucous membranes and skin, while gentle lymphatic support assists movement of excess fluid and waste. Light nutritive compounds provide mild mineral support without overstimulating digestion. This combination reduces irritation and congestion while promoting steady comfort and balance.

---

## Primary Uses

Soothes eczema, rashes, itching, and inflamed skin
Supports lymphatic flow and mild detoxification
Eases constipation and digestive "heat"
Provides gentle nourishment (vitamins/minerals)
Helps clear mild respiratory congestion

---

## Scientific Backing

Early studies support anti-inflammatory, antifungal, and wound-healing activity. Saponins contribute to cooling/moistening effects; flavonoids and minerals support tissue repair. Traditional use aligns with emerging research for dermatitis/itch relief, lymphatic congestion, digestive irritation, and gentle detoxification.

---

## Forms Available

Fresh or dried herb (poultice, compress)
Infused oils, salves, creams
Tinctures and glycerites
Tea
Fresh leaves (edible—salads, soups, smoothies)

---

## How to Use (Dosage & Methods)

- **Tea:** 1–2 tsp dried herb per cup; steep 10 min; drink 1–2× daily.
- **Tincture:** 2–4 mL up to 2× daily for inflammation, lymph stagnation, or mild edema.
- **Topical:** Apply fresh poultice or Chickweed salve to hot/itchy skin 1–3× daily.
- **Food Use:** Add fresh Chickweed to meals for cooling, mineral-rich nourishment.

---

## Shelf Life / Potency After Preparation

**Shelf Life:** Dried herb ~1 year · Oils/salves 6–12 months (refrigerate for longest life) · Tinctures 3–5 years
**Potency:** Fresh poultice is strongest immediately · Oils/salves stay effective through shelf life · Tea best within 24 hrs refrigerated · Tincture is the most stable internal form

---

## Caution Level — ▨ Caution

Generally very safe. Large internal doses may cause loose stools due to cooling nature. Avoid concentrated extracts during pregnancy. Source from clean soil (can absorb contaminants). Use with awareness if allergic to Caryophyllaceae family.

---

## 🚹 🚺 Gender-Specific Safety (GS)

● **Men:** Supports skin clarity, lymph flow, digestion, and weight balance; large doses may loosen stools temporarily.
● **Women:** Helpful for PMS bloating, heat, and water retention; supports skin/lymph/digestion; safe in moderate daily use.
● **Pregnancy / Nursing:** Safe in mild tea or food amounts. Avoid strong tinctures/medicinal dosing except under professional guidance.

---

## ⌛ Expected Results

Skin calming: 1–5 days
Constipation relief: 1–2 days

Congestion easing: 3–5 days
Lymphatic clarity & cooling: 5–10 days

---

## DIY Recipe — Chickweed Cooling Poultice

Crush a handful of fresh Chickweed and apply directly to itchy, inflamed, or hot skin. Leave on 20–30 minutes; repeat 2–3× daily.

---

## Same / Similar Results

● Calendula • ● Plantain Leaf • ● Red Clover • ● Marshmallow Root • ● Burdock Root

---

## Herbal Reflections of Chickweed

Chickweed brings cool moisture to what feels hot, itchy, and overworked. It calms inflammation, hydrates dry tissues, and gently moves stagnation without force. Where Calendula warms and repairs and Plantain draws and cleanses, Chickweed cools and soothes—quietly refreshing overheated systems.

★ **Herbal Confidence Index:** 🌿 🌿 🌿 🌿

*(4/5 green stars — gentle, cooling demulcent; excellent for skin irritation, lymph flow, and inflammation with high safety and nourishing qualities.)*

# FEVERFEW

★★★★

*Tanacetum parthenium*

**Feverfew** is a bitter, daisy-like herb long used to prevent migraines, ease fever, and calm inflammatory pain. It can reduce headache frequency and intensity, soothe menstrual cramping, and settle inflamed joints while offering mild digestive and antispasmodic support. Herbalists often use it as a preventive daily ally for those prone to recurring migraines.

Treasured since antiquity and named for its historic use in reducing fevers, Feverfew has been a staple of European herbalism for centuries. Its bitter leaves continue to bridge folk tradition and modern migraine research alike.

---

🌿 **Core Herbal Category — Feverfew**

**Primary Core: Anti-Inflammatory & Pain Support** with (parthenolide-rich, migraine-preventive principles that calm inflammatory and vascular pain pathways)

**Secondary Cores:** Migraine Support · Women's Health · Digestive Support

---

## How It Works

Feverfew works primarily through parthenolide, a sesquiterpene lactone that inhibits inflammatory prostaglandins and reduces excessive constriction and dilation of blood vessels in the brain—one of the key mechanisms behind migraine pain. Its anti-inflammatory action also calms irritated joints and eases menstrual cramping. These combined effects are most noticeable when taken preventively and consistently over time.

---

## Primary Uses

Reduces frequency and severity of migraine headaches
Eases fever and inflammatory pain
Soothes menstrual cramping
Calms inflamed, arthritic joints
Settles mild digestive upset and bloating
Supports overall inflammatory balance

---

## Scientific Backing

Clinical research on Feverfew, particularly standardized extracts high in **parthenolide**, supports its traditional use for migraine prevention, with several trials showing reduced headache frequency and severity. Studies also note anti-inflammatory activity relevant to *arthritic* joint discomfort, plus antispasmodic and mild antimicrobial effects. Constituents such as **sesquiterpene lactones** contribute to its vascular, anti-inflammatory, and antispasmodic actions.

---

## Forms Available

Dried leaf
Fresh leaf (traditionally chewed, though bitter)
Capsules or standardized parthenolide extract
Tinctures
Teas or infusions

---

## How to Use (Dosage & Methods)

• **Tea/Infusion:** 1 tsp dried leaf steeped 10 minutes; drink 1× daily as a preventive.
• **Capsules:** 100–300 mg standardized **parthenolide** extract once daily for migraine prevention.
• **Tincture:** 1–2 mL up to 2× daily for pain and inflammatory support.
• **Fresh leaf:** 1–2 small leaves daily (traditional use; very bitter and may cause mouth sores in sensitive individuals).

---

## Shelf Life / Potency After Preparation

**Shelf Life:** Dried leaf 1–2 yrs · Capsules 1–2 yrs · Tinctures 3–5 yrs (cool/dark)
**Potency:** Fresh leaf is most potent; dried leaf loses strength gradually · Standardized capsules provide the most reliable parthenolide dosing · Tincture provides steady long-term dosing

---

## Caution Level — ▨ Caution

Avoid abrupt discontinuation after long-term daily use; **"post-feverfew syndrome"** (rebound headache, joint pain, anxiety) has been reported. Avoid during pregnancy. Use caution with blood-thinning medications. Fresh leaf may cause mouth ulcers or irritation in sensitive individuals. **Avoid if allergic to ragweed or other Asteraceae-family plants.**

---

## Gender-Specific Safety (GS)

● **Men:** Supports migraine prevention, joint comfort, and inflammatory balance. Generally well tolerated at standard doses.

● **Women:** Widely used for migraine prevention and menstrual cramp relief. Generally well tolerated; use moderately.

● **Pregnancy / Nursing:** Avoid. Traditional emmenagogue and uterine-stimulant use; insufficient safety data.

## Expected Results

Migraine frequency reduction: noticeable after 4–6 weeks of consistent use
Fever/inflammatory relief: within hours
Joint comfort: cumulative with consistent use
Menstrual cramp relief: within the same cycle

## DIY Recipe — Feverfew Migraine-Prevention Tea

Steep 1 tsp dried Feverfew leaf in 1 cup hot water for 10 minutes. Add honey and lemon to offset the bitterness. Drink 1× daily as a preventive; not intended for acute migraine relief.

## Same / Similar Results

● Butterbur • ● Willow Bark • ● Ginger • ● Skullcap • ● Turmeric

## Herbal Reflections of Feverfew

Feverfew is patience expressed as prevention—bitter, steady, and unglamorous in its daily discipline. It does not chase down pain that has already arrived; it quietly forestalls the storm before it builds. Where willow bark and other analgesics answer pain after the fact, Feverfew works upstream, reminding us that some of the deepest relief comes from consistency rather than rescue.

**Herbal Confidence Index:**

*(4/5 green stars — a well-studied, time-tested migraine-preventive herb; most effective as a daily long-term ally rather than an acute remedy.)*

# COLTSFOOT

★★★

*Tussilago farfara*

**Coltsfoot** is a soothing respiratory herb used to calm coughs, loosen mucus, and ease bronchial irritation and sore throat. It is especially valued for dry, irritated, or inflamed airway conditions, offering gentle relief during colds, flu recovery, and lingering chest congestion. Used for centuries in European traditions (as tea or smoke), its name reflects its purpose: "Tussilago" comes from *tussis* (cough). With early-blooming yellow flowers, Coltsfoot remains a classic symbol of springtime lung renewal.

---

**Core Herbal Category — Coltsfoot**
**Primary Core: Respiratory System Support** with (soothing demulcent action that calms irritated airways)
**Secondary Cores:** Demulcent · Expectorant · Anti-Inflammatory

---

## How It Works

Coltsfoot coats irritated respiratory tissues with mucilage, easing dryness, inflammation, and cough-trigger irritation. This moistening action also helps loosen sticky mucus and supports more comfortable breathing. Mild anti-inflammatory activity further calms bronchial soreness. Its action is protective and soothing rather than stimulating, making it best for dry, irritated, or inflamed cough patterns.

---

## Primary Uses

Relieves dry, irritating, or lingering coughs
Soothes bronchial inflammation and soreness
Eases hoarseness and throat irritation
Mild expectorant support for chest congestion

---

## Scientific Backing

Contains mucilage, flavonoids, zinc, and polysaccharides that soothe airway tissues and support expectoration. **Important:** Coltsfoot naturally contains **pyrrolizidine alkaloids (PAs)** that may stress the liver. **PA-free extracts exist and are the preferred option** for internal use.

---

## Forms Available

Dried leaf tea (short-term use only)
Cough syrups or lozenges
Tinctures (**PA-free recommended**)
Warm poultices for throat or chest

---

## How to Use (Dosage & Methods)

**Tea:** 1 tsp dried leaf per cup; steep 10 min. Drink 1–2× daily for **up to 5–7 days**.
**Tincture:** 1–2 mL up to 2× daily; **short-term only** (prefer PA-free).
**Cough Syrup:** Mix cooled tea with honey; take 1 tsp as needed.
**Topical:** Apply a warm compress of infused leaf to chest or throat for irritation.

---

## Shelf Life / Potency After Preparation

**Shelf Life:** Dried leaf 1–2 yrs · Syrups/lozenges 6–12 mos · Tea best within 12 hrs · PA-free tincture 3–5 yrs
**Potency:** Tea is mild/short-acting · Syrups provide moderate soothing · Tinctures are stronger but limited by safety profile

---

## Caution Level — ▨ Caution

Internal use should be **short-term (5–7 days)**. Prefer **PA-free extracts**. Avoid if you have liver disease. Avoid for children, pregnancy, and breastfeeding. Do not combine with other PA-containing herbs. Use the minimum effective dose.

---

## Gender-Specific Safety

● **Men:** Helpful for stubborn dry cough and seasonal chest irritation; **short-term internal use only**.
● **Women:** Useful for throat strain, bronchial irritation, and lingering post-cold cough; avoid extended/high-dose use.
● **Pregnancy / Nursing:** Not recommended. Choose safer options such as **Marshmallow Root, Mullein, Slippery Elm**.

---

## Expected Results

Cough relief: 1–2 doses
Throat soothing: within 24 hours

Bronchial comfort: 2–3 days
Congestion clearing: 2–4 days

---

## DIY Recipe — Coltsfoot Soothing Tea

Steep 1 tsp Coltsfoot leaf + 1 tsp Licorice Root + a pinch of Marshmallow leaf in 1 cup hot water for 10 minutes. Drink once daily for up to 5 days.

---

## Same / Similar Results

Mullein · Marshmallow Root · Slippery Elm · Lobelia · Horehound

---

## Herbal Reflections of Coltsfoot

Coltsfoot brings relief like early spring—softly and steadily—cushioning tired airways and easing the burden of a lingering cough. Yet it also asks for restraint. Used wisely and briefly (preferably PA-free), it can be a gentle ally for irritated lungs and stubborn dryness.

**Herbal Confidence Index:** *(3/5)*

A reliable short-term respiratory soother with real benefits, but limited by safety concerns due to pyrrolizidine alkaloids.

# COMFREY

★★★

*Symphytum officinale*

**Comfrey** is a powerful "knitbone" herb used **externally** to speed recovery from sprains, bruises, strains, and joint pain. It supports rapid tissue repair and helps reduce swelling and discomfort—making it one of the most effective topical herbs for musculoskeletal recovery when used short-term and with strict boundaries.

Historically respected across Europe and Asia, Comfrey's reputation comes largely from **allantoin**, a tissue-repair compound that promotes cell regeneration. Because Comfrey also contains **pyrrolizidine alkaloids (PAs)** that can harm the liver, its best use is **topical, on unbroken skin only**.

---

🌿 **Core Herbal Category — Comfrey**

**Primary Core: Lymphatic & Skin Support** with (rapid regenerative principles that support cell renewal)

**Secondary Cores:** Musculoskeletal · Anti-Inflammatory

---

## How It Works

Comfrey accelerates repair through **allantoin**, supporting faster regeneration of skin and connective tissue. Used topically, it can reduce inflammation and swelling while strengthening injured areas (muscles, tendons, ligaments). Because PAs present internal risk—and can be absorbed through damaged skin—Comfrey is kept **external and controlled**.

---

## Primary Uses

- Speeds healing of sprains, strains, and bruises
- Helps reduce swelling and inflammation
- Soothes sore joints and overuse injuries
- Supports minor abrasions/irritations (**external only; intact skin**)

## Scientific Backing

Topical Comfrey preparations have evidence for reducing pain and improving recovery in acute injuries (especially sprains and bruising). Key constituents include **allantoin**, **rosmarinic acid**, and tannins.

⚠ **Safety limitation:** Comfrey contains **PAs**—liver-toxic if ingested and potentially risky on broken skin or with prolonged heavy topical exposure.

## Forms Available

- Salves, creams, ointments (topical)
- Leaf poultice / compress
- Infused oil

---

## How to Use (Dosage & Methods)

- **Topical cream/salve:** Apply to **unbroken skin** 1–3× daily for **up to 7–10 days**.
- **Poultice:** Rehydrate dried leaf (or use fresh), apply to intact skin 20–30 minutes, 1–2× daily.
- **Warm compress:** Strong tea (1–2 tbsp dried leaf in hot water); apply cloth 15–20 minutes.

**Rule:** *External use only. Never apply to open wounds.*

---

## Shelf Life / Potency After Preparation

**Shelf Life:** Dried leaf/root ~1 year · Infused oil 12–18 months · Salves ~1 year · Poultice use immediately

**Potency:** Strongest within first 6–9 months; gradually declines thereafter.

---

## Caution Level — ● Supervision Required

- **Do not ingest** Comfrey (PA risk).
- Use **only on intact skin**, **short-term**, and on **small areas**.
- Avoid prolonged/repeated heavy use, large-area application, or use with liver disease.
- **Avoid in pregnancy and breastfeeding** unless specifically directed by a qualified clinician.

---

## Gender-Specific Safety

**Men:** Excellent for injury recovery **externally**; keep use short-term and small-area. Avoid broken skin.

**Women:** Helpful for bruising, strains, postpartum muscle soreness (**external only**). Same strict limits.

● **Pregnancy / Nursing:** Avoid internal use entirely. If used topically, keep to **small-area, short-term** only under professional guidance.

---

## Expected Results

Pain & swelling: 24–48 hours

Bruise improvement: 2–4 days

Sprain/strain recovery support: 3–7 days

---

## DIY Recipe — Comfrey Healing Salve

Infuse dried Comfrey leaf in olive oil 2–3 weeks; strain and thicken with beeswax.
Apply gently to sore joints, bruises, and sprains.
⚠ Do **not** use on broken skin or internally.

---

## Same / Similar Results

● Arnica • ● Calendula • ● St. John's Wort • ● Plantain • ● White Willow Bark

---

## Herbal Reflections of Comfrey

Comfrey is restoration with speed—remarkable for external tissue repair where bruises, strains, and joint soreness need quick support. Yet it's also a boundary herb: powerful, effective, and **not** meant for casual internal use. Used wisely—short-term and on intact skin—Comfrey remains one of the most valuable topical healers in herbal medicine.

★ **Herbal Confidence Index:** 🌿 🌿 🌿 *(3/5)*
Fair; Limited-Use Herb — unmatched for external repair, restricted by PA safety limits.

# CORDYCEPS

★★★★★

*Cordyceps sinensis*

**Cordyceps** is a premier tonic used to build energy, strengthen the lungs, and enhance stamina and endurance. It supports immune resilience, recovery after illness, and long-term vitality—often chosen when fatigue is deep, breathing feels weak, or the body needs sustainable strength without harsh stimulation.

Revered in Traditional Chinese Medicine and once reserved for royalty, Cordyceps became famous for restoring endurance in harsh mountain environments. Modern cultivated forms are widely available and retain its reputation as a high-level vitality builder.

---

🌿 **Core Herbal Category — Cordyceps**
**Primary Core: Adaptogens** with (vitality-building principles that enhance stress resilience)
**Secondary Cores:** Respiratory · Energy · Endurance · Immune

---

## How It Works

Cordyceps supports how the body **produces and uses cellular energy**, improving oxygen efficiency and stamina—especially through lung and adrenal support. It may enhance ATP output and improve fatigue recovery while helping regulate stress response (adaptogenic action). Benefits build **gradually** with consistent use.

---

## Primary Uses

- Increases energy, stamina, and endurance
- Strengthens lungs and oxygen efficiency
- Supports immune resilience and recovery
- Supports libido and reproductive vitality
- Assists blood-sugar balance and fatigue resistance

---

## Scientific Backing

Cordyceps contains **cordycepin, adenosine, and beta-glucan polysaccharides** linked to energy metabolism, immune modulation, and performance support. Studies suggest benefits for aerobic performance, fatigue reduction, inflammation balance, glucose metabolism, and respiratory function—consistent with its long-standing tonic use.

---

## Forms Available

• Powdered extract (capsules/drinks)
• Dual-extraction products
• Tinctures / liquid extracts
• Whole dried fungus for decoctions

---

## How to Use (Dosage & Methods)

• **Capsules/Powder:** 500–1,500 mg daily.
• **Tea/Decoction:** Simmer 1–2 tsp dried Cordyceps 10–15 minutes, 1–2× daily.
• **Tincture:** 2–3 mL, 1–2× daily for lung/immune support.
**Use Note:** Best with consistent daily use over several weeks.

---

## Caution Level — ▨ Caution

Generally well tolerated. High doses may feel overstimulating in sensitive individuals. Use caution with autoimmune conditions or immunomodulating/hormone-related medications. Avoid in pregnancy/nursing unless supervised (limited data).

---

## Gender-Specific Safety

● **Men:** Supports stamina, libido, lung capacity, and endurance; helpful for fatigue recovery. Consider cycles (6–8 weeks on, 1–2 weeks off).

● **Women:** Supports energy recovery, circulation, and vitality. Use moderate dosing; caution with hormone-related medications.

● **Pregnancy / Nursing:** Use only with professional guidance; prefer food-like amounts or gentler adaptogens.

---

## Expected Results

Energy lift: 5–7 days
Breathing/respiratory strength: 1–2 weeks
Endurance + immune support: 3–6 weeks

---

## DIY Recipe — Cordyceps Energy Tea

Simmer 1 tsp Cordyceps powder in 1½ cups water for 10–15 minutes; strain and drink daily.
Optional: ginger or honey.

---

## Same / Similar Results

● Reishi · ● Ginseng · ● Eleuthero · ● Ashwagandha · ● Schisandra

---

## Shelf Life / Potency After Preparation

**Shelf Life:** Dried/powder/capsules 2–3 years · Tinctures 4–5 years · Brewed tea best within 24 hours refrigerated

**Potency:** Dried forms hold strong potency for years; alcohol extracts preserve peak strength longest.

---

## Herbal Reflections of Cordyceps

Cordyceps teaches endurance without strain—an energy that grows from breath, recovery, and steady resilience. It doesn't push like a stimulant; it strengthens the foundation so the body can do more with less fatigue. For depleted lungs, overworked systems, or long-haul vitality building, Cordyceps stands as one of the most dependable allies.

🌟 **Herbal Confidence Index:** 🌿 🌿 🌿 🌿 🌿 *(5/5)*

Premier energy-and-lung tonic; exceptionally effective and reliable for stamina and recovery.

# CORN SILK

★★★★

*Zea mays*

**Corn Silk** is the fine, thread-like strands from the top of corn ears. Traditionally used in Native American and Chinese herbal systems, it's prized as a **gentle urinary soother** that supports the **bladder, kidneys, and comfortable elimination**. It's especially useful when the urinary tract feels irritated, inflamed, or "hot," and when fluid retention needs a mild, non-draining diuretic.

Corn Silk's strength is its **soft, demulcent calm**—it helps the body release excess fluid while easing irritation rather than pushing harsh stimulation.

---

🌿 **Core Herbal Category — Corn Silk**

**Primary Core: Kidney & Urinary Support** with (soothing demulcent action that calms urinary irritation)

**Secondary Cores:** Urinary · Kidney · Anti-Inflammatory

---

## How It Works

Corn Silk increases gentle urine flow while coating and calming the bladder and urinary lining. Its mucilaginous compounds help reduce burning, urgency, and inflammation so elimination feels smoother and less reactive. This dual action supports waste removal **without stripping** the system.

---

## Primary Uses

- Supports urinary tract comfort and flow
- Soothes bladder irritation and inflammation
- Helps reduce mild water retention and puffiness
- Supportive during UTI-prone periods (as a soothing ally)
- May mildly support blood pressure via fluid balance

---

## Scientific Backing

Corn Silk contains flavonoids, plant sterols, potassium salts, and volatile compounds associated with **anti-inflammatory**, **antioxidant**, and **mild diuretic** effects. Research and traditional use support its role in promoting healthy urinary flow and easing irritation, with a gentle electrolyte profile when used in normal tea amounts.

---

## Forms Available

- Dried corn silk (tea/infusion)
- Tincture or liquid extract
- Capsules / powder
- Glycerite

---

## How to Use (Dosage & Methods)

- **Tea:** 1–2 tsp dried Corn Silk per cup; steep 10–15 minutes. Drink 1–3× daily.
- **Tincture:** 2–4 mL up to 3× daily for stronger soothing/diuretic support.
- **Capsules/Powder:** 300–500 mg, 1–2× daily (follow product directions).

---

## Caution Level — ● Safe

Corn Silk is typically very gentle. Use caution if you:

- have a **corn allergy**
- take **prescription diuretics**, **blood thinners**, or certain **heart meds**
- have **low potassium** or are prone to electrolyte imbalance

Stop if rash/itching occurs.

---

## Gender-Specific Safety

● **Men:** Excellent for urinary comfort and **prostate-related irritation patterns**; no hormonal effects.

● **Women:** Great for urinary discomfort and PMS-related bloating; safe as a daily tea.

● **Pregnancy / Nursing:** Generally safe as **mild tea** for occasional swelling/irritation. Avoid high-dose extracts unless supervised.

---

## Expected Results

Urinary irritation relief: 1–3 days
Diuretic / fluid balance: within 3–7 days
Preventive comfort support: builds with consistent use

---

## DIY Recipe — Corn Silk Soothing Tea

1–2 tsp dried Corn Silk in 1 cup hot water; steep 10 minutes.
Drink 1–2× daily. Optional: lemon or honey.

---

## Same / Similar Results

● Dandelion Leaf · ● Cleavers · ● Nettle Leaf · ● Horsetail · ● Uva Ursi *(stronger; short-term only)* · ● Juniper Berry

## Shelf Life / Potency After Preparation

• Dried Corn Silk: ~1 year airtight
• Tea: best within 24 hours refrigerated
• Tincture/Glycerite: 3–5 years
**Potency note:** tea is best fresh; tinctures hold strength long-term.

---

## Herbal Reflections of Corn Silk

Corn Silk heals by gentleness—cooling irritation, easing urgency, and restoring comfort to the urinary pathways without draining the body. It reminds us that the best medicine isn't always force; sometimes the softest remedy brings the steadiest relief.

⭐ **Herbal Confidence Index:** 🌿 🌿 🌿 🌿 *(4/5)*
Mild but highly effective urinary demulcent; exceptionally safe and reliable for bladder/kidney comfort.

# CRAMP BARK

★★★★

*Viburnum opulus*

**Cramp Bark** is a traditional antispasmodic used to relieve smooth-muscle tension in the uterus, digestive tract, and musculoskeletal system. It is most commonly applied for menstrual cramping, uterine spasm, and tension-related pain where tissues are locked into contraction rather than inflamed or damaged. Its effects are calming and releasing without producing sedation.

Long used in Native American and European herbal traditions, Cramp Bark supports the body by easing involuntary muscle tightening and restoring normal rhythmic movement. It is best suited for episodic use during acute cramping or tension states rather than continuous daily administration.

---

🌿 **Core Herbal Category — Cramp Bark**

**Primary Core: Reproductive & Women's Health Support** with (relaxing principles that ease smooth-muscle contraction)

**Secondary Cores:** Women's Health · Musculoskeletal · Pain Relief

---

## How It Works

Cramp Bark relaxes involuntary muscle contraction—especially in the uterus and other smooth muscle tissue—by calming neuromuscular signaling that drives spasm. This reduces cramping intensity, eases radiating pain, and helps the body return to normal rhythmic function. It supports release rather than sedation.

---

## Primary Uses

- Eases menstrual cramps and uterine tension
- Relieves smooth-muscle spasms (digestive cramping)
- Helps reduce muscle tightness linked to stress/tension
- Supports comfort during PMS pain patterns

---

## Scientific Backing

Cramp Bark contains coumarins, flavonoids, and other constituents associated with smooth-muscle relaxation and mild analgesic effects. Evidence and long-standing traditional use support its role as a reliable antispasmodic for menstrual and tension-related discomfort.

---

## Forms Available

- Tincture (often most effective)
- Decoction/tea (bark preparations)
- Glycerite (gentler option)
- Capsules (product-dependent)

---

## How to Use (Dosage & Methods)

- **Decoction:** Simmer 1–2 tsp dried bark in 1 cup water for 10–15 minutes; drink 1–2× daily during cramping.
- **Tincture:** 2–4 mL up to 3× daily as needed.
- **Capsules:** 300–500 mg, 1–2× daily as needed (follow label).

---

## Caution Level — ▨ Caution

Generally safe at standard doses.

- May **lower blood pressure**—use caution with antihypertensive meds or dizziness.
- Avoid if you're sensitive to heavy relaxation/sedation.
- **Avoid during pregnancy** unless supervised.

---

## Gender-Specific Safety

● **Women:** Excellent for menstrual cramping and uterine tension. Avoid during pregnancy and use caution if trying to conceive without practitioner guidance.

● **Men:** Useful for tension-related muscle tightness and spasm patterns; no hormonal effects.

● **Pregnancy / Nursing:** Not recommended in pregnancy. During nursing, use only with professional guidance.

---

## Expected Results

Menstrual cramp relief: 15–45 minutes
Muscle spasm support: same day
Reduced tension pattern: 1–2 days

---

## DIY Recipe — Cramp-Ease Blend (Tincture)

Combine equal parts **Cramp Bark** + **MOTHERWORT** tincture.
Optional: add a small amount of **Valerian** for stronger relaxation.
Take 30–60 drops in water every 4–6 hours as needed.

---

## Same / Similar Results

● Motherwort · ● Wild Yam · ● Valerian · ● Chamomile · ● Black Cohosh

---

## Shelf Life / Potency After Preparation

• Dried bark: 2–3 years airtight
• Tincture: 4–6 years (strongest, most consistent)
• Glycerite: ~2 years
• Tea/decoction: best within 12–18 hours refrigerated

---

## Herbal Reflections of Cramp Bark

Cramp Bark is relief through release—an herb that helps the body unclench where pain has taken hold. It comforts without forcing, restoring rhythm to muscles and tissues that have tightened under stress, hormones, or strain. In menstrual pain especially, it serves as a steady ally: calm, effective, and deeply respected.

**Herbal Confidence Index:** *(4/5)*
Reliable antispasmodic for menstrual cramps and tension spasms; excellent effectiveness with strong overall safety when used properly.

# DANDELION ROOT

★★★★★

*Taraxacum officinale*

**Dandelion Root** is a classic liver-and-digestive tonic that helps stimulate bile flow, improve sluggish digestion, and support steady detoxification. It's also valued for gentle diuretic support, fluid balance, and metabolic clarity—making it one of the most dependable herbs for seasonal resets and long-term vitality. Though often dismissed as a weed, Dandelion has earned respect worldwide as a resilient, nourishing cleanser that supports the body's natural elimination pathways.

---

🌿 **Core Herbal Category — Dandelion Root**
**Primary Core: Liver & Detoxification Support** with (bile-stimulating cleansing support)
**Secondary Cores:** Digestive · Diuretic · Hormonal · Bitter

---

## How It Works

Dandelion Root increases bile production and supports bile flow from the liver and gallbladder, which improves fat digestion and helps the body move metabolic waste more efficiently. Its mild diuretic action supports fluid release and reduces internal "congestion." By improving liver clearance and digestive tone, it can also support hormonal balance and skin clarity. Its action is **steady and food-like**, not harsh.

---

## Primary Uses

- Stimulates bile flow and digestive efficiency
- Supports liver detoxification and metabolic clarity
- Helps reduce water retention and puffiness
- Supports clearer skin through internal elimination
- Prebiotic support for gut flora and blood-sugar steadiness

---

## Scientific Backing

Dandelion Root contains **inulin** (prebiotic fiber), **sesquiterpene lactones** (bitter digestive stimulants), and **flavonoids/phenolic compounds** associated with antioxidant and liver-supportive activity. Research and traditional use support its **digestive bitter**, **mild diuretic**, and **anti-inflammatory** actions.

## Forms Available

- Dried root (decoction)
- Powder (capsules / blends)
- Tincture / liquid extract
- Roasted root (coffee substitute)

## How to Use (Dosage & Methods)

- **Decoction:** Simmer 1–2 tbsp chopped root in 2 cups water for 15–20 minutes. Drink 1–2× daily.
- **Tincture:** 2–4 mL up to 3× daily for digestion and steady detox support.
- **Capsules/Powder:** 500–1,000 mg, 1–2× daily.
- **Roasted Root Coffee:** Daily beverage use for gentle long-term support (not a "strong detox" approach).

## Caution Level — ◍ Caution

Generally very safe, but use caution if you have:
- **Gallstones**, bile duct obstruction, or acute gallbladder flare
- **Active ulcers / severe reflux** (bitters can aggravate some people)
- **Asteraceae allergy** (ragweed/daisy family sensitivity)

**Medication note:** Use caution with **lithium** and **prescription diuretics**; discuss with a clinician if applicable.

## Gender-Specific Safety

● **Men:** Excellent for digestion, liver clearance, and fluid balance; no hormonal stimulation.

● **Women:** Supports estrogen clearance via liver pathways; useful for PMS bloating and skin congestion.

● **Pregnancy / Nursing:** Food-level and mild tea use is typically acceptable. Avoid high-dose "detox dosing" unless supervised.

## Expected Results

Digestive lift (bitters): 30–90 minutes (often same day)
Fluid balance: 3–7 days
Liver/skin clarity: 1–2 weeks (continues improving with consistent use)

## DIY Recipe — Gentle Liver Support Decoction

Simmer: **Dandelion Root + Burdock Root** (equal parts) for 20 minutes.
Optional: add a pinch of Peppermint after simmering. Drink daily for 7–14 days.

---

## Same / Similar Results

● Burdock Root · ● Milk Thistle · ● Yellow Dock · ● Artichoke Leaf · ● Oregon Grape Root

---

## Shelf Life / Potency After Preparation

- Dried root: 2–3 years airtight
- Powder: 12–18 months
- Tincture: 4–6 years
- Roasted root: 1–2 years
- Decoction: best within 24–36 hours refrigerated

---

## Herbal Reflections of Dandelion Root

Dandelion Root proves that humble medicine can be profound. Its bitterness awakens digestion and bile flow, while its nourishment supports the very organs doing the cleansing. Unlike aggressive detox approaches, Dandelion works with the body's rhythms—clearing while replenishing—restoring momentum when the system feels heavy, stagnant, or overloaded.

⭐ **Herbal Confidence Index:** 🌿 🌿 🌿 🌿 🌿 *(5/5)*
Cornerstone liver + digestive bitter; exceptionally safe, food-like, and deeply effective for steady detox support.

# DAMIANA

★★★★

*Turnera diffusa*

**Damiana** is an aromatic nervine traditionally used to support mood balance, ease nervous tension, and promote healthy libido. It is most often applied when emotional stress, fatigue, or low mood contribute to reduced vitality or diminished sexual interest. Its effects are gently uplifting and relaxing rather than stimulating.

Long valued in Mesoamerican herbal traditions, Damiana supports the nervous system by easing tension while maintaining mental clarity. It is best suited for short-to-moderate use during periods of stress, emotional strain, or recovery, rather than continuous daily use.

---

🌿 **Core Herbal Category — Damiana**

**Primary Core: Nervous System Support (Nervines)** with (uplifting principles that relax and brighten mood)

**Secondary Cores:** Libido · Circulatory · Hormonal

---

## How It Works

Damiana gently relaxes stress-driven nervous tension while improving emotional tone. By reducing performance anxiety and mental tightness, it can help libido return more naturally. Mild circulatory support may enhance pelvic blood flow and sensory responsiveness. It's not a sedative—more of a **soft uplift** that works best with consistent use.

---

## Primary Uses

- Supports libido and sensual vitality
- Eases anxiety and mild low mood
- Helps reduce stress-related sexual inhibition
- Supports PMS mood tension and emotional irritability
- Promotes relaxed circulation and warmth

---

## Scientific Backing

Damiana contains flavonoids and aromatic compounds studied for **mood support**, **nervine relaxation**, and potential **sexual-function support** (especially where stress is a major factor). Evidence is still developing, but traditional use is strong and consistent across cultures.

## Forms Available

- Dried leaf (tea)
- Tincture / liquid extract
- Capsules / powdered leaf
- Included in libido and mood formulas

## How to Use (Dosage & Methods)

- **Tea:** 1–2 tsp dried leaf; steep 10 minutes. Drink 1–2× daily.
- **Tincture:** 2–4 mL up to 2× daily.
- **Capsules:** 400–500 mg, 1–2× daily (follow label).

**Best results:** 7–14 days of consistent use for mood + libido patterns.

## Caution Level — Caution

Generally safe in moderate amounts.

- Avoid high doses late in the day if prone to **insomnia**.
- Use caution with **blood-sugar medications** (may add mild lowering effects in some people).
- Avoid during **pregnancy** due to limited safety data.

Stop if headaches, irritability, or digestive upset occurs.

## Gender-Specific Safety

**Men:** Supports libido, confidence, and relaxed mood without hormonal forcing.

**Women:** Supports libido and emotional warmth; helpful for PMS mood tension and stress patterns.

**Pregnancy / Nursing:** Avoid in pregnancy; during nursing, avoid concentrated dosing unless supervised.

## Expected Results

Nervous relaxation: 30–60 minutes
Mood lift: 1–3 days
Libido support: 1–2 weeks consistent use

## DIY Recipe — Damiana Warmth Tea

Steep 1 tsp Damiana in 1 cup hot water for 10 minutes.
Optional: add **cinnamon** or **raw cacao** for warmth and synergy.

## Same / Similar Results

Maca · Muira Puama · Ginseng · Ashwagandha · Shatavari

---

## Shelf Life / Potency After Preparation

- Dried leaf: 1–2 years airtight
- Powder: ~1 year
- Tincture: 4–6 years
- Prepared tea: best within 24 hours refrigerated

---

## Herbal Reflections of Damiana

Damiana restores warmth—of mood, of confidence, of connection. It doesn't force desire; it removes the nervous tension that blocks it. Where some tonics push energy, Damiana harmonizes emotion and body, helping intimacy feel natural again. It reminds us that vitality often returns when the mind softens and the heart reopens.

**Herbal Confidence Index:** *(4/5)*

Trusted mood-and-libido nervine; effective, gentle, and best for stress-linked libido and emotional dullness.

# DANDELION LEAF

★★★★★

*Taraxacum officinale var. officinale*

**Dandelion Leaf** is a mineral-rich diuretic used to support kidney function, fluid balance, and gentle detoxification. Unlike harsh water-draining agents, it promotes urinary elimination while replenishing potassium and trace minerals, helping prevent depletion. It is commonly used for mild edema, skin congestion, and metabolic sluggishness associated with fluid retention.

Traditionally gathered in European and North American herbal practice as a spring tonic, Dandelion Leaf supports steady daily elimination and renewal. Its action is balancing rather than forceful, making it appropriate for short- to moderate-term use or gentle seasonal support.

---

**🌿 Core Herbal Category — Dandelion Leaf**
**Primary Core: Nutritional & Tonic Support** with (mineral-rich principles that gently rebuild and cleanse)
**Secondary Cores:** Urinary · Liver · Digestive

---

**How It Works**
Dandelion Leaf increases gentle urine flow while preserving electrolytes, especially potassium. Its bitter-green compounds support digestion and liver efficiency, aiding waste clearance without strain. This allows fluid release and metabolic support to occur together.

---

### 🌱 Primary Uses

- Supports fluid balance and reduces puffiness
- Aids kidney filtration and urinary comfort
- Supports liver and digestive function
- Replenishes minerals during gentle cleansing
- Promotes skin clarity through improved elimination

---

### 🔬 Scientific Backing

Dandelion Leaf contains flavonoids, phenolic compounds, and potassium salts linked to diuretic and antioxidant activity.
Research supports increased urination without potassium loss, aligning with its traditional use for fluid balance and spring cleansing.

---

### 💊 Forms Available

- Fresh or dried leaf (tea/infusion)

• Powder (daily blends)
• Capsules or tablets

---

### How to Use (Dosage)

• Tea/Infusion: 1–2 tsp dried leaf per cup; steep 10–15 minutes, 1–3× daily
• Fresh Leaf: Culinary use in salads or cooked dishes
• Capsules/Powder: 500–1,000 mg, 1–2× daily
Maintain adequate hydration during use.

---

### Caution Level: Caution

Generally safe and well tolerated.
Avoid with bile duct obstruction, acute gallbladder issues, severe kidney disease, or Asteraceae allergy.
Use caution alongside prescription diuretics or lithium.

---

### Gender-Specific Safety

Men:
Supports kidney and urinary balance without hormonal stimulation.
Women:
Helpful for fluid shifts, PMS-related bloating, and skin congestion.
Pregnancy / Nursing:
Safe in culinary or mild tea amounts; avoid concentrated dosing.

---

### Expected Results

• Reduced water retention: 24–48 hours
• Urinary comfort: 2–5 days
• Skin clarity and metabolic lightness: 1–2 weeks
• Mineral support: cumulative with regular use

---

### DIY Recipe — Mineral Detox Tea

Steep 1 tbsp Dandelion Leaf with 1 tsp Nettle Leaf in hot water for 10–15 minutes.
Drink 1–2× daily.

---

### Same / Similar Results

Nettle Leaf · Cleavers · Parsley · Red Clover · Burdock Root

---

### Shelf Life / Potency After Preparation

• Dried Leaf: 1–2 years, airtight storage
• Powder: ~1 year
• Prepared Tea: Best within 24 hours refrigerated

---

💭 **Herbal Reflections of Dandelion Leaf**

Dandelion Leaf teaches release without loss. It clears excess while quietly restoring what the body depends on to stay strong. In this balance of letting go and replenishing, it reminds us that true cleansing supports vitality rather than stripping it away.

---

🌟 **Herbal Confidence Index:** 🌿 🌿 🌿 🌿 🌿 **(5 / 5 green stars)**

Cornerstone nutritive diuretic—potassium-preserving, reliable, and exceptionally safe for steady fluid balance and gentle cleansing.

# ANNATTO

★★★

*Bixa orellana*

**Annatto** is a tropical plant with a long history of use by Indigenous Amazonian cultures, where its bright red-orange seeds were applied to the skin to protect against sun, infection, and environmental stress, and used to color the body for ritual, identity, and healing. This same pigment carried medicinal value—helping calm irritation and support tissue resilience. Medicinally, Annatto is best known for skin support, gentle tissue protection, and antioxidant nourishment. Its key compounds—**carotenoids** and **tocotrienols**—act as natural cellular defenders. Carotenoids help shield skin and tissues from heat, sun, and oxidative damage, while tocotrienols (a potent form of vitamin E) support cell integrity, circulation, and liver protection. Annatto's strength lies not in forceful stimulation, but in protection, making it especially useful for skin care and mild internal support.

---

### 🌿 Core Herbal Category — Annatto

Primary Core: **Lymphatic & Skin Support** with (protective antioxidant principles that support cellular integrity)
Secondary Cores: Circulatory · Digestive · Liver · Antioxidant

---

**How It Works**
Annatto supports healing primarily through antioxidant protection. Its carotenoids (bixin/norbixin) and tocotrienols help reduce oxidative stress that slows tissue recovery and contributes to inflammation. Topically, this protection can calm irritation and support a cleaner healing environment. Internally, its antioxidant profile may support healthy lipids and metabolic balance, but its strongest traditional use remains skin-focused and supportive rather than "powerfully regenerative."

---

**Primary Uses**
- Soothes skin irritation and supports wound comfort (topical)
- Provides antioxidant support and inflammation reduction
- Supports cardiovascular and liver wellness (mild supportive use)
- Traditional digestive support
- May support balanced blood sugar in some individuals

---

**Scientific Backing**
Annatto contains bixin, norbixin, and tocotrienols—compounds studied for antioxidant and anti-inflammatory activity. Research supports protective effects against oxidative stress and suggests potential benefits for lipid balance and metabolic markers, while traditional use strongly supports topical soothing and skin protection.

---

**Forms Available**
• Leaf infusion (internal or external wash)
• Seed paste / infused oil / salves (topical)
• Capsules or tocotrienol supplements

---

**How to Use (Dosage & Methods)**
• Tea/Infusion: Steep 1–2 tsp dried Annatto leaf in hot water for 10–15 minutes; drink 1× daily.
• Capsules/Supplements: 300–500 mg, 1–2× daily (follow label).
• Topical: Apply Annatto-infused oil or seed paste 1–2× daily for irritation.
Use consistently for 1–2 weeks to evaluate skin and digestive support.

---

**Caution Level — ● Caution**
• May trigger allergy/sensitivity in some individuals (including those sensitive to food colorants).
• Use caution with low blood pressure or antihypertensive medication.
• Stop if rash, itching, or respiratory irritation occurs.

---

**Gender-Specific Safety: SAFE**
● Men: Supports antioxidant defense and mild cardiovascular wellness; helpful topically for minor irritation.
● Women: Useful for skin clarity and gentle liver-supportive antioxidant tone at food/tea levels.
● Pregnancy / Nursing: Food-level use is generally acceptable. Avoid concentrated supplements/strong extracts due to limited safety data.

---

**Expected Results**
• Skin soothing: 1–3 days (topical use)
• Reduced irritation / improved comfort: 2–7 days
• Cardiovascular/metabolic support: 3–6 weeks (consistent use)

---

**DIY Recipe — Annatto Leaf Skin Wash**
Boil 1 tbsp dried Annatto leaves in 2 cups water, then simmer 10 minutes.
Cool, strain, and use as a gentle wash for irritated skin. Use within 24–48 hours refrigerated.

---

**Same / Similar Results**
● Calendula · ● Turmeric · ● Gotu Kola · ● Milk Thistle

---

**Shelf Life / Potency After Preparation**
• Dried leaves: 1–2 years
• Seeds: 2–3 years
• Powdered pigment: ~1 year airtight
• Prepared wash: 24–48 hours refrigerated

---

**Herbal Reflections of Annatto**
Annatto reminds us that protection is a form of healing. Its medicine is less about force and more about shielding—reducing the oxidative "static" that keeps tissues irritated and slow to recover. It's a quiet ally for skin comfort and gentle internal support, carrying the warmth of tradition and the strength of antioxidant defense in the same bright color.

**Herbal Confidence Index**: 🌿 🌿 🌿 (3/5)
Steady antioxidant + topical support herb—useful and culturally significant, strongest for skin comfort and protection, milder for internal tonic power.

# SWEET CICELY

★★★★

*Myrrhis odorata*

**Sweet Cicely** is a fragrant, old-world digestive and respiratory herb valued for its gentle anise-like sweetness and calming influence. Long cultivated in monastery gardens and rural apothecaries, it was traditionally used to ease indigestion, coughs, and fatigue while softening bitter remedies. Both medicinal and culinary, Sweet Cicely is best known as a "comfort herb" — restoring appetite, easing tension, and bringing harmony to sensitive systems.

---

**Core Herbal Category — Sweet Cicely**
**Primary Core: Digestive System Support** with (gentle carminative principles that ease discomfort)
**Secondary Cores:** Respiratory · Nervine

---

## How It Works

Sweet Cicely gently relaxes the digestive tract, helping relieve gas, cramping, and post-meal discomfort without stimulating heat or irritation. Aromatic carminative compounds support smooth digestion, while mild nervine action calms tension that can aggravate digestive upset. Subtle expectorant effects offer light respiratory comfort during colds or seasonal transitions. Its action is soft, balancing, and well suited for sensitive constitutions.

---

## Primary Uses

- Relieves gas, bloating, and mild indigestion
- Soothes throat and chest irritation during colds
- Supports appetite and digestion during recovery
- Gently sweetens herbal blends and bitter formulas
- Provides mild mood and adrenal support

---

## Scientific Backing

Sweet Cicely contains essential oils rich in anethole, along with coumarins and aromatic compounds associated with:

- Carminative and antispasmodic activity
- Light expectorant effects

• Antioxidant and anti-inflammatory support
Research aligns with its traditional use for digestive comfort, respiratory ease, and gentle emotional uplift.

---

## Forms Available

• Dried leaves or root (tea / decoction)
• Tincture
• Syrups and herbal honeys
• Culinary herb or natural sweetener

---

## How to Use (Dosage & Methods)

• **Tea:** Steep 1 tsp dried leaf or ½ tsp crushed root in 8 oz hot water for 10 minutes
• **Tincture:** 1–2 mL, up to 3× daily
• **Culinary:** Add to teas, tonics, or foods for digestive and mood support

---

## Expected Results

• Digestive relief: 30–60 minutes
• Throat or cough comfort: 1–2 days
• Appetite and strength restoration: 3–5 days

---

## ⚠ Caution Level — Safe

Very safe in tea and culinary amounts
Use moderation with long-term heavy use if on anticoagulants (coumarin content)
Well tolerated by adults and children

---

## Gender-Specific Safety

**Men:** Supports digestion, calm focus, and gentle respiratory comfort
**Women:** Helpful for PMS bloating, mild fatigue, and appetite recovery
**Pregnancy / Nursing:** Safe in culinary and light tea use; avoid strong tinctures late in pregnancy

## DIY Recipe — Sweet Digestive Tea

• 1 tsp Sweet Cicely
• ½ tsp Fennel
• ½ tsp Lemon Balm
Steep 10 minutes after meals for gas, tension, and sluggish digestion.

---

## 🔄 Same / Similar Results

● Fennel · ● Anise Seed · ● Chamomile · ● Lemon Balm · ● Licorice Root

---

## 📦 Shelf Life / Potency After Preparation

• Dried leaf: ~1 year (airtight)
• Dried root: 1–2 years
• Tincture: 4–5 years
• Syrup / honey: 6–12 months (refrigerated)
• Culinary blends: 6–12 months for peak flavor

---

## 💬 Herbal Reflections of Sweet Cicely

Sweet Cicely teaches that medicine does not need bitterness to be effective. Favored by monks and household healers alike, it softens tension, uplifts the spirit, and restores ease to digestion and breath. Where stronger herbs push, Sweet Cicely comforts — bringing warmth, sweetness, and balance to bodies recovering from stress, illness, or seasonal strain.

⭐ **Herbal Confidence Index:** 🌿 🌿 🌿 🌿 (4/5)

*Safe, aromatic digestive and respiratory ally; especially valued for its gentleness, versatility, and ability to soften stronger formulas.*

# PASSION FLOWER

★★★★★

*Passiflora incarnata*

**Passionflower** is a calming nervine traditionally used to quiet racing thoughts, ease anxious rumination, and support natural sleep without heavy sedation. Indigenous North American tribes first used the vine to settle the nerves and calm the mind, and it later became a respected European evening tea for restlessness and insomnia.

Unlike stronger sedatives, Passionflower gently relaxes both mental and physical tension, making it especially helpful for those who feel "tired but wired." Modern research supports its long-standing use, showing that its flavonoid compounds help calm nervous overactivity and support smoother sleep onset and continuity without dependence.

---

🌿 **Core Herbal Category — Passion Flower**

**Primary Core: Nervous System Support (Nervines)** with (sedating principles that quiet nervous overactivity)

**Secondary Cores:** Sleep · Anxiety · Muscle Relaxation

---

## How It Works

Passionflower calms excessive nervous-system activity, helping the body shift out of heightened alertness. Its sedative nervine compounds reduce mental restlessness and muscle tension without suppressing normal function. Rather than forcing sleep, it gently encourages relaxation and emotional settling, supporting natural sleep onset and continuity.

---

## Primary Uses

- Supports sleep onset and continuity
- Reduces anxious rumination and evening restlessness
- Provides gentle daytime calm in low doses

---

## Scientific Backing

Contains flavonoids (including vitexin) and harmala alkaloids that support GABA activity and reduce nervous overstimulation. Studies show reduced sleep latency, improved sleep depth, and better emotional regulation with consistent use.

## 💊 Forms Available

• Tincture (fast-acting)
• Tea / infusion
• Capsules (standardized extracts)

---

## 🥄 How to Use (Dosage & Methods)

• Tea: 1–2 tsp dried herb per cup; steep 10 minutes, 1–2× daily
• Tincture: 1–2 mL up to 3× daily
• Capsules: 300–500 mg, 1–2× daily
• Bedtime: Take 30–60 minutes before sleep
Pairs well with Lemon Balm, Skullcap, or Magnolia.

---

## ⚠ Caution Level — ▨ Caution

• May enhance sedatives or sleep medications
• Avoid driving after use
• Use caution with antidepressants or benzodiazepines
• Avoid during pregnancy (mild uterine effects)

---

## 🚹 🚺 Gender-Specific Safety

● Men: Calms overthinking, improves sleep quality without daytime dullness
● Women: Eases hormonally influenced anxiety and perimenopausal sleep issues
● Pregnancy / Nursing: Avoid during pregnancy; caution while nursing

---

## ⌛ Expected Results

• Mental quieting: few nights to 1 week
• Sleep improvement: 1–2 weeks
• Daytime calm (low dose): same day to 3 days

---

## 🛠 DIY — Bedside Passiflora Tincture

1–2 mL tincture in water, 30–60 minutes before bed
Optional blend: Lemon Balm or Magnolia Bark
Reduce dose if morning grogginess occurs.

---

## 🔄 Same / Similar Results

● Lemon Balm · ● Magnolia · ● Valerian · ● Jatamansi · ● Mulungu · ● Chamomile · ● Kava (short-term) ● Lavender

---

## 📦 Shelf Life / Potency

• Dried herb: 1–2 years
• Tincture: 4–6 years
• Capsules: ~2 years
• Tea: best within 24 hours

---

## 💬 Herbal Reflections

Passionflower is a tender remedy for a restless mind. Rather than forcing sedation, it invites unwinding—allowing sleep to emerge naturally. Used consistently, it teaches the nervous system to soften, release tension, and rest.

---

### ⭐ Herbal Confidence Index

🌿 🌿 🌿 🌿 🌿

*(5/5 — cornerstone nervine; exceptionally safe and effective for anxiety and sleep without dependency.)*

# DONG QUAI

★★★★

*Angelica sinensis*

**Dong Quai**, often called the "Queen of Women's Herbs," is a traditional Chinese root used for centuries to nourish blood, improve circulation, and support menstrual and hormonal balance. Historically valued for restoring strength after depletion, it was used for irregular cycles, pelvic tension, and recovery following childbirth.

Rather than acting quickly, Dong Quai works gradually—warming, nourishing, and harmonizing the reproductive system over time. Its role is long-term balance, not short-term symptom suppression.

---

🌿 **Core Herbal Category — Dong Quai**

**Primary Core: Reproductive & Women's Health Support** with (blood-nourishing principles that regulate menstrual cycles)

**Secondary Cores**: Circulatory · Hormonal · Nervine · Postpartum

---

## How It Works

Dong Quai nourishes and gently moves the blood, restoring circulation to pelvic and reproductive tissues. It supports balanced uterine tone and regular flow rather than stimulation. Improved blood quality eases cycle discomfort and supports postpartum recovery, while mild nervine effects calm hormonally driven emotional tension.

---

## Primary Uses

- Balances irregular or uncomfortable menstrual cycles
- Reduces cramping and pelvic tension
- Supports menopausal transition
- Nourishes blood (fatigue, pallor, postpartum weakness)
- Enhances pelvic and systemic circulation
- Eases emotional stagnation
- Supports postpartum recovery (when appropriate)

---

## Scientific Backing

Contains ferulic acid, ligustilide, polysaccharides, and volatile oils that support circulation, smooth-muscle relaxation, and mild estrogen modulation. Research supports reduced cramping, improved circulation, blood nourishment, and benefits for menopausal mood and thermal balance.

---

## Forms Available

- Dried root (tea/decoction)
- Powder
- Capsules / tablets
- Tincture
- Extracts and combined formulas

---

## How to Use

- Capsules/Tablets: 400–600 mg, 1–2× daily
- Tincture: 1–2 mL up to 2× daily
- Tea/Decoction: 1–2 tsp root, simmer 10–15 minutes, 1× daily

Best used in cycles (3–6 weeks on, 1–2 weeks off).
Avoid during heavy menstrual flow.

---

## Expected Results

- Menstrual comfort: 1–2 cycles
- Hormonal steadiness: 2–4 weeks
- Circulation & vitality: 2–6 weeks
- Postpartum support: gradual over 4–8 weeks (with guidance)

---

## ⚠ Caution Level — ◍ Moderate / Use With Guidance

Avoid or use cautiously with:

- Heavy bleeding
- Blood thinners
- Hormone-sensitive conditions
- Upcoming surgery (stop 2 weeks prior)
- Diarrhea or loose stools
- Acute infections or fever

## Gender-Specific Safety

● Men: Generally safe but not primary; avoid high doses with blood thinners
● Women: Excellent for cycles and perimenopause; avoid during heavy bleeding
● Pregnancy / Nursing: Avoid; may stimulate uterine activity

---

## Same / Similar Results

Black Cohosh · Vitex · Peony Root · Schisandra · Red Clover · Motherwort

---

## Shelf Life / Potency

- Dried root: 2 years
- Powder: ~1 year
- Tincture: 3–5 years
- Capsules: 1–2 years
- Decoction: use within 48 hours

---

## DIY — Dong Quai Hormonal Balance Tea

1 tsp Dong Quai
1 tsp Peony Root
Optional ginger slice
Simmer 10–12 minutes; drink during non-bleeding days.

---

## Herbal Reflections

Dong Quai is quiet strength—warming, nourishing, and harmonizing. It restores rhythm to cycles and steadiness to vitality through balance rather than force, reminding us that deep healing often comes through slow restoration.

## Herbal Confidence Index

🌿🌿🌿🌿

*(4/5 — foundational reproductive and circulatory tonic; powerful, time-tested, and safe when used with awareness.)*

# Devil's Claw

★★★★

*Harpagophytum procumbens*

**Devil's Claw** is a traditional African joint and pain-relief herb valued for easing inflammation, stiffness, and mobility limitations in arthritis, gout, and chronic back pain. Indigenous healers of southern Africa relied on its bitter roots to relieve pain, fever, and digestive weakness—uses later confirmed by modern clinical study. Slow-building but dependable, Devil's Claw is best suited for long-term musculoskeletal support rather than quick, numbing relief.

---

**Core Herbal Category — Devil's Claw**

**Primary Core: Anti-Inflammatory & Pain Support** with (anti-inflammatory principles that reduce pain and improve joint mobility)

**Secondary Cores:** Pain Relief · Anti-Inflammatory · Digestive · Circulatory

---

### How It Works

Devil's Claw reduces inflammatory signaling in joints, muscles, and connective tissue, easing swelling, stiffness, and pain over time. Its iridoid compounds calm inflammatory pathways rather than masking sensation, allowing gradual restoration of flexibility and comfort. Mild circulatory and digestive stimulation support nutrient delivery and absorption. Effects are cumulative, making consistent use essential.

---

### Primary Uses

- Relieves joint pain and stiffness (arthritis, gout)
- Reduces chronic back and musculoskeletal pain
- Supports tendon and ligament recovery
- Aids muscle recovery after exertion
- Provides mild digestive stimulation

---

### Scientific Backing

Devil's Claw contains **harpagoside**, an iridoid glycoside shown to reduce inflammation and pain.

Human studies demonstrate:

- Reduced osteoarthritis pain
- Improved joint mobility

• Meaningful relief in chronic lower-back pain
• Best outcomes with sustained use

---

## 💊 Forms Available

• Dried root (decoction)
• Capsules or standardized extracts
• Powdered root
• Tincture or liquid extract

---

## 🍵 How to Use (Dosage & Methods)

• **Capsules:** 600–1,000 mg standardized extract (1–3% harpagoside), 1–2× daily
• **Tincture:** 2–4 mL, 2–3× daily
• **Decoction:** Simmer 1–2 tsp dried root in 1 cup water for 10–15 minutes (very bitter)
• **Timing:** Expect noticeable effects after 1–3 weeks of consistent use

---

## ⚠ Caution Level — 🟠 Caution

• May irritate stomach lining; avoid with ulcers or severe GERD
• Use caution with gallstones, blood thinners, diabetes medications, or NSAIDs
• Avoid during pregnancy (mild uterine effects)
• Discontinue if digestive discomfort worsens

---

## 👨 👩 Gender-Specific Safety

🔵 **Men:**
Excellent for chronic joint strain, back pain, and work-related stiffness. Non-hormonal; suitable for long-term use if digestion tolerates bitterness.
🟣 **Women:**
Helpful for inflammatory joint pain and stiffness. May cause stomach sensitivity at higher doses.
🔴 **Pregnancy / Nursing:**
Avoid due to uterine-stimulating potential and limited safety data.

---

## ⌛ Expected Results

• Pain or stiffness relief: 7–14 days
• Improved mobility: 2–4 weeks
• Best results with ongoing use and gentle movement

---

## 🛠 DIY Recipe — Joint-Support Decoction

Simmer equal parts:

• Devil's Claw root
• Turmeric
• Ginger
Use 1 tbsp blend in 2 cups water; simmer 20 minutes. Drink 1–2× daily.

---

## 🔄 Same / Similar Results

Turmeric · Boswellia · Willow Bark · Meadowsweet · Yucca Root

---

## Shelf Life / Potency After Preparation

• Dried root: 2 years
• Powder: ~1 year (bitterness fades with potency)
• Tincture: 4–5 years
• Decoction: use within 24 hours (refrigerated)
• Capsules: typically 2 years

## Herbal Reflections of Devil's Claw

Devil's Claw heals through persistence, not force. Its bitterness signals a medicine that works slowly but deeply—softening inflammation and restoring movement over time. Unlike fast-acting pain herbs, it rebuilds comfort gradually, rewarding patience with steadier mobility and reduced stiffness.

**Herbal Confidence Index:**

*(4/5 — dependable long-term anti-inflammatory and joint-support herb; clinically validated and effective when used consistently, but limited by digestive sensitivity in some users.)*

# ANDROGRAPHIS

★★★★

*Andrographis paniculata*

**Andrographis** is a bitter, fast-acting immune herb used to shorten the severity and duration of colds, flu, and respiratory infections while strengthening overall immune defense. Long known in Ayurveda and Traditional Chinese Medicine as the "King of Bitters," it was traditionally used to clear heat, reduce fever, and combat infection. Modern research confirms its effectiveness in acute illness, making Andrographis a reliable short-term ally for immune challenges rather than long-term tonic use.

---

**Core Herbal Category — Andrographis**
**Primary Core: Immune System Support** with (strong defensive and pathogen-inhibiting action)
**Secondary Cores:** Antiviral · Anti-Inflammatory · Respiratory · Liver & Detoxification

---

## How It Works

Andrographis activates immune defenses that help identify and suppress pathogens early in infection. Its bitter compounds support antiviral and antimicrobial activity while moderating excessive inflammation. At the same time, it assists liver detox pathways, helping the body clear metabolic waste generated during immune response. This dual action supports faster recovery without prolonged inflammatory strain. Best results occur when used early or during acute illness.

---

## Primary Uses

• Shortens colds, flu, and upper respiratory infections
• Strengthens immune resilience under stress
• Reduces inflammatory congestion in lungs and digestion
• Supports liver detox during illness

---

## Scientific Backing

Andrographis contains **andrographolides**, compounds shown to be antiviral, antibacterial, and anti-inflammatory.
Clinical studies demonstrate:

- Reduced duration and severity of URTIs
- Lower fever, cough, congestion, and fatigue
- Improved immune response efficiency
- Reduced mucosal inflammation

---

## 💊 Forms Available

- Standardized extract capsules or tablets
- Tincture / liquid extract
- Tea or decoction (extremely bitter)

---

## How to Use (Dosage & Methods)

- **Capsules/Tablets:** 300–600 mg standardized extract (10–30% andrographolides), 1–2× daily
- **Tincture:** 1–2 mL up to 3× daily during illness
- **Tea:** 1 tsp dried herb simmered 10 minutes; 1–2× daily

**Timing:** Most effective at first sign of infection for 3–7 days

---

## ⚠ Caution Level — Caution

- May cause stomach upset or fatigue in sensitive individuals
- Avoid during pregnancy or while trying to conceive
- Use caution with immune-suppressants, anticoagulants, or blood-pressure medications
- Intended for short-term use; avoid long continuous cycles

---

## Gender-Specific Safety

**Men:**

Supports immune strength and detoxification without hormonal effects. Useful during physical or seasonal stress.

**Women:**

Aids immune recovery and liver-based detox. High doses may slightly increase menstrual flow.

**Pregnancy / Nursing:**

Avoid due to uterine effects and limited safety data.

---

## ⌛ Expected Results

- Cold/flu symptom reduction: 3–5 days
- Energy recovery: 1–2 weeks
- Best outcomes with rest, hydration, and consistent dosing

---

## 🛠 DIY Recipe — Immune Support Tea

1 tsp Andrographis
½ tsp Licorice Root
1 tsp Peppermint
Steep 10 minutes; drink warm during illness.

---

## 🔄 Same / Similar Results

● Echinacea · ● Elderberry · ● Astragalus

---

## 📦 Shelf Life / Potency After Preparation

- Dried herb: 1–2 years
- Capsules/Tablets: ~2 years
- Tincture: 4–6 years
- Prepared tea: 24 hours refrigerated

---

## 💬 Herbal Reflections of Andrographis

Andrographis is sharp, bitter, and direct—medicine that wastes no time. It excels when the body is under attack, clearing heat and restoring strength with precision. Though not gentle enough for constant use, it remains one of the most dependable short-term immune defenders in herbal medicine.

⭐ **Herbal Confidence Index:**

🌿 🌿 🌿 🌿

*(4/5 — potent short-term immune and antiviral herb; highly effective when used early and appropriately, but best used intermittently due to strength.)*

# BACOPA

★★★★

*Bacopa monnieri*

**Bacopa** is a traditional brain and nerve tonic used to enhance memory, focus, and emotional steadiness while protecting the nervous system from stress and fatigue. Known in Ayurveda as **Brahmi**, it was prized by scholars and meditators for sharpening intellect while calming the mind. Rather than stimulating the brain, Bacopa strengthens cognitive resilience gradually, making it a trusted long-term herb for mental clarity and emotional balance.

---

**Core Herbal Category — Bacopa**
**Primary Core: Nervous System Support (Nervines)** with (cognitive-nourishing principles that strengthen mental clarity)
**Secondary Cores:** Adaptogen · Memory · Emotional Balance

---

## How It Works

Bacopa nourishes and protects nerve cells while supporting communication between neurons. Its compounds enhance antioxidant activity in brain tissue, reducing mental fatigue and stress-related cognitive decline. Over time, this neuroprotective action improves memory retention, learning capacity, and emotional steadiness. Effects build gradually, making consistent use essential.

---

## Primary Uses

- Improves memory, focus, and concentration
- Reduces anxiety and nervous tension
- Supports long-term brain and nerve health
- Assists attention and learning challenges
- Promotes calm sleep and mental clarity

---

## Scientific Backing

Bacopa's active compounds (**bacosides A & B**) have been shown to:
- Improve memory retention and recall
- Enhance processing speed and learning
- Support neuron communication
- Reduce oxidative stress in brain tissue

Clinical studies confirm benefits after several weeks of consistent use.

---

## 💊 Forms Available

• Dried herb (tea or infusion)
• Tincture / liquid extract
• Capsules or tablets (standardized bacosides)
• Powder (traditionally taken with warm milk or ghee)

---

## How to Use (Dosage & Methods)

• **Capsules/Powder:** 300–450 mg standardized extract daily (take with food)
• **Tincture:** 2–5 mL, 1–2× daily
• **Tea:** 1 tsp dried herb simmered 10 minutes; drink 1× daily
**Consistency:** Full benefits appear after 4–6 weeks of daily use

---

## ⚠ Caution Level — Caution

• May cause mild nausea, fatigue, or digestive upset initially
• Avoid during pregnancy
• Use caution with thyroid or antidepressant medications
• Start low and increase gradually

---

## Gender-Specific Safety

**Men:**
Enhances focus, memory, and stress resilience without overstimulation. Suitable for long-term cognitive support.

**Women:**
Supports mood stability and clarity during hormonal transitions. Generally safe in moderate, long-term use.

**Pregnancy / Nursing:**
Avoid during pregnancy. Nursing: mild tea only with professional guidance.

---

## ⌛ Expected Results

• Calm focus: 1–2 weeks
• Memory and learning gains: 4–8 weeks
• Sleep improvements: 3–7 days

---

## DIY Recipe — Bacopa Brain Tea

1 tsp dried Bacopa

1 cup boiling water
Steep 10–15 minutes; drink once daily.

---

## 🔄 Same / Similar Results

● Gotu Kola · ● Lion's Mane · ● Ginkgo Biloba · ● Ashwagandha · ● Rhodiola

---

## 📦 Shelf Life / Potency After Preparation

• Dried herb: ~1 year
• Powder: 6–9 months
• Capsules/Tablets: 1–2 years
• Tincture: 4–5 years
• Prepared tea: 24 hours refrigerated

---

## 💬 Herbal Reflections of Bacopa

Bacopa refines the mind through steadiness rather than force. It quiets mental noise while strengthening clarity, teaching the nervous system to function with calm precision. Its wisdom lies in patience—rewarding consistent use with sharper memory, balanced mood, and lasting cognitive resilience.

⭐ **Herbal Confidence Index:**

🌿 🌿 🌿 🌿

*(4/5 — classic Ayurvedic brain tonic; safe, effective, and deeply supportive of long-term memory, focus, and emotional balance.)*

# BETONY

★★★★

*Stachys officinalis*

**Betony** is a classic Old-World nervine used to relieve tension headaches, calm nervous anxiety, and steady digestion under stress. Valued since Roman times—when it was said to belong in every garden—it became a trusted remedy for headaches, digestive upset, and nervous exhaustion throughout medieval Europe. Today, Betony remains a gentle, grounding herb for restoring balance when stress shows up in the head, gut, or mood.

---

🌿 **Core Herbal Category — Betony**
**Primary Core: Nervous System Support (Nervines)** with (grounding principles that ease tension and steady the nerves)
**Secondary Cores:** Digestive · Headache Relief · Respiratory · Mood Support

---

## How It Works

Betony gently calms the nervous system while releasing tension held in the head, neck, and digestive tract. Its grounding nervine action quiets overstimulation that often underlies headaches, anxiety, and stress-related digestive upset. Mild bitter and aromatic compounds support circulation and digestion, helping tension resolve rather than migrate.

---

## Primary Uses

- Relieves tension headaches and migraines
- Calms nervous tension and mild anxiety
- Eases gas, bloating, and stress-related digestive upset
- Supports respiratory comfort and seasonal irritation
- Provides mild anti-inflammatory and circulatory support

---

## Scientific Backing

Modern clinical research is limited, but extensive European herbal tradition documents Betony's use for nervous tension, headaches, digestive upset, and throat irritation. Its tannins contribute astringent and anti-inflammatory effects, while volatile oils provide gentle nervine support—aligning with its long reputation as a "head, stomach, and spirit" herb.

## Forms Available

• Dried leaf (tea or blends)
• Tincture / liquid extract
• Capsules or powdered extracts
• External compress (tea applied topically)

---

## How to Use (Dosage & Methods)

• **Tea:** 1–2 tsp dried leaf steeped 10–15 minutes; drink 1–3× daily
• **Tincture:** 2–4 mL up to 3× daily
• **Topical:** Apply cooled tea to temples or tense muscles
*Best results with several days of steady use.*

---

## Caution Level — Mild Caution

Generally very safe.
Use caution with low blood pressure or antihypertensive medication.
Pregnancy/nursing: light tea only.
Excessive doses may cause mild dizziness or fatigue.

---

## Gender-Specific Safety

**Men:** Reduces stress-related headaches and digestive tightness without sedation.
**Women:** Helpful for PMS-related headaches, digestive strain, and emotional tension.
**Pregnancy/Nursing:** Avoid concentrated doses; light tea only with guidance.

---

## Expected Results

• Headache or anxiety relief: 30–60 minutes
• Digestive improvement: 2–3 days of consistent use

---

## DIY Recipe — Headache Relief Tea

1 tsp Betony
1 tsp Chamomile
½ tsp Lemon Balm

Steep 10 minutes; drink at headache onset or for gentle relaxation.

## 🔄 Same / Similar Results

Lemon Balm · Chamomile · Skullcap · Peppermint · Passionflower

---

## 📦 Shelf Life & Potency

- Dried leaf: 1–2 years
- Powder: 6–9 months
- Tincture: 4–5 years
- Prepared tea: 24 hours refrigerated

---

## 💬 Herbal Reflections of Betony

Betony is a quiet stabilizer—grounding the nerves, easing the gut, and lifting tension without sedation. It restores clarity where stress has tightened the system, reminding us that calm often comes not from force, but from gentle rebalancing.

---

**Herbal Confidence Index:** 🌿 🌿 🌿 🌿

*(4/5 — steady grounding nervine; effective for tension headaches, stress digestion, and nervous imbalance.)*

# BLADDERWRACK

★★★★

*Fucus vesiculosus*

**Bladderwrack** is a mineral-rich sea herb traditionally used to nourish the thyroid, support metabolism, and restore trace nutrients often missing from modern diets. Collected for centuries along European coastlines, it served as both food and medicine—valued for its iodine content, digestive-soothing fibers, and whole-body nourishment. Today, Bladderwrack remains a foundational nutritive for thyroid-linked fatigue, sluggish metabolism, and mineral depletion.

---

**Core Herbal Category — Bladderwrack**
**Primary Core: Nutritional & Tonic Support** with (iodine-rich principles that support thyroid nourishment)
**Secondary Cores:** Metabolic · Digestive · Mineral-Building

---

### How It Works

Bladderwrack supplies bioavailable iodine and trace minerals that nourish the thyroid and support healthy metabolic signaling. This supports energy regulation without forcing hormone output. Its mucilaginous fibers soothe the digestive tract and improve nutrient absorption, allowing metabolic balance through nourishment rather than stimulation.

---

### Primary Uses

- Supports healthy thyroid hormone production
- Provides iodine and trace minerals
- Supports metabolism and energy balance
- Soothes digestive lining
- May ease joint stiffness linked to inflammation

---

### Scientific Backing

Bladderwrack is among the most researched seaweeds for thyroid support due to its iodine content. Key compounds include fucoidan (anti-inflammatory, antioxidant), alginic acid (digestive-soothing and binding), and iodine (essential for thyroid hormone synthesis). Research supports its role in iodine-deficiency hypothyroid patterns and gentle detox support.

---

## 🖋 Forms Available

- Dried whole herb
- Powder
- Capsules or tablets
- Tincture
- Seaweed or mineral blends

---

## How to Use (Dosage & Methods)

- **Capsules/Powder:** 400–600 mg, 1–2× daily
- **Tea/Infusion:** 1 tsp dried herb steeped 10 minutes, 1× daily
- **Tincture:** 1–2 mL, 1–2× daily

*Use moderately; avoid long-term high dosing.*

---

## ⚠ Caution Level — Caution

High iodine content may alter thyroid function in sensitive individuals.
Avoid with hyperthyroidism or iodine sensitivity.
Do not combine with thyroid medication unless supervised.
Not recommended during pregnancy or breastfeeding.

---

## Gender-Specific Safety

**Men:** Supports thyroid-related energy and metabolism; use moderate doses.

**Women:** May assist mild hypothyroid patterns; avoid prolonged or high-dose use without guidance.

**Pregnancy/Nursing:** Avoid due to fetal/infant thyroid risk.

---

## ⌛ Expected Results

- Metabolic/thyroid support: 7–14 days
- Energy, skin, hair improvements: 3–4 weeks

---

## 🛠 DIY Recipe — Mineral Sea Soup

Simmer 1 tbsp Bladderwrack in 3 cups water for 10 minutes.
Stir in miso and vegetables; enjoy warm for mineral nourishment.

## 🔄 Same / Similar Results

⚪ Kelp · ⚪ Irish Moss · ⚪ Dulse · ⚪ Sea Lettuce · ⚪ Nettle Leaf

---

## 📦 Shelf Life & Potency

- Dried herb: 1–2 years
- Powder: 6–12 months
- Tincture: 4–5 years
- Prepared tea: 24 hours refrigerated

---

## 💬 Herbal Reflections of Bladderwrack

Bladderwrack is nourishment from the sea—slow, steady, and foundational. Rather than pushing the body, it rebuilds what is missing, restoring metabolic rhythm through mineral balance and gentle support.

---

⭐ **Herbal Confidence Index:** 🌿 🌿 🌿 🌿
*(4/5 — mineral-rich thyroid nutritive; highly effective when used intelligently, unsuitable for iodine-sensitive individuals.)*

# Motherwort

★★★★

*Leonurus cardiaca*

**Motherwort** is a classic heart-and-nervine herb used to calm anxiety, ease stress-related palpitations, and support emotional and hormonal balance. Long valued as a "wort for mothers," it has been relied on in European herbalism to steady the emotional and physical heart during menstruation, menopause, and postpartum recovery. Bitter yet grounding, Motherwort is especially helpful when emotional strain expresses itself through the heart or nervous system.

---

### Core Herbal Category — Motherwort

**Primary Core: Nervous System Support (Nervines)** *(heart-calming principles that ease emotional tension)*

**Secondary Cores:** Women's Health · Circulatory · Hormonal

---

## How It Works

Motherwort gently calms the nervous system while relaxing cardiac and smooth muscle tissue. Its bitter nervine compounds reduce emotional agitation and stress-related palpitations without heavy sedation. This calming effect also supports uterine comfort, making it especially useful when emotional stress affects the heart or reproductive system.

---

### Primary Uses

- Calms anxiety and emotional agitation
- Supports heart rhythm and stress-related palpitations
- Eases menstrual cramping and PMS tension
- Supports menopausal mood balance

---

### Scientific Backing

Contains alkaloids such as **leonurine**, associated with mild sedative, antispasmodic, and anti-arrhythmic effects. Traditional and emerging research supports its use in women's health and stress-related cardiovascular support.

---

### Forms Available

- Tea / infusion

- Tincture
- Capsules
- Women's health blends

---

## How to Use

- **Tea:** 1–2 tsp per cup, steep 10–15 min; up to 2 cups daily
- **Tincture:** 1–2 mL, up to 3× daily
  Best used in **small, consistent doses**.

---

## Caution Level — Caution

- Avoid during pregnancy
- Use caution with heart, thyroid, or sedative medications
- May lower blood pressure in sensitive individuals

---

## Gender-Specific Safety

- **Men:** Supports stress-related palpitations and nervous tension
- **Women:** Excellent for PMS, menopause, and emotional steadiness
- **Pregnancy/Nursing:** Avoid during pregnancy; postpartum use only with guidance

---

## Expected Results

- Emotional calming: 30–60 minutes
- Heart steadiness: 1–3 weeks
- Hormonal tension relief: 5–7 days

---

## Same / Similar Results

Passionflower · Lemon Balm · Dong Quai · Blue Vervain

---

## 💬 Herbal Reflections

Motherwort is a steadying presence — calming the heart, softening emotional overload, and restoring rhythm during times of transition. Its medicine is quiet but dependable, offering strength without force.

⭐ **Herbal Confidence Index:** 🌿 🌿 🌿 🌿

*(4/5 — trusted cardiac and women's nervine; highly effective for emotional and heart-centered tension.)*

# Cat's Claw

★★★★

*Uncaria tomentosa*

**Cat's Claw** is a traditional Amazonian vine used to strengthen immunity, reduce chronic inflammation, and support joint and digestive health. Long revered in South American medicine, it is valued not for rapid stimulation but for its ability to **modulate** immune response over time. Its claw-shaped thorns reflect its nature — gripping steadily and restoring resilience through patience and consistency.

---

🌿 **Core Herbal Category — Cat's Claw**
**Primary Core: Immune System Support** *(modulating principles that strengthen balanced immune response)*
**Secondary Cores:** Anti-Inflammatory · Joint · Digestive · Antioxidant

---

## How It Works

Cat's Claw supports immune regulation rather than overstimulation. Its alkaloids help immune responses activate appropriately and resolve efficiently, reducing chronic inflammation while supporting tissue repair — especially in joints and the gut. Benefits build gradually with consistent use.

---

🌱 **Primary Uses**

- Reduces chronic joint inflammation and pain
- Supports immune recovery after infection
- Assists autoimmune and inflammatory balance
- Protects gut lining and digestive integrity

---

🔬 **Scientific Backing**
Contains **pentacyclic oxindole alkaloids (POAs)** associated with immune modulation and anti-inflammatory activity. Research supports benefits in arthritis, oxidative stress reduction, immune recovery, and gastrointestinal protection.

---

### Forms Available

- Decoction (inner bark)
- Tincture
- Capsules / tablets
- Powder

---

### How to Use

- **Decoction:** 1 tsp bark in 2 cups water, simmer 15–20 min
- **Capsules:** 250–500 mg, 2–3× daily
- **Tincture:** 1–2 mL, 2–3× daily
  **Best used in cycles:** 2–3 weeks on, 1 week off.

---

### Caution Level — Caution

- Avoid during pregnancy or breastfeeding
- Consult provider if autoimmune disease or immunosuppressants are present
- May cause mild digestive upset

---

### Gender-Specific Safety

- **Men:** Excellent for inflammation and immune recovery
- **Women:** Supports immune and joint balance; avoid during pregnancy
- **Pregnancy/Nursing:** Do not use

---

### Expected Results

- Immune balance: 1–2 weeks
- Joint comfort: 2–3 weeks
- Digestive repair: 3–4 weeks

---

### Same / Similar Results

Boswellia · Devil's Claw · Ashwagandha · Pau d'Arco

---

### Herbal Reflections of Cat's Claw

Cat's Claw works through patience rather than force. It does not push the immune system into overreaction, but instead encourages discernment—strengthening response while calming excess. In long-term inflammation or immune fatigue, it supports recovery by restoring balance at the roots rather than chasing symptoms. Its lesson is endurance: healing that unfolds steadily, guided by rhythm, restraint, and respect for the body's limits.

---

**Herbal Confidence Index:** (4 / 5 green stars)

Powerful immune-modulating vine — especially well suited for long-term inflammatory and immune support when used cyclically.

# YARROW

★★★★★

*Achillea millefolium*

**Yarrow** is one of the most ancient and respected healing herbs in human history, famously associated with Achilles, who used it to treat battlefield wounds. Valued for its ability to stop bleeding, regulate inflammation, and restore balance, Yarrow has served as both a first-aid remedy and a deeper systemic healer for thousands of years.
Beyond wound care, it has long been used for fevers, colds, menstrual discomfort, digestive upset, and circulatory imbalance. Often described as a "boundary herb," Yarrow helps regulate flow — slowing excess bleeding, encouraging perspiration during fever, and steadying overstimulation — protecting vitality during times of stress.

---

🌿 **Core Herbal Category — Yarrow**
**Primary Core: Immune System Support** *(fever-regulating and defensive-balancing action)*
**Secondary Cores:** Circulatory · Wound Healing · Digestive · Women's Health · Foundational / Systemic Support

---

## How It Works

Yarrow supports balanced immune response by improving circulation and peripheral blood flow, allowing heat and immune activity to distribute and resolve rather than stagnate. Its diaphoretic action helps normalize fevers, while bitter and aromatic compounds reduce congestion and inflammatory tension. Astringent and styptic properties tighten tissues and slow bleeding, making Yarrow effective both internally and externally. The result is efficient immune activation followed by proper resolution.

---

🌱 **Primary Uses**

- Stops minor external bleeding and supports wound closure
- Helps break fevers through gentle sweating
- Eases colds, flu, and sinus congestion
- Relieves menstrual cramps and heavy or "flooding" menses
- Supports healthy circulation and mild blood-pressure balance
- Soothes digestive cramping and gas

---

### Scientific Backing

Yarrow contains flavonoids, sesquiterpene lactones, tannins, and volatile oils that:

- Provide anti-inflammatory and antispasmodic effects
- Tone tissues (astringent action)
- Promote circulation and perspiration (diaphoretic)
- Support platelet aggregation and wound repair
  Both traditional and modern herbal practice recognize Yarrow as a key first-aid and fever-management herb.

---

### Forms Available

- Dried aerial parts (tea, infusion, compress)
- Tincture / liquid extract
- Powder (capsules or blends)
- Fresh plant poultice for minor cuts and scrapes

---

### How to Use (Dosage & Methods)

**Tea / Infusion:**
1–2 tsp dried herb per cup; steep 10–15 min. Drink 1–3× daily for fever, colds, or menstrual support.
**Fever Blend:**
Combine Yarrow with Elderflower and Peppermint; drink warm every 2–3 hours at onset.
**Tincture:**
1–2 mL, up to 3× daily for circulation, fever, or menstrual regulation.
**Topical:**
Apply strong tea or fresh-crushed leaves as a compress or poultice to slow bleeding and support wound closure.

---

### ⚠ Caution Level — Caution: Use with Care

- Avoid internal use during pregnancy (mild emmenagogue)
- Use caution with blood-thinning medications or bleeding disorders
- Possible sensitivity in those allergic to the Asteraceae family

- Rare skin sensitivity with long-term high dosing
  Discontinue if rash, itching, or unusual bruising occurs.

---

**Gender-Specific Safety**

**Men:**
Safe for wound care, fever support, circulation, and muscle soreness.

**Women:**
Helpful for heavy or irregular menses and pelvic congestion. Avoid heavy use if cycles are already very light.

**Pregnancy / Nursing:**
Pregnancy: Avoid internal use.
Nursing: Light tea for colds may be acceptable with guidance; avoid strong or prolonged dosing.

---

**Expected Results**

- Fever and cold relief: 1–3 days
- Styptic effect (topical): within minutes
- Menstrual comfort: same cycle with consistent use
- Circulatory balance: 1–3 weeks

---

**DIY Recipe — Yarrow Fever & First-Aid Tea**

- 1 tsp Yarrow
- 1 tsp Elderflower
- ½ tsp Peppermint
  Steep 10–15 minutes. Drink warm every few hours at fever onset or 1–2× daily for menstrual discomfort.

---

**Same / Similar Results**

Elderflower · Plantain Leaf · Chamomile · Shepherd's Purse · Goldenrod

---

**Shelf Life & Potency**

- Dried herb: 1–2 years
- Tincture: 4–6 years

- Capsules/powder: 1–2 years
- Prepared tea: 24 hours refrigerated
- Compress/wash: 24–48 hours refrigerated

---

💭 **Herbal Reflections of Yarrow**

Yarrow is a guardian of boundaries — governing the flow of blood, heat, and tension. Where Calendula soothes and Comfrey knits, Yarrow decides when to move and when to contain.

From ancient battlefields to modern homes, it remains a steady ally in moments of crisis, teaching the body — and the spirit — how to conserve strength, restore order, and heal with clarity.

🌟 **Herbal Confidence Index:** 🌿 🌿 🌿 🌿 🌿

*(5/5 — cornerstone first-aid and immune-balancing herb; exceptional for wounds, fevers, and menstrual regulation when used respectfully.)*

# COSTUS ROOT

★★★

*Saussurea costus*

**Costus Root** is a warming, aromatic herb long valued in Ayurveda and Traditional Chinese Medicine for clearing stagnation in the lungs, digestion, and skin. Traditionally used for bronchial congestion, bloating, and inflammatory skin conditions, it is known for its penetrating nature and ability to restore movement where heaviness has set in.

Its warming action makes it especially useful for damp, sluggish conditions marked by mucus, gas, or inflammatory congestion. While potent, it works best when used carefully and in moderate doses.

---

**Core Herbal Category — Costus Root**

**Primary Core:** Digestive System Support with (warming principles that restore digestive balance)

**Secondary Cores:** Respiratory · Circulatory · Skin & Tissue Repair

---

## How It Works

Costus Root works by warming and stimulating digestion, improving bile flow and relieving gas and stagnation. Its aromatic compounds dry excess mucus, supporting clearer breathing and bronchial comfort. This warming, moving action helps restore circulation and immune responsiveness without harsh purging.

---

**Primary Uses**

- Relieves bronchial congestion and cough
- Eases bloating, gas, and sluggish digestion
- Soothes inflammatory skin conditions
- Supports menstrual and circulatory movement

---

**Scientific Backing**

Costus Root contains sesquiterpene lactones, flavonoids, and phenolic acids known for:

- Anti-inflammatory effects
- Bronchodilating activity
- Antimicrobial and antioxidant action
- Digestive stimulation

Modern findings align closely with its traditional role in respiratory, digestive, and skin support.

---

### Forms Available

- Dried root chips or powder
- Capsules
- Tincture
- Infused oil
- Essential oil (external only)

---

### How to Use

- Decoction: Simmer 1 tsp root in 2 cups water for 15–20 minutes
- Capsules: 250–500 mg, 1–2× daily
- Tincture: 1–2 mL up to 3× daily
- Topical: Diluted oil for rashes or inflammation

Essential oil is external only.

---

### Caution Level — Caution

- Avoid during pregnancy
- Not recommended with gallstones or active ulcers
- May irritate stomach if taken on empty stomach
- Essential oil must always be diluted

---

### Gender-Specific Safety

**Men:** Supports digestion, lungs, and circulation; avoid excessive long-term use.

**Women:** Traditionally used for cramps and congestion; avoid strong extracts.

**Pregnancy / Nursing:** Avoid internal use.

---

### Expected Results

- Digestive relief: same day
- Respiratory easing: 1–3 days
- Skin improvement: 7–10 days

---

### DIY Recipe — Costus Respiratory Decoction

Simmer:

- 1 tsp Costus Root
- 1 tsp Mullein
- ½ tsp Licorice Root

Reduce by half; sip warm 1–2× daily.

---

### Same / Similar Results

Mullein · Licorice Root · Coltsfoot · Turmeric

---

### Shelf Life

- Dried root: 2–3 years

• Powder: 1–2 years
• Tincture: 4–6 years
• Infused oil: 1 year
• Decoction: 24 hours refrigerated

---

### Herbal Reflections of Costus Root

Costus Root carries the signature of movement and release. Its warmth does not rush the body but patiently loosens what has grown heavy, damp, or stuck — whether in the breath, the skin, or the digestive fire. Where stagnation dulls vitality, Costus reintroduces circulation and clarity, reminding the body how to breathe, warm, and move again. It teaches that healing often begins not by adding force, but by restoring flow.

---

### Herbal Confidence Index

*(3/5 — effective warming digestive and respiratory herb; valuable but requires careful dosing and sourcing.)*

# *GOLDENROD*

★★★★★

*Solidago virgaurea*

**Goldenrod** is a bright, late-summer flowering herb often blamed for seasonal allergies—yet it is actually one of the classic herbs used to **reduce allergy symptoms**, clear sinus pressure, and calm irritated mucous membranes. Revered in both Native American and European folk medicine, Goldenrod has also been widely used as a **urinary tract tonic**, supporting kidney flow, reducing inflammation, and helping the body release excess fluid without harsh depletion. Goldenrod shines as a steady, balancing herb for the **urinary and respiratory systems**—helping the body "let go" of what is stuck: inflammation, congestion, and fluid retention. It is especially useful for people who feel puffy, congested, and sluggish during allergy season or urinary irritation cycles.

---

🌿 **Core Herbal Category — Goldenrod**
**Primary Core: Kidney & Urinary Support** with (gentle diuretic and tissue-toning principles that support kidney function)
**Secondary Cores:** Anti-Inflammatory · Respiratory · Immune

---

## How It Works

Goldenrod works by gently increasing urine flow while toning and soothing the tissues of the urinary tract, helping flush metabolic waste without causing depletion. Its mild anti-inflammatory action calms irritation in the kidneys and bladder, making elimination more comfortable. At the same time, its astringent and antihistamine-like effects help calm overreactive mucous membranes in the sinuses and throat. The overall effect is clearing and strengthening—supportive enough for longer-term maintenance.

---

## 🏵 Primary Uses

- Relieves seasonal allergies, hay fever, and sinus congestion
- Mild diuretic for water retention and swelling
- Supports urinary tract and kidney comfort (irritation/UTI tendency)
- Soothes sore throat and mild cough
- Promotes wound healing and tissue repair (topical)

---

## 🧪 Scientific Backing

Goldenrod contains quercetin, kaempferol, saponins, and phenolic acids that contribute to:

- Antihistamine and anti-inflammatory activity
- Diuretic and urinary-toning effects
- Antimicrobial support

Modern herbal research supports Goldenrod's usefulness for urinary tract inflammation and immune/mucosal balance, aligning with its traditional role in allergy relief and urinary comfort.

---

## 💊 Forms Available

- Dried flowering tops (tea/infusion)
- Tincture / liquid extract
- Capsules or powdered herb
- Topical wash or poultice

---

## How to Use (Dosage & Methods)

**Tea / Infusion:** Steep 1–2 tsp dried tops in 1 cup hot water for 10–15 minutes; drink 2–3× daily for urinary support or allergies.

**Tincture:** 1–2 mL up to 3× daily for fluid balance or inflammation.

**Topical:** Cooled infusion applied to wounds, irritated skin, or inflamed areas.

**Hydration Note:** Pair with adequate water intake to support kidney flushing.

Avoid strong diuretic use during acute kidney inflammation.

---

## ⚠ Caution Level — Caution

- Use caution with kidney disease
- Those with Aster-family allergies should use care
- Overuse may cause dryness, mild dehydration, or dizziness
- Discontinue if headache, excessive dryness, or irritation develops

## Gender-Specific Safety

**Men:** Supports urinary flow, reduces fluid retention after exertion, and eases sinus pressure. Safe in tea or tincture doses with good hydration.

**Women:** Helps reduce water retention and post-menstrual bloating; supports urinary comfort and allergy-season sinus pressure.

**Pregnancy / Nursing:** Avoid concentrated tinctures or strong diuretic dosing; light tea only with guidance.

---

## ⌛ Expected Results

- Allergy relief / sinus easing: 1–3 days
- Urinary comfort: 2–5 days
- Water retention reduction: 3–7 days
- Topical healing: 2–4 days
- Full systemic benefit: 1–2 weeks

---

## 🛠 DIY Recipe — Goldenrod & Nettle Allergy Tea

- 1 tsp Goldenrod
- 1 tsp Nettle Leaf
- ½ tsp Peppermint

Steep 10–15 minutes; drink 1–2× daily during allergy season.

---

## 🔄 Same / Similar Results

● Nettle Leaf · ● Dandelion Leaf · ● Parsley · ● Cleavers · ● Plantain Leaf

---

## 📦 Shelf Life / Potency After Preparation

- Dried herb: 1–2 years
- Tincture: 4–6 years
- Capsules: 1–2 years
- Topical washes: 24–48 hours refrigerated
- Prepared tea: 24 hours refrigerated

## 💬 Herbal Reflections of Goldenrod

Goldenrod embodies late-summer renewal—clearing heaviness from the body: congestion, inflammation, swelling, and sinus pressure. Misunderstood as an allergen, it is often a **natural ally against allergy misery**, supporting the body's ability to drain, calm, and reset. Goldenrod reminds us that healing often comes through release—letting go of what the body no longer needs.

---

### ⭐ Herbal Confidence Index

🌿 🌿 🌿 🌿 🌿

*(5/5 — cornerstone urinary and allergy-support herb; exceptionally reliable for kidney-toning, fluid balance, and mucous-membrane calming when used with good hydration.)*

# *NETTLE LEAF*

★★★★★

*Urtica dioica*

**Nettle Leaf** is a **deeply nutritive restorative herb** traditionally used to rebuild depleted systems while gently supporting detoxification and inflammatory balance. Long valued across Europe, Asia, and North America, Nettle acts primarily on the **blood, kidneys, joints, and immune system**, supplying the body with a dense spectrum of minerals, vitamins, and chlorophyll. Unlike stimulating tonics, Nettle strengthens through **gradual replenishment**, making it especially useful for fatigue, allergies, joint discomfort, anemia tendencies, and long-term vitality support. Its rare ability to **cleanse while rebuilding** has earned it a reputation as one of the most dependable foundational herbs in Western herbalism.

---

🌿 **Core Herbal Category — Nettle Leaf**

**Primary Core: Nutritional & Tonic Support** with (mineral-rich principles that rebuild and restore depleted systems)

**Secondary Cores:** Urinary Support · Anti-Inflammatory · Respiratory Support · Circulatory · Foundational / Systemic Support

---

## How It Works

Nettle Leaf works by delivering a broad range of bioavailable minerals, vitamins, and chlorophyll that nourish the blood, connective tissues, and metabolic systems. This deep nourishment strengthens resilience rather than producing quick stimulation. Its mild diuretic action supports kidney filtration and waste elimination, while anti-inflammatory compounds help modulate allergic and inflammatory responses. Over time, this steady rebuilding improves energy, joint comfort, immune balance, and overall tissue strength.

---

🌱 **Primary Uses**

- Eases arthritis and joint inflammation
- Relieves hay fever and seasonal allergies
- Strengthens hair, skin, and nails
- Supports kidney and urinary tract health
- Replenishes iron, minerals, and trace nutrients

---

🧪 **Scientific Backing**

Nettle Leaf contains flavonoids, lectins, phenolic compounds, minerals, and chlorophyll shown to:

• Modulate histamine response (natural antihistamine)
• Inhibit inflammatory pathways (COX-1 & COX-2)
• Support urinary detoxification
• Improve mineral status and blood quality
• Provide antioxidant and tissue-building effects

Supported by studies in *Journal of Ethnopharmacology*, *Phytomedicine*, and *Planta Medica*.

---

### Forms Available

• Loose dried leaf (tea or long infusion)
• Capsules
• Tincture
• Freeze-dried leaf
• Powdered extract

---

### How to Use (Dosage & Methods)

**Tea:**
1–2 tsp dried leaf per cup; steep 10–15 minutes; drink 1–3× daily

**Capsules:**
300–500 mg up to 3× daily

**Tincture:**
1–2 mL in water, 2–3× daily

**Strong Mineral Infusion:**
¼ cup dried leaf per quart of hot water; steep 4–8 hours; sip through the day

---

### Caution Level — Caution

Generally well tolerated.
• Mild diuretic effect may increase urination
• Avoid high doses during pregnancy unless guided
• May interact with blood-pressure, diabetic, or diuretic medications
• Fresh leaves sting — handle carefully
• Long-term use is safe with adequate hydration

---

### Gender-Specific Safety

**Men — Safe**
Supports prostate health, circulation, joint comfort, and energy.

**Women — Safe**
Excellent for mineral replenishment, hair/skin health, and menstrual fatigue.

**Pregnancy / Nursing — Generally Safe**
Often used as a mineral tonic; use regularly only with guidance due to diuretic action.

---

### Expected Results

• Allergy relief: 3–7 days

• Energy & mineral replenishment: 1–2 weeks
• Joint comfort: 2–3 weeks
• Hair & skin strengthening: 3–4 weeks

---

### 🛠 DIY Recipe — Nettle Hair Strength Tonic

Steep 2 tbsp dried Nettle Leaf in 2 cups hot water for 30 minutes.
Strain and apply to scalp daily.

---

### 🔄 Same / Similar Results

● Dandelion Leaf · ● Red Clover · ● Burdock Root · ● Yellow Dock · ● Alfalfa Leaf

---

### Shelf Life / Potency After Preparation

• Dried leaf: 1–2 years
• Tincture: 4–6 years
• Capsules/powder: 1–2 years
• Prepared tea: 24 hours refrigerated

---

### 💬 Herbal Reflections of Nettle Leaf

Once its sting is removed, Nettle becomes one of the most generous herbs in nature. It rebuilds quietly, strengthening blood, joints, immunity, and resilience over time. Few plants match its ability to nourish while restoring balance — a true cornerstone herb.

---

### ⭐ Herbal Confidence Index

🌿 🌿 🌿 🌿 🌿

*(5/5 green stars — cornerstone nutritive and restorative herb; exceptionally safe and effective.)*

# *Lamb's Ear*

★★★★

*Stachys byzantina*

**Lamb's Ear** is a **topical first-aid herb** historically used to protect wounds, stop minor bleeding, and support surface healing. Known as "woundwort," its soft, absorbent leaves were applied directly to injuries on ancient battlefields, serving as natural bandages long before modern gauze or antiseptics. Lamb's Ear acts primarily on the **skin and superficial tissues**, offering cushioning, moisture control, and mild antimicrobial protection. Its value lies in **gentle external care**, making it ideal for cuts, scrapes, burns, and irritated skin.

---

🌿 **Core Herbal Category — Lamb's Ear**

**Primary Core: Lymphatic & Skin Support** with (soft, absorbent principles that protect and support healing)

**Secondary Cores:** Astringent · Antimicrobial · Wound Care

---

## How It Works

Lamb's Ear works by creating a soft, protective barrier over damaged skin, shielding wounds from friction, excess moisture, and environmental exposure. Its mild astringent and antimicrobial compounds support clean healing while reducing irritation and minor inflammation. The leaf's absorbent texture helps control oozing and moisture imbalance, allowing tissues to repair naturally without disturbance.

---

🌱 **Primary Uses**

- Stops minor bleeding
- Cushions and protects wounds
- Soothes cuts, scrapes, burns, and irritated skin
- Reduces surface inflammation and redness
- Absorbs moisture from damp or oozing wounds

---

🧪 **Scientific Backing**

Lamb's Ear contains tannins, flavonoids, and antibacterial compounds shown to:

- Reduce surface bacterial growth
- Support wound contraction
- Provide moisture-absorbing protection

These findings mirror its long-standing use as a battlefield dressing and first-aid plant.

---

### Forms Available

- Fresh leaves (natural bandage)
- Dried leaf (wash or poultice)
- Powdered leaf (wound dusting)
- Infused oil or healing salve

---

### How to Use (Dosage & Methods)

**Natural Bandage:**
Apply clean, fresh leaves directly to minor wounds.
**Poultice:**
Crush fresh leaves and apply to irritated skin.
**Herbal Wash:**
Steep 1–2 tbsp dried leaf; cool and apply with cloth.
*(Primarily external use.)*

---

### Caution Level — Generally Safe

- Safe for most individuals when used externally
- Do not use on deep puncture wounds or severe infections
- Rare skin sensitivity possible
- Avoid internal use

---

### Gender-Specific Safety

**Men — Safe**
Excellent for cuts, scrapes, and minor bleeding.
**Women — Safe**
Soothes chafing, burns, and irritated skin.
**Pregnancy / Nursing — Safe (Topical)**
Avoid internal use.

---

### Expected Results

- Stops bleeding: immediate
- Skin calming: minutes
- Redness reduction: 1–2 days
- Minor wound healing: 2–4 days

---

### DIY Recipe — Lamb's Ear Battlefield Poultice

Crush 2–3 fresh leaves until moist.
Apply directly to wound for 15–20 minutes.

---

### Same / Similar Results

Plantain Leaf · Yarrow · Comfrey Leaf · Calendula · Aloe Vera

---

### Shelf Life / Potency After Preparation

- Fresh leaves: use immediately
- Dried leaf: 1 year
- Infused oil: 1 year refrigerated
- Salve: 6–12 months

---

### Herbal Reflections of Lamb's Ear

Lamb's Ear reminds us that some of the most effective healing is quiet and protective rather than forceful. Its soft, silvery leaves offer comfort, shielding the skin while the body does its natural work of repair. Long before modern bandages, this humble plant served as a guardian on wounds and weary skin alike. Lamb's Ear reflects a timeless truth of herbal medicine: healing often begins with gentleness, presence, and care.

---

### Herbal Confidence Index

*(4/5 green stars — excellent topical healer; limited internal use.)*

# BAYBERRY

★★★★

*Myrica cerifera*

**Bayberry** is a **warming astringent and mucus-drying tonic** used when tissues feel **lax, soggy, and congested**—especially in the throat, sinuses, gums, and upper respiratory tract. It is chosen for people who tend toward chronic dampness: lingering congestion, thick mucus, weak mucous membranes, or slow recovery from seasonal illness.

This is not a soothing "comfort herb." Bayberry **tightens and restores tone**, improves surface circulation, and helps the body clear excess secretions. Because it is strong and drying, it is best used **short-term** or paired with moistening herbs when dryness is a concern.

---

### Core Herbal Category — Bayberry

Primary Core: **Digestive System Support** with (astringent, warming principles that tone and stimulate digestion)

**Secondary Cores:** Respiratory Support · Circulatory & Cardiovascular Support · Astringent

---

### How It Works

Bayberry works by **astringing mucous membranes**, reducing excess secretions and improving tissue tone. Its warming action increases local circulation, helping tissues recover faster and resist recurring congestion. This makes it useful for chronic catarrh, sore throat patterns, and gum weakness—especially in cold, damp constitutional states.

---

### Primary Uses

- Tightens and strengthens gums, throat, and mucous membranes
- Helps dry thick mucus and reduce chronic congestion
- Supports circulation in low-vitality states
- Supports digestion where lax tissue and sluggish tone are present

---

### Scientific Backing

Bayberry is rich in **tannins and resinous compounds** associated with:

- antimicrobial action
- astringent tissue tightening
- mucus reduction and membrane support

Its traditional classification as a warming stimulant astringent aligns strongly with its phytochemical profile.

---

### Forms Available

- Dried root bark (cut/powder)
- Tincture / liquid extract
- Gargle or mouth rinse
- Decoction (short simmer)
- Poultice (topical)

---

### How to Use (Dosage & Methods)

Tincture: 1–2 mL up to 3× daily (short-term)
Decoction: ½–1 tsp bark per cup; simmer 10–15 minutes; up to 2× daily
Powder: ¼–½ tsp in warm water/honey 1–2× daily
Pairing Rule: Combine with Marshmallow, Licorice, or Slippery Elm if dryness is an issue.
Avoid pregnancy.

---

### Caution Level — Caution

- Overuse may cause nausea (high tannins)
- Avoid long-term use if constipation-prone or overly dry
- Avoid during pregnancy
- Use cautiously during high fever/heat states

---

### Gender-Specific Safety

Men: Helpful for chronic congestion, gum weakness, and sluggish digestion. Best short-term or blended.

Women: Traditional postpartum use exists, but avoid during pregnancy; strong astringency requires moderation.

Pregnancy / Nursing: Avoid in pregnancy. Postpartum use only with guidance.

---

### Expected Results

- Throat/gum tone: 1–3 days
- Congestion drying: 1–3 days
- Digestive "tone" improvement: several days

---

### DIY Recipe — Bayberry Throat & Sinus Decoction

Simmer ½ tsp Bayberry bark in 1 cup water 10–12 minutes.
Add ½ tsp Marshmallow Root and steep 10 minutes (balances dryness).
Sip warm once daily for 2–5 days.

---

### Same / Similar Results

Myrrh · Goldenseal · Cayenne · Yarrow

---

### Shelf Life / Potency After Preparation

- Dried bark: 2–3 years

• Tincture: 4–6 years
• Powder: 1 year
• Tea/decoction: 24 hours refrigerated

---

## 💬 Herbal Reflections of Bayberry

Bayberry carries the signature of early American herbalism — bold, warming, and unapologetically strengthening. It was relied upon in times when illness stemmed from cold, dampness, and exhaustion, offering restoration through tone, circulation, and resilience. Its astringency tightens what has become lax, while its warmth revives tissues weakened by stagnation or chronic congestion.

Bayberry reminds us that healing sometimes requires fortification rather than soothing, movement rather than rest. It stands as a reminder that vitality is restored not only through nourishment, but through renewed structural strength.

---

### 🌟 **Herbal Confidence Index**

🌿 🌿 🌿 🌿

(4/5 green stars — reliable astringent and circulatory stimulant; exceptionally effective but requires moderate, thoughtful use due to strong tannin profile.)

---

# *LINDEN FLOWER*

★★★★

*Tilia cordata*

**Linden Flower** is a **gentle nervous-system relaxer** that calms stress, softens emotional tension, and helps the body "unclench." It is chosen when anxiety shows up in the body as restlessness, tension headaches, stress, indigestion, or difficulty settling into sleep. Unlike heavier sedatives, Linden relaxes without dulling, making it ideal for people who need calm but still want clarity.

Linden also supports the **respiratory tract during colds and feverish states** by promoting mild sweating and soothing irritated tissues. Its medicine is broad but subtle: it reduces stress load, eases circulatory tension, and helps the body move out of fight-or-flight and back into repair.

---

🌿 **Core Herbal Category — Linden Flower** Primary Core: Nervous System Support (Nervines) with (gentle calming principles that ease tension and promote relaxation)
Secondary Cores: Cardiovascular Support · Respiratory Support · Anti-inflammatory

---

**How It Works**

Linden works through mild sedative and antispasmodic compounds that reduce stress signaling and relax tension in the nervous system. It also supports gentle vasodilation, which can ease pressure-related headaches and promote a calmer circulatory state. During colds, its diaphoretic action helps the body release heat while its mucilage soothes irritated throat and upper airway tissues.

---

🌱 **Primary Uses**

- Calms anxiety, restlessness, and nervous tension
- Supports sleep onset and nighttime settling
- Eases tension headaches and stress palpitations
- Supports colds/fever through gentle sweating
- Soothes throat irritation and cough tightness

---

🔬 **Scientific Backing**

Linden contains flavonoids, volatile oils (including farnesol), and mucilage associated with:

- mild anxiolytic/sedative activity
- antispasmodic calming effects
- throat and tissue soothing

Traditional European monographs (including Commission E) support Linden for nervous tension and cold/flu discomfort.

---

### Forms Available
• Tea / infusion (dried flowers)
• Tincture or liquid extract
• Glycerite (kid-friendly)
• Herbal bath / steam

---

### How to Use (Dosage & Methods)
Tea: 1–2 tsp per cup; steep 10–15 min; 1–3× daily
Tincture: 2–4 mL up to 3× daily
Bath/Steam: add a handful of flowers for relaxation or sinus comfort
Blend Tip: Combine with Chamomile or Lemon Balm for sleep; with Elderflower for colds.

---

### Caution Level — Safe
• May mildly lower blood pressure in sensitive individuals
• Use caution if prone to dizziness or very low BP
• Avoid excessive long-term high dosing in serious heart disease unless guided

---

### Gender-Specific Safety
Men: Helps reduce stress load and tension headaches; supports circulatory relaxation.
Women: Excellent for anxiety, sleep settling, and stress digestion; very well tolerated.
Pregnancy / Nursing: Light tea is generally acceptable; avoid heavy daily dosing without guidance.

---

### Expected Results
• Calm/relaxation: same day to 1–2 days
• Sleep improvement: 3–5 nights
• Cold/fever comfort: 1–3 days
• Stress digestion: 5–7 days

---

### DIY Recipe — Linden Night-Settle Tea
• 1 tsp Linden • 1 tsp Chamomile • ½ tsp Lemon Balm
Steep 10–15 minutes. Drink 30–60 minutes before bed.

---

### Same / Similar Results
Chamomile · Lemon Balm · Passionflower · Skullcap

---

### Shelf Life / Potency After Preparation
• Dried flowers: 1–2 years
• Tincture: 4–6 years

• Glycerite: 2–3 years
• Prepared tea: 24 hours refrigerated

---

💭 **Herbal Reflections of Linden Flower**

Linden carries the kind of calm that feels safe—softening the nervous system, easing tension from the chest and belly, and returning the body to rest. It teaches that relaxation is not weakness; it is the doorway through which repair enters. In both stress and sickness, Linden helps the body release what it is gripping so healing can begin.

---

**Herbal Confidence Index**

🌿🌿🌿🌿

(4/5 green stars — highly reliable gentle nervine; deeply effective for calming stress, easing tension, soothing the respiratory tract, and improving sleep without heaviness.)

# MEADOWSWEET

★★★★★

*Filipendula ulmaria*

**Meadowsweet** is a fragrant, cream-flowered meadow plant traditionally gathered in bloom for its cooling, stomach-protective qualities and gentle fever relief. Meadowsweet supports digestion, pain modulation, and inflammation control by buffering excess acidity while delivering natural salicylates that reduce discomfort without irritating the stomach. Its tannins and mucilage protect digestive tissues, making it especially useful for acid reflux, gastritis, fevers, and inflammatory pain where gentleness and effectiveness are both required.

---

🌿 **Core Herbal Category — Meadowsweet**

**Primary Core: Anti-Inflammatory & Pain Support** with (salicylate-rich principles that reduce inflammation and ease pain)

**Secondary Cores:** Anti-inflammatory · Urinary Support · Pain Modulation

---

### How It Works

Meadowsweet works by coating and protecting irritated digestive tissues while naturally moderating inflammation through plant-based salicylates. Unlike synthetic aspirin, its compounds reduce pain and fever without damaging the stomach lining. This dual action allows inflammation control while maintaining digestive comfort and tissue integrity.

---

🌱 **Primary Uses**

- Relieves acid reflux, heartburn, and gastritis
- Eases fevers, headaches, and mild inflammatory pain
- Supports digestive comfort and spasm reduction
- Calms urinary irritation with mild diuretic action

---

### Scientific Backing

Meadowsweet contains salicylates, flavonoids, tannins, and mucilage. Research confirms its ability to reduce pain and fever while protecting gastric tissue — a property that directly inspired the development of aspirin but without aspirin's gastrointestinal irritation.

---

### Forms Available

- Dried flowers or leaves (tea)
- Tincture / liquid extract
- Capsules or powder
- Topical washes

---

### How to Use

- **Tea:** 1–2 tsp dried herb per cup; steep 10–15 min; 2–3× daily
- **Tincture:** 2–4 mL up to 3× daily
- **Capsules:** 300–500 mg, 2–3× daily

---

### Caution Level — Safe

- Avoid if allergic to aspirin (salicylates)
- Not recommended for children with viral illness
- Use moderately during pregnancy

---

### Gender-Specific Safety

- **Men:** Supports joint comfort, digestion, and fever reduction
- **Women:** Helpful for reflux, headaches, and menstrual discomfort
- **Pregnancy/Nursing:** Occasional tea only; avoid concentrated extracts

---

### ⏳ Expected Results

- Digestive relief: 1–3 days
- Pain/fever relief: within hours
- Inflammation reduction: 1–2 weeks

---

–

### 🔄 Same / Similar Results

● Willow Bark · ● Chamomile · ● Licorice Root · ● Peppermint

---

### 💬 Herbal Reflections of Meadowsweet

Meadowsweet stands as a rare example of strength paired with kindness. Where pain relief often comes with irritation or harshness, this herb offers comfort while protecting the very tissues it serves. Its sweet fragrance and cooling nature remind us that healing does not need to be forceful to be effective. Meadowsweet teaches that true relief arises when the body is supported gently, allowing balance and calm to return naturally.

### ⭐ Herbal Confidence Index

🌿 🌿 🌿 🌿 🌿

*(5/5 — cornerstone digestive and anti-inflammatory herb; exceptional safety and reliability.)*

# *Yellow Dock*

★★★★

*Rumex crispus*

**YELLOW DOCK** is a deep-rooted perennial traditionally harvested for its mineral-rich taproot and bitter properties that support elimination and blood quality.
Yellow Dock functions as a slow, restorative cleanser that improves bile flow, enhances digestion, and supports iron absorption. Rather than forcing detoxification, it restores elimination efficiency over time, making it valuable for skin issues, fatigue, and sluggish digestion linked to internal congestion.

---

🌿 **Core Herbal Category — Yellow Dock**
**Primary Core: Liver & Detoxification Support** with (restorative principles that improve elimination and tissue tone)
**Secondary Cores:** Digestive · Liver · Mild Laxative

---

## How It Works

Yellow Dock gently stimulates bile production and intestinal movement while delivering minerals that support blood and tissue repair. Its bitter compounds improve digestive signaling, allowing waste to clear efficiently without harsh purging.

---

🌱 **Primary Uses**

- Supports liver detoxification
- Improves iron absorption
- Eases sluggish bowels
- Clears chronic skin congestion

---

🧪 **Scientific Backing**
Contains anthraquinones, tannins, and mineral compounds shown to stimulate bile

flow, improve elimination, and support antimicrobial balance when used moderately.

---

### Forms Available

- Dried root (decoction)
- Tincture
- Capsules or powder

---

### How to Use

- **Tincture:** 1–2 mL, 2–3× daily
- **Decoction:** 1 tsp root simmered 20 min
- **Capsules:** 400–500 mg up to 2× daily

---

### Caution Level — Caution

- Excess may loosen stools
- Avoid during pregnancy
- Not for long-term high-dose use

---

### Gender-Specific Safety

- **Men:** Supports detox and energy balance
- **Women:** Helpful for skin and iron support
- **Pregnancy/Nursing:** Avoid internal use

---

### Expected Results

- Improved elimination: 2–4 days
- Skin clarity: 2–3 weeks

- Iron support: 3–5 weeks

---

### Same / Similar Results

Burdock Root · Dandelion Root · Nettle Leaf

---

### Herbal Reflections of Yellow Dock

Yellow Dock works quietly and deeply, earning its place as a long-term restorative rather than a dramatic cleanser. Its deep root mirrors its action — drawing minerals upward while encouraging the body to release waste through steady, improved elimination. Unlike harsher detoxifiers, it cleanses while nourishing, supporting blood quality and tissue repair alongside detoxification.

Yellow Dock teaches that renewal does not need urgency to be effective. Its medicine reflects the value of patience, balance, and steady internal housekeeping as foundations of lasting vitality.

---

### Herbal Confidence Index

*(4/5 — reliable detox and iron-support root when used thoughtfully.)*

---

# CHANCA PIEDRA

★★★★

*Phyllanthus niruri*

**Chanca Piedra**, meaning "Stone Breaker," is a small tropical herb traditionally used to clear urinary and biliary blockages.
Chanca Piedra supports kidney, liver, and gallbladder function by relaxing smooth muscle tissue and discouraging mineral buildup. Its actions promote freer elimination, reduced inflammation, and improved detoxification when paired with proper hydration.

---

### Core Herbal Category — Chanca Piedra

**Primary Core:** Kidney & Urinary Support with (relaxing principles that ease flow and reduce obstruction)
**Secondary Cores:** Liver · Antispasmodic · Detox

---

### How It Works

Chanca Piedra relaxes urinary tract muscles, reducing spasms and resistance while supporting bile flow and detox pathways. This discourages stone formation and eases passage without force.

---

### Primary Uses

- Supports kidney stone prevention
- Eases urinary irritation
- Supports gallbladder and liver function

---

### Scientific Backing

Studies show reduced calcium-oxalate stone formation, improved ureter relaxation, antiviral activity, and liver enzyme normalization.

---

### 💊 Forms Available

- Tea or decoction
- Tincture
- Capsules

---

### 📏 How to Use

- **Tea:** 1–2 tsp per cup, 2× daily
- **Tincture:** 2–4 mL up to 2× daily
- **Capsules:** 400–600 mg, 2× daily

---

### ⚠️ Caution Level — 🟡 Caution

- May lower blood pressure
- Avoid during pregnancy
- Use in cycles, not continuously

---

### 🚹 🚺 Gender-Specific Safety

- 🟢 **Men:** Supports urinary comfort and stone prevention
- 🟡 **Women:** Helpful for UTIs and gallbladder support
- 🔴 **Pregnancy/Nursing:** Avoid

---

### ⏳ Expected Results

- Urinary relief: 3–7 days
- Stone support: 1–2 weeks
- Liver support: 2–3 weeks

### 🔄 Same / Similar Results

● Corn Silk · ● Hydrangea Root · ● Marshmallow Root

---

### 💬 Herbal Reflections of Chanca Piedra

Chanca Piedra has earned its reputation as a remover of blockages, both physical and systemic. Long valued in South American medicine, it supports the body's ability to release what has hardened, stagnated, or obstructed natural flow. Its action is not aggressive, but persistent — softening resistance so elimination can occur without trauma.

Symbolically, Chanca Piedra reflects the body's capacity for release and renewal when supported with patience and consistency. It reminds us that healing often comes not from force, but from allowing what no longer serves to gently pass.

---

### ⭐ Herbal Confidence Index

🌿🌿🌿🌿

*(4/5 — powerful urinary and detox herb when used in hydrated, time-limited cycles.)*

# Chaste Tree Berry (Vitex)

★★★★

*Vitex agnus-castus*

**Chaste Tree Berry,** commonly known as Vitex, is one of the most respected herbs for supporting women's hormonal balance. Used since ancient Greek and Roman times, it was traditionally relied upon to regulate menstrual cycles, ease PMS symptoms, and support reproductive health.
Unlike hormone replacement therapies, Vitex works indirectly by encouraging the body's own endocrine rhythm. Its steady, cumulative action makes it especially valuable for long-term hormonal regulation involving fertility, cycle irregularity, or menopausal transition.

---

### 🌿 Core Herbal Category — Chaste Tree

**Primary Core: Endocrine & Hormonal Support** with (regulating principles that normalize feedback signaling)
**Secondary Cores:** Nervine Support · Reproductive Support · Mood Balance

---

### How It Works

Chaste Tree works by influencing pituitary signaling that governs hormone release and balance. Rather than supplying hormones, it helps normalize communication within the endocrine feedback loop, particularly prolactin regulation. Over time, this stabilizes cyclical hormone fluctuations and reduces strain on hormonal regulation systems.

---

### 🌱 Primary Uses

- Regulates irregular menstrual cycles
- Eases PMS symptoms (mood swings, breast tenderness, cramps)
- Supports fertility and healthy ovulation
- Relieves menopausal discomfort
- Reduces hormonal acne

---

### Scientific Backing

Vitex contains diterpenes that act on dopaminergic pathways of the pituitary gland, helping reduce excess prolactin and support luteal-phase progesterone balance.

Commission E and modern clinical research support its use for PMS, PMDD, fertility support, hormonal acne, and menopausal transition symptoms.

---

### 💊 Forms Available

- Dried berries (tea or tincture)
- Capsules / standardized tablets
- Liquid tincture or extract

---

### 📏 How to Use (Dosage)

Capsules/Tablets: 300–600 mg once daily (morning dosing preferred)
Tincture: 1–2 mL once daily in the morning
Tea: 1–2 tsp crushed berries simmered 10 minutes; once daily
Vitex works gradually — allow 2–3 months for full benefit.

---

### ⚠️ Caution Level — 🟡 Caution

- Avoid during pregnancy
- Use cautiously with hormonal contraceptives, IVF medications, or HRT
- Temporary cycle shifts may occur during the first 1–2 months

---

### 🚹 🚺 Gender-Specific Safety

🟡 **Men:** Generally neutral; long-term use not recommended
🟢 **Women:** Premier endocrine herb for long-term hormonal balance
🔴 **Pregnancy / Nursing:** Avoid completely

---

### ⏳ Expected Results

- PMS relief: 1–2 cycles
- Cycle regularity & fertility support: 2–3 months
- Hormonal acne improvement: 1–2 months

---

### 🛠 DIY Recipe — Hormone-Balancing Tea

- 1 tsp crushed Chaste Tree berries
- 1 tsp Raspberry Leaf
- ½ tsp Chamomile

Steep 10 minutes; drink daily.

---

### 🔄 Same / Similar Results

🟢 Raspberry Leaf · 🟢 Black Cohosh · 🟡 Dong Quai · 🟢 Maca Root · 🟢 Ashwagandha

---

### Shelf Life / Potency

• Dried berries: 2–3 years
• Tincture: 4–6 years
• Capsules/tablets: 1–2 years

---

### Herbal Reflections of Chaste Tree Berry

Chaste Tree Berry teaches patience and cooperation with the body's natural rhythms. Rather than forcing change, it restores balance by guiding hormonal communication back into harmony. Its slow, dependable action reflects an important truth of endocrine healing — lasting regulation comes through consistency, timing, and respect for the body's internal intelligence.

---

### Herbal Confidence Index

*(4/5 — premier hormonal-balancing herb; clinically supported, safe for long-term use in women, and highly effective when used consistently.)*

---

# BEE BALM

★★★★

*Monarda didyma*

Bee Balm, also known as Oswego Tea, is a North American aromatic herb traditionally used for digestive discomfort, respiratory congestion, and mild infections. Native American tribes valued it both as a medicinal tea and as a calming remedy that lifted the spirit during illness.
Its strength lies in its warming aromatic oils, which support digestion, clear congestion, and provide antimicrobial protection. Bee Balm is equally suited for internal use as a tea and external use for skin or respiratory support.

---

**Core Herbal Category — Bee Balm**
**Primary Core: Digestive System Support** with (aromatic warming principles that stimulate and regulate digestion)
**Secondary Cores:** Antimicrobial · Respiratory Support · Nervine Support

---

### How It Works

Bee Balm stimulates digestive signaling through volatile oils that increase secretions and motility. These same compounds exhibit antimicrobial and antispasmodic effects, helping reduce internal congestion and digestive stagnation while supporting respiratory clearance.

---

**Primary Uses**

- Relieves cold, flu, and respiratory congestion
- Eases indigestion, gas, and bloating
- Supports skin and oral infections
- Calms mild anxiety and tension

---

**Scientific Backing**

Bee Balm contains thymol, carvacrol, geraniol, and rosmarinic acid, compounds shown to inhibit bacteria, reduce spasms, and calm inflammation.
Historically brewed as Oswego Tea, it served as a primary antimicrobial and digestive

remedy in early American herbal practice.

---

### Forms Available

- Tea (dried leaves or flowers)
- Tincture or extract
- Infused oil or salve
- Steam inhalation

---

### How to Use (Dosage)

Tea: 1–2 tsp per cup; steep 10–15 minutes; drink 1–2× daily
Tincture: 2–4 mL up to 3× daily
Steam: Inhale vapors 5–10 minutes for congestion

---

### Caution Level — Safe / Mild Caution

- Avoid internal use of concentrated essential oil
- Use moderately with thyroid imbalance
- Discontinue if stomach irritation occurs

---

### Gender-Specific Safety

**Men:** Supports digestion and respiratory clarity
**Women:** Helpful for cramps, digestion, and stress
**Pregnancy / Nursing:** Light tea acceptable; avoid strong extracts

---

### Expected Results

- Digestive comfort: within hours
- Respiratory relief: 1–3 days
- Emotional calm: same day

---

### DIY Recipe — Bee Balm Steam

Add a handful of dried Bee Balm to hot water; inhale 10 minutes.

---

### Same / Similar Results

Thyme · Oregano · Lemon Balm · Chamomile · Echinacea

---

### Shelf Life

- Dried herb: 1–2 years
- Tincture: 4–6 years
- Infused oil/salve: 1 year

---

### 💭 Herbal Reflections of Bee Balm

Bee Balm carries warmth, clarity, and reassurance. Its aromatic presence clears congestion not only in the lungs and digestion, but also in the nervous system. Traditionally relied upon as a household remedy, it reminds us that healing does not always require complexity — sometimes it begins with warmth, fragrance, and gentle stimulation that restores comfort and ease.

---

### 🌟 Herbal Confidence Index

🌿🌿🌿🌿

*(4/5 — dependable aromatic healer; effective for digestion, respiratory support, and mild infections while remaining gentle enough for regular use.)*

# SWEET WOODRUFF

★★★

*Galium odoratum*

**Sweet Woodruff** is a fragrant woodland herb long used in European tradition to promote calm, ease mild digestive tension, and support restful sleep. Its signature "new-mown hay" aroma comes largely from **coumarin**, which is also the reason this herb is best used in **short, moderate cycles**.
Historically placed in spring tonics, wreaths, and sleep sachets, Sweet Woodruff carries a reputation for gentle renewal. Today it remains a mild nervine and light lymphatic mover—useful when stress, tension, or seasonal fatigue needs soft support rather than strong sedation.

---

🌿 **Core Herbal Category — Sweet Woodruff**
**Primary Core: Nervous System Support (Nervines)** with (mild relaxing principles that ease tension and promote calm)
**Secondary Cores:** Circulatory Support · Lymphatic Support · Mild Diuretic

---

## How It Works

Sweet Woodruff calms mild nervous excitability through gentle relaxing compounds that reduce tension signaling. It also supports subtle fluid movement through light lymphatic and diuretic action, helping the body feel less "stuck" or heavy. The combined effect is quiet relaxation with mild systemic clearing.

---

🌱 **Primary Uses**
• Promotes relaxation and restful sleep
• Calms nervous tension and mild stress
• Supports digestion and liver "sluggishness" patterns
• Eases mild headaches and menstrual discomfort
• Gentle circulatory and fluid-movement support

---

🧪 **Scientific Backing**
Sweet Woodruff contains coumarin, flavonoids, and tannins associated with mild

relaxing, digestive, and supportive cleansing actions. Formal clinical trials are limited; however, phytochemical research and long-standing European use support its role as a **mild nervine and digestive ally**. Its coumarin content explains why **long-term daily dosing is discouraged**.

---

### Forms Available

- Dried leaves/flowers (tea, sachets, wine flavoring)
- Tincture or liquid extract
- Sleep sachets / herbal pillows (aromatic use)

---

### How to Use (Dosage)

Tea/Infusion: 1 tsp dried herb in 1 cup hot water; steep 5–10 minutes; drink once nightly

Tincture: 1–2 mL before bed as needed

Sachet/Pillow: dried herb near pillow for gentle aromatherapy

Use short-term (1–2 weeks). Avoid long-term daily use due to coumarin accumulation.

---

### Caution Level — Caution

- Avoid high doses or long-term daily use (coumarin may trigger headache, nausea, or liver irritation)
- Not recommended during pregnancy
- Use caution with blood thinners / anticoagulants
- Best used intermittently and moderately

---

### Gender-Specific Safety

**Men:** Helpful for stress tension and occasional sleep difficulty; use short-term.

**Women:** Useful for PMS irritability and mild cramping; avoid strong extracts during pregnancy.

**Pregnancy / Nursing:** Avoid tinctures/strong infusions; if used at all, only very weak occasional tea under guidance.

---

### Expected Results

- Relaxation / sleep support: within the first few nights
- Digestive easing: same day to 2 days
- "Detox / fluid movement" support: 2–3 weeks (if used intermittently, not continuously)

---

### DIY Recipe — Sweet Woodruff Dream Pillow

Fill a small pouch with: Sweet Woodruff + Chamomile + Lavender.

Place near the pillow to support calm and reduce nighttime tension.

### Same / Similar Results

Chamomile · Lemon Balm · Skullcap · Linden Flower

### Shelf Life / Potency After Preparation

• Dried herb: 1 year
• Tincture: 3–5 years
• Sachets/pillows: 1–2 years (kept dry)
• Prepared tea: 24 hours refrigerated

### Herbal Reflections of Sweet Woodruff

Sweet Woodruff is the kind of herb that does not announce itself loudly—it settles in quietly, like evening air through an open window. Its fragrance alone carries a message of rest, and its medicine follows that same pattern: gentle support when the nervous system is overworked and the body feels subtly burdened. It reminds us that some remedies are meant to be used like seasons—briefly, wisely, and with respect—so the calm they offer remains clean, soft, and renewing.

### Herbal Confidence Index

*(3/5 — gentle calming and digestive herb; effective for mild restlessness and tension, but limited by coumarin content and best used short-term in moderate doses.)*

# GOTU KOLA

★★★★★

*Centella asiatica*

**Gotu Kola** is a low-growing, water-loving herb long revered in Ayurveda and Traditional Chinese Medicine for its steadying influence on the mind and nerves. Rather than stimulating, it is known for cultivating clarity, focus, and calm together—earning a reputation as a tonic for longevity, contemplation, and balanced awareness.
Native to Asia and tropical regions, Gotu Kola was traditionally used by monks, scholars, and healers to support prolonged mental effort and emotional steadiness. Its distinction lies in its dual role: quietly strengthening circulation and connective tissue while nurturing cognitive resilience without agitation.

---

**Core Herbal Category — Gotu Kola**

**Primary Core: Cardiovascular System Support** with (restorative principles that strengthen connective tissue and microcirculation)

**Secondary Cores:** Nervine Support · Cognitive Support · Wound Support

---

**How It Works**

Gotu Kola works by improving microcirculation and reinforcing connective tissue integrity. Its triterpenoid compounds support collagen production and vascular tone, enhancing efficient blood flow. Improved circulation nourishes nerves and tissues, supporting repair without overstimulation.

---

**Primary Uses**

- Improves memory, focus, and concentration
- Supports wound healing and skin repair
- Strengthens veins and circulation
- Calms nervous tension and supports sleep onset
- Promotes gentle rejuvenation and resilience

---

**Scientific Backing**

Gotu Kola contains triterpenoid saponins (asiaticoside, madecassoside) linked to

collagen synthesis and microvascular strength.
Clinical studies support its role in venous insufficiency, scar recovery, anxiety reduction, and mild cognitive support.
Traditional systems classify it as a longevity tonic that harmonizes mental clarity with emotional calm.

---

### Forms Available

- Tea / infusion
- Capsules / powder
- Tincture / extract
- Topical creams / gels

---

### How to Use (Dosage)

- Tea/Infusion: 1–2 tsp dried leaf per cup; steep 10–15 minutes, 1–2× daily
- Capsules/Powder: 400–600 mg standardized extract or 1–2 g whole herb daily
- Tincture: 2–4 mL up to 2× daily

Use consistently for several weeks for cognitive, circulatory, and nerve support.

---

### Caution Level: Caution

Generally well tolerated; high doses may cause mild headache or skin sensitivity.
Avoid during pregnancy or with liver conditions without guidance.
Periodic breaks are advised with long-term use.

---

### Gender-Specific Safety

Men:
Supports clarity, circulation, and stress recovery; no known hormonal effects.
Women:
Supports emotional balance, skin integrity, and gentle calm; discontinue if dizziness occurs.
Pregnancy / Nursing:
Limited safety data—use only with professional supervision.

---

### Expected Results

- Mental focus & calm: 1–2 weeks

• Circulation & vein support: 3–6 weeks
• Skin healing & repair: 2–4 weeks
• Overall resilience: ≈ 1 month

---

🛠 **DIY Recipe — Gotu Kola Brain Tonic Tea**
1 tsp Gotu Kola leaf + 1 tsp Ginkgo + ½ tsp Peppermint.
Steep 10 minutes; drink once daily.

---

🔄 **Same / Similar Results**
🟢 Ginkgo
🟢 Bacopa
🟢 Ashwagandha
🟢 Lemon Balm

---

🧴 **Shelf Life / Potency After Preparation**
• Dried Leaf: 1–2 years, cool and dark storage
• Tincture: 4–5 years
• Tea: Up to 24 hours refrigerated
• Topicals: 6–12 months

---

💬 **Herbal Reflections of Gotu Kola**
Gotu Kola teaches steadiness rather than speed, offering clarity that arises from balance instead of stimulation. It supports the long view—quietly reinforcing mind and tissue over time. In this way, it remains a companion for those seeking resilience, presence, and sustainable vitality.

---

⭐ **Herbal Confidence Index:** 🌿 🌿 🌿 🌿 🌿 **(5 / 5 green stars)**
Cornerstone Herb — exceptionally reliable for cognition, circulation, skin repair, and nervous-system balance.

# WATERCRESS

★★★★

*Nasturtium officinale*

**Watercress** is a peppery, nutrient-dense streamside green traditionally used as a **spring-renewal tonic**—supporting digestion, gentle cleansing, and mineral repletion. Best used as food, it offers "clean energy" by pairing nourishment with mild detox support.
For centuries it was gathered to rebuild strength after winter, valued for its crisp bite, mineral richness, and refreshing effect on appetite, circulation, and overall vitality.

---

### 🌿 Core Herbal Category — Watercress

**Primary Core: Liver & Detoxification Support** with (nutrient-dense principles that support cleansing and renewal)

**Secondary Cores:** Digestive Support · Mineral Support · Antioxidant

---

## How It Works

Watercress supports renewal by supplying **bioavailable micronutrients** and plant compounds that assist normal detox pathways and metabolic efficiency. Its mild bitter/peppery principles stimulate digestive signaling, while antioxidant constituents help lower oxidative burden during periods of "cleaning out." The net effect is **cleansing that doesn't deplete**—it rebuilds while it refreshes.

---

### 🌱 Primary Uses

- Nutrient-dense rebuilding tonic (especially post-winter)
- Supports antioxidant and detox pathways
- Helps clear excess mucus / respiratory "catarrh" patterns
- Mild diuretic support for kidneys and bladder
- Encourages cardiometabolic balance

---

### 🧪 Scientific Backing

Watercress provides concentrated vitamins/minerals and antioxidant compounds, including glucosinolate-derived constituents such as PEITC, associated with support for phase II detox enzyme activity and oxidative balance. Research on leafy greens consistently links nutrient-dense greens with benefits for vascular health, inflammation modulation, and metabolic support.

---

### Forms Available

• Fresh leaves (food/salads)
• Juice / smoothies
• Pesto / green sauces
• Powder / capsules
• Tincture or extract (less common)

---

### How to Use (Dosage)

Fresh greens: ½–1 cup daily in salads/sandwiches/soups (add at the end)
Juice/tonic: small handful blended with lemon + apple, 3–4× weekly
Warm infusion: steep 1 tbsp fresh chopped leaves 5 minutes; sip for mild respiratory cleansing
Best used fresh/raw when possible. Wash thoroughly before eating.

---

### Caution Level — Safe

• Generally safe as a food and tonic
• Use moderation with active ulcers or kidney inflammation (peppery compounds may irritate)
• Avoid large medicinal doses during pregnancy
• Wash well (especially if wild-harvested)

---

### Gender-Specific Safety

**Men:** Supports circulation, metabolic balance, and mild cleansing; safe as daily food.

**Women:** Restorative for energy and skin clarity; supports gentle liver/digestive tone; safe as food.

**Pregnancy / Nursing:** Safe as food; avoid concentrated extracts or heavy medicinal dosing.

---

### Expected Results

• Digestive "lightness": several days
• Respiratory/mucus reduction: 3–7 days
• Circulatory & cleansing support: 1–2 weeks
• Skin tone & vitality: 2–3 weeks

---

### Shelf Life / Potency After Preparation

• Fresh leaves: 3–5 days refrigerated (potency drops quickly)
• Powder: ~1 year airtight, cool/dry
• Tincture: 3–4 years
• Fresh juice: best within 24 hours refrigerated

---

### DIY Recipe — Watercress Spring Pesto

Blend: 2 cups watercress + ½ cup nuts/seeds + 1 clove garlic + lemon + olive oil + pinch of salt.
Use on soups, fish, grains, or roasted vegetables for a cleansing mineral boost.

---

### Same / Similar Results

Arugula · Dandelion Leaf · Parsley · Nasturtium

---

### Herbal Reflections of Watercress

Watercress is the taste of "wake up"—bright, peppery, and alive. It reminds us that some of the strongest medicines don't arrive in a bottle; they arrive as food that restores the body's baseline. Its gift is simple but profound: it clears heaviness without draining strength, and it nourishes while it refreshes. Watercress teaches that renewal is often built from small, consistent choices—clean greens, clean flow, and the quiet return of energy.

---

### Herbal Confidence Index

*(4/5 — excellent nutrient-dense cleansing food-herb with broad safety; reliable for gentle detox support, circulation, and vitality when used consistently as part of diet.)*

# SWEET VIOLET

★★★★

*Viola odorata*

**Sweet Violet** is a cooling, softly fragrant woodland herb long cherished in European folk medicine for its ability to soothe irritation, calm congestion, and restore gentle balance to the body. Its heart-shaped leaves and delicate purple flowers have made it a symbol of tenderness and quiet healing for centuries. Traditionally used for dry coughs, sore throats, inflamed skin, and swollen glands, Violet has always been valued where tissues are dry, tight, or overheated. From the physicians of ancient Greece to medieval herbalists, Sweet Violet was relied upon to ease lung congestion, cool fevers, and calm melancholy. Its reputation grew not from forceful action, but from its consistent ability to comfort — gently supporting the lymphatic system, softening inflammation, and inviting rest and emotional ease.

---

**Core Herbal Category — Sweet Violet**

**Primary Core: Lymphatic & Skin Support** with (cooling, moistening principles that promote gentle fluid movement)

**Secondary Cores:** Respiratory Support · Anti-inflammatory · Skin Support

---

## How It Works

Sweet Violet works by encouraging lymphatic flow through cooling, demulcent compounds that soften tissues and mobilize stagnant fluids. Its mucilage coats and protects irritated membranes, while mild anti-inflammatory constituents calm overactive pathways. Together, these actions support gentle clearance and relief without stimulating or depleting the system.

---

**Primary Uses**

- Relieves dry coughs, sore throat, and mild bronchitis
- Soothes inflamed or irritated skin
- Supports lymphatic drainage and swollen glands
- Promotes mild relaxation and deeper rest
- Acts as a gentle digestive demulcent

---

**Scientific Backing**

Sweet Violet contains mucilage, flavonoids, and mild salicylate-like compounds that account for its soothing, expectorant, anti-inflammatory, and cooling properties.

European herbal tradition consistently recognizes Violet for calming irritated respiratory tissue, cooling inflamed skin, easing lymphatic stagnation, and supporting emotional quiet during periods of stress or heat.

---

### Forms Available

- Tea / syrup
- Tincture / glycerite
- Infused oil / salve
- Fresh poultice

---

### How to Use (Dosage)

- **Tea/Infusion:** 1–2 tsp dried leaf/flower per cup; steep 10–15 minutes. Drink 1–2× daily.
- **Syrup:** 1–2 tsp, 2–3× daily for dry coughs or throat irritation (gentle enough for children).
- **Poultice:** Apply crushed fresh leaves to minor skin irritation or lymphatic swelling.

Use consistently over several days for best results.

---

### Caution Level — Safe

- Generally safe for adults and children
- Avoid excessive use of concentrated tinctures (possible mild nausea)
- Those sensitive to salicylates should use with awareness
- Safe for short-term daily use as tea or syrup

---

### Gender-Specific Safety

**Men:** Helps ease tension-related coughs, chest tightness, and seasonal congestion. Gentle enough for daily use.

**Women:** Traditionally used for lymphatic tenderness, skin dullness, and mild PMS irritability. Cooling and calming.

**Pregnancy / Nursing:** Safe as tea or syrup; avoid strong tinctures unless professionally guided.

---

### Expected Results

- Throat & cough soothing: same day–3 days
- Skin & lymphatic comfort: 1–2 weeks
- Respiratory ease & relaxation: several days
- Digestive soothing: within hours

---

### DIY Recipe — Violet Honey Cough Syrup

Steep fresh or dried Violet leaves and flowers in warm honey for 1–2 hours; strain.
Take 1 tsp as needed for dry cough, sore throat, or chest irritation.

---

### Same / Similar Results

Marshmallow · Plantain Leaf · Mullein · Chamomile

---

### 🪨 Shelf Life / Potency After Preparation

• Dried leaves & flowers: ~1 year (airtight, cool, dark)
• Violet honey/syrup: 6–12 months refrigerated
• Tincture or glycerite: 3–5 years
• Infused oil/salve: 6–9 months

---

### 💭 Herbal Reflections of Sweet Violet

Sweet Violet heals through gentleness. It does not push or force release, but instead softens what has grown tight — in the lungs, the lymph, the skin, and the heart. Where dryness irritates and heat inflames, Violet cools and comforts, reminding the body how to rest and breathe again. Its quiet nature teaches an enduring lesson: some of the most effective medicines are those that soothe rather than stimulate. Sweet Violet stands as a reminder that tenderness itself can be profoundly restorative.

---

### 🌟 Herbal Confidence Index

🌿 🌿 🌿 🌿 🌿

**Cornerstone Herb** — exceptionally gentle, safe, and effective for respiratory comfort, lymphatic balance, and skin soothing.

# CILANTRO

★★★★

*Coriandrum sativum*

**Cilantro** is cherished around the world for its cooling, cleansing nature and bright, aromatic flavor. More than a culinary delight, **it soothes digestion, eases bloating, and gently stimulates the appetite. Both traditional wisdom and emerging research suggest that Cilantro may help support the body's natural detox pathways**—assisting in the safe elimination of certain heavy metals when paired with a wholesome diet. **Rich in antioxidants and mild antimicrobial compounds,** it serves as a refreshing ally for the digestive tract and a calming companion during heat, irritation, or spicy meals.

---

## *Core Herbal Category — Cilantro*

**Primary Core: Liver & Detoxification Support** with (binding principles that assist removal of unwanted residues)
**Secondary Cores:** Digestive Support · Antioxidant · Mineral Support

---

### *How It Works*

Cilantro works by binding and mobilizing unwanted residues so they can be carried out through normal elimination pathways. Its aromatic compounds stimulate digestive and metabolic activity, supporting efficient processing. Antioxidant activity reduces oxidative stress during detoxification. This supports gradual internal clearing without forcing elimination.

---

## Primary Uses

- Eases gas, bloating, and post-meal heaviness
- Supports natural detoxification pathways
- Provides cooling relief for digestive heat and irritation
- Offers gentle antimicrobial and antioxidant support

---

## Scientific Backing

Cilantro contains aromatic aldehydes, flavonoids, and phenolic acids that contribute to its carminative, antioxidant, and mild antimicrobial effects.
Research on heavy-metal detoxification is promising but inconsistent; however, strong evidence supports Cilantro's role in digestive comfort, oxidative balance, and microbial modulation.

Across many traditional systems, Cilantro straddles the line between food and medicine, offering cooling, digestive, and cleansing benefits.

---

## Forms Available

- Fresh leaves / juice
- Pesto or chutney
- Tincture / glycerite
- Powder / capsules

---

## How to Use (Dosage)

- Fresh Herb: Add ¼–½ cup fresh chopped Cilantro to meals daily for digestive ease, detox support, and blood-sugar balance.
- Tea/Infusion: Steep 1–2 tsp fresh or dried leaf in hot water for 10 minutes; drink 1–2× daily for mild digestive or cooling benefits.
- Tincture/Extract: 1–2 mL, 2× daily as part of a cleansing or gentle detox protocol.

Most effective when used consistently in food or tea over several days to weeks.

---

## Caution Level: Safe

Generally safe for everyday culinary and tea use.
Rarely, high doses or concentrated extracts may cause mild digestive or skin sensitivity.
Individuals allergic to Apiaceae-family plants should use caution.
Safe in normal culinary amounts during pregnancy and breastfeeding.

---

## Gender-Specific Safety

**Men:**

Helps reduce heaviness from rich meals, supports gentle liver cleansing, improves breath freshness, and enhances post-meal comfort. Beneficial for mild metabolic sluggishness or cholesterol imbalance. Safe for daily use.

**Women:**

Supports clearer skin and hormonal steadiness by easing digestive heat and enhancing liver balance. Helps with digestive spasms, PMS bloating, and fluid retention. Safe in food form; tinctures should be moderate during pregnancy.

**Pregnancy / Nursing:**

Safe in moderate culinary amounts.
Avoid large medicinal doses or essential oil preparations.

---

## Expected Results

- Digestive comfort & reduced bloating: same day
- Cooling & detox support: 1–2 weeks
- Skin & metabolic clarity: 2–3 weeks
- Improved appetite & energy balance: several days

## 🛠 DIY Recipe — Cooling Cilantro Chutney

Blend Cilantro, lemon juice, fresh ginger, a pinch of cumin, and sea salt.
Serve over bowls, salads, rice, or tacos to lighten heavy meals and support digestion.

---

## 🔄 Same / Similar Results

- Parsley
- Fennel
- Mint
- Lemon Balm

---

## Shelf Life / Potency After Preparation

• Fresh Cilantro (refrigerated): 5–7 days; potency drops quickly once chopped.
• Dried Leaf: 6–9 months; flavor and medicinal strength decline faster than many herbs.
• Tincture / Glycerite: 3–5 years; preserves digestive and cooling actions well.
• Chutney / Pesto: 3–5 days refrigerated; freezes well for up to 2 months.

---

## 💬 Herbal Reflections of Cilantro

There is a refreshing honesty in Cilantro's medicine — a cool green clarity that cuts through stagnation and awakens the body to its own rhythm again. Its leaves soothe the gut, lighten the spirit, and soften the internal heat that comes from stress, rich foods, or long days.

Beloved around the world, Cilantro stands as proof that healing often begins in the simplest places: the garden bed, the dinner plate, the familiar flavors that both nourish and cleanse. With each taste, it invites the body back to ease.

---

## ⭐ Herbal Confidence Index: 🌿🌿🌿🌿 (4 / 5 green stars)

Excellent digestive and detox-supporting herb — gentle, versatile, and most effective when used fresh and consistently as part of a cleansing diet.

# Guaraná

★★★★

*Paullinia cupana*

Guaraná is an Amazonian climbing plant whose seeds have long been valued by Indigenous peoples for stamina, alertness, and mental endurance. Unlike many stimulants, its naturally bound caffeine is released more slowly, giving Guaraná a reputation for steady, controlled energy rather than abrupt stimulation.
Native to the Amazon Basin, Guaraná was traditionally roasted, ground, and prepared as a tonic by the Mawé and Guarani peoples to sustain long hunts and demanding rituals. Its identity has always centered on endurance and clarity, setting it apart from coffee-like stimulants that act quickly but fade fast.

---

🌿 **Core Herbal Category — Guaraná**

**Primary Core: Nervous System Support (Nervines)** with (stimulating principles that enhance alertness and sustained energy)

Secondary Cores: Cognitive Support · Adaptogenic Support · Metabolic Support

---

**How It Works**

Guaraná works by stimulating the central nervous system through caffeine bound to tannins and other compounds. This binding slows absorption, producing a longer-lasting and smoother stimulatory effect. Neural activation increases focus and wakefulness while supporting physical drive without rapid depletion.

---

🌱 **Primary Uses**

- Increases energy, focus, and reaction time
- Supports exercise performance and fatigue resistance
- Aids appetite control and elevates mood
- Provides occasional headache relief when paired with analgesics

---

🔬 **Scientific Backing**

Guaraná seeds contain caffeine alkaloids, polyphenols, and saponins responsible for

stimulant and antioxidant activity.
Clinical studies associate standardized extracts with improved alertness, attention, and reaction time.
Its traditional use for stamina aligns with its unusually high and stable natural caffeine content.

---

**Forms Available**

- Powdered seed / extract
- Capsules
- Energy drinks / bars (standardized preparations)

---

**How to Use (Dosage)**

- Capsules/Tablets: 200–400 mg standardized extract once in the morning
- Powder: ½–1 tsp mixed into food or drinks; begin with smaller amounts
- Tea/Infusion: ½ tsp powder steeped 10 minutes; once daily

Avoid late-day use to prevent sleep disruption.

---

**Caution Level: Caution**

Use moderately—Guaraná is highly concentrated in caffeine.
Excess intake may cause jitteriness, insomnia, anxiety, or elevated heart rate.
Avoid combining with other stimulants.
Not advised during pregnancy, breastfeeding, or for those with cardiac conditions.

---

**Gender-Specific Safety**

Men:
Supports stamina, focus, and physical output. Avoid high doses if prone to hypertension or tension headaches.

Women:
Supports energy and clarity during fatigue. Best used earlier in the day to avoid overstimulation.

Pregnancy / Nursing:
Avoid due to caffeine concentration.

---

### ⏳ Expected Results

• Energy & mental focus: 30–60 minutes
• Exercise performance: ≈ 30 minutes before activity
• Mood & motivation lift: same day (2–4 hours)
• Reduced fatigue: ≈ 1 week of consistent use

---

### 🛠 DIY Recipe — Smooth Energy Mix

Blend ¼–½ tsp Guaraná powder into a smoothie with cacao or banana.
Increase slowly based on tolerance.

---

### 🔄 Same / Similar Results

🟢 Yerba Mate
🟢 Green Tea / Matcha
🟢 Cola Nut
🟣 Rhodiola

---

### 📦 Shelf Life / Potency After Preparation

• Powdered Seed: 1–2 years, airtight and dry
• Capsules: 1–2 years, cool storage
• Tincture/Extract: 4–5 years
• Prepared Drinks: 1–2 days refrigerated

---

### 💭 Herbal Reflections of Guaraná

Guaraná represents focused power rather than excess, offering alertness that is deliberate and sustained. It reminds the user that stimulation is most effective when paired with restraint. In honoring balance, Guaraná reflects the endurance of the forest itself—steady, potent, and meant to be respected.

---

### 🌟 Herbal Confidence Index: 🌿 🌿 🌿 🌿 (4 / 5 green stars)

Natural stimulant and endurance enhancer — highly effective for alertness and stamina when used with moderation.

# Indian Gooseberry (Amla)

★★★★★

*Phyllanthus emblica*

Indian Gooseberry, commonly known as Amla, is a small sour fruit revered in Ayurveda as a foundational tonic for balance, resilience, and longevity. Cooling and deeply nourishing, it is distinguished by its ability to strengthen vitality while remaining gentle enough for daily, long-term use.

Used for thousands of years in India, Amla was traditionally planted near homes and temples as a symbol of health and endurance. Best known as the central ingredient in Triphala, it is valued not for stimulation but for its capacity to restore equilibrium across digestion, immunity, and metabolic function.

---

**🌿 Core Herbal Category — Indian Gooseberry**

Primary Core: Liver & Detoxification Support with (rejuvenating principles that restore balance and cellular resilience)

Secondary Cores: Digestive Support · Immune Support · Antioxidant

---

**How It Works**

Indian Gooseberry works by supporting detoxification while simultaneously replenishing tissues. Its antioxidant and polyphenol compounds protect cells from oxidative stress while improving metabolic efficiency. This dual action allows cleansing and restoration to occur together without depletion.

---

**🌱 Primary Uses**

- Strengthens immunity and antioxidant defenses
- Supports digestion and nutrient assimilation
- Promotes liver and cardiovascular health
- Enhances skin integrity and hair vitality

---

### Scientific Backing

Amla contains vitamin C, tannins, ellagic acid, and flavonoids linked to antioxidant and anti-inflammatory activity.

Research supports benefits for lipid balance, glycemic regulation, liver protection, and oxidative stress reduction.

These findings align with its traditional classification as a Rasayana herb for longevity and cellular renewal.

---

### Forms Available

- Powder (alone or in Triphala)
- Fresh fruit / juice
- Capsules
- Tincture / extract

---

### How to Use (Dosage)

- Powder: ½–1 tsp daily in warm water or juice
- Capsules/Tablets: 500–1,000 mg standardized extract, 1–2× daily
- Juice: 1–2 tbsp diluted in water, preferably on an empty stomach

Suitable for long-term use; commonly paired with Triphala or Turmeric.

---

### Caution Level: Safe

Generally safe for routine daily use.

May cause mild digestive sensitivity in those unaccustomed to sour herbs.

Avoid combining with large doses of iron supplements due to tannins.

---

### Gender-Specific Safety

Men:

Supports stamina, antioxidant balance, liver health, and hair vitality; safe for regular use.

Women:

Supports skin clarity, hair strength, and gentle hormonal balance through cooling action.

Pregnancy / Nursing:

Safe in dietary amounts; avoid concentrated extracts unless professionally guided.

⌛ **Expected Results** • Digestive balance & energy: 1–2 weeks • Immune & skin support: 2–4 weeks • Hair strength & vitality: 1–2 months

---

🛠 **DIY Recipe — Amla Hair Mask** Mix 2 tbsp Amla powder with yogurt or warm water. Apply to scalp for 20–30 minutes, then rinse.

---

🔄 **Same / Similar Results** ● Triphala ● Hibiscus ● Gotu Kola ● Neem

---

📦 **Shelf Life / Potency After Preparation** • Powder: 1–2 years, airtight storage • Fresh Fruit / Juice: 3–5 days refrigerated • Tincture / Extract: 4–6 years • Prepared Paste: 24–48 hours refrigerated

---

💬 **Herbal Reflections of Amla**

Amla reflects the power of quiet nourishment rather than forceful intervention. It restores by cooling excess, strengthening what is depleted, and supporting balance over time. As a daily companion rather than an acute remedy, it embodies the Ayurvedic principle that longevity is built through consistency, moderation, and renewal from within.

---

⭐ **Herbal Confidence Index:** 🌿 🌿 🌿 🌿 🌿 **(5 / 5 green stars)**

Cornerstone Ayurvedic herb — exceptionally reliable for digestion, immunity, detox balance, and long-term vitality.

# WILD LETTUCE

★★★

*Lactuca virosa*

**Wild Lettuce** is a traditional nervine valued for calming restlessness, easing mild pain, and supporting natural sleep. Its bitter white latex, known as lactucarium, earned the nickname "lettuce opium," not for narcotic effects, but for its ability to quiet the nervous system without intoxication.

In European folk medicine, Wild Lettuce was commonly used for insomnia, headaches, coughs, and nervous agitation. During the 19th century it was carried by herbalists as a gentler alternative to stronger sedatives, prized for inviting rest rather than forcing it—a role it still fills today.

---

### 🌿 Core Herbal Category — Wild Lettuce

**Primary Core: Nervous System Support (Nervines)** with (sedative principles that quiet nerve signaling and reduce tension)

Secondary Cores: Pain Modulation · Sleep Support · Antispasmodic

---

### How It Works

Wild Lettuce works by reducing nerve excitability through mild sedative and analgesic compounds. It dampens pain signaling and relaxes muscular tension, allowing the nervous system to downshift. This supports relaxation and rest without heavy suppression.

---

### 🌱 Primary Uses

- Supports natural sleep and evening relaxation
- Relieves mild to moderate pain and muscle tension
- Eases coughs and chest irritation

---

### 🧪 Scientific Backing

Wild Lettuce contains sesquiterpene lactones, including lactucin and lactucopicrin, associated with sedative, antitussive, and analgesic activity.

While modern clinical studies are limited, extensive ethnobotanical records document its use for restlessness, tension, cough, and nighttime discomfort.
Its current use remains focused on gentle nervous calming rather than strong sedation.

---

### Forms Available

- Dried leaves
- Tincture (leaf or latex extract)
- Capsules or powder
- Syrups or herbal cough blends

---

### How to Use (Dosage)

- Tea/Infusion: 1–2 tsp dried leaf per cup; steep 10–15 minutes, once in the evening
- Tincture: 1–2 mL in water, once or twice in the evening
- Capsules/Powder: 300–500 mg in late afternoon or evening

Use the lowest effective dose; avoid daytime use due to sedation.

---

### Caution Level: Caution

Use responsibly; excessive doses may cause dizziness, nausea, or vivid dreams.
Not recommended during pregnancy or breastfeeding.
Avoid use in individuals with low blood pressure.
Do not combine with strong sedatives or sleep medications.

---

### Gender-Specific Safety

Men:
Supports relaxation and sleep without hormonal effects; avoid alert activities after use.
Women:
Useful for stress-related insomnia and mild cramping; keep tincture doses modest.
Pregnancy / Nursing:
Not recommended; safer alternatives include Chamomile, Lemon Balm, or Linden.

---

### Expected Results

- Relaxation & sleep support: 30–90 minutes
- Mild pain & cough relief: within hours
- Nervous-system support: after several evenings of use

### 🛠 DIY Recipe — Evening Calm Blend

Combine Wild Lettuce, Passionflower, and Skullcap tinctures in equal parts.
Take 1–2 mL before bed.

---

### Same / Similar Results

**California Poppy · Passionflower · Valerian · Hops · Skullcap**

---

### Shelf Life / Potency After Preparation

- Dried Leaves: 1–2 years, airtight storage
- Tincture: 4–6 years
- Capsules/Powder: 1–2 years
- Syrups: 6–12 months refrigerated

---

### Herbal Reflections of Wild Lettuce

Wild Lettuce offers relief by softening tension rather than overpowering it. It encourages rest by creating space for calm, making it well suited for those sensitive to stronger sedatives. In its quiet way, it reminds us that rest is most lasting when it is gently invited.

---

### Herbal Confidence Index: 🌿 🌿 🌿 (3 / 5 green stars)

Traditional nervine and mild sedative—moderately effective for tension, restlessness, and minor pain when used with care.

# WITCH HAZEL

★★★★

*Hamamelis virginiana*

**Witch Hazel** is a classic North American shrub valued for its firming, cooling influence on skin and veins. Long trusted for calming irritation, swelling, and minor bleeding, it stands apart for its precise astringent action that tones tissues without harshness. Indigenous peoples used Witch Hazel leaves and bark as a wound remedy, knowledge later adopted into Eclectic and early American medicine. By the 19th century, distilled Witch Hazel became a household staple, a role it still holds today as a dependable first-aid and skin-care ally.

---

### 🌿 Core Herbal Category — Witch Hazel

**Primary Core: Lymphatic & Skin Support** with (tightening principles that strengthen tissue tone and reduce excess fluid)

Secondary Cores: Circulatory Support · Skin Support · Anti-inflammatory

---

### How It Works

Witch Hazel works by tightening tissues and constricting superficial blood vessels through potent astringent compounds. This reduces excess fluid, irritation, and minor bleeding while improving tissue tone. The action restores firmness and support without blocking circulation.

---

### 🌱 Primary Uses

- Relieves hemorrhoids and varicose veins
- Soothes irritated, inflamed, or weepy skin
- Supports healing of minor cuts, bruises, and insect bites

---

### 🧪 Scientific Backing

Witch Hazel bark and leaves contain hamamelitannins, flavonoids, and volatile oils responsible for astringent and anti-inflammatory effects.

Clinical use and historical literature support its value for swollen veins, hemorrhoids,

bruising, and topical irritation.
Distilled Witch Hazel remains widely used for pore tightening, puffiness reduction, and skin soothing.

---

### Forms Available

- Distilled extract / hydrosol
- Decoction of bark or leaf
- Ointments, creams, and compresses

---

### How to Use (Dosage)

- Topical Hydrosol: Apply with a cotton pad to affected areas 2–3× daily
- Compress: Apply a chilled Witch Hazel–soaked cloth for 10–15 minutes
- Internal Decoction (short-term): 1–2 tsp dried bark simmered in 1 cup water; use infrequently

Topical use is preferred; internal use should be brief and supervised.

---

### Caution Level: Safe

Generally well tolerated, especially topically.
Internal use should be short-term due to high tannin content.
Avoid strong alcohol preparations on very sensitive or broken skin.

---

### Gender-Specific Safety

Men:
Useful for razor irritation, bruising, swollen veins, and post-activity inflammation.
Women:
Valuable for hemorrhoids, varicose veins, and postpartum perineal care; topical use preferred.
Pregnancy / Nursing:
Safe topically; avoid internal preparations or high-alcohol extracts.

---

### Expected Results

- Itching or puffiness relief: minutes after topical application
- Hemorrhoid or vein support: noticeable improvement in 3–7 days
- Skin tone refinement: 1–2 weeks of consistent use

### 🛠 DIY Recipe — Cooling Witch Hazel Compress

Soak a cotton pad in chilled Witch Hazel hydrosol mixed with a small amount of aloe gel.
Apply for 10 minutes to calm heat and swelling.

---

### 🔄 Same / Similar Results

● Horse Chestnut · ● Yarrow · ● Oak Bark · ● Calendula · ● Aloe Vera

---

### Shelf Life / Potency After Preparation

- Distilled Hydrosol: 1–2 years unopened; 6–12 months opened, refrigerated
- Dried Bark or Leaf: 1–2 years, cool and dry storage
- Homemade Decoction: 5–7 days refrigerated
- Ointments / Creams: 6–12 months

---

### 💬 Herbal Reflections of Witch Hazel

Witch Hazel restores boundaries by reinforcing what has become overworked or irritated. Its strength lies in precision—tightening and calming without aggression. Quietly reliable, it remains a reminder that effective healing often comes from steady, supportive restraint rather than force.

---

### 🌟 Herbal Confidence Index: 🌿 🌿 🌿 🌿 (4 / 5 green stars)

Cornerstone topical herb — safe, dependable, and highly effective for skin and vein support.

# COUCH GRASS

★★★

*Elymus repens*

**Couch Grass** is a cooling, moisture-rich herb long valued for calming irritation in the urinary tract and restoring comfort to the bladder and prostate. Rather than forcing elimination, it soothes inflamed tissues and supports steady, strain-free urinary flow, making it especially suitable for sensitive or reactive systems.

In traditional European herbalism, Couch Grass earned a reputation as one of the safest remedies for cystitis, kidney gravel, and chronic urinary irritation. Often paired with Corn Silk or Marshmallow Root, it was trusted for long-term use, valued more for reliability and gentleness than for dramatic or aggressive action.

---

### 🌿 Core Herbal Category — Couch Grass

Primary Core: **Kidney & Urinary Support** with (soothing demulcent principles that promote gentle fluid clearance)

Secondary Cores: Lymphatic Support · Digestive Support · Anti-inflammatory

---

### How It Works

Couch Grass works by coating and calming irritated urinary tissues while mildly increasing urine flow. Its demulcent compounds reduce friction and inflammation along mucous membranes. This supports waste clearance without overstimulation, allowing congestion and irritation to ease gradually.

---

### 🌱 Primary Uses

- Eases bladder irritation and cystitis
- Supports prostate comfort and urinary frequency
- Provides gentle cooling and mild diuretic support

---

### 🔬 Scientific Backing

Couch Grass rhizome contains mucilage, triticin polysaccharides, and silica that contribute to its soothing and anti-inflammatory effects.

Historical European and North American texts document its use for cystitis, kidney gravel, prostate irritation, and chronic bladder sensitivity.
Its profile favors long-term tissue support rather than acute antimicrobial action.

---

### Forms Available

- Decoction (rhizome)
- Tincture or liquid extract
- Capsules or teas

---

### How to Use (Dosage)

- Decoction: Simmer 1 tbsp rhizome in 2 cups water for 15–20 minutes; drink 1 cup 2× daily
- Tincture: 2–3 mL up to 2× daily in water
- Capsules: 500–1,000 mg 2× daily

Use for 1–3 weeks during irritation, alongside adequate hydration.

---

### Caution Level: Safe

Exceptionally well tolerated with no known toxicity.
Maintain hydration due to mild diuretic action.
Suitable for extended use in moderate amounts.

---

### Gender-Specific Safety

Men:
Supports urinary flow and prostate comfort without hormonal effects; suitable for steady use.

Women:
Soothes bladder sensitivity and mild water retention; pairs well with Corn Silk or Marshmallow Root.

Pregnancy / Nursing:
Generally safe as a mild tea; avoid concentrated extracts unless professionally advised.

---

### Expected Results

- Reduced irritation and burning: 2–4 days

• Improved urinary flow and comfort: 1–2 weeks
• Ongoing soothing support: with consistent daily use

---

### 🛠 DIY Recipe — Soothing Couch Grass Tea

Simmer 1 tbsp Couch Grass rhizome in 2 cups water for 15 minutes.
Add Corn Silk and steep 10 more minutes; strain and drink warm.

---

### 🔄 Same / Similar Results

● Corn Silk · ● Marshmallow Root · ● Cleavers · ● Uva Ursi (short-term only)

---

### 📦 Shelf Life / Potency After Preparation

• Dried Rhizome: 1–2 years, airtight storage
• Tincture / Liquid Extract: 4–6 years
• Capsules / Powder: ~1 year for best mucilage potency
• Prepared Decoction: 48–72 hours refrigerated

---

### 💬 Herbal Reflections of Couch Grass

Couch Grass works quietly, restoring comfort through patience rather than force. It supports healing by reducing irritation and allowing tissues to recover at their own pace. In this way, it reflects the principle that lasting relief often comes from gentleness, consistency, and respect for the body's need to cool and soften.

---

### ⭐ Herbal Confidence Index: 🌿 🌿 🌿 🌿 (4 / 5 green stars)

Dependable urinary demulcent—especially effective for long-term bladder comfort, kidney flow, and gentle detox support.

# CORNFLOWER

★★★

*Centaurea cyanus*

**Cornflower** is a gentle, cooling herb best known for soothing delicate tissues, especially the eyes and skin. Traditionally prepared as washes or compresses, its vivid blue petals were trusted to calm redness, puffiness, and irritation without harshness, making it a staple for sensitive conditions.

Gathered from European grain fields and midsummer gardens, Cornflower was valued as much for clarity and comfort as for beauty. Its role has always been restorative rather than forceful—supporting lymphatic movement, cooling excess heat, and easing mild tension wherever tissues feel overworked or inflamed.

---

🌿 **Core Herbal Category — Cornflower**

**Primary Core: Lymphatic & Skin Support** with (cooling principles that encourage gentle fluid movement)

**Secondary Cores:** Urinary Support · Eye Support · Anti-inflammatory

---

**How It Works**

Cornflower works by cooling overheated tissues while gently encouraging lymphatic flow. This helps reduce puffiness, congestion, and localized inflammation. Mild diuretic and astringent actions support balanced fluid distribution without drying.

---

🌱 **Primary Uses**

- Soothes red, puffy, irritated eyes
- Calms inflamed or sensitive skin
- Supports gentle lymphatic drainage
- Provides mild digestive bitter support
- Offers light nervine cooling for tension

---

### Scientific Backing

Cornflower petals contain flavonoids, anthocyanins, and tannins associated with cooling and anti-inflammatory effects.

European pharmacopoeias historically listed Cornflower for topical eye care, noting its ability to reduce puffiness and calm irritation.

Internal use remains lightly supported, with strongest evidence rooted in traditional topical application.

---

### Forms Available

- Dried petals (tea or infusion)
- Hydrosol
- Tincture
- Infused oils or skin preparations

---

### How to Use (Dosage)

- Tea/Infusion: 1 tsp dried petals per cup; steep 10 minutes (mild internal use)
- Eyewash/Compress: Prepare a strong infusion, strain thoroughly, and use cooled
- Hydrosol: Mist over eyelids or irritated skin 1–3× daily
- Skin Care: Add infusion to lotions or toners

---

### Caution Level: Safe

Non-irritating when properly strained and prepared.
Do not allow plant particles into the eyes.
Internal use should remain light due to limited systemic research.

---

### Gender-Specific Safety

Men:
Safe for tired eyes, mild skin inflammation, and gentle lymphatic support.

Women:
Helpful for puffy eyes, sensitive skin, and mild swelling related to heat or cycles.

Pregnancy / Nursing:
Safe in mild tea or compress form; avoid concentrated internal use.

---

⌛ **Expected Results**

• Eye comfort: minutes to hours after topical use
• Reduced redness and puffiness: 1–3 days
• Digestive or lymphatic support: 1–2 weeks with gentle internal use

---

🛠 **DIY Recipe — Cornflower Eye Compress**

Steep 1 tsp dried petals in ½ cup hot water for 10 minutes.
Strain finely, cool completely, and apply with cotton pads for 5–10 minutes.

---

🔄 **Same / Similar Results**

● Eyebright · ● Chamomile · ● Calendula · ● Borage

---

📦 **Shelf Life / Potency After Preparation**

• Dried Petals: 1–2 years, airtight storage
• Infusion/Eyewash: 24–48 hours refrigerated
• Hydrosol: 6–12 months refrigerated after opening
• Tincture: 4–6 years
• Infused Oil: 6–9 months refrigerated

---

💬 **Herbal Reflections of Cornflower**

Cornflower heals through softness rather than correction. It calms where tissues are overstimulated and restores comfort where sensitivity dominates. In its quiet clarity, it reminds us that gentle care often brings the most lasting relief.

---

⭐ **Herbal Confidence Index:** 🌿 🌿 🌿 **(3 / 5 green stars)**

Gentle cooling herb—highly reliable for eye and skin soothing, with limited depth as a systemic internal remedy.

# BEET ROOT

★★★★

*Beta vulgaris*

**Beet Root** is a deeply nourishing root long used to support circulation, vitality, and steady endurance. Valued as both food and medicine, it stands out for strengthening blood flow while replenishing minerals—working through nourishment rather than stimulation.

Used for centuries across Europe and the Middle East, Beet Root earned respect for supporting strength during fatigue and recovery. Its defining character lies in restoration: improving oxygen delivery and metabolic efficiency while remaining gentle enough for regular, dietary use.

---

### 🌿 Core Herbal Category — Beet Root

**Primary Core: Cardiovascular System Support** with (nutrient-rich principles that enhance blood flow and vitality)

**Secondary Cores:** Liver Support · Detoxification Support · Endurance Support

---

### How It Works

Beet Root increases nitric oxide availability, allowing blood vessels to relax and circulation to improve. Its mineral and antioxidant content supports blood quality and oxygen delivery. Enhanced flow improves tissue nourishment and metabolic efficiency, supporting sustained cardiovascular performance.

---

### 🌱 Primary Uses

- Improves blood flow and circulation
- Supports heart health and healthy blood pressure
- Aids liver detoxification and methylation
- Enhances stamina and exercise endurance
- Supports red blood cell function

---

### 🔬 Scientific Backing

Beet Root contains dietary nitrates, betaine, betalains, folate, and polyphenols

associated with vascular elasticity and nitric oxide production.
Human studies support benefits for blood pressure reduction, oxygen efficiency, exercise performance, and liver support.
Its betaine content contributes to methylation and metabolic balance.

---

### 💊 Forms Available

- Fresh root (raw, cooked, or juiced)
- Powdered root (smoothies or capsules)
- Fermented beet kvass
- Extracts or tinctures (less common)

---

### 💉 How to Use (Dosage)

- Juice: Blend raw beet with other vegetables or fruit; use several times weekly
- Powder: 1–2 tsp daily in water, smoothies, or capsules
- Cooked Root: Include regularly as a food
- Kvass: 2–4 oz daily

Food-based use is preferred for steady support.

---

### ⚠️ Caution Level: ● Safe

Generally safe as food or supplement.
May cause harmless red coloration of urine or stool.
Moderate intake if prone to kidney stones due to oxalates.

---

### 🚹 🚺 Gender-Specific Safety

● Men:
Supports stamina, circulation, and heart health; suitable for regular dietary use.
● Women:
Supports vitality, circulation, and liver-related hormonal balance; safe in food and powder forms.
● Pregnancy / Nursing:
Safe in normal food amounts; avoid concentrated extracts unless advised.

---

### ⏳ Expected Results

• Circulation & stamina: 7–14 days
• Blood pressure support: 1–2 weeks
• Liver and metabolic support: 2–3 weeks

---

### 🛠 DIY Recipe — Beet–Lemon Juice

Blend 1 raw beet with water and lemon; drink several times weekly.

---

### 🔄 Same / Similar Results

● Dandelion Root · ● Hawthorn Berry · ● Nettle Leaf · ● Milk Thistle · ● Cayenne

---

## 📦 Shelf Life / Potency After Preparation

• Fresh Root: 2–3 weeks refrigerated
• Fresh Juice: Best within 24 hours refrigerated
• Powder: 1–2 years airtight storage
• Kvass: 1–2 months refrigerated
• Tincture/Extract: 4–6 years

---

### 💬 Herbal Reflections of Beet Root

Beet Root restores through nourishment rather than force. It strengthens circulation by feeding the blood and supporting steady flow, not by pushing the system. In its simplicity, it reflects the principle that vitality grows when the body is supplied, balanced, and allowed to work efficiently.

---

### ⭐ Herbal Confidence Index: 🌿 🌿 🌿 🌿 (4 / 5 green stars)

Nutritive circulatory herb—reliable for endurance, vascular support, and gentle detox when used regularly as food or supplement.

# CASSIA BARK

★★★

*Cinnamomum cassia*

**Cassia Bark** is a bold, warming spice-herb valued for stimulating digestion, improving circulation, and supporting metabolic balance. Hotter and more pungent than Ceylon cinnamon, it carries stronger aromatic oils that give it a more assertive medicinal character and pronounced antimicrobial strength.
Used for thousands of years in Traditional Chinese Medicine and Ayurveda, Cassia was prescribed to dispel internal cold, invigorate sluggish digestion, and move stagnation in the blood. Its identity rests in heat and motion—an herb chosen when warmth, activation, and forward movement are needed.

---

### 🌿 Core Herbal Category — Cassia Bark

**Primary Core: Digestive System Support** with (warming aromatic principles that stimulate digestive activity)
**Secondary Cores:** Antimicrobial · Circulatory Support · Carminative

---

### How It Works

Cassia Bark stimulates digestive secretions through warming volatile compounds that increase motility and reduce stagnation. Its aromatic constituents support microbial balance during digestion. Improved circulation enhances nutrient delivery and metabolic efficiency. Together, these actions promote warmth, movement, and digestive clarity.

---

### 🌱 Primary Uses

• Supports blood sugar balance
• Stimulates sluggish digestion
• Improves circulation and warms the body
• Eases menstrual discomfort
• Provides antimicrobial support

---

### 🔬 Scientific Backing

Cassia contains cinnamaldehyde, coumarin, and eugenol associated with warming,

antimicrobial, and circulatory effects.
Studies indicate benefits for insulin sensitivity, post-meal blood sugar control, and broad-spectrum antimicrobial activity.
Due to higher coumarin content than Ceylon cinnamon, long-term high-dose use should be moderated.

---

### Forms Available

- Bark sticks or chips
- Powder
- Capsules
- Essential oil (topical use only; dilute)

---

### How to Use (Dosage)

- Tea/Decoction: Simmer a small piece of bark or ½ tsp powder in 1 cup water for 10–15 minutes, 1–2× daily
- Culinary Powder: ¼–½ tsp added to meals or warm drinks
- Tincture: 1–2 mL up to 2× daily (short-term use)
- Topical: Diluted essential oil for fungal skin issues

---

### Caution Level: Caution

Use moderately; avoid high daily doses for extended periods due to coumarin content.
Those pregnant or with liver conditions should prefer Ceylon cinnamon.
Essential oil must be diluted and not taken internally.

---

### Gender-Specific Safety

Men:
Supports digestion, circulation, and metabolic balance; avoid high-dose extracts.
Women:
Helpful for coldness, bloating, and menstrual sluggishness; keep tincture use moderate.
Pregnancy / Nursing:
Light culinary or mild tea use only; avoid concentrated preparations.

---

### ⏳ Expected Results

- Digestive warmth and activation: 30–60 minutes
- Circulatory or metabolic support: 1–2 weeks of steady use

---

### 🛠 DIY Recipe — Cassia Circulation Tea

Simmer 1 Cassia stick with ½ tsp Ginger in 2 cups water for 15 minutes.
Optional: add Clove or Orange Peel.

---

### 🔄 Same / Similar Results

Ceylon Cinnamon · Ginger · Clove · Fennel · Cardamom

---

### 📦 Shelf Life / Potency After Preparation

- Whole Bark: 3–4 years, airtight storage
- Powder: 1–2 years
- Tincture/Extract: 4–6 years
- Essential Oil: 3–4 years, sealed and protected from light
- Prepared Tea: 24–48 hours refrigerated

---

### 💬 Herbal Reflections of Cassia Bark

Cassia teaches the value of warmth when life slows or cools too far. It restores movement—of digestion, blood, and energy—by rekindling inner fire. Used with respect, it reminds us that strength is most effective when applied deliberately rather than excessively.

---

### ⭐ Herbal Confidence Index: 🌿 🌿 🌿 🌿 (4 / 5 green stars)

Potent warming and antimicrobial spice—highly effective for digestive sluggishness, circulation, and metabolic support when used mindfully.

# SWEET ANNIE

★★★★★

*Artemisia annua*

***Sweet Annie,** also known as Qing Hao or Sweet Wormwood, is a fragrant cooling herb long valued for clearing heat, supporting immune response, and restoring balance during persistent infection or fever. Native to Asia but now cultivated worldwide, it is distinguished from other Artemisia species by its lightness, sweet aroma, and targeted strength rather than harsh bitterness.*

*For centuries, Sweet Annie was prepared as a simple infusion in Chinese medicine to relieve malarial fevers and epidemic heat conditions. Its identity shifted dramatically in the modern era with the discovery of artemisinin, yet the herb itself remains respected not as a blunt weapon, but as a precise, time-tested cleanser that bridges classical herbalism and contemporary science.*

---

🌿 **Core Herbal Category — Sweet Annie Primary Core: Immune System Support** with (bitter aromatic principles that disrupt unwanted organisms) **Secondary Cores:** Antimicrobial · Liver Support · Fever Support

---

**How It Works** Sweet Annie works by interfering with the metabolic processes of unwanted organisms through its bitter aromatic constituents. These compounds enhance immune recognition while limiting overactivation. Concurrent liver-supportive actions assist in processing metabolic byproducts generated during immune clearance. This allows effective cleansing without exhausting the system.

---

🌱 **Primary Uses** • Antimalarial and antiparasitic support • Helps clear persistent infections and fevers • Supports liver detoxification during immune stress • Reduces inflammation linked to heat conditions

---

🔬 **Scientific Backing** Sweet Annie contains artemisinin, a sesquiterpene lactone internationally recognized for its role in malaria treatment and validated through WHO-endorsed clinical research. Additional studies and traditional data support its broad antimicrobial and antifungal activity, as well as immune-modulating effects. Complementary phytochemicals—including flavonoids and volatile oils—contribute to its heat-clearing and detoxifying profile.

---

**Forms Available** • Dried aerial parts (tea or infusion) • Capsules or standardized extracts • Tincture • Essential oil (external use only)

---

**How to Use** • Tea/Infusion: Steep 1 tsp dried Sweet Annie in 1 cup hot water for 10–15 minutes. Drink 1× daily for short-term immune or fever support (up to 7 days). • Tincture: 1–2 mL in water, up to 2× daily for short courses under guidance. • Capsules/Extracts: Follow product dosing; use cyclically rather than continuously. Avoid internal use of essential oil or prolonged high-dose regimens.

---

**Caution Level:** **Caution** Not for long-term or high-dose use; may irritate digestion or affect liver enzymes if overused. Avoid during pregnancy and breastfeeding. Always distinguish Sweet Annie (Artemisia annua) from Wormwood (Artemisia absinthium), which is stronger and more toxic.

---

**Gender-Specific Safety** Men: Appropriate for short immune-support or fever-clearing courses. Avoid prolonged use or combining with multiple strong detox herbs. Women: Traditionally used for fever and detox recovery; best limited to brief, supervised use due to liver-stimulating potential. Pregnancy / Nursing: Avoid entirely due to possible uterine and metabolic effects.

---

**Expected Results** • Fever or infection support: 2–7 days • Liver and detox support: within 1 week of short-term use

---

**Anti-Parasite Tonic** Simmer 1 tsp Sweet Annie, ½ tsp Black Walnut Hull, and ½ tsp Clove in 2 cups water for 15 minutes. Strain and drink once daily for 5–7 days only.

---

**Same / Similar Results** Wormwood · Black Walnut · Clove · Pau d'Arco · Garlic

---

**Shelf Life / Potency After Preparation** • Dried aerial parts: 1–2 years airtight, protected from light • Tincture / extract: 4–6 years • Capsules / powder: ~1 year for best potency • Tea / infusion: Best within 24 hours refrigerated

---

**Herbal Reflections of Sweet Annie** Sweet Annie stands at the meeting point of ancient insight and modern precision. It demonstrates how a humble field herb can hold targeted power when used with restraint and understanding.

*Its lesson is not force, but accuracy—clearing what does not belong while preserving balance. In this way, Sweet Annie reminds us that the most effective medicine often*

*works quietly, briefly, and with great respect for the body's own intelligence.*

---

⭐ ***Herbal Confidence Index:*** 🌿🌿🌿🌿🌿 *Cornerstone antimicrobial and immune herb — highly effective when used short-term and cyclically; powerful, validated, and deserving of disciplined application.*

# BLACK SEED

★★★★★

*Nigella sativa*

**Black Seed** is a revered medicinal seed known for strengthening immunity, easing respiratory conditions, and supporting metabolic balance. Used continuously for more than 2,000 years across Ancient Egypt, Islamic medicine, and Ayurveda, it earned the title "the Blessed Seed" for its broad and dependable healing reach. Its primary bioactive compound, thymoquinone, delivers antioxidant, anti-inflammatory, and immune-modulating effects that strongly validate its traditional uses.
More than a single-target remedy, Black Seed harmonizes multiple systems at once—supporting the lungs, digestion, circulation, joints, and detox pathways simultaneously. Both restorative and preventive, it stands among the world's most trusted natural medicines. Across cultures, Black Seed symbolizes protection, balance, and vitality—a true **Cornerstone Herb** of holistic health.

---

🌿 **Core Herbal Category — Black Seed Oil**

**Primary Core: Immune System Support** with (broad-acting protective principles that strengthen resistance)

**Secondary Cores:** Anti-inflammatory · Antioxidant · Digestive Support

---

**How It Works**

Black Seed Oil supports immune signaling pathways that enhance recognition and response to stressors. Its active compounds reduce excessive inflammatory signaling while preserving protective immune function. Strong antioxidant activity limits oxidative stress during immune engagement. Together, these actions strengthen resilience without overstimulation or depletion.

---

🌱 **Primary Uses**

- Immune and inflammation support
- Promotes respiratory ease
- Aids digestive comfort
- Nourishes skin and hair
- Balances joints and metabolism
- Supports cardiovascular and liver health

---

### Scientific Backing

Black Seed contains thymoquinone, a bioactive compound shown to exhibit antioxidant, anti-inflammatory, antihypertensive, and immunomodulatory effects.
Clinical trials demonstrate benefits for blood sugar regulation, lipid balance, and respiratory function, while preclinical studies suggest hepatoprotective and anticancer potential.
Long valued in Middle Eastern and Ayurvedic medicine, Black Seed is now widely recognized for its broad-spectrum systemic benefits.

---

### Forms Available

• Cold-pressed oil
• Capsules / softgels
• Whole or ground seeds
• Topical oil
• Powder

---

### How to Use

• **Oil (internal):** ½–1 tsp cold-pressed oil daily; may be mixed with honey or warm water for respiratory or immune support
• **Seeds (culinary):** ½–1 tsp whole or lightly toasted seeds sprinkled over food or brewed as tea
• **Capsules:** 500–1,000 mg, 1–2× daily (follow label guidance)
• **Topical:** Apply a small amount to joints, scalp, or skin; patch-test first

---

### Caution Level: Caution

Generally safe in food-level amounts. Excessive intake of concentrated oil may irritate digestion or lower blood pressure.
Avoid high doses during pregnancy or when using hypotensive medications.

---

### Gender-Specific Safety

**Men:**

Supports immune strength, metabolism, and stamina without hormonal disruption. Safe for daily use in small amounts; excessive dosing may cause digestive upset or transient hypotension.

**Women:**
Supports hormonal balance, skin clarity, menstrual comfort, and hair health. Safe in culinary or moderate supplemental use; avoid excessive dosing.

**Pregnancy / Nursing:** Small culinary amounts are generally acceptable. Avoid medicinal doses of oil or capsules during pregnancy. Nursing use should remain food-level only.

---

**Expected Results** • Respiratory ease: 3–7 days • Skin & scalp improvement: 1–2 weeks • Joint comfort: 2–4 weeks • Metabolic & blood-sugar balance: 4–8 weeks

---

**DIY Recipe — Black Seed Immunity Tonic** Mix ½ tsp Nigella sativa oil with 1 tsp honey and a pinch of turmeric. Take each morning to support immunity and inflammation balance.

---

**Same / Similar Results** Turmeric · Ashwagandha · Garlic · Goldenseal · Elderberry

---

**Shelf Life / Potency After Preparation** Cold-pressed oil: 1–2 years (dark glass; refrigerate after opening) Capsules: 1–2 years (cool, dry storage) Tincture / extract: 4–6 years Homemade infused oil: 6–12 months refrigerated Refrigeration after opening strongly preserves thymoquinone potency

---

**Herbal Reflections of Black Seed**
Black Seed carries the weight of legend and the precision of science. Revered as Habbatul Barakah—the Seed of Blessing—it bridges ancient prophetic medicine, Egyptian healing traditions, and modern clinical validation.
What distinguishes Black Seed is not force, but orchestration. It calms inflammation, strengthens immunity, and restores metabolic rhythm without overriding the body's intelligence. Compared to sharper immune stimulants like Oregano Oil or Echinacea, Black Seed offers endurance rather than urgency.
Small in size yet vast in influence, it reminds us that healing does not always arrive loudly. Sometimes it arrives as balance—steady, patient, and deeply sustaining.

---

**Herbal Confidence Index:**
Cornerstone immune and restorative seed — exceptionally effective, broadly protective, and remarkably safe when used consistently; one of the most historically validated herbs in the world.

# BALLOON FLOWER

★★★★

*Platycodon grandiflorus*

**Balloon Flower** root is a classic East Asian respiratory herb valued for soothing sore throats, easing coughs, and clearing stubborn phlegm from the upper chest. Gentle yet effective, it relieves hoarseness, laryngitis, and congestion without overdrying or heavy sedation, making it suitable for daytime use and for people who rely heavily on their voice.

In Traditional Chinese Medicine, Jie Geng is known as a "messenger herb," prized for its ability to guide remedies directly to the lungs and throat. Used for over a thousand years in teas, syrups, and lozenges, it remains a trusted household remedy across East Asia for seasonal coughs and lingering throat irritation—respected as much for its strategic role in formulas as for its direct relief.

---

### 🌿 Core Herbal Category — Balloon Flower

**Primary Core: Respiratory System Support** with (expectorant principles that loosen and move congestion)

**Secondary Cores:** Immune Support · Anti-inflammatory · Digestive Support

---

### How It Works

Balloon Flower works by thinning thick mucus and gently stimulating its expulsion from the respiratory tract. Its saponins calm inflamed tissues while improving clearance of secretions. Reduced irritation allows airflow to normalize. This restores comfortable breathing and throat function.

---

### 🌱 Primary Uses

- Sore throat, hoarseness, laryngitis
- Phlegmy or congested coughs
- Bronchitis and upper-chest congestion
- Support for sensitive or reactive airways

---

### 🔬 Scientific Backing

Balloon Flower root contains platycodins, triterpenoid saponins shown to reduce mucus thickness, promote expectoration, and calm inflammation (preclinical).

Classical East Asian medical texts document its long-standing use for sticky phlegm, throat pain, and coughs that linger after colds or infection.

---

### Forms Available

- Dried root (tea or decoction)
- Syrups or lozenges
- Capsules
- Tincture or liquid extract

---

### How to Use (Dosage)

**Tea/Decoction:** Simmer 1 tsp dried root in 2 cups water for 15–20 minutes; drink 1–2 cups daily.
**Syrups/Lozenges:** Use as directed for throat strain or cough.
**Tincture/Extract:** 1–2 mL up to 3× daily for congestion or cough.
**Children:** Use a weaker tea (½ tsp root per 2 cups water).

---

### Caution Level: Safe

Generally well tolerated in moderate herbal amounts.
Excessive dosing may cause mild nausea or stomach upset.
Avoid concentrated extracts during pregnancy or breastfeeding.
Those with sensitive digestion should begin with small amounts.

---

### Gender-Specific Safety

**Men:**
Supports throat comfort and phlegm clearance, especially for smokers, teachers, or those exposed to pollutants. Safe for short-term daily use during respiratory irritation.
**Women:**
Soothes coughs and sore throats during colds or seasonal congestion. Suitable for gentle, repeated tea use when needed.
**Pregnancy / Nursing:**
Use cautiously. Mild tea for short-term throat discomfort may be acceptable; avoid tinctures or high doses due to limited safety data.

---

### Expected Results

- Throat comfort and easier mucus release: 3–5 days

• Faster relief when taken at the first sign of throat irritation

🛠 **DIY Recipe — Throat-Soothing Balloon Flower Tea**

1 tsp Balloon Flower root + 1 tsp Licorice Root + 1 tsp Marshmallow Root in 2 cups water.

Simmer 15 minutes, strain, and sip warm. Honey optional.

🔄 **Same / Similar Results**

● Mullein · ● Marshmallow Root · ● Licorice Root · ● Elecampane · ● Coltsfoot

⏳ **Shelf Life / Potency After Preparation**

• Dried root: up to 2 years airtight and dry
• Tincture / extract: 4–6 years
• Capsules / powder: 1–2 years
• Prepared tea or decoction: 24–48 hours refrigerated

💬 **Herbal Reflections of Balloon Flower**

Balloon Flower is the quiet opener of breath and voice. It clears what is stuck, soothes what is irritated, and restores ease without force. As a guiding herb, it directs relief upward to the throat and lungs, reminding us that gentle precision often brings the most reliable healing.

---

⭐ **Herbal Confidence Index:** 🌿 🌿 🌿 🌿 (4 / 5 green stars — a gentle, dependable respiratory herb with exceptional value for throat irritation, phlegm clearing, and voice support)

# CELANDINE

★★★

*Chelidonium majus*

**Celandine** is a powerful bitter liver herb traditionally used to stimulate bile flow, ease upper-abdominal tension, and relieve spasmodic digestive discomfort. Known for its vivid yellow sap and pronounced bitterness, it has been employed when meals feel "stuck" beneath the ribs, often accompanied by nausea, cramping, or colicky pain. Across Greco-Roman, European monastic, and later Eclectic traditions, Celandine was regarded as a remedy of last resort—used when gentler bitters proved insufficient. Modern herbalism continues to respect its effectiveness while emphasizing restraint, precision, and short-term use due to its narrow safety margin.

---

### 🌿 Core Herbal Category — Celandine

**Primary Core: Liver & Detoxification Support** with (strong bitter principles that stimulate bile movement)

**Secondary Cores:** Digestive Support · Antispasmodic · Nervine Support

---

### How It Works

Celandine stimulates bile secretion through potent bitter alkaloids, increasing internal movement within the liver and gallbladder. Its antispasmodic action relaxes tension in smooth muscle, reducing resistance to bile flow. This combination allows congested digestion to release without mechanical force. Used carefully, it restores motion where stagnation dominates.

---

### 🌱 Primary Uses

- Sluggish bile flow and upper-GI stagnation
- Spasmodic digestive discomfort beneath the ribs
- Traditional short-term topical use for warts

---

### 🧪 Scientific Backing

Celandine contains isoquinoline alkaloids (including chelidonine and sanguinarine) with documented cholagogue and antispasmodic activity.

Clinical and pharmacological literature note a narrow therapeutic window, reinforcing the need for professional oversight with internal use.

---

**Forms Available**

• Tincture (drop-dose, supervised)
• Standardized capsules (practitioner-guided)
• Fresh latex for warts (topical only, brief use)

---

**Caution Level: Use Only Under Professional Supervision**

Contains potent alkaloids that may irritate the gastrointestinal tract or stress the liver if misused.

Internal use must be limited in dose and duration.

Avoid entirely during pregnancy, breastfeeding, liver disease, or bile duct obstruction.

Topical latex should be applied sparingly to intact skin for very short periods only.

---

**Gender-Specific Safety**

**Men:**

May ease biliary congestion or upper-abdominal tightness in very small, supervised doses. Prolonged or excessive use increases risk of liver irritation.

**Women:**

Historically used for gallbladder-related digestive tension. Safe only in short, guided courses; higher doses may provoke nausea or cramping.

**Pregnancy / Nursing:**

Not recommended. Alkaloids may affect uterine activity and fetal or infant liver function.

---

**Expected Results**

• Digestive and biliary ease: days to 1–2 weeks (short courses only)
• Topical wart response: variable with cautious, repeated application

---

**DIY Recipe — Guided Liver Support Blend** (professional oversight required)

1 mL Celandine tincture + 1 mL Dandelion Root + 1 mL Milk Thistle in water, once daily for a brief, supervised course.

---

### 🔄 Same / Similar Results

Goldenseal · Dandelion Root · Milk Thistle

### ⏳ Shelf Life / Potency After Preparation

- Dried herb: 1–2 years airtight
- Tincture / extract: 4–6 years
- Capsules / powder: ~1 year
- Fresh latex: use immediately; potency fades rapidly
- Prepared decoction: discard after 24 hours

---

### 💭 Herbal Reflections of Celandine

Celandine teaches the discipline of restraint. Its bright sap and sharp bitterness remind the herbalist that some medicines demand humility as much as knowledge. When used lightly and with respect, it can unlock deep stagnation; when misused, it cautions against force. In this balance lies its lesson—that true healing depends not on strength alone, but on precision.

---

### 🌟 Herbal Confidence Index: 🌿 🌿 🌿

Potent bile-moving and antispasmodic herb — effective for stubborn stagnation when carefully guided, but limited by a narrow safety window requiring professional supervision.

# PLANTAIN LEAF

★★★★★

*Plantago major*

**Plantain Leaf** is a classic first-aid herb valued for drawing out toxins, calming heat, and accelerating tissue repair. Used fresh or dried, it soothes irritated skin and mucous membranes, helping ease bites, stings, cuts, burns, rashes, sore throats, coughs, reflux, ulcers, and urinary irritation through its cooling, demulcent nature.

Common across Europe, Asia, and North America, Plantain earned the name "the green bandage" for its everyday reliability. From medieval herbals to Indigenous practice and modern clinical use, it has remained a household remedy—abundant, accessible, and consistently effective.

---

### 🌿 Core Herbal Category — Plantain Leaf

**Primary Core: Lymphatic & Skin Support** with (drawing and soothing principles that assist tissue clearance)

**Secondary Cores:** Astringent · Skin Support · Anti-inflammatory

---

### How It Works

Plantain Leaf draws excess fluid and irritants from tissues while coating and calming inflamed surfaces. Mild astringency improves tissue tone and containment. Anti-inflammatory compounds reduce reactive signaling. Together, these actions support steady lymphatic movement and local recovery.

---

### 🌱 Primary Uses

- Wounds, bites, stings, and minor burns
- Demulcent support for throat, lungs, and GI tract
- Heartburn and ulcer soothing
- Drawing poultice for splinters, toxins, and irritation

---

### 🧪 Scientific Backing

Plantain's mucilage and allantoin support tissue repair and regeneration.

Iridoids and flavonoids provide anti-inflammatory and antimicrobial actions supported by modern herbal research.

---

### Forms Available

• Fresh or dried leaf (tea, poultice)
• Salves and creams
• Tincture / extract
• Capsules

---

### How to Use

• **Tea:** Steep 1–2 tsp dried leaf in 1 cup hot water for 10–15 minutes; drink 1–3× daily for throat, reflux, or urinary irritation.
• **Poultice:** Crush fresh leaves or mix powdered leaf with warm water; apply to bites, cuts, or stings for 15–30 minutes.
• **Tincture:** 1–2 mL up to 3× daily for internal soothing or bladder support.
• **Salves/Oils:** Apply topically for skin repair, irritation, or minor burns.

---

### Caution Level: Generally Safe

Rare allergies may occur in those sensitive to Plantaginaceae.
Mild blood-thinning effects warrant monitoring with anticoagulants.
Harvest only from clean, pesticide-free areas.
Safe for children in reduced doses.

---

### Gender-Specific Safety

**Men:**

Supports wound healing, digestion, throat comfort, and urinary ease. Safe for daily use; no hormonal effects.

**Women:**

Soothes urinary irritation, digestive upset, menstrual bloating, and inflamed tissues. Suitable for daily tea or topical use.

**Pregnancy / Nursing:**

Generally safe in mild tea or topical form. Avoid strong tinctures unless professionally guided.

---

### Expected Results

• Throat and GI soothing: within hours

• Skin repair: 1–3 days with regular use

---

### 🛠 DIY Recipe — Plantain Skin-Soother Salve

Infuse ½ cup dried Plantain in ½ cup olive oil over low heat for 2 hours.
Strain, melt in 1 tbsp beeswax, and jar.

---

### 🔄 Same / Similar Results

● Calendula · ● Comfrey · ● Mullein · ● Marshmallow Root · ● Slippery Elm

---

### ⏳ Shelf Life / Potency After Preparation

• Dried leaf: 1–2 years airtight, protected from moisture and light
• Tincture / extract: 4–6 years
• Capsules / powder: ~1 year (mucilage declines gradually)
• Infused oil: 9–12 months refrigerated
• Prepared tea: best within 24 hours refrigerated

---

### 💬 Herbal Reflections of Plantain Leaf

Plantain is quiet medicine—cooling, steady, and dependable. It draws out what irritates and restores what is injured without force or drama.
Its lesson is accessibility: profound healing can be simple, nearby, and consistent. In the small moments of care—a sting, a scratch, a sore throat—Plantain shows how gentleness, applied well, becomes strength.

---

### ⭐ Herbal Confidence Index: 🌿 🌿 🌿 🌿 🌿

Cornerstone wound-healing and anti-inflammatory herb — exceptionally safe, versatile, and indispensable for tissue repair, toxin drawing, and mucous membrane soothing.

# Parsley

★★★★

*Petroselinum crispum*

**PARSLEY** is a nutrient-dense kidney ally and gentle diuretic that eases water retention, freshens breath, and supports smooth digestion. Rich in flavonoids (notably apigenin), vitamin K, vitamin C, folate, and essential minerals, it functions as a daily detox herb that supports urinary flow, light liver clearance, and vascular tone—all while remaining easy to use in food.

For bloating, mild hypertension, or morning puffiness, Parsley gently encourages fluid movement without harsh depletion. Its culinary familiarity makes it ideal for long-term, low-dose use, which is where this humble herb quietly excels.

From ancient Greek and Roman traditions to European kitchen gardens, Parsley has been chewed, sipped, and juiced for urinary support, breath freshening, and menstrual regularity. It embodies food as medicine—accessible, reliable, and safe for consistent use in most adults.

Modern herbalists still rely on Parsley in gentle detox and daily vitality protocols, often pairing it with Dandelion Leaf, Nettle, or Celery for sustained fluid balance without electrolyte loss.

---

🌿 **Core Herbal Category — Parsley**

**Primary Core: Kidney & Urinary Support** with (stimulating yet mineral-balanced principles that increase fluid clearance)

**Secondary Cores:** Digestive Support · Mineral Support · Antioxidant

---

### *How It Works*

Parsley increases urinary flow, assisting the kidneys in clearing excess fluid and metabolic waste. Its mineral content helps maintain electrolyte balance during elimination, while mild digestive stimulation improves upstream processing. Together, these actions promote clean elimination without depletion or strain.

---

🌱 **Primary Uses**

- Kidney and urinary support; mild diuretic for water retention
- Digestive comfort and breath freshening
- Light liver and hormonal support

• Antioxidant and vascular tone support

---

### Scientific Backing

Parsley contains apigenin, polyphenols, vitamin C, and volatile oils associated with anti-inflammatory, carminative, and diuretic effects.

Research indicates Parsley increases urinary output without significant electrolyte loss and provides supportive cardiometabolic and antioxidant benefits.

---

### How to Use (Dosage)

- **Tea:** 1–2 tsp fresh or dried leaf, steep 10–12 minutes
- **Capsules / Powder:** 500–1000 mg daily
- **Juice:** 1–2 tbsp fresh Parsley juice
- **Parsley Seed:** Much stronger — use only in small, guided doses

**Forms Available:** Fresh leaf · Dried leaf · Seed · Tincture / liquid extract · Capsule or powder

---

### Expected Results

- Diuretic and digestive lightness: 1–2 days
- Gentle detox or hormonal tone: 1–2 weeks

---

### Caution Level: Caution

- Safe in food or tea amounts; avoid large medicinal doses
- Avoid concentrated extracts during pregnancy (uterine stimulation)
- Those with active kidney inflammation or severe renal disease should limit intake
- Maintain adequate hydration during detox use

---

### Gender-Specific Safety (GS)

**Men:** Safe — supports bladder and kidney function, digestion, and breath freshness. Avoid high-dose tinctures.

**Women:** Safe — helps reduce bloating, mild menstrual discomfort, and fluid retention.

**Pregnancy/Nursing:** Caution — culinary amounts are safe; avoid parsley seed or concentrated preparations.

---

### Same / Similar Results

Dandelion Leaf — diuretic + liver support

Nettle Leaf — kidney + mineral support

Cilantro — detox + chelation

Parsley Seed — stronger diuretic
Celery Leaf — fluid balance + gentle detox
Juniper Berry — warming diuretic + urinary stimulant

---

**DIY Recipe — Parsley Kidney Cleanse Tea**

- 2 tsp fresh chopped Parsley
- ½ tsp Lemon Peel
- ½ tsp Dandelion Leaf

Steep 10 minutes in 1½ cups boiling water.
Drink daily for 5–7 days for fluid balance and gentle detox.

---

**Shelf Life / Potency After Preparation**

- Dried leaf: 1–2 years (airtight, cool, dark)
- Tincture / extract: 4–5 years
- Capsules / powder: best within 1 year
- Parsley-infused oil: 6–9 months (refrigerated)
- Fresh juice: best within 24 hours

---

**Herbal Reflections of Parsley**

Parsley is often underestimated because of its familiarity, yet beneath its humble appearance lies a herb of quiet power. It clears stagnation, refreshes the kidneys, sweetens the breath, and renews vitality through steady, nourishing support.
In small, consistent doses, Parsley teaches the value of subtle restoration—healing that unfolds through rhythm, nourishment, and balance rather than force. It reminds us that detoxification is a gradual journey, and some of the most effective medicine grows close to home.

---

**Herbal Confidence Index:**

(4/5 green stars — refreshing digestive and kidney-supportive herb; highly effective for gentle detoxification, breath freshening, and easing bloating, though milder than deeper-acting diuretics.)

# CRANBERRY

★★★★

*Vaccinium macrocarpon*

**Cranberry** is a premier urinary preventive that helps reduce recurrent UTIs by stopping bacteria—especially E. coli—from adhering to the bladder wall. Rather than acting as a harsh antimicrobial, it shifts the urinary terrain, supporting bladder comfort while its tart polyphenols also contribute antioxidant benefits for vessels and gums. This makes Cranberry especially effective between flare-ups, where consistency matters more than force.

A revered North American native, Cranberry was used by Indigenous peoples for urinary issues, wound care, and nourishment long before becoming a colonial staple. Modern standardized extracts focusing on PACs (type-A proanthocyanidins) translate centuries of practice into dose-reliable prevention, placing Cranberry among the rare herbs where clinical evidence and tradition strongly align.

---

### 🌿 Core Herbal Category — Cranberry

**Primary Core: Kidney & Urinary Support** with (anti-adhesion principles that prevent unwanted attachment)

**Secondary Cores:** Antioxidant · Circulatory Support · Oral Health

---

### How It Works

Cranberry delivers compounds that interfere with the ability of unwanted organisms to adhere to urinary tract surfaces. This reduces colonization and allows normal urine flow to flush material out more effectively. Antioxidant activity protects delicate tissues from irritation during clearance. Prevention occurs through mechanical interruption rather than direct suppression.

---

### 🌱 Primary Uses

- Prevents recurrent UTIs (anti-adhesion activity)
- Supports bladder and kidney comfort
- Antioxidant support for vessels and gums
- Complements hydration and D-mannose in urinary programs

---

### Scientific Backing

• Type-A proanthocyanidins (PACs) block E. coli from attaching to uroepithelial cells
• Clinical trials show reduced UTI recurrence at ~36 mg PACs/day
• Polyphenols contribute anti-inflammatory, vascular, and oral-gum support

---

### How to Use (Dosage)

• Juice: 4–8 oz/day of unsweetened cranberry juice
• Capsules/Tablets: Standardized to ~36 mg PACs/day
• Dried Fruit: 1–2 tbsp/day (unsweetened)
• Tincture/Extract: 2–4 mL up to 2× daily as part of a urinary wellness plan

---

### Forms Available — Cranberry

• Fresh or dried berries · Unsweetened juice · Capsules / standardized extract · Powder · Tincture

---

### Expected Results

• Urinary comfort: 1–3 days
• Reduction in UTI recurrence: 2–4 weeks
• Antioxidant / gum support: several days to 2 weeks

---

### Caution Level: Safe

• Generally safe long-term in food or supplement form
• High amounts may cause mild GI upset
• May increase urinary oxalates—use moderation if prone to kidney stones
• May interact with warfarin; monitor as needed
• Choose unsweetened juice or standardized PAC products for therapeutic use

---

### Gender-Specific Safety

Men: Supports urinary tract and prostate comfort via anti-adhesion effects

Women: Highly effective for preventing recurrent UTIs with consistent use

Pregnancy / Nursing: Moderate juice or capsule use generally regarded as safe; avoid excessive intake

---

### Same / Similar Results

Dandelion Leaf · Goldenrod · Parsley · Uva Ursi (short-term only)

---

### DIY Recipe — Cranberry UTI Prevention Drink

1 cup unsweetened cranberry juice

½ fresh lemon
1 tsp honey (optional)
Mix and sip throughout the day; increase hydration for best results.

---

🧴 🧴 **Shelf Life / Potency After Preparation**

- Dried berries: ~1 year airtight
- Capsules/Tablets: 2–3 years
- Unsweetened juice: 7–10 days refrigerated after opening
- Frozen berries: 8–12 months
- Tincture/Extract: 4–5 years

---

💭 **Herbal Reflections of Cranberry**

Cranberry teaches the quiet strength of prevention. It does not overpower microbes or inflame tissues; it simply makes imbalance harder to establish. Through steady use, it protects by shaping terrain rather than fighting battles.

For those prone to recurring UTIs, Cranberry becomes a daily guardian—proactive, consistent, and supported by both tradition and science. Its lesson is simple and enduring: true healing often lies in what we prevent, not only in what we correct.

---

🌟 **Herbal Confidence Index:** 🌿 🌿 🌿 🌿

(4/5 — cornerstone preventive urinary herb; highly effective for reducing UTI recurrence through anti-adhesion action, exceptionally safe for long-term use.)

# SCHISANDRA

★★★★★

*Schisandra chinensis*

**Schisandra** is an adaptogenic "five-flavor" berry that sharpens focus, steadies stress responses, and protects the liver while supporting respiratory tone and healthy energy. It enhances mental clarity, sustained endurance, mood stability, and skin vitality—energizing without jitters and calming without sedation. This makes it ideal for cyclical stress, demanding schedules, and recovery protocols where resilience matters more than stimulation.

Used traditionally to "secure the essence," Schisandra has been relied upon for centuries in Traditional Chinese Medicine to strengthen the lungs, brighten the eyes, and preserve vitality. Hunters and messengers historically used it to reduce fatigue and sharpen night vision. Its name—five-flavor fruit—reflects its harmonizing action across multiple organ systems.

From classical imperial formulas to modern wellness routines, Schisandra remains a longevity tonic prized for endurance, clarity, graceful aging, and stable performance under pressure.

---

**Core Herbal Category — Schisandra**

**Primary Core: Adaptogens** with (balancing principles that stabilize stress response and nervous output)

**Secondary Cores:** Liver Support · Endurance Support · Cognitive Support · Respiratory Support

---

## *How It Works*

Schisandra regulates stress-response signaling, helping the body maintain equilibrium under physical and mental demand. Its lignans support coordinated adrenal and nervous system activity while protecting the liver during metabolic stress. The result is steadier energy, improved focus, and sustained resilience without overstimulation.

---

**Primary Uses**

- Adaptogenic support for stress resilience and steady energy
- Enhances mental clarity and concentration
- Protects and supports liver function

• Strengthens respiratory tone and endurance
• Aids athletic recovery and stamina

---

### Scientific Backing

Schisandra's lignans—schisandrin, schizandrol, and gomisin—demonstrate antioxidant, hepatoprotective, and neuro-supportive effects.

Studies show:

• improved endurance and oxygen utilization
• enhanced stress adaptation and cortisol modulation
• measurable cognitive support
• liver-enzyme balancing and detox support

---

### How to Use (Dosage)

• **Tea/Decoction:** 1–2 tsp dried berries, simmer 15–20 minutes, 1–2× daily
• **Capsules/Powder:** 500–1,000 mg up to 2× daily
• **Tincture:** 2–4 mL, 2–3× daily
• **Chewed berries:** 3–6 berries for mild stimulation and clarity

---

### Expected Results

• Energy & vitality: 5–7 days
• Mental clarity & focus: 1–2 weeks
• Stress adaptation: 2–3 weeks
• Liver support: 3–4 weeks
• Endurance & recovery: 10–14 days

---

### Caution Level: Use With Awareness

• May influence CYP450 liver-enzyme metabolism—use caution with liver-processed medications
• Avoid in acute liver disease or uncontrolled hypertension
• Excessive dosing may cause restlessness or heartburn
• Pregnancy/Nursing: avoid concentrated forms; light tea only under guidance

---

### Gender-Specific Safety

**Men:** Supports stamina, focus, stress resilience, and liver protection
**Women:** Supports energy, mood balance, liver clarity, and skin vitality
**Pregnancy/Nursing:** Light tea only with guidance; avoid tinctures

---

### Forms Available

- Dried berries (tea/decoction)
- Powder (capsules or smoothies)
- Tincture / extract
- Classical TCM formulas

---

**Same / Similar Results**

Ginseng · Rhodiola · Ashwagandha · Goji Berry

---

**DIY Recipe — Schisandra Vitality Tea**

- 1 tsp Schisandra berries
- 1 tsp Goji berries
- ½ tsp Licorice root

Simmer in 2 cups water for 15 minutes. Sip warm for clarity and sustained vitality.

---

**Shelf Life / Potency After Preparation**

- Dried berries: 2–3 years (airtight, cool)
- Tincture/extract: 5–6 years
- Powder: 1–2 years
- Prepared tea: 48 hours refrigerated
- Frozen berries: 10–12 months

---

**Herbal Reflections of Schisandra**

Schisandra builds clarity and calm at the same time—sharpening the mind without agitation and steadying the nerves without sedation. Where Ginseng excites and Ashwagandha soothes, Schisandra harmonizes.

It teaches that true performance is not force, but coordination—when systems communicate smoothly, vitality becomes effortless.

**Herbal Confidence Index:**

(5/5 green stars — cornerstone adaptogenic and liver-protective herb; exceptionally effective for resilience, stamina, cognitive clarity, and long-term vitality.)

# CHICKPEA

★★★★

*Cicer arietinum*

**Chickpea** is a restorative **food-herb** that builds strength, steadies energy, and nourishes the blood with plant protein, fiber, iron, and magnesium. As a nutritive tonic, it supports satiety, healthy glycemic control, and digestive regularity while supplying B-vitamins and minerals that underpin cardiovascular and neuromuscular function. Rather than fast, drug-like actions, Chickpea excels at slow, structural improvements—smoother digestion, steadier energy, and improved lipid balance when used as a daily staple. Proper soaking, cooking, or sprouting improves digestibility and mineral availability.

With roughly 7,000 years of cultivation across the Middle East and South Asia, Chickpea anchors cuisines and healing traditions alike. In Ayurveda and Unani practice, it is associated with strength, fertility, and digestive balance, appearing in porridges, stews, and convalescent diets. Its cultural longevity reflects a simple truth: reliable nourishment builds durable health.

---

🌿 **Core Herbal Category — Chickpea**

**Primary Core: Nutritional & Tonic Support** with (protein- and fiber-rich principles that build steady nourishment)

**Secondary Cores:** Digestive Support · Metabolic Support · Cardiovascular Support

---

### *How It Works*

Chickpea supplies dense plant protein, complex carbohydrates, and minerals that support tissue repair and energy production. Its soluble fiber slows digestion, stabilizing blood sugar and improving nutrient absorption efficiency. This results in sustained nourishment that strengthens baseline function over time.

---

🌱 **Primary Uses**

- Nutritive tonic for strength and stamina
- Supports digestion and healthy gut flora
- Helps regulate blood sugar and cholesterol
- Plant protein for tissue repair and recovery
- Traditional support for women's vitality and lactation

---

### Scientific Backing

Chickpeas are rich in protein, fiber, folate, iron, magnesium, and saponins. Regular intake is associated with improved glycemic control, lower LDL cholesterol, increased satiety, and gradual micronutrient repletion.

---

### Forms Available

- Cooked beans
- Roasted snacks
- Flour (baking, flatbreads)
- Sprouted chickpeas

---

### How to Use

- Cooked: ½–1 cup daily with meals
- Flour: replace up to 25–30% of other flours
- Sprouted: ¼–½ cup daily for improved digestibility

---

### Caution Level: Safe

- May cause gas or bloating if undercooked or overconsumed
- Use caution with legume allergies
- Avoid raw or undercooked beans (lectins)
- Separate from iron or zinc supplements by a few hours

---

### Gender-Specific Safety

**Men:** Supports protein intake, metabolic health, and cardiovascular function.

**Women:** Supports iron status, digestion, and energy, especially during menstruation or recovery.

**Pregnancy / Nursing:** Highly nourishing when well-cooked; reduce if digestive discomfort occurs.

---

### Expected Results

- Digestive comfort and satiety: immediate with meals
- Blood sugar and cholesterol balance: 4–8 weeks
- Energy and nourishment: cumulative with steady intake

---

### DIY Recipe — Chickpea Nutritive Stew

Simmer soaked chickpeas with onion, carrot, celery, garlic, and bay leaf until tender. Finish with olive oil and parsley.

---

### 🔄 Same / Similar Results

● Lentils · ● Mung Beans · ● Black Beans · ● Quinoa

---

### 💬 Herbal Reflections of Chickpea

Chickpea embodies food as medicine—quiet, reliable, and deeply nourishing. Its strength lies not in dramatic effects, but in gradual restoration of energy, digestion, and metabolic balance. Used consistently, it reinforces the foundation on which vitality depends.

---

### ⭐ Herbal Confidence Index: 🌿 🌿 🌿 🌿

(4/5 green stars — dependable nutritive food-herb; highly effective for long-term strength, blood-sugar balance, and metabolic resilience rather than acute medicinal action.)

# BLACK HOREHOUND

★★

*Ballota nigra*

**Black Horehound** is a **nervine-digestive** herb used to relieve nausea, motion sickness, and the "nervous stomach" pattern where anxiety, dizziness, or overstimulation disturb digestion. Its bitter, aromatic compounds provide antispasmodic and mild sedative effects that can calm queasiness linked to stress or travel. Though pungent and unpalatable, it becomes useful when gentler carminatives are insufficient.

European folk medicine employed Black Horehound for seasickness, vertigo, hysteria, and unsettled digestion, often blending it with Lemon Balm, Skullcap, or Chamomile to soften its sharpness. While overshadowed by White Horehound, historical herbals consistently document its niche role in nervous nausea and balance disturbances.

---

**Core Herbal Category — Black Horehound**

**Primary Core: Nervous System Support (Nervines)** with (bitter calming principles that steady nerve signaling)

**Secondary Cores:** Digestive Support · Antispasmodic · Mild Sedative

---

### *How It Works*

Black Horehound calms overactive nerve signaling while reducing spasmodic responses that trigger nausea and dizziness. Its bitter compounds modulate sensory input from the gut and inner-balance pathways, while mild sedative action steadies the nervous system without suppression. Together, these effects restore equilibrium in stress-related digestive upset.

---

**Primary Uses**

- Nausea and motion sickness
- Nervous stomach patterns
- Vertigo and dizziness
- Mild anxiety with digestive upset

---

**Scientific Backing**

Black Horehound contains diterpenes, phenolic acids, and volatile oils associated with antiemetic, antispasmodic, and mild sedative effects. Formal clinical trials are limited, but traditional literature documents centuries of use for nervous nausea and balance disturbances.

---

### Forms Available

- Dried herb (tea)
- Tincture / liquid extract
- Capsules

---

### How to Use

- Tea: 1 tsp dried herb per cup; steep 10 minutes. Blend with Lemon Balm or Chamomile.
- Tincture: 1–2 mL up to 3× daily; often combined with Skullcap or Motherwort.
- Capsules: Follow product directions; less common due to bitterness.

---

### Caution Level: Caution

- Large doses may worsen nausea or cause dizziness
- Avoid during pregnancy and breastfeeding
- Use cautiously in dopamine-related conditions
- Best used short-term and in blends

---

### Gender-Specific Safety

**Men:** Useful for motion sickness or nervous digestive upset; short-term use only.

**Women:** Helpful for anxiety-related nausea; avoid prolonged or high-dose use.

**Pregnancy / Nursing:** Not recommended except for rare, weak tea under professional guidance.

---

### Expected Results

- Nausea and vertigo relief: 30–90 minutes
- Nervous-digestive patterns: improved within 3–7 days

---

### DIY Recipe — Anti-Nausea Infusion

Blend 1 tsp Black Horehound with 1 tsp Lemon Balm. Steep 10 minutes. Sip slowly.

---

### Same / Similar Results

Lemon Balm · Chamomile · Skullcap · Valerian

---

### Herbal Reflections of Black Horehound

Black Horehound is a problem-solver, not a pleasure herb. Its bitterness mirrors its purpose—addressing stubborn nausea and nervous imbalance when more agreeable remedies fall short. Used judiciously and blended well, it earns a quiet place as a situational ally rather than a daily tonic.

---

**Herbal Confidence Index:**

(2/5 green stars — situational anti-nausea nervine; occasionally helpful for motion sickness
and nervous tension, but limited by taste, narrow use-case, and safer modern alternatives.)

# CHICORY ROOT

★★★★

*Cichorium intybus*

**Chicory Root** is a gentle liver and digestive tonic that stimulates bile flow, eases post-meal discomfort, and supports regularity through its prebiotic fiber (inulin). As a food-grade bitter, it promotes smoother digestion, helps balance lipids, and nourishes the gut microbiome—benefits that build steadily with consistent use. Well known as a caffeine-free coffee alternative, roasted chicory has long bridged kitchen and clinic, offering daily metabolic and digestive support without strain.

---

### Core Herbal Category — Chicory Root

**Primary Core: Digestive System Support** with (bitter tonic principles that stimulate bile flow and digestion)

**Secondary Cores:** Liver Support · Prebiotic Support · Metabolic Support

---

### How It Works

Chicory activates bitter receptors that increase bile and digestive secretions, improving fat breakdown and nutrient uptake. Inulin feeds beneficial gut bacteria, supporting microbial balance and regular elimination. Together, these actions enhance digestive efficiency and metabolic tone.

---

### Primary Uses

- Digestive bitters; bile stimulation
- Mild regularity support
- Prebiotic gut nourishment
- Gentle liver/gallbladder support

---

### Scientific Backing

Inulin supports Bifidobacterium and Lactobacillus growth and is associated with improved bowel function, glycemic control, and lipid markers. Bitter principles contribute to bile flow and hepatoprotective effects.

---

### Forms Available
• Roasted root (beverage) · Cut/dried root (tea) · Capsules · Tincture

---

### How to Use (Dosage)
• Roasted beverage: 1 tsp per cup, steep 10–15 min
• Tea: 1 tsp cut root per cup, simmer 10 min
• Capsules/extract: 500–1,000 mg, 1–2× daily

---

### Caution Level: Caution
• Excess may cause gas/bloating (inulin)
• Asteraceae allergy awareness
• Seek advice with gallstones or bile duct obstruction
• Use modest amounts in pregnancy; avoid strong extracts

---

### Gender-Specific Safety
**Men:** Supports digestion, liver tone, and cholesterol; safe in food/beverage use
**Women:** Aids digestion and skin clarity via liver support; safe for daily use
**Pregnancy/Nursing:** Small food amounts acceptable; avoid strong preparations

---

### Expected Results
• Digestive comfort: 3–7 days
• Prebiotic/metabolic support: several weeks

---

### DIY — Chicory Tonic
1 tsp roasted chicory per cup boiling water; steep 10–15 min; 1–2× daily.

---

### Same / Similar Results
Dandelion Root · Burdock Root · Milk Thistle · Artichoke Leaf

---

### Shelf Life / Potency
• Roasted powder: ~1 year · Dried root: up to 18 months · Tincture: 3–5 years · Tea: 24 hours refrigerated

---

### Herbal Reflections of Chicory Root
Chicory heals quietly through repetition—waking digestion, feeding the microbiome, and

supporting the liver day by day. It is where food meets function, turning simple ritual into steady balance.

---

***Herbal Confidence Index:*** *(4 / 5), food-grade digestive tonic; effective for bile flow, liver support, and gentle detox with long-term use.*

# GAMBIR

★★★

*Uncaria gambir*

**Gambir** is a powerful astringent used to tighten tissues, reduce minor bleeding, and calm inflamed mucosa—especially in the mouth, throat, and gut. Rich in catechins and tannins, it acts quickly to firm lax or weepy tissues, making it useful for gum irritation, canker sores, diarrhea, and minor skin lesions when used briefly and diluted. Its strength demands restraint; Gambir excels as a targeted tool, not a daily tonic.

---

**Core Herbal Category — Gambir**

**Primary Core: Lymphatic & Skin Support** with (intense tightening principles that strengthen tissues)

**Secondary Cores:** Anti-inflammatory · Digestive Support · Skin Support

---

**How It Works**

High tannins contract surface proteins, reducing excess moisture and minor bleeding while stabilizing irritated tissues. This rapid tightening restores containment and comfort when laxity or seepage is present.

---

**Primary Uses**

- Oral/gum astringent (rinses, paints)
- Minor bleeding or weepy skin
- Short-term diarrhea support (supervised)

---

**Scientific Backing**

Catechins and tannins account for antioxidant, antimicrobial, and anti-inflammatory effects; activity against oral pathogens is documented.

---

**Forms Available**

- Powder · Extract · Chewable cube · Mouth rinse

---

**How to Use (Dosage)**

- **Oral rinse:** ¼ tsp powder in 1 cup warm water; swish 30 sec, spit; up to 2× daily
- **Internal (short-term):** 300–500 mg extract in divided doses (guided)

• **Topical:** Weak paste to small areas, 1–2 min, then rinse

---

⚠ **Caution Level:** ● **Caution**

• Strong astringent—use sparingly and diluted
• May cause constipation, dry mouth, or stomach irritation if overused
• Avoid in pregnancy/nursing; caution with iron or anticoagulants
• Limit duration to prevent nutrient binding

---

**Gender-Specific Safety**

● **Men:** Short-term use for oral/GI needs; avoid prolonged courses

● **Women:** Helpful for mouth/gum irritation; watch iron status

● **Pregnancy/Nursing:** Avoid except under professional supervision

---

**Expected Results**

• Oral/gum relief: 1–3 days
• Diarrhea tightening: 1–2 doses
• Weepy skin: 1–2 applications

---

**DIY — Gambir Gum Rinse**

¼ tsp powder in 1 cup warm water; swish and spit; up to 2× daily.

---

**Same / Similar Results**

● Oak Bark · ● Myrrh · ● Calendula · ● Chamomile

---

**Shelf Life / Potency**

• Powder/cubes: up to 2 years airtight · Extract/tincture: 3–5 years · Rinse: 24 hours

---

**Herbal Reflections of Gambir**

Gambir is medicine of precision—firm, fast, and restrained. Used briefly and thoughtfully, it restores tone and integrity where tissues have grown lax.

---

**Herbal Confidence Index:** (3 / 5)

Strong, targeted astringent; effective short-term for oral and weepy conditions, best used sparingly due to tannin intensity.

# OAK BARK

★★★★

*Quercus robur*

**Oak Bark** is a classic astringent used to tighten lax tissues, reduce minor bleeding, and calm inflamed skin and mucosa. Its dense tannin content makes it especially useful for hemorrhoids, weeping eczema, minor wounds, mouth ulcers, sore throats, and short-term diarrhea support. Traditionally prepared as decoctions, washes, and compresses, Oak Bark has served as a household remedy across Europe and beyond for centuries, prized for its firming and protective qualities.

---

### 🌿 Core Herbal Category — Oak Bark

**Primary Core: Lymphatic & Skin Support** with (firm tightening principles that restore tissue tone and containment)

**Secondary Cores:** Anti-inflammatory · Digestive Support · Skin Support

---

### *How It Works*

Oak Bark delivers high levels of tannins that bind to surface proteins, causing tissues to contract and strengthen. This reduces excess moisture, irritation, and minor seepage while improving structural integrity. Its action restores firmness without blocking normal tissue function.

---

### 🌱 Primary Uses

- Astringent for skin, gums, throat, hemorrhoids
- Anti-diarrheal (brief internal use)
- Anti-inflammatory wash or soak

---

### 🔬 Scientific Backing

Tannins provide antimicrobial, hemostatic, and anti-inflammatory effects. Evidence supports topical use for dermatitis, minor wounds, and oral conditions. Internal use should remain short-term.

---

### 💊 Forms Available

Dried bark · Tea/decoction · Tincture/extract · Powder · Compress/soak

---

### How to Use (Dosage)

• **Topical rinse/compress:** 1–2 tsp chopped bark per cup water; simmer 10–15 min; use 1–3× daily
• **Internal (short-term):** 2–4 oz diluted decoction 1–2× daily for 1–3 days (guided)
• **Sitz bath:** ½ cup strong decoction added to warm bath; soak 10–20 min

---

### Caution Level: Caution

Strong astringent. Prolonged internal use may irritate digestion or reduce nutrient absorption. Use internally only for short durations. External applications are generally safe when properly diluted.

---

### Gender-Specific Safety

**Men:** Effective for skin, gum irritation, hemorrhoids, and short-term diarrhea. Avoid extended internal use.

**Women:** Useful for vaginal irritation, hemorrhoids, and inflamed skin externally. Keep internal use brief.

**Pregnancy/Nursing:** Avoid internal use. External rinses, baths, or compresses are generally safe.

---

### Expected Results

• Topical improvement: 2–3 days
• GI tightening: 1–4 days (short-term use)

---

### DIY Recipe — Oak Bark Skin Compress

Boil 1 Tbsp dried bark in 1 cup water for 10 minutes. Cool, soak cloth, and apply to affected area.

---

### Same / Similar Results

Gambir · Myrrh · Calendula · Plantain Leaf

---

### Shelf Life / Potency

• Dried bark: up to 3 years
• Tincture/extract: 5+ years
• Prepared decoction: use within 24–48 hours refrigerated

---

### Herbal Reflections of Oak Bark

Oak Bark is a disciplined remedy—best applied in short, purposeful courses when tissues need firming and protection. It restores boundaries, calms inflammation, and reinforces structure without excess force.

---

**Herbal Confidence Index:** 🌿 🌿 🌿 🌿

(4/5 green stars — strong, reliable astringent; highly effective for tightening tissues and calming inflammation, best used short-term or topically due to concentrated tannins.)

# MYRRH

★★★★★

*Commiphora myrrha*

**Myrrh** is a powerful resinous astringent and antiseptic used to cleanse infected tissue, speed wound granulation, and support oral health. Its resin acids and sesquiterpenes provide antimicrobial, anti-inflammatory, and tissue-tightening actions valuable for gingivitis, mouth ulcers, sore throats, weeping skin infections, and slow-healing wounds. Strong and stimulating by nature, Myrrh is best applied topically or in mouth rinses, with internal use reserved for short, expert-guided courses.

---

### 🌿 Core Herbal Category — Myrrh

**Primary Core: Antimicrobial Support** with (resinous antimicrobial principles that tighten and protect tissues)

**Secondary Cores:** Antimicrobial · Wound Support · Digestive Support

---

### *How It Works*

Myrrh's resin compounds create a protective, tightening layer over tissues while limiting microbial growth. This reduces seepage, irritation, and inflammation as tissues stabilize. The combined astringent and antiseptic action supports clean, controlled healing.

---

### 🌱 Primary Uses

- Oral health: gums, ulcers, sore throat rinses
- Antiseptic wound care
- Local inflammation and infection
- Digestive or respiratory stagnation (short, supervised internal use)

---

### 🧪 Scientific Backing

Resin acids and sesquiterpenes demonstrate antimicrobial, anti-inflammatory, and wound-healing activity. Clinical use supports topical and oral applications.

---

### Forms Available

Resin · Powder · Tincture/extract · Capsules · Essential oil (diluted) · Mouth rinse

---

### How to Use (Dosage)

- **Mouth rinse:** ½ tsp tincture in ½ cup warm water; swish and spit, up to 2× daily
- **Topical:** Diluted resin in salves or oils; apply sparingly to clean wounds
- **Internal:** 10–30 drops tincture in water, short-term only under guidance

---

### Caution Level: Caution

Very strong resin. Excess use may irritate digestion. Can stimulate uterine activity. Avoid during pregnancy and breastfeeding. Use cautiously with blood thinners or antidiabetic medications. Limit to short courses.

---

### Gender-Specific Safety

**Men:** Effective for oral health, wound care, and digestive stagnation when used briefly.

**Women:** Helpful for antimicrobial and tissue-firming needs; avoid during pregnancy.

**Pregnancy/Nursing:** Avoid internal use entirely. Mild external use only under guidance.

---

### Expected Results

- Oral/wound improvement: 2–4 days
- Gum conditions: 7–10 days with regular application

---

### DIY Recipe — Myrrh Mouth Rinse

1 tsp Myrrh tincture + ½ cup warm water. Swish 30–60 seconds and spit. Use short-term only.

---

### Same / Similar Results

Frankincense · Goldenseal · Oak Bark · Thuja · Calendula

---

### Shelf Life / Potency

- Resin: 10+ years
- Tincture: 5+ years
- Prepared rinse: 24–48 hours refrigerated

---

### Herbal Reflections of Myrrh

Myrrh is a guardian herb—cleansing, firming, and protective. It is not gentle medicine, but precise medicine, best used where boundaries have been breached and integrity must be restored.

---

🌟 **Herbal Confidence Index:** 🌿 🌿 🌿 🌿 🌿 5/5 green stars — cornerstone antiseptic and wound-healing resin, dependable and effective
when used with respect for dose and duration.)

# *SPILANTHES*

★★★★★

*Acmella oleracea*

**Spilanthes**, often called the **"Toothache Plant"** or **"Electric Daisy,"** is a vivid sensory herb prized for its rapid numbing, immune-activating, and circulatory effects. When chewed, the flower produces a distinctive tingling that increases salivation and local blood flow—an action traditionally used for oral discomfort and early immune support.
Rather than a long-term tonic, Spilanthes excels as an **onset-stage herb**, valued for waking up sluggish tissues and quickly rallying local defenses when the body needs to respond fast.

---

### *Core Herbal Category — Spilanthes*

**Primary Core: Immune System Support** (stimulating principles that activate local defense response)
**Secondary Cores:** Circulatory Support · Lymphatic Support · Digestive Support

---

### *How It Works*

Spilanthes rapidly stimulates sensory nerve endings, increasing local circulation and immune signaling. This activation enhances lymphatic movement and brings defensive cells to surface tissues. The result is fast, localized immune engagement without prolonged stimulation.

---

### *Primary Uses*

- Numbs oral discomfort and supports oral hygiene
- Primes immune response at onset
- Stimulates microcirculation (topical adjunct)
- Encourages appetite and digestion in bitters

---

### Scientific Backing

Spilanthes contains alkamides—particularly **spilanthol**—associated with sialagogue activity, mild anesthetic effects, and immunomodulation. Both traditional and modern herbal practice consistently report rapid oral effects and immune-supportive benefits when used at the earliest signs of challenge.

---

### *Forms Available*

- Fresh flower or leaf (chewed)
- Tincture / liquid extract (fresh preferred)
- Topical oil or liniment
- Bitters blends

---

### *How to Use*

- **Fresh flower/leaf:** Chew ½–1 flower for oral numbing and salivation
- **Tincture:** 20–40 drops in water, up to 2× daily
- **Mouth rinse:** 30–40 drops tincture in ½ cup water; swish and spit
- **Topical:** Infused oil for circulation or minor muscle aches

---

### *Expected Results*

- Oral numbing/tingle: within minutes
- Immune-onset support: 1–3 days with early use
- Digestive stimulation: immediate in bitters

---

### ⚠ Caution Level: Caution

- Tingling and numbing are expected; discontinue if irritation persists
- Avoid application on open mouth lesions unless guided
- Possible sensitivity in Asteraceae (ragweed/daisy family)
- Limited pregnancy and lactation data—avoid large internal doses

---

### Gender-Specific Safety

**Men:** Safe — supports gum health, immune onset, and circulation

**Women:** Safe — effective for oral care and lymphatic tone

**Pregnancy/Nursing:** Caution — mild topical use only; avoid strong internal dosing

---

### *Same / Similar Results*

*Clove · Echinacea · Ginger*

---

### Herbal Reflections of Spilanthes

Spilanthes doesn't whisper — it **signals**.
Its electric tingle announces movement, moisture, and response, reminding the body how to react when defenses lag. This is an alert herb, sharp and decisive, best used briefly to wake things up and then step aside.

---

### Herbal Confidence Index:

*(5/5 green stars — a vibrant immune and oral-health tonic, renowned for its numbing action, lymphatic activation, and unmistakable "electric daisy" spark.)*

# PUMPKIN SEED

★★★★★

*Cucurbita pepo*

**Pumpkin Seed** is a deeply nourishing food-medicine known for strengthening the urinary system, supporting prostate health, and restoring foundational vitality. Rich in zinc, essential fatty acids, and plant sterols, it rebuilds depleted tissues rather than forcing stimulation.
Gentle enough for lifelong use, Pumpkin Seed excels as a **long-term ally**, supporting bladder tone, hormonal balance, and steady reproductive health in both men and women.

---

### *Core Herbal Category — Pumpkin Seed*

**Primary Core: Reproductive & Women's Health Support** (rebuilding principles that nourish urinary and prostate tissues)
**Secondary Cores:** Urinary Support · Endocrine Support · Mineral Support

---

### *How It Works*

Pumpkin Seed supports the body through its rich concentration of minerals, fatty acids, and plant sterols that nourish the urinary and reproductive systems. Its natural oils help maintain healthy prostate and bladder function while supporting smooth urinary flow and tissue tone. Zinc and trace nutrients strengthen immune and hormonal balance, while gentle anti-inflammatory compounds soothe irritated tissues. Rather than acting as a fast stimulant, Pumpkin Seed works gradually by rebuilding strength, lubrication, and stability in the urinary tract and surrounding tissues.

---

### *Primary Uses*

- Supports prostate health and urinary flow
- Nourishes reproductive tissues
- Assists hormonal balance with aging
- Strengthens bladder tone and pelvic support

• Provides zinc-rich nutritional vitality

---

## Scientific Backing

Pumpkin Seed contains **phytosterols, zinc, linoleic acid, and antioxidants** that support prostate and urinary health. Clinical and observational studies associate Pumpkin Seed and its oil with improved urinary flow, prostate comfort, and reduced oxidative stress in reproductive tissues.

---

## *Forms Available*

- Raw whole seeds
- Roasted seeds (food-grade)
- Ground seed powder
- Cold-pressed Pumpkin Seed oil
- Capsules (seed or oil)

---

## *How to Use*

- **Whole seeds:** 1–2 Tbsp daily, raw or lightly roasted
- **Ground powder:** 1 Tbsp daily in food
- **Oil:** 1–2 tsp daily with meals
- **Capsules:** Typically 1,000–2,000 mg daily

---

## ⚠ Caution Level: Safe

- Extremely well tolerated
- Rare digestive upset with excessive intake
- Safe for long-term daily use
- No known toxicity in food or medicinal use

---

## Gender-Specific Safety

**Men:** Highly beneficial for prostate and urinary comfort

**Women:** Supports bladder tone and nutritional balance

**Pregnancy/Nursing:** ● Safe in food-level amounts

---

### ⌛ *Expected Results*

- Urinary comfort: 1–2 weeks
- Prostate support: 3–6 weeks
- Hormonal nourishment: gradual, cumulative
- Vitality support: ongoing with regular use

---

### 🛠 DIY Recipe — Pumpkin Seed Prostate Blend

- 1 Tbsp ground Pumpkin Seed
- 1 tsp ground Flaxseed
- ½ tsp Cinnamon

Mix into oatmeal or a smoothie once daily.

---

### *Same / Similar Results*

● Saw Palmetto · ● Pygeum · ● Parsley · ● Flaxseed · ● Tongkat Ali

---

### 💬 Herbal Reflections of Pumpkin Seed

Pumpkin Seed teaches a quiet lesson in strength.
It does not force energy or provoke sensation; it rebuilds patiently from the inside out. Its medicine is steady, grounding, and restorative — a reminder that lasting vitality grows from nourishment, not urgency.

---

### ★ Herbal Confidence Index: 🌿 🌿 🌿 🌿 🌿

(5/5 green stars — cornerstone nutritive herb for prostate and urinary health; exceptionally safe, effective, and suitable for lifelong use.)

# *FIG LEAF*

★★★

*Ficus carica*

**Fig Leaf** is a gentle metabolic and respiratory ally traditionally used to steady blood sugar, soften inflammatory patterns, and calm irritated tissues. Taken as a tea or light extract, it supports balanced glucose handling when paired with diet and movement, while also offering soothing benefits for digestion, skin, and the bronchial system. Topically, it has been used for eczema, dermatitis, and inflamed skin.
Mediterranean and Middle-Eastern household medicine valued the leaf—often overshadowed by the fruit—as a quiet but reliable support for metabolic, respiratory, and dermal balance. Modern interest reflects this same wisdom: sustainable, non-forcing support that complements (not replaces) clinical care.

---

**Core Herbal Category — Fig Leaf**
**Primary Core: Endocrine & Hormonal Support** with (cooling, regulatory action that steadies glucose handling and metabolic rhythm)
**Secondary Cores:** Digestive Support · Skin & Tissue Repair · Respiratory Support · Anti-inflammatory

---

### *How It Works*

Fig Leaf works by cooling metabolic and inflammatory excess, helping the body regulate blood sugar more smoothly. Its compounds support insulin sensitivity and reduce digestive irritation, easing metabolic strain. This cooling, calming influence extends to respiratory tissues and inflamed skin, making Fig Leaf a systemic harmonizer rather than a stimulant.

---

**Primary Uses**

- Supports healthy blood sugar balance
- Soothes digestive irritation and bloating
- Calms coughs and mild bronchial tension
- Reduces inflammatory skin responses
- Offers gentle antimicrobial and antioxidant support

---

**Scientific Backing**

Fig Leaf contains flavonoids, tannins, psoralen, and phenolic compounds associated with improved insulin sensitivity, reduced post-meal glucose spikes, and anti-inflammatory activity. Studies suggest Fig Leaf tea may lower insulin requirements in some individuals and support wound-healing and skin repair when used topically.

---

### How to Use (Dosage)

- **Tea:** 1 tbsp dried leaf simmered 10 minutes; 1–2 cups daily
- **Capsules:** 300–600 mg, 1–2× daily
- **Tincture:** 1–2 mL, up to 3× daily
- **Topical:** Strong decoction applied 2–3× daily to skin

---

### Expected Results

- Digestive calming: 1–2 days
- Blood sugar support: 1–2 weeks
- Respiratory easing: same day to several days
- Skin improvement: 3–7 days

---

### Caution Level: Caution

- May lower blood sugar — monitor with medication
- Possible photosensitivity in fair skin
- Avoid excessive topical use on sun-exposed areas
- Not suitable for fig-latex allergy

---

### Gender-Specific Safety (GS)

**Men:** Safe — metabolic and respiratory support without hormonal effects

**Women:** Safe — helpful for digestion, skin, and metabolic balance

**Pregnancy/Nursing:** Mild caution — light tea acceptable; avoid concentrates

---

### Same / Similar Results

Mulberry Leaf · Olive Leaf · Plantain Leaf · Bay Leaf · Nettle Leaf

---

### DIY Recipe — Fig Leaf Balancing Tea

1 tbsp dried Fig Leaf · 2 cups water
Simmer 10–12 minutes. Drink once or twice daily.

---

### Herbal Reflections of Fig Leaf

Fig Leaf is quiet medicine. It doesn't push or provoke — it steadies. Cooling, softening, and patient, it restores rhythm where excess and irritation have crept in. Like shade under a fig tree, its strength is subtle, protective, and enduring.

---

🌟 **Herbal Confidence Index:** 🌿🌿🌿🌿
(4/5 — dependable, gentle metabolic and inflammatory regulator; best for steady, long-term balance rather than acute intervention.)

# *GIANT HYSSOP*

★★★★

*Agastache rugosa*

**Giant Hyssop** is an aromatic nervine-carminative that calms anxiety, eases digestive tension, and gently supports the lungs. Its sweet licorice-mint profile relaxes cramping, gas, and stress-related digestive upset, making it ideal for teas, syrups, and infused honey during colds or emotional strain.
Long used by Indigenous traditions and later adopted into herbal practice, Giant Hyssop bridges comfort and clarity — soothing without sedation and uplifting without stimulation. Its gentle nature makes it well suited for repeated, family-friendly use.

---

### 🌿 Core Herbal Category — Giant Hyssop

**Primary Core: Nervous System Support (Nervines)** with (calming aromatic action that relaxes the nerves while easing digestive tension)
**Secondary Cores:** Digestive Support · Respiratory Support · Immune Support

---

## *How It Works*

Giant Hyssop works by calming the nervous system while relaxing smooth muscle tension in the digestive tract. Its aromatic oils reduce stress-driven gut spasm, support comfortable breathing, and gently lift mood. By easing nervous overload, it indirectly supports immune resilience and respiratory comfort.

---

### 🌱 Primary Uses

- Calms anxiety and emotional tension
- Relieves gas, cramping, and digestive discomfort
- Soothes coughs and mild respiratory irritation
- Supports immune balance during stress

---

### 🧪 Scientific Backing

Giant Hyssop contains volatile oils and flavonoids with antioxidant, antifungal, mild sedative, and anti-inflammatory properties. Research supports its traditional use for digestive relaxation, mood calming, and microbial defense.

---

### 💊 How to Use (Dosage)

- **Tea:** 1–2 tsp dried herb per cup; steep 10 min; 1–3× daily

• **Tincture:** 1–2 mL up to 3× daily
• **Infused Honey/Syrup:** By spoon or in warm water for cough or tension

---

⚠ **Caution Level:** ● **Safe**
Generally very gentle. Use moderation with concentrated preparations. Mint-family sensitivities possible. During pregnancy, stick to light tea or culinary use.

---

**Gender-Specific Safety (GS)**
**Men:** ● Safe — excellent for stress-related digestion and breathing
**Women:** ● Safe — supports calm mood, digestion, and restful sleep
**Pregnancy/Nursing:** ● Mild caution — avoid strong tinctures

---

**Expected Results**
• Digestive calming: 30–60 minutes
• Respiratory comfort: several days of regular use

---

**Same / Similar Results**
● Lemon Balm · ● Chamomile · ● Lavender · ● Skullcap · ● Anise Seed

---

**Herbal Reflections of Giant Hyssop**
Giant Hyssop is comfort you can breathe. It loosens what's knotted, settles what's anxious, and invites the body back into ease. Aromatic, gentle, and reassuring, it reminds us that calm can be fragrant and effective at the same time.

---

**Herbal Confidence Index:**
(4/5 — reliable, calming, and versatile; especially valuable for stress-linked digestion and mild respiratory tension.)

# COPTIS ROOT

★★★★

*Coptis chinensis*

**Coptis Root** (Huang Lian) is one of the most intensely bitter and antimicrobial herbs in traditional medicine. Rich in berberine, it is used for acute digestive infections, ulcers, inflammatory gut conditions, and heat-driven metabolic imbalance. Small doses exert strong effects, making it a precision herb rather than a daily tonic.
Across Chinese, Tibetan, and Japanese medicine, Coptis was reserved for clearing "toxic heat" — infections, fevers, liver congestion, and inflammatory skin eruptions — and was almost always paired with gentler herbs to moderate its force. Its reputation endures as a decisive intervention herb when inflammation and microbial overgrowth are entrenched.

---

### Core Herbal Category — Coptis Root

**Primary Core:** Digestive System Support with (intense bitter, heat-clearing action that suppresses microbial overgrowth and cools inflammatory digestive fire)
**Secondary Cores:** Liver & Detoxification · Metabolic & Blood Sugar Support · Immune Support

---

### *How It Works*

Coptis Root works by powerfully cooling inflammatory heat and inhibiting pathogenic microbes in the gut. Its berberine content suppresses bacterial and fungal overgrowth, reduces intestinal irritation, and improves bile flow. This cooling action extends to the liver and metabolic system, helping regulate blood sugar and dampen immune overactivation. It is most effective when inflammation is sharp, hot, and infectious in nature.

---

### Primary Uses

- Acute bacterial or fungal gut infections
- Ulcers, gastritis, inflammatory diarrhea
- Liver heat and toxin overload
- Feverish or heat-based skin eruptions
- Short-term metabolic flare support (blood sugar, lipids)

---

### Scientific Backing

Coptis Root is among the richest herbal sources of **berberine**, extensively studied for antimicrobial, anti-inflammatory, glucose-regulating, and liver-protective effects. Research supports its use for H. pylori, infectious diarrhea, insulin resistance, and inflammatory skin conditions, with clear evidence that **dose and duration must be limited**.

---

### How to Use (Dosage)

- **Decoction:** ½–1 tsp dried root simmered 15–20 min in 2 cups water (short-term only)
- **Tincture:** 10–30 drops, 1–2× daily for 3–10 days (guided use recommended)
- **Capsules:** 300–500 mg per dose with meals (follow product guidance)

---

### Expected Results

- Digestive relief: 1–3 days
- Heat clearing / skin improvement: 3–7 days
- Metabolic support (monitored): 1–2 weeks

---

### Caution Level: Caution

- High-potency berberine herb — **short-term use only**
- Avoid during pregnancy or breastfeeding
- May interact with diabetic, blood-pressure, or antibiotic medications
- Not suitable for cold, weak, or underweight constitutions
- Overuse may suppress beneficial gut flora

---

### Gender-Specific Safety (GS)

**Men:** Caution — effective for acute gut and metabolic flare-ups; avoid long-term use

**Women:** Caution — useful for inflammatory skin or liver heat; avoid preconception and nursing

**Pregnancy/Nursing:** Avoid — berberine crosses placenta and breast milk

---

### Same / Similar Results

Goldenseal · Oregon Grape · Barberry · Licorice Root · Dandelion Root

---

### Herbal Reflections of Coptis Root

Coptis does not negotiate — it corrects. Bitter, exacting, and uncompromising, it steps in when heat and infection have overstayed their welcome. This is an herb of boundaries and discipline, reminding us that strong medicine works best when used briefly, precisely, and with respect.

---

### Herbal Confidence Index:

(4/5 — exceptionally effective antimicrobial and heat-clearing herb with strong clinical backing, but narrow margins that demand precision and restraint.)

# ACORUS (Sweet Flag)

★★

*Acorus calamus*

**Acorus,** also known as Sweet Flag, is an aromatic marsh root traditionally used to stimulate digestion, sharpen mental clarity, and clear stagnant mucus. Its warming, penetrating nature made it valuable for sluggish digestion, mental fog, and ritual focus — but also demanded careful handling.

Used across Ayurvedic, Native American, and East Asian traditions, Acorus occupied a dual role as both medicine and ceremonial ally. Modern safety concerns surrounding **β-asarone** have narrowed its internal use, reinforcing its place as a **specialized, supervised herb rather than a daily remedy**.

---

### Core Herbal Category — Acorus

**Primary Core: Digestive System Support** with *(warming, aromatic action that sharpens awareness and mobilizes stagnant digestion)*

**Secondary Cores:** Cognitive Clarity · Respiratory Clearing · Ritual / Spiritual Support

---

## How It Works

Acorus works by stimulating the nervous system and digestive tract through aromatic volatile oils. These compounds increase circulation, awaken mental alertness, reduce digestive stagnation, and loosen thick mucus. Because its action is sharp and penetrating, benefits appear quickly — but only at **very low, carefully controlled doses**.

---

### Primary Uses

- Mental fog, sluggish focus (short-term)
- Digestive stagnation, gas, bloating
- Mucus congestion in lungs or sinuses
- Ritual grounding and clarity practices

---

### Scientific Backing

Acorus contains volatile oils (asarone, eugenol, shyobunone) with antispasmodic, carminative, and nervine effects. However, **β-asarone** has demonstrated neurotoxic and carcinogenic potential in animal studies, leading to strict limitations on internal use and the exclusion of high-asarone Asian strains.

---

### How to Use (Dosage)

- **Tea (short-term):** ¼–½ tsp root per cup; simmer 10 min (verified low-asarone only)

• **Tincture:** 1–3 *drops* (not droppers), 1–2× daily — professional supervision required
• **Aromatic use:** Incense, sachet, or external applications preferred

---

⌛ **Expected Results**
• Digestive stimulation: 30–90 minutes
• Mental clarity: 45–60 minutes
• Mucus clearing: same day to 24 hours

---

⚠ **Caution Level: ● Supervision Required**
• **β-asarone toxicity is the primary concern**
• Avoid Asian triploid strains entirely
• Avoid during pregnancy, nursing, seizures, liver or neurological conditions
• Not for daily or long-term internal use
• Essential oil is **external only**

---

**Gender-Specific Safety (GS)**
**Men:** ● Caution — short-term digestive or cognitive use only
**Women:** ● Caution — avoid frequent or internal use
**Pregnancy/Nursing:** ● Avoid — uterine stimulation and neurotoxicity risk

---

**Same / Similar Results**
● Gotu Kola · ● Lemon Balm · ● Bacopa · ● Eleuthero · ● Rhodiola

---

**Herbal Reflections of Acorus**
Acorus sharpens the edge of awareness. Its presence is immediate — clarifying, penetrating, and grounding — but it insists on discipline. This is not a comfort herb; it is a threshold herb, reminding us that clarity sometimes comes with limits and responsibility.

---

**Herbal Confidence Index:**
*(2/5 — culturally significant and functionally effective, yet narrowly usable today due to safety constraints. Potent, purposeful, and reserved for rare, well-defined situations.)*

# SARSAPARILLA

★★★★

*Smilax officinalis*

**Sarsaparilla** is a classic "blood purifier," long relied on for skin conditions, joint inflammation, and detoxification. Its active compounds bind circulating toxins, reduce inflammatory burden, and support liver and immune function. It is especially valued for chronic skin eruptions such as eczema, psoriasis, and acne, where internal congestion needs gradual clearing rather than suppression.

Deeply rooted in folk and Western herbalism, Sarsaparilla rose to prominence in the 19th century as both a medicine and a tonic drink, even inspiring early root beer formulas. Across cultures, it earned a reputation as a rejuvenator — steady, detoxifying, and strengthening rather than stimulating.

---

### Core Herbal Category — Sarsaparilla

**Primary Core: Liver & Detoxification Support** with (blood-cleansing, eliminative action that assists toxin and inflammatory waste removal)

**Secondary Cores:** Hormonal & Endocrine Support · Musculoskeletal Support · Skin & Tissue Repair · Men's Vitality · Foundational / Systemic Support

---

### How It Works

Sarsaparilla supports liver-based detoxification and blood cleansing, helping escort inflammatory and metabolic waste out of the body. Its saponins bind circulating toxins, reducing internal congestion that often manifests as skin eruptions or joint discomfort. By lowering toxic load, it indirectly supports hormonal balance and immune clarity. The result is gradual restoration of skin, joints, and overall vitality through steady internal cleanup rather than force.

---

### Primary Uses

- Promotes clearer skin (eczema, acne, psoriasis)
- Relieves joint pain, stiffness, and rheumatic patterns
- Supports detoxification and "blood purification"
- Assists hormonal balance and endocrine strain
- Strengthens liver, kidney, and immune function

---

### Scientific Backing

Sarsaparilla contains saponins, flavonoids, and plant sterols shown to bind endotoxins and support immune-mediated detoxification. Research supports its use for inflammatory skin conditions, arthritis, and metabolic detox support, with antioxidant and mild hormone-modulating effects noted in modern studies.

---

### Forms Available

- Dried root (tea, decoction, powder)
- Tinctures and fluid extracts
- Capsules and blended formulas

---

### How to Use (Dosage)

- **Tea/Decoction:** 1 Tbsp dried root per 2 cups water; simmer 15 minutes; drink 1–2 cups daily
- **Tincture:** 1–2 mL up to 3× daily
- **Capsules/Powder:** 300–600 mg, 1–2× daily per label

---

### Caution Level: Safe

Generally well tolerated in tea or tonic form. High doses may cause mild stomach upset due to saponins. Those with kidney conditions or using diuretics should moderate use. May increase absorption of certain medications; avoid combining with prescriptions without guidance. Use in cycles (3–4 weeks on, 1 week off) for sustained detox support.

---

### Gender-Specific Safety

- **Men:** Supports stamina, hormone balance, and skin health; safe for long-term tonic use
- **Women:** Helpful for PMS-related congestion, menopausal skin issues, and liver support
- **Pregnancy/Nursing:** Gentle tea only; avoid concentrated extracts

---

### Expected Results

- Skin clarity: 7–10 days
- Energy improvement: 10–14 days

- Hormonal balance: 2–3 weeks
- Joint relief & detox: 3–4 weeks
- Overall vitality: 1–2 months

---

🛠 **DIY Recipe — Sarsaparilla Detox Decoction**
Simmer 1 Tbsp dried Sarsaparilla root in 2 cups water for 15 minutes.
Drink 1 cup daily for gentle detox and skin support.

---

🔄 **Same / Similar Results**
🟤 Burdock Root · 🟤 Dandelion Root · ⚪ Licorice Root · 🟤 Yellow Dock

---

🧪 **Shelf Life / Potency**

- Dried root: up to 2 years (airtight, cool storage)
- Tincture: 4–5 years
- Powder: best within 1 year
- Decoction: refrigerate; use within 48 hours

---

💬 **Herbal Reflections of Sarsaparilla**
Sarsaparilla moves like a slow river through the body — steady, cleansing, transformative. It doesn't force change; it encourages release, allowing strength to rebuild. Long honored as a tonic for the weathered and overburdened, it teaches that real healing comes from consistency, not intensity.
🌟 **Herbal Confidence Index:** 🌿 🌿 🌿 🌿
*(4/5 green stars — trusted restorative and blood purifier; effective, gentle, and well suited for sustained detox and skin support.)*

# *SAW PALMETTO*

★★★★★

*Serenoa repens*

**Saw Palmetto** is one of the most respected herbs for men's prostate and urinary health, with deep roots in Native American medicine of the southeastern United States. The dark berries were traditionally used to maintain urinary flow, reproductive vitality, and hormonal balance, particularly with aging.

Modern herbal practice recognizes Saw Palmetto as a cornerstone remedy for benign prostatic hyperplasia (BPH). Rather than forcing hormonal suppression, it works by gently moderating excess androgen activity, calming inflammation, and supporting healthy bladder emptying — making it both effective and well tolerated.

---

**Core Herbal Category — Saw Palmetto**

**Primary Core: Kidney & Urinary Support** with (prostate-toning, urinary-flow–supporting action that improves bladder emptying and pelvic outlet function)

**Secondary Cores:** Endocrine & Hormonal Regulation · Anti-Inflammatory & Pain Modulation · Foundational Regulation & Terrain Support

---

**How It Works**

Saw Palmetto gently inhibits excess conversion of testosterone into dihydrotestosterone (DHT), a primary contributor to prostate enlargement. This modulation reduces prostate congestion without suppressing healthy hormone levels. Its fatty acids and sterols also calm inflammation in prostate and urinary tissues, easing pressure and irritation. Together, these actions restore comfort, flow, and long-term reproductive stability.

---

**Primary Uses**

- Supports prostate size and comfort
- Improves urinary flow and reduces nighttime urination
- Helps balance testosterone and DHT activity
- Supports bladder tone and emptying
- Promotes long-term male reproductive health

---

### Scientific Backing

Saw Palmetto berries contain fatty acids and phytosterols shown to inhibit 5-alpha-reductase activity, reduce prostate inflammation, and improve urinary function. Clinical literature (including *Journal of Urology* and *Phytotherapy Research*) demonstrates meaningful symptom relief for BPH, often comparable to pharmaceutical options with fewer side effects.

---

### Forms Available

- Standardized berry extract (capsules/softgels)
- Whole dried berries
- Liquid extract / tincture

---

### How to Use (Dosage)

- **Capsules/Softgels:** 160 mg standardized extract, 1–2× daily
- **Tincture:** 1–2 mL up to 2× daily
  *Note: Benefits are cumulative; consistent daily use is essential.*

---

### Caution Level: Safe

Generally well tolerated. Mild digestive upset may occur in sensitive individuals. Avoid during pregnancy or breastfeeding. Consult a practitioner if using hormone-modulating medications.

---

### Gender-Specific Safety

- **Men:** Excellent long-term support for prostate health and urinary strength
- **Women:** Occasionally used for androgen-related concerns under guidance
- **Pregnancy/Nursing:** Not recommended

---

### Expected Results

- Improved urinary flow: 2–4 weeks
- Reduced nighttime urination: 3–6 weeks
- Prostate comfort: 1–3 months
- Long-term maintenance: ongoing use

### 🛠 DIY Recipe — Prostate Support Blend

- 2 parts Saw Palmetto
- 1 part Pumpkin Seed
- 1 part Nettle Leaf
- ½ part Pygeum
  Encapsulate or decoct; use daily.

---

### Same / Similar Results

Pumpkin Seed · Pygeum · Nettle Leaf · Horsetail · Maca Root

---

### Shelf Life / Potency

- Dried berries: 2–3 years
- Capsules/softgels: ~2 years
- Tincture: 4–6 years

---

### Herbal Reflections of Saw Palmetto

Saw Palmetto represents quiet strength and endurance. It restores balance where time has created pressure, supporting function without disruption. For men seeking longevity rather than quick fixes, it stands as a steady guardian — reliable, patient, and deeply supportive.

**Herbal Confidence Index:** 🌿 🌿 🌿 🌿 🌿

*(5/5 green stars — cornerstone prostate herb; exceptionally reliable, clinically validated, and safe for long-term use.)*

# HOPS

★★★★

*Humulus lupulus*

**Hops**, the flowering cone of the hop plant, is best known in brewing but has long been treasured in herbal medicine for its calming, sedative, and digestive effects. It eases anxiety, restlessness, and sleep disturbance, while its bitter qualities help downshift stress-related digestive tension. This dual nervine–bitter action makes Hops especially useful when mental agitation and digestive upset occur together.

Since the Middle Ages, hops have been stuffed into pillows for insomnia and brewed into tonics for nervous tension. Modern herbalists continue to rely on Hops for anxiety, menopausal discomfort, and sleep support, reflecting its enduring versatility and reliability.

---

### Core Herbal Category — Hops

**Primary Core: Nervous System Support (Nervines)** with (sedative, calming action that quiets nervous excitation and supports restorative sleep)

**Secondary Cores:** Digestive Support · Women's Health · Musculoskeletal Support · Hormonal & Endocrine Support

---

### How It Works

Hops works by calming nervous system overactivity, making it effective for restlessness, anxiety, and sleep disruption. Its bitter-sedative compounds slow neural signaling and relax muscle tension, preparing the body for rest. In the digestive tract, its bitter action helps down-regulate stress-induced digestive disturbance. Hops also gently influences hormonal signaling, which can be supportive during menopausal transition. Overall, it restores nighttime recovery and nervous-system calm rather than forcing sedation.

---

### Primary Uses

- Promotes natural sleep and relaxation
- Calms anxiety, stress, and irritability
- Offers gentle menopausal support
- Acts as a digestive bitter to settle stress-related digestion

---

### Scientific Backing

Hops contains volatile oils, flavonoids, and bitter acids that interact with GABA receptors to produce sedative effects. Research supports its role in reducing sleep latency, easing nervous tension, and mildly modulating estrogen activity — particularly useful during menopause.

---

### Forms Available

- Dried flowers (tea, pillows, sachets)
- Tinctures and extracts
- Capsules (standardized)
- Aromatic sleep pillows

---

### How to Use (Dosage)

- **Tea:** 1 tsp dried flowers per cup; steep 10 minutes; drink before bed
- **Tincture:** 1–2 mL up to 3× daily
- **Pillow/Sachet:** Place near head at bedtime for calming aroma

---

### Caution Level: Safe

Generally safe in moderate amounts. Avoid combining with alcohol or prescription sedatives, as effects may be amplified. Prolonged high intake may mildly lower libido in men due to phytoestrogens. Avoid concentrated use during pregnancy or breastfeeding.

---

### Gender-Specific Safety

- **Men:** Supports sleep, digestion, and nervous calm; prolonged high doses may mildly reduce libido
- **Women:** Especially helpful for sleep disturbance, anxiety, and menopausal irritability
- **Pregnancy/Nursing:** Avoid concentrated forms; mild tea or pillows used sparingly

---

### Expected Results

- Nervous relaxation: 30–60 minutes
- Improved sleep quality: 3–5 nights

- Digestive tension relief: 1–2 days
- Mood steadiness: 5–7 days

---

🛠 **DIY Recipe — Hops Bedtime Tea**
1 tsp dried Hops + 1 tsp Chamomile + 1 cup hot water
Steep 10 minutes. Sip 30 minutes before bed.

---

🔄 **Same / Similar Results**
● Valerian · ● Passionflower · ● Lemon Balm · ● Black Cohosh

---

**Shelf Life / Potency**

- Dried flowers: 1–2 years (airtight, cool, dark storage)
- Tincture: 4–5 years
- Capsules/powder: best within 1 year
- Sleep pillows: replace every 9–12 months

---

💬 **Herbal Reflections of Hops**
Hops is the herb of quiet evenings. It softens the edges of a restless mind and gently lowers the body toward rest. Its bitterness grounds excess energy, while its aroma carries calm into the nervous system. Hops doesn't knock the body out — it teaches it how to let go.

⭐ **Herbal Confidence Index:** 🌿🌿🌿🌿
*(4/5 green stars — a dependable sedative-bitter; highly effective for sleep, anxiety, and menopausal ease with a long record of safe traditional use.)*

# FENUGREEK

★★★

*Trigonella foenum-graecum*

**Fenugreek** is a warming, nutritive herb that supports blood sugar balance, digestion, and hormonal health in both men and women. Its golden seeds are valued for stabilizing metabolism, lowering cholesterol, and enhancing milk production in nursing mothers. Rich in fiber, iron, and diosgenin, Fenugreek strengthens digestion while gently rebuilding depleted systems.

Used since ancient Egypt and throughout Ayurvedic and Mediterranean traditions, Fenugreek has long been regarded as a tonic for endurance, recovery, and metabolic strength. Its maple-like aroma and food-medicine nature place it firmly at the intersection of nourishment and therapy.

---

## 🌿 Core Herbal Category — Fenugreek

**Primary Core: Endocrine & Hormonal Support** with (warming, nutritive action that stabilizes glucose and supports hormonal balance)

**Secondary Cores:** Digestive Support · Women's Health · Cardiovascular Support · Nutritive & Restorative

---

## 🌿 How It Works

Fenugreek slows glucose absorption and improves insulin sensitivity, helping stabilize blood sugar and energy levels. Its mucilaginous fibers soothe the digestive tract and improve nutrient assimilation. This nutritive support strengthens hormonal balance, particularly during lactation or recovery. Fenugreek also supports circulation and lipid metabolism, acting as a warming, rebuilding metabolic tonic rather than a stimulant.

---

## 🌱 Primary Uses

- Supports lactation and postpartum recovery
- Regulates blood sugar and insulin sensitivity
- *Lowers LDL cholesterol*
- Soothes digestion and stimulates appetite
- *Supports menstrual and hormonal balance*

---

## Scientific Backing

Fenugreek contains saponins, fiber, alkaloids, iron, amino acids, and diosgenin associated with improved blood sugar control, enhanced milk production, cholesterol reduction, digestive mucosal healing, and improved metabolic efficiency. Clinical research supports its use in diabetes care, digestion, and lactation.

---

## Forms Available

- *Whole seeds*
- *Powdered seeds*
- *Capsules / standardized extracts*
- *Tinctures*
- *Teas and digestive blends*

---

## How to Use (Dosage)

- **Tea:** 1 tsp crushed seeds; steep 10 minutes; drink 1–2× daily
- **Capsules:** 300–600 mg extract, 1–2× daily
- **Powder:** ¼–½ tsp mixed into food or warm water daily
- **Culinary:** Added to soups, stews, and curries
- ***Tincture:*** *1–2 mL up to 2× daily*

---

## Expected Results

- *Digestive comfort: 2–4 days*
- Blood sugar / cholesterol support: 2–4 weeks
- *Lactation increase: 24–72 hours*
- *Hormonal stamina: 2–3 weeks*

---

## Caution Level: Caution

May lower blood sugar — monitor with diabetic medications. High doses can cause gas or digestive upset. Avoid during pregnancy unless supervised. May slightly alter breast-milk flavor. Use caution with legume allergies.

---

## Gender-Specific Safety

- **Men:** Supports stamina, metabolism, and digestion
- **Women:** Helpful for PMS, fatigue, and hormonal balance
- **Pregnancy/Nursing:** Avoid concentrated extracts during pregnancy; nursing use acceptable under guidance

---

## Same / Similar Results

Fennel Seed · Cinnamon · Dong Quai · Milk Thistle

---

## DIY Recipe — Fenugreek Digestive Tea

1 tsp crushed Fenugreek seeds
1 cup boiling water
Steep 10 minutes; sip after meals.

---

## Shelf Life / Potency

- *Whole seeds: up to 2 years*
- *Powder: ~1 year*
- *Capsules: 18–24 months*
- *Tincture: 4–6 years*
- Prepared tea: refrigerate; use within 48 hours

## Herbal Reflections of Fenugreek

Fenugreek nourishes where the body has been depleted. It warms, steadies, and rebuilds without urgency. Its medicine unfolds through consistency — soothing digestion, stabilizing energy, and restoring rhythm. Fenugreek reminds us that strength is often grown slowly, seed by seed.

**Herbal Confidence Index:**

(4/5 green stars — a deeply nourishing metabolic and hormonal balancer; versatile and reliable, best used mindfully and in moderation.)

# ELECAMPANE

★★★★

*Inula helenium*

**Elecampane** is a tall, golden-flowered plant famous for deep lung support. Its aromatic root is a **warming expectorant** that helps loosen stubborn, stuck mucus and restore strength when the chest feels congested, heavy, or "weak." Herbalists still reach for it for bronchitis patterns, chronic cough, and recovery after long colds. It also carries a gentle bitter edge that can wake up sluggish digestion.

The Greeks and Romans valued Elecampane in wines and tonics, and European folklore linked it to the sun—"bringing light" into damp, burdened lungs. That tradition holds up: Elecampane remains a classic respiratory builder when congestion lingers.

---

### Core Herbal Category — Elecampane

**Primary Core: Respiratory System Support** with (warming expectorant action that clears deep mucus while strengthening lung tissue)

**Secondary Cores:** Digestive Support · Immune Support · Musculoskeletal & Pain-Relief

---

### How It Works

Elecampane supports the lungs by warming and thinning thick mucus so it can move up and out more easily. Its aromatic constituents help open stuck, damp congestion while its tissue-toning action supports the bronchi as they recover from irritation. The root also contains inulin and bitter principles that improve digestive function and microbial balance—important because digestion and mucus production often track together in traditional practice. Overall, Elecampane is a "deep-clearing + rebuilding" lung herb: it clears what's lodged and strengthens what's been strained.

---

### Primary Uses

- Clears deep congestion and thick phlegm
- Supports bronchitis patterns and chronic cough
- Strengthens respiratory weakness after illness
- Calms irritated airways when mucus is heavy
- Gently stimulates appetite and digestion

---

### Scientific Backing

Elecampane contains **inulin** and sesquiterpene lactones (including **alantolactone/isoalantolactone**) associated with expectorant, antimicrobial, and anti-inflammatory effects in research. Inulin also supports beneficial gut flora. The evidence base is more traditional/preclinical than large clinical trials, but it aligns well with its long-standing use for thick mucus and post-infectious lung drag.

---

### Forms Available

- Dried root (tea/decoction)
- Syrups (often with honey)
- Tincture / liquid extract
- Powder (for decoctions)

---

### How to Use (Dosage)

- **Decoction:** ½–1 tsp dried root per cup; simmer 15 minutes; 1–2 cups daily
- **Tincture:** 1–2 mL up to 3× daily (short-term)
- **Syrup:** 1 tsp as needed for cough/congestion

---

### Expected Results

- Chest loosening/clearer cough: 1–3 days
- Mucus movement: same week
- Lung tone and stamina: 1–2 weeks
- Full rebuilding after chronic congestion: 2–4 weeks

---

### Caution Level: Caution

Generally safe in moderate amounts, but high doses may cause nausea or stomach upset. Use caution with **Asteraceae** allergies. Avoid strong dosing in pregnancy. If you're prone to very "dry" coughs with little mucus, use modestly and consider blending with moistening herbs.

---

### Gender-Specific Safety (GS)

- **Men:** Safe — excellent for thick mucus and sluggish digestion; avoid excess if sensitive stomach

- **Women:** 🟢 Safe — supportive for post-cold recovery and damp congestion; stop if nausea occurs
- **Pregnancy / Nursing:** 🟡 Caution — avoid strong tinctures/high daily doses; light tea only under guidance

---

🔄 **Same / Similar Results**
🟢 Mullein · 🟢 Thyme · 🟢 Osha Root · 🟡 Licorice Root

---

🛠 **DIY Recipe — Elecampane Honey Cough Syrup**
1 tbsp dried Elecampane root + 1 cup water
Simmer 20 minutes → strain → add ½ cup honey
Take 1 tsp for cough, mucus, or chest tightness.

---

🧴 **Shelf Life / Potency After Preparation**

- Dried root: ~2 years
- Tincture: 3–5 years
- Honey syrup: up to 6 months (refrigerated)
- Powder: ~1 year (airtight)

---

💬 **Herbal Reflections of Elecampane**
Elecampane feels like sunlight in the lungs. It doesn't just hush a cough — it **pulls the old weight up and out** and then helps the chest stand tall again. When the lungs feel damp, tired, and "stuck," Elecampane brings warmth, movement, and backbone. It's a patient worker: not flashy, just dependable—one of those roots that restores breath the way a good heater restores a cold room.
⭐ **Herbal Confidence Index:** 🌿 🌿 🌿 🌿
*(4/5 green stars — trusted deep-mucus expectorant and lung rebuilder; especially valuable for lingering congestion and winter chest weakness. Slightly intense/warming, best used in measured courses.)*

# CRANESBILL

★★★

*Geranium maculatum*

**Cranesbill** (Wild Geranium) is a deeply grounding woodland astringent prized for tightening, toning, and repairing tissues. Rich in tannins, it's traditionally used for diarrhea, irritated gut lining, minor bleeding, sore gums/throat, and for external use on wounds, weepy skin, and hemorrhoids. It's one of those "restore the boundary" herbs—excellent when tissues feel too loose, too leaky, or too inflamed.

Native American healers and early settlers relied on it as a steady astringent tonic—simple, direct, and effective. Today it remains a precision herb for flare-ups that need containment and calm.

---

### Core Herbal Category — Cranesbill

**Primary Core: Digestive System Support** with (strong astringent action that tightens, tones, and restores irritated mucosal tissues)

**Secondary Cores:** Skin & Tissue Repair · Urinary & Kidney Support · Musculoskeletal & Pain-Relief

---

### How It Works

Cranesbill works through high tannin content that binds to surface proteins and **tightens relaxed or irritated tissues**. This reduces excess fluid loss, slows minor bleeding, and calms inflamed mucosa—especially in the digestive tract during diarrhea or irritation. The same sealing, toning action helps protect skin and wound surfaces externally, supporting cleaner healing. In short: Cranesbill restores structure where tissues have become raw, leaky, or overreactive.

---

### Primary Uses

- Short-term diarrhea support; gut lining "tone"
- Minor bleeding support (situational)
- Gum/throat irritation (gargle/rinse)
- Wounds, weepy skin, hemorrhoids (external)
- Urinary/mucosal irritation (short courses)

---

### Scientific Backing

Cranesbill contains **tannins** and related compounds (including gallic-acid–type constituents) associated with astringent, antimicrobial, and anti-inflammatory effects. Evidence supports the general mechanism of mucosal tightening and reduction of secretion/bleeding typical of strong tannin herbs.

---

### Forms Available

- Dried root (tea/infusion)
- Tincture
- Capsules/powder
- External rinse/compress preparations

---

### How to Use (Dosage)

- **Infusion:** 1–2 tsp dried root per cup; steep 15–20 minutes; up to 2–3× daily (short-term)
- **Tincture:** 30–60 drops up to 2× daily
- **Powder (external):** small amount on minor cuts (clean first)
- **Gargle:** cooled tea for gums/throat

---

### Caution Level: Safe to Mild Caution

Strong tannins can cause constipation or stomach discomfort if overused. Use caution with anemia/low iron status or if you're taking anticoagulants. Best used **short-term** for flare-ups rather than daily long-term.

---

### Gender-Specific Safety

- **Men:** Safe short-term; good for GI/urinary irritation; no hormonal concerns
- **Women:** Safe short-term; may help heavy-flow patterns situationally; avoid long daily strong decoctions
- **Pregnancy / Nursing:** Caution — light tea only if needed; avoid strong daily use; external use generally fine

---

⏳ **Expected Results**

- Diarrhea/irritation: often within 1–2 doses
- Gum/throat calming: 1–3 days
- Wound/weeping skin: visible improvement in 1–3 days

---

🛠 **DIY Recipe — Soothing Mouth Rinse**

1 tsp Cranesbill root + ½ tsp Sage in 1 cup boiling water
Steep 15 minutes → strain → cool → rinse 2–3× daily.

---

🔄 **Same / Similar Results**

Agrimony · Witch Hazel · Plantain Leaf · Marshmallow Root · Slippery Elm

---

**Shelf Life / Potency After Preparation**

- Dried root: 2–3 years (airtight)
- Tincture: 4–5 years
- Powder: best within 1 year
- Prepared tea/rinse: 24 hours refrigerated
- Poultice: prepare fresh

---

## 💬 Herbal Reflections of Cranesbill

Cranesbill is a *quiet closer*. When the body feels too open—too leaky, too raw, too irritated—this herb draws a clean line and restores order. It's not a hype herb; it's a *boundary herb*. The kind you respect for doing exactly what it's supposed to do: calm the mess, seal the edges, and let the tissues recover in peace.

⭐ **Herbal Confidence Index:** 🌿 🌿 🌿 🌿

*(4/5 green stars — reliable tissue-toning astringent; excellent for short-term GI flare-ups, gum/throat irritation, and external wound support. Best used in measured courses due to strong tannins.)*

# BITTER MELON

★★★★

*Momordica charantia*

Bitter Melon — also called bitter gourd or karela — is a tropical vine used as both **food and strong metabolic medicine**, best known for helping regulate blood sugar. Its fruit (and sometimes leaf) carries compounds that support glucose handling, cool "metabolic heat," and sharpen digestion through its bitter tonic effect. In traditional systems it's a cleanser: taken in cycles to restore balance when sugar, appetite, weight, or liver sluggishness start drifting.
For centuries it has been a staple in Ayurvedic and Chinese traditions for diabetes patterns, digestion, and cleansing. Its sharp bitterness is part of the medicine: it signals the body to wake up metabolic pathways and reduce excess.

---

### 🌿 Core Herbal Category — Bitter Melon

**Primary Core:** Endocrine & Hormonal Support with (cooling, insulin-sensitizing action that supports glucose metabolism and energy balance)
**Secondary Cores:** Digestive Support · Liver & Detoxification · Immune Support · Hormonal & Endocrine Support

---

### 🌿 How It Works

Bitter Melon supports blood sugar balance by improving how cells take up and use glucose and by helping the body respond more efficiently to insulin signals. Its bitter compounds also stimulate digestive secretions, which can improve appetite regulation and metabolic rhythm after meals. The herb's cooling, anti-inflammatory tone helps reduce "metabolic heat" — the inflammatory stress that can burden the pancreas and liver during blood sugar instability. Overall, Bitter Melon acts like a metabolic reset herb: it tightens regulation, cools excess, and helps the system handle sugar with less strain.

---

### 🌱 Primary Uses

- Supports healthy blood sugar patterns
- Stimulates digestion and appetite signaling (bitter tonic)
- Supports liver function and cleansing routines
- Helps reduce inflammatory/oxidative stress load
- Used traditionally during metabolic "sluggishness" cycles

---

### Scientific Backing

Bitter Melon contains compounds such as **charantin** and **polypeptide-p**, often cited in research for hypoglycemic activity. Human studies show mixed-to-moderate benefit in type 2 diabetes patterns, with outcomes depending on preparation, dose, and duration. It also shows antioxidant and liver-supportive activity in broader research—useful context, but dosing must be conservative.

---

### Forms Available

- Fresh fruit (culinary) / dried slices
- Tea (fruit and sometimes leaf)
- Capsules/tablets (extracts)
- Tincture / liquid extract
- Fresh juice (most intense)

---

### How to Use (Dosage)

- **Tea:** 1 tsp dried fruit/leaf simmered 10–15 minutes; 1 cup daily (cycle use)
- **Capsules/Tablets:** 500–1000 mg daily (follow label; start low)
- **Juice:** 1–2 oz fresh juice daily (strong—use caution)
- **Culinary:** sauté/steam; salt soak reduces bitterness

---

### Expected Results

- Blood sugar effect: within hours to a few days (monitor)
- Appetite/digestive signaling: 30–60 minutes
- Metabolic "trend" improvement: 1–2 weeks (with diet consistency)

---

### Caution Level: Caution

- Can significantly lower blood sugar—use caution with insulin or diabetes meds
- Avoid in pregnancy (uterine stimulation/hypoglycemia risk)

- Not recommended while breastfeeding (bitter compounds; limited data)
- High doses may cause GI upset/diarrhea
- Best used **in cycles**, not endlessly

---

**Gender-Specific Safety (GS)**

- **Men:** Caution — helpful for metabolic regulation; avoid excess or if prone to low blood sugar / on meds
- **Women:** Caution — supports metabolic balance and skin clarity; avoid high doses if hypoglycemic
- **Pregnancy / Nursing:** Avoid — pregnancy contraindicated; nursing not recommended

---

**Same / Similar Results**

Gymnema · Berberine herbs (Oregon Grape/Barberry) · Cinnamon · Dandelion Root · Fenugreek

---

**DIY Recipe — Metabolic Bitter Tea**

Blend Bitter Melon + Dandelion Root + Ceylon Cinnamon (1 tsp total).
Steep 10–12 minutes. Drink before meals for digestion + blood-sugar support.

---

**Shelf Life / Potency After Preparation**

- Dried fruit/leaf: 1–2 years (airtight)
- Capsules/Tablets: 2–3 years (check expiration)
- Tincture/Extract: 4–5 years (cool, dark)
- Fresh juice: 24 hours refrigerated
- Prepared tea: 12–24 hours refrigerated

---

**Herbal Reflections of Bitter Melon**

Bitter Melon has swagger — the kind that doesn't smile first. It's blunt medicine with a clear message: **get your balance back.** Where sweeter herbs persuade, Bitter Melon corrects. It's the tough coach of the metabolic world—effective, honest, and best respected in short, disciplined rounds. If you can handle the bitterness, it rewards you with clarity.

🌟 **Herbal Confidence Index:** 🌿 🌿 🌿 🌿

*(4/5 green stars — potent metabolic regulator with strong traditional use and real modern interest; highly effective when used wisely, but its glucose-lowering strength demands careful dosing and monitoring.)*

# EYEBRIGHT

★★★★

*Euphrasia officinalis*

**Eyebright** is a gentle astringent herb that soothes irritated eyes while calming allergy-driven congestion in the sinuses, nose, and throat. It restores balance to overactive mucous membranes, making it especially useful for itchy, watery eyes, hay fever, post-nasal drip, and eye strain caused by pollen or screens.

What distinguishes Eyebright is its precision — it works simultaneously on ocular and upper-respiratory tissues, offering focused relief without sedation. Mild yet effective, it is best suited for short-term, situational use when clarity and comfort are needed.

---

## 🌿 Core Herbal Category — Eyebright

**Primary Core: Respiratory System Support herb** with *(upper-respiratory and ocular astringent action that tones inflamed mucous membranes)*

**Secondary Cores:** Skin & Tissue Repair herb · Immune Support herb · Circulatory & Cardiovascular herb

---

## 🌿 How It Works

Eyebright works by tightening and toning irritated mucous membranes, particularly in the eyes, sinuses, and upper respiratory tract. Its astringent compounds help reduce excess discharge and calm inflammation, improving clarity and comfort. By stabilizing capillary integrity, it supports healthy circulation to delicate eye tissues. Its immune-modulating action helps ease allergy-driven irritation. Overall, Eyebright acts as a precision herb for restoring tone and clarity to sensitive respiratory and eye tissues.

---

## 🌱 Primary Uses

- Supports eye clarity; soothes itchy, watery eyes
- Relieves sinus pressure, congestion, and post-nasal drip
- Helps with seasonal allergies / hay fever
- Calms inflamed mucous membranes (eyes, nose, throat)

---

## Scientific Backing

Eyebright contains aucubin, tannins, and flavonoids that contribute to its anti-inflammatory and astringent actions. Preliminary research suggests benefit in allergic conjunctivitis, eye strain, and allergic rhinitis. Antioxidant glycosides help support capillary strength and mucosal comfort.

---

## Forms Available

- Dried herb (tea)
- Tinctures and liquid extracts
- Sterile commercial eyewash formulas

---

## How to Use (Dosage)

- Tea: 1–2 tsp dried herb per cup boiling water; steep 10 minutes, strain
- Tincture: 1–2 mL (30–40 drops) up to 3× daily
- Eyewash: Only use professionally prepared sterile solutions — *never homemade for direct eye application*

---

## Caution Level: Safe to Caution (Mild)

General: Gentle and appropriate for most people as tea or diluted tincture.

Eye Use: Only use sterile, commercial eyewash formulas.

Avoid use with contact lenses, after recent eye surgery, or during active eye infection unless guided by a professional.

Pregnancy / Nursing: Mild tea may be acceptable; avoid strong tinctures due to limited systemic data.

---

## Gender-Specific Safety

- **Men:** Safe and effective for eye strain, sinus issues, and seasonal allergies. No hormonal concerns.
- **Women:** Helpful for eye fatigue, sinus congestion, and puffiness around the eyes due to mild astringency. Safe in tea or diluted tincture form.
- **Pregnancy / Nursing:** Mild tea or sterile eyewash likely safe. Avoid internal tinctures or

concentrated extracts.

---

### ⏳ Expected Results

- Eye comfort & reduced irritation: 1–3 days
- Allergy / sinus relief: ~1 week
- Mucous membrane soothing: 5–7 days with consistent use

---

### 🛠 DIY Recipe — Eye-Soothing Compress

1 tsp Eyebright + ½ tsp Chamomile
Steep in 1 cup boiling water for 10 minutes
Strain thoroughly and cool completely
Soak a clean cloth and place over closed eyes for 10–15 minutes

---

### 🔄 Same / Similar Results

**Bilberry · Goji Berry · Chamomile · Nettle Leaf · Goldenseal**

---

### ⏳ Shelf Life / Potency After Preparation

- Tincture: 3–5 years in cool, dark storage
- Dried herb / tea: 1–2 years before potency declines
- Sterile eyewash: Use before expiration; discard within 30 days after opening
- Prepared tea: Use within 12–24 hours refrigerated

---

### 💬 Herbal Reflections of Eyebright

Eyebright lives up to its name — a herb of clarity, precision, and renewal. It works quietly and specifically, restoring comfort without dulling the senses. Acting like a gentle lens-cleaner for the body, it clears irritation and brings lightness where strain once lingered.

Its strength lies in restraint: Eyebright dries what is excessive, calms what is inflamed, and restores balance without force. For moments when vision — physical or perceptual — feels clouded, Eyebright offers steady, focused relief.

---

**Herbal Confidence Index:** 🌿🌿🌿🌿🌿 ***(5 / 5 green stars** — cornerstone eye and sinus-support herb; precise, reliable, and well-tolerated, honored for centuries for its gentle yet effective relief.)*

# GINKGO BILOBA

★★★★★

***Ginkgo biloba***

**Ginkgo Biloba** is a circulatory and cognitive-support herb used to enhance memory, focus, and blood flow to the brain and extremities. It is especially valued for supporting mental clarity under cognitive load, easing tinnitus and vertigo, and warming cold hands and feet through improved microcirculation.

Rather than acting as a stimulant, Ginkgo supports steady neurological performance by improving oxygen and nutrient delivery to nerve tissue. Its benefits develop gradually, making it best suited for consistent, medium- to long-term use.

As one of the oldest living tree species on Earth, Ginkgo has endured for over 200 million years and was revered in Chinese temple gardens as a symbol of longevity and resilience. Modern clinical research has reinforced this legacy, placing Ginkgo among the most extensively studied botanicals for cognitive and vascular health.

---

### Core Herbal Category — Ginkgo Biloba

**Primary Core: Cardiovascular System Support** herb with *(microcirculatory-enhancing action that improves blood flow to the brain and peripheral tissues)*

**Secondary Cores:** Nervines (Nervous System Support) herb · Immune Support herb · Nutritive & Restorative herb

---

### How It Works

Ginkgo Biloba works by improving microcirculation, particularly to the brain, enhancing oxygen and nutrient delivery to nerve tissues. Its flavonoids and terpene lactones protect neurons and blood vessels from oxidative stress, supporting cognitive clarity and memory retention. By strengthening vascular tone and capillary integrity, Ginkgo supports sensory processing, balance, and peripheral circulation. Overall, it functions as a circulatory intelligence herb that sustains brain and nerve vitality over time.

---

### Primary Uses

- Supports memory, concentration, and mental alertness

- Assists with age-related cognitive decline
- Improves circulation to brain, hands, and feet
- Helps tinnitus, vertigo, and sensory imbalance
- Provides antioxidant protection for neurons

---

**Scientific Backing**

Ginkgo contains flavone glycosides and terpene lactones shown to enhance cerebral blood flow and provide neuroprotective effects. Large-scale reviews, including Cochrane analyses, support its benefit for cognition and peripheral circulation when standardized extracts are used.

---

**Forms Available**

- Standardized capsules or tablets
- Tinctures and liquid extracts
- Dried leaf (tea form)

---

**Caution Level:** Caution

- May thin blood — avoid combining with anticoagulants or antiplatelet medications unless supervised
- Discontinue 5–7 days before surgery
- Possible mild headache, nausea, or dizziness when initiating use
- Avoid during pregnancy and breastfeeding due to limited safety data
- Avoid strong extracts if seizure disorder or epilepsy is present

---

**Gender-Specific Safety**

- **Men:** Supports circulation, memory, and cognitive stamina. Safe for moderate long-term use with medication awareness.

- **Women:** Helpful for brain fog, circulation, and menopausal cognitive dips. Pause before surgery or when using blood thinners.
- **Pregnancy / Nursing:** Avoid concentrated supplements; not recommended near delivery or during heavy menstrual flow.

---

**Expected Results**

- Mental clarity & circulation support: **1–2 weeks**
- Cognitive & memory improvement: **4–6 weeks**
- Tinnitus / vertigo relief: **4–8 weeks**
- Peripheral warmth (hands, feet): **3–5 weeks**

Ginkgo works cumulatively — slow, steady improvement through enhanced circulation.

---

**DIY Recipe — Brain-Boost Tea**

1 tsp Ginkgo
1 tsp Gotu Kola
½ tsp Rosemary
Steep 10 minutes; drink mid-morning.

---

**Same / Similar Results**

Gotu Kola · Bacopa · Rhodiola · Rosemary · Ashwagandha

---

**Shelf Life / Potency After Preparation**

- Tincture: 4–5 years (cool, dark storage)
- Dried leaf / tea: 1–2 years
- Capsules/tablets: 2–3 years

- ☕☕ Prepared tea: Use within 12–24 hours refrigerated

---

💭 **Herbal Reflections of Ginkgo Biloba**

Ginkgo is the herb of endurance and flow. It strengthens by restoring movement — of blood, oxygen, and thought — rather than forcing stimulation. Its medicine unfolds slowly, sharpening awareness while supporting warmth and vitality throughout the body.

For those feeling mentally taxed, forgetful, or dulled by time, Ginkgo offers renewal through consistency. Like its ancient leaves, its power lies not in urgency, but in patience.

---

⭐ **Herbal Confidence Index:** 🌿 🌿 🌿 🌿 🌿

*(5 / 5 green stars — cornerstone circulatory and cognitive herb; exceptionally well-studied and effective for improving memory, focus, and vascular health with long-term reliability.)*

# CORIANDER

★★★

*Coriandrum sativum*

**Coriander** is a gentle digestive-support herb used to relieve gas, bloating, and digestive stagnation while supporting mild detoxification. Its aromatic seeds stimulate digestive enzymes, calm cramping, and assist balanced blood sugar and cholesterol patterns.
Distinct from harsher digestive stimulants, Coriander cools excess heat without weakening digestion, making it especially useful after heavy meals or during cleansing phases.
With more than 3,000 years of use across the Mediterranean, Middle East, and South Asia, Coriander has long bridged kitchen and clinic. Ancient physicians praised it for "sweetening the belly," and modern use continues to explore its supportive role in metabolic balance and gentle detoxification.

---

### Core Herbal Category — Coriander

**Primary Core: Digestive System Support herb** with *(aromatic carminative action that relieves gas, supports digestion, and restores digestive comfort)*
**Secondary Cores:** Liver & Detoxification herb · Metabolic & Blood Sugar Support herb · Immune Support herb · Nutritive & Restorative herb

---

### How It Works

Coriander works by gently stimulating digestive activity while calming spasms and gas, improving digestive efficiency. Its aromatic compounds reduce inflammation and stagnation, easing discomfort after meals. Coriander also supports liver detoxification pathways, assisting metabolic waste clearance and contributing to balanced blood sugar and lipid metabolism. Overall, it functions as a food-grade medicinal herb that restores digestive and metabolic harmony.

---

### Primary Uses

- Relieves bloating, gas, and indigestion
- Supports gentle detoxification

- Assists blood sugar and cholesterol balance
- Provides mild liver and anti-inflammatory support

---

### 📊 Scientific Backing

Coriander's linalool-rich essential oils support GI motility and digestive comfort. Studies suggest glycemic and lipid improvements, antioxidant activity, and possible metal-binding support in detox protocols.

---

### Forms Available

- Whole or ground seeds
- Powdered spice
- Tinctures and fluid extracts

---

### ⚙ How to Use

- **Tea:** 1 tsp crushed seeds per cup hot water; steep 10–15 minutes
- **Tincture:** 1–2 mL up to 3× daily before meals
- **Culinary:** Add seeds to meals; chewing after eating aids digestion
- **Topical:** Diluted essential oil only — never undiluted

---

### ⚠ Caution Level: Safe to Caution (Mild)

- Safe in culinary amounts and mild tea
- Strong tinctures or essential oil may cause mild digestive upset
- May slightly lower blood pressure — use caution if hypotensive
- Never apply undiluted essential oil
- Pregnancy / Nursing: Culinary use acceptable; avoid therapeutic doses

### Gender-Specific Safety

- **Men:** Eases gas and digestive tension; supports gentle detox and metabolic balance.
- **Women:** Helps bloating, fluid retention, and hormone-related digestive discomfort.
- **Pregnancy / Nursing:** Safe in food and mild tea; avoid tinctures and essential oil.

### Expected Results

- Digestive relief: **30–60 minutes**
- Detoxification support: **1–2 weeks**
- Blood sugar / lipid support: **days to weeks**

### DIY Recipe — Coriander Digestive Tea

1 tsp crushed Coriander seeds
½ tsp Fennel
¼ tsp Cumin
Steep 10 minutes; sip after meals.

### Same / Similar Results

Fennel · Cilantro Leaf · Cumin · Dandelion Root · Milk Thistle

### Shelf Life / Potency After Preparation

- Whole seeds: 2–3 years
- Ground powder: Best within 1 year
- Tincture: 3–5 years

- Essential oil: 2–3 years unopened or refrigerated

---

💭 **Herbal Reflections of Coriander**

Coriander is the quiet harmonizer. It restores flow where digestion feels heavy and calms excess without force. Its medicine is subtle, fragrant, and steady — easing discomfort while reestablishing balance.

Though modest in strength, Coriander's value lies in refinement. It reminds us that gentle corrections often sustain the body better than dramatic interventions.

---

🌟 **Herbal Confidence Index:** 🌿 🌿 🌿

*(3 / 5 green stars — reliable and safe digestive and detox-support herb; best used as a supportive ally alongside stronger therapeutic herbs.)*

# BLACK WALNUT HULL

★★★★

*Juglans nigra*

**Black Walnut Hull** is a powerful cleansing herb traditionally used to address intestinal parasites, fungal overgrowth, and stubborn microbial imbalance. Rich in juglone and tannins, it acts decisively—clearing unwanted organisms while tightening and toning tissues that have become overly permissive to invasion. Because of its strength, Black Walnut Hull is best reserved for **short, intentional protocols**, not continuous or casual use.

Applied externally, it has long been respected for persistent fungal conditions such as ringworm, where its antimicrobial action helps restore balance to compromised skin. Internally or externally, its value lies in precision rather than duration.

A mainstay of Indigenous and early American herbal medicine, the green hulls of Black Walnut earned a reputation as a serious cleanser. Traditionally used for intestinal worms, candida patterns, and fungal skin or oral issues, it was often paired with Wormwood and Clove in classic parasite-clearing formulas. Its enduring place in herbalism reflects both its effectiveness **and** the discipline required to use it responsibly.

---

**Core Herbal Category — Black Walnut Hull**

**Primary Core: Antimicrobial Support** herb with (juglone-driven action that disrupts parasitic and fungal overgrowth and limits pathogenic environments)

**Secondary Cores:** Digestive Support herb · Liver & Detoxification herb · Skin & Tissue Repair herb

---

### *How It Works*

Black Walnut Hull works by interfering with the metabolic activity of parasites, fungi, and certain microbes. Its juglone content creates an inhospitable environment for overgrowth, while its high tannin content tightens and tones intestinal tissues, reducing conditions that favor infestation. This dual antimicrobial and astringent action supports digestive cleansing and assists liver detoxification pathways. When applied topically, the same properties helprestore balance to fungal-affected skin. Overall, Black Walnut Hull functions as a

**precision cleanser** for pathogen-driven imbalance.

---

### 🌱 Primary Uses

• Intestinal parasites and worms (short-term protocols only)
• Antifungal support (candida patterns, ringworm, stubborn skin fungi)
• Digestive cleansing and microbial rebalancing
• Oral and topical cleansing applications

---

### Scientific Backing

Black Walnut Hull contains juglone, a naphthoquinone compound shown to disrupt parasitic and fungal metabolism. Its tannins contribute strong astringent, antimicrobial, and tissue-toning effects. Both traditional use and modern herbal research support its role as an antiparasitic and antifungal agent when used briefly and deliberately.

---

### Forms Available

• Liquid tincture or extract
• Dried hull powder or capsules
• Topical tincture washes or salves

---

### How to Use (Dosage & Method)

**Internal Use — Short-Term Only:**
• Tincture: 15–20 drops in water, 1–2× daily for **no more than 2–3 weeks**
• Powder/Capsules: Follow label dosing within guided cleansing cycles
**Topical Use:**
• Diluted tincture applied with a cotton swab to fungal skin areas
• Avoid broken, inflamed, or highly sensitive skin
**Traditional Parasite Protocol:**
• Commonly paired with Wormwood and Clove
• Always used in **cycles with rest periods**, never continuously

---

### ⚠️ Caution Level: Caution

• Potent herb — prolonged or excessive use may irritate the gastrointestinal lining
• Use **only in short cycles** to avoid microbiome disruption
• Avoid with nut allergies, active liver disease, thyroid disorders, or chronic GI inflammation

• Topical use may temporarily stain skin
• 🔴 **Avoid entirely during pregnancy and breastfeeding**

---

### 🚹 🚺 Gender-Specific Safety (GS)

**Men:** 🟡 Caution — Effective for short-term cleansing and fungal issues; avoid extended use.
**Women:** 🟡 Caution — Useful for candida or fungal imbalance in **7–14 day cycles only**; avoid with hormone-sensitive conditions unless professionally guided.
**Pregnancy / Nursing:** 🔴 Avoid — Do not use internally; topical use only under professional supervision.

---

### ⏳ Expected Results

• Parasite reduction: 3–7 days
• Digestive relief and microbial balance: 1–2 weeks
• Fungal skin improvement: 2–3 weeks
• Full protocol effect: 2–3 weeks on, followed by a rest period

---

### 🛠 DIY Preparation — Traditional Anti-Parasite Tonic

(Short-term use only)
• 20 drops Black Walnut tincture
• 10 drops Wormwood tincture
• 5 drops Clove tincture
Dilute in water and take 2× daily for **up to 14 days** only.
🔄 **Same / Similar Results** 🟢 Wormwood · 🟢 Clove · 🟢 Neem Leaf · 🟢 Oregano Oil · 🟢 Garlic

---

### 🧴 Shelf Life / Potency After Preparation

• Tincture: 4–6 years
• Powder/Capsules: Best within 2 years
• Topical preparations: 2–3 years if properly stored and uncontaminated

---

### 🌙 Herbal Reflections of Black Walnut Hull

Black Walnut Hull is the herb of boundaries. It clears what does not belong and reinforces the body's internal lines of defense. Firm, dark, and uncompromising, it restores order where invasion has taken hold.
Its medicine demands respect—used briefly, deliberately, and with purpose. In that discipline lies its power: not continuous force, but a decisive reset that leaves clarity and

balance in its wake.

⭐ **Herbal Confidence Index:** 🌿 🌿 🌿 🌿 (4 / 5 green stars — a powerful antiparasitic and antifungal herb, highly effective when used in short, controlled cycles with proper caution and rest periods.)

# OREGANO OIL

★★★★

*Origanum vulgare*

**Oregano Oil** is a high-potency antimicrobial used for acute bacterial, viral, and fungal infections. Concentrated in carvacrol and thymol, it acts quickly by disrupting microbial cell membranes, making it most appropriate for short, targeted use rather than long-term supplementation.

Because of its intensity, Oregano Oil is reserved for situations where gentler herbs are insufficient and must always be diluted and cycled carefully.

Rooted in Mediterranean herbal tradition, oregano served kitchens and sickrooms alike—used for respiratory illness, digestive upset, and food preservation. Modern distillation intensified its power, increasing effectiveness while requiring greater discipline in dosing. It remains a go-to remedy when swift antimicrobial action is needed.

---

### Core Herbal Category — Oregano Oil

**Primary Core: Immune System Support herb** with *(high-potency antimicrobial action that suppresses pathogenic bacteria, fungi, and viruses)*

**Secondary Cores:** Respiratory Support herb · Digestive Support herb · Skin & Tissue Repair herb

---

### How It Works

Oregano Oil works by rapidly disrupting pathogenic microorganisms, puncturing microbial membranes and inhibiting replication. This action supports immune control during acute infection. In the respiratory system, it assists airway defense and microbial clearance. In the digestive tract, it helps rebalance dysbiosis when used briefly. Externally, proper dilution allows it to restore healthy skin microbial balance.

---

### Primary Uses

- Acute bacterial, viral, and fungal infections
- Colds, flu, bronchitis, and sinus congestion

- Digestive imbalance and microbial overgrowth
- Topical support for ringworm and fungal rashes

---

📊 **Scientific Backing**

Oregano Oil is rich in carvacrol and thymol, phenolic compounds shown to damage microbial cell membranes. Research supports activity against Candida, resistant bacteria (including MRSA), and respiratory pathogens, alongside antioxidant and anti-inflammatory effects.

---

💉 **Forms Available**

- Essential oil (must be diluted)
- Pre-diluted capsules or softgels
- Topical salves, sprays, and blends

⚙ **How to Use**

**Internal (Diluted & Short-Term Only):**

- Essential oil: 2–4 drops diluted in 1 tsp carrier oil
- Capsules: Follow label dosing, typically 1–2 daily for 7–10 days

**Topical (Always Diluted):**

- 1–2 drops essential oil in 1 tsp carrier oil
- Apply 1–2× daily to fungal areas

**Inhalation:**

- 1–2 drops in steaming water
- Inhale vapor for sinus and lung support

---

⚠ **Caution Level:** ⚪ Caution

- Must always be diluted

- High doses may irritate stomach or disrupt gut flora
- Avoid during pregnancy and breastfeeding
- May interact with thyroid medication or iron absorption
- Long-term use may reduce beneficial microbes

---

### Gender-Specific Safety

- **Men:** Effective for acute infections; avoid prolonged use.
- **Women:** Useful for yeast and sinus infections; keep cycles short.
- **Pregnancy / Nursing:** Avoid completely.

---

### Expected Results

- Infection relief: **2–5 days**
- Respiratory clarity: **3–7 days**
- Yeast/digestive balance: **1–2 weeks**

---

### DIY Recipe — Oregano Immune Guard

- 2 drops Oregano essential oil
- 1 tsp olive oil
  Take once daily for up to 7 days.

---

### Same / Similar Results

Thyme Oil · Garlic · Olive Leaf · Echinacea · Black Walnut Hull

---

### Shelf Life / Potency After Preparation

- Essential oil (undiluted): 3–5 years

- Capsules/Softgels: 2–3 years
- Topical blends: 12–18 months

---

**Herbal Reflections of Oregano Oil**

Oregano Oil is fire with purpose. It burns through stagnation, clears infection, and restores strength where the body has been overrun. Its medicine is bold, fast, and unmistakable.

Yet its true lesson is restraint. Used briefly and wisely, it heals decisively. Used carelessly, it overwhelms. In Oregano Oil, power and discipline walk hand in hand.

**Herbal Confidence Index:**

*(4 / 5 green stars — potent natural antimicrobial; highly effective for acute infections, requiring strict dilution and short-term use.)*

# SLIPPERY ELM

★★★★★

*Ulmus rubra*

**Slippery Elm** (*Ulmus rubra*) is one of nature's most comforting healers — a soft, soothing balm for the body's most delicate linings. **Harvested from the inner bark of the red elm tree, it forms a gentle mucilage that coats, protects, and restores irritated tissues from throat to intestine.** Revered by Native American healers and early physicians alike, **Slippery Elm was used for wounds, sore throats, ulcers, and recovery after illness, offering nourishment as much as relief. Its mild, food-like nature makes it safe for children, elders, and those weakened by chronic conditions.**

**When blended with warm water, its powdered bark transforms into a silky tonic that calms inflammation, eases reflux, and rebuilds strength from within** — a reminder that true healing often begins with comfort and care.

---

## Core Herbal Category — Slippery Elm

**Primary Core: Digestive System Support herb** with (mucilaginous demulcent action that coats, soothes, and protects irritated digestive tissues)

**Secondary Cores:** Respiratory Support herb · Skin & Tissue Repair herb · Immune Support herb

---

## How It Works

Slippery Elm works by **forming a soothing mucilage that coats inflamed or irritated tissues**, protecting them from further irritation. In the digestive tract, this action **calms inflammation and supports healing of the gut lining**. When used for the throat and lungs, it **soothes dry, irritated mucous membranes**, easing cough and discomfort. Its protective coating helps reduce **inflammatory stress**, allowing tissues to repair more efficiently. Overall, Slippery Elm acts as a **gentle, deeply soothing tissue-protective herb**.

---

### Primary Uses

- Soothes sore throats and dry coughs
- Calms acid reflux, gastritis, and ulcers

• Protects mucous membranes of throat, gut, and urinary tract
• Aids recovery during illness, weakness, or convalescence
• Used as a poultice for wounds and inflamed skin

---

## Scientific Backing

Slippery Elm's mucilage polysaccharides form a protective gel over irritated tissues. Studies in Pharmacognosy Reviews confirm its benefits for GERD, sore throat, and IBD. It offers both symptom relief and regenerative effects and has shown to support tissue healing in inflamed mucosal linings.
Note: Slippery Elm may reduce medication absorption — separate by at least 2 hours.

---

## *Forms Available*

• Powder (most versatile)
• Capsules
• Tea bags
• Lozenges
• Salves or tinctures for external use

---

## *How to Use*

**Tea / Infusion:** Mix 1 tsp powdered bark into warm (not boiling) water; stir until smooth. Drink 1–3× daily for throat or digestive support
**Capsules:** 400–500 mg, 2–3× daily
**Lozenges:** Use as needed for cough or sore throat
**Poultice:** Combine powder with warm water to create a paste; apply to wounds, burns, or inflamed skin

---

## ⚠ Caution Level: Safe to Caution (Mild)

Widely regarded as gentle, safe, and soothing when mixed with water.
Take at least 1–2 hours apart from medications or supplements to avoid delayed absorption.
Use only the **inner bark** — outer bark may irritate or cause nausea.
**Pregnancy/Nursing:** Generally safe, but should be discussed with a professional due to limited clinical studies.
Always mix powder with sufficient liquid to prevent throat irritation.

---

## Gender-Specific Safety

**Men:** Excellent for acid reflux, sore throats, and gut inflammation. Safe for long-term use due to food-like nature. Ideal for soothing damage after digestive flare-ups or during stress.
**Women:** Supports digestive comfort and mucosal protection. Helpful during stress-related

stomach upset or during convalescence. Safe during menstruation; may assist with mild nausea relief.

⚪ **Pregnancy / Nursing:** Slippery Elm is widely used in food-like doses for sore throats and reflux during pregnancy. However, due to a lack of extensive modern research, internal use during pregnancy should be discussed with a qualified professional. Always avoid dehydrated powder without liquid.

---

## *Expected Results*

• Throat and cough relief: **within 30 minutes**
• Digestive healing: **1–3 weeks** of regular use
• Skin soothing (poultice): **hours to days**

---

## DIY Recipe — Slippery Elm Soothing Digestive Drink

Mix together:
• 1 tsp Slippery Elm powder
• ½ tsp Cinnamon
• 1 tsp Honey
Add to warm water until smooth. Sip slowly after meals or at bedtime for digestive or throat relief.

---

## Same/Similar Results

- Marshmallow Root
- Licorice Root
- Aloe Vera (inner gel)
- Plantain Leaf
- Mullein Leaf

---

## Shelf Life / Potency After Preparation

- **Powdered Bark:** 1–2 years in airtight container, stored in cool, dark place
- **Capsules:** 2–3 years (check label for expiry)
- **Lozenges/Teas:** 18–24 months sealed
- **Mixed Slurry:** Use within 24 hours or refrigerate up to 48 hours

---

## 💬 Herbal Reflections of Slippery Elm

Slippery Elm is gentle strength embodied. Unlike harsh remedies, it nurtures and heals with its protective mucilage, restoring tissues while providing nourishment. For sore throats, ulcers, or recovery after illness, it offers comfort that feels like a warm blanket for the body.
Its softness belies its power: many herbalists rank it alongside Marshmallow and Licorice as part of the "holy trinity" of mucosal healers. Its versatility, safety, and soothing touch make it indispensable in any herbal medicine cabinet, especially in times of weakness, illness, or stress.

---

## ★ Herbal Confidence Index: 🌿 🌿 🌿 🌿 🌿

(5/5 green stars — **cornerstone demulcent and nutritive digestive-healing herb**; exceptionally safe and effective for soothing sore throats, ulcers, and irritated tissues, restoring comfort and strength to the entire digestive tract with gentle, nourishing relief.)

# *LEMON BALM*

★★★★★

*Melissa officinalis*

**Lemon Balm** is one of the most trusted calming herbs in Western herbal medicine, prized for its ability to gently soothe the nervous system while simultaneously supporting digestion, mood, and immune balance. A member of the mint family with a soft lemon scent, it has been used for centuries to ease anxiety, lift melancholy, calm digestive discomfort, and support restful sleep. Unlike stronger sedatives, Lemon Balm works by **settling the nervous system without dulling the mind**. It is equally valued for emotional tension, stress-related digestive upset, and immune weakness linked to exhaustion. Its gentle yet broad action makes it one of the most versatile and widely applicable herbs in the book.

---

## *Core Herbal Category — Lemon Balm*

**Primary Core: Nervous System Support (Nervines) (Nervous System Support) herb** with (calming, uplifting action that soothes the nerves while restoring emotional balance)
**Secondary Cores:** Digestive Support herb · Immune Support herb · Hormonal & Endocrine Support herb · Respiratory Support herb

---

## *How It Works*

Lemon Balm works by gently calming nervous system overactivity, easing anxiety, restlessness, and emotional tension. Its aromatic compounds help lift mood while relaxing digestive stress, especially when emotions disrupt digestion. This calming influence supports sleep readiness by quieting mental overstimulation. Lemon Balm also supports immune resilience, particularly during stress-related depletion. Overall, it acts as a nervous-system harmonizer that restores calm, clarity, and rhythmic balance.

---

### *Primary Uses*

- Calms anxiety, nervous tension, and restlessness
- Eases stress-related digestive upset and cramping
- Supports mood balance and emotional resilience
- Promotes relaxation and sleep readiness
- Supports immune health during stress or exhaustion

---

### Scientific Backing

Lemon Balm contains rosmarinic acid, flavonoids, polyphenols, and volatile oils that contribute to its calming, antiviral, and digestive-supportive effects. Research published in Phytomedicine, Journal of Ethnopharmacology, and Nutrients indicates Lemon Balm may:

- Reduce anxiety and nervous agitation
- Improve sleep quality and relaxation
- Calm digestive spasms and bloating
- Support immune response during viral stress
- Improve cognitive calm without sedation

Clinical studies support its traditional use for stress-related symptoms, mild insomnia, digestive discomfort, and nervous system regulation.

### Forms Available

- Fresh or dried leaf
- Tea / infusion
- Tincture / liquid extract
- Capsules or powdered leaf
- Topical balm (for stress or cold sores)

### How to Use (Dosage & Methods)

**Tea / Infusion**

Steep 1–2 teaspoons dried leaf in hot water for 10–15 minutes.
Drink 1–3× daily for calm or digestion.

**Tincture**

1–2 mL up to 3× daily for stress, anxiety, or digestive tension.

**Capsules**

400–600 mg once or twice daily.

### Caution Level — Safe

- Extremely gentle and well tolerated
- Safe for long-term use
- May slightly reduce thyroid activity at very high doses (use moderately if hypothyroid)

### Gender-Specific Safety

**Men:**

Supports stress resilience, digestive calm, and emotional balance without sedation.

**Women:**

Highly supportive for anxiety, mood shifts, stress-related digestion, and sleep readiness.

**Pregnancy / Nursing:**
Generally regarded as safe in tea and moderate tincture doses.

---

**Expected Results**
- Calming effect: 30–60 minutes
- Digestive relief: 1–3 days
- Sleep readiness: 3–7 days
- Emotional balance: 1–2 weeks

---

**DIY Recipe — Lemon Balm Calm Tea**
- 1 tsp Lemon Balm
- ½ tsp Chamomile
- ½ tsp Peppermint

Steep 10–15 minutes; drink in the evening or during stress.

---

**Same / Similar Results**
Chamomile · Passionflower · Lavender · Skullcap · Peppermint Lavender

---

**Shelf Life / Potency After Preparation**
- Dried leaf: 1–2 years
- Tincture: 3–5 years
- Prepared tea: 24 hours refrigerated
- Fresh leaf: use within several days refrigerated

---

**Herbal Reflections of Lemon Balm**
Lemon Balm carries a quiet intelligence — it does not overpower, sedate, or force change. Instead, it reminds the body how to return to calm on its own terms. In times of emotional overload, digestive distress, or nervous exhaustion, it offers reassurance rather than suppression.
Its gentle presence across so many systems speaks to its role as a true balancing herb. Lemon Balm teaches that healing does not always come through strength — sometimes it comes through softness, consistency, and care.

---

**Herbal Confidence Index**
(5/5 green stars — cornerstone calming herb; exceptionally safe, broadly effective, and indispensable for nervous system, digestive, and stress-related support.)

# EUROPEAN MISTLETOE

★★★

*Viscum album*

**European Mistletoe** is a specialized cardiovascular and nervous-system balancing herb used to support blood-pressure rhythm, vascular tone, and stress-driven tension patterns. It does not "push" the system like a stimulant; instead, it is known for regulatory, calming influence—best suited for carefully guided use in properly prepared forms only.

Because the raw plant (especially berries) can be toxic and dosing precision matters, European Mistletoe belongs in the category of **professional-supervision herbs**, not casual home experimentation.

Long revered in European folk medicine—and famously honored by ancient Druids as sacred—Mistletoe has remained a plant of paradox: revered for deep balancing effects, yet respected for its narrow safe range. In modern Europe, standardized preparations have also been used in supervised settings within integrative medical traditions. Its story, across centuries, is one of **precision, restraint, and respect**.

---

### Core Herbal Category — European Mistletoe

**Primary Core: Cardiovascular System Support** herb with *(regulatory action that supports balanced blood pressure and vascular tone without overstimulation)*

**Secondary Cores:** Nervines (Nervous System Support) herb · Immune Support herb · Musculoskeletal & Pain-Relief herb

---

### How It Works

European Mistletoe works by gently influencing vascular tone and cardiovascular rhythm, helping the body trend toward balance rather than forcing constriction or dilation. Its calming constituents also reduce stress-driven nervous-system overactivity, which can contribute to cardiovascular strain. Through this nervous–vascular coordination, it supports steadier circulation and a calmer "pressure response." Additionally, it may influence immune signaling, which can help reduce systemic stress load. Overall, it functions as a **regulatory, balancing herb** whose benefits depend on **correct preparation and careful dosing**.

### 🌱 Primary Uses

- Supports balanced blood pressure patterns (guided use only)
- Helps calm stress-related cardiovascular tension
- Supports nervous-system settling and sleep rhythm (in supervised protocols)
- Used in specialized, supervised European preparations for immune balance

---

### Scientific Backing

European Mistletoe contains lectins, viscotoxins, flavonoids, and polysaccharides that have been studied for effects on immune signaling and cardiovascular regulation. In some European integrative-care contexts, **standardized mistletoe extracts** are used under clinical supervision, primarily to support wellbeing and symptom burden in complex cases. These applications are **not** interchangeable with home use, and self-preparation is not considered safe due to variability and toxicity risk.

---

### Forms Available

- Dried herb for **cold infusion only** (guided use)
- Standardized oral extracts (professional-grade)
- Injectable extracts (clinical settings only; region-dependent)

---

### How to Use (Dosage & Methods)

**Cold Infusion (Traditional Method — Not Hot Tea):**

- 1 tsp dried herb in 1 cup cool water
- Steep 8–12 hours (overnight), strain
- Sip **once daily** only under guidance

**Tincture / Extract:**

- Use **only** professional-standard products
- Dose varies widely by preparation and case—must be guided

❌ **Never** self-prepare from fresh plant.
❌ **Never** ingest berries.
❌ **Never** use "wild harvested" homemade extracts.

---

⚠️ **Caution Level:** 🔴 Supervision Required

- Raw plant (especially berries) can be toxic
- Avoid during pregnancy and breastfeeding
- May interact with blood-pressure medications, cardiac medications, immune therapies
- Use only properly prepared standardized products or guided cold infusion

---

🚹 🚺 **Gender-Specific Safety**

⚪ **Men:** Potentially supportive for stress-related cardiovascular tension **only with professional guidance**; avoid unsupervised use.
⚪ **Women:** May be used in supervised protocols for circulatory rhythm and nervous tension; **not self-prepared.**
🔴 **Pregnancy / Nursing: Strictly avoid.**

---

⏳ **Expected Results**

- Nervous-system settling: 30–90 minutes (when appropriate form is used)
- Circulation/blood-pressure pattern support: 1–3 weeks (supervised use)
- Systemic balance / vitality support: 2–6 weeks (protocol-dependent)

---

🫖 **DIY Recipe — Cold Mistletoe Heart Infusion (Guided Use Only)**
**Ingredients:** 1 tsp dried European Mistletoe · 1 cup cool water
**Directions:** Cover and steep 8–12 hours → strain → sip once daily

**Note:** Use only under guidance from a trained professional.

---

### Same / Similar Results

- Hawthorn Berry
- Motherwort
- Linden Flower
- Olive Leaf
- Valerian *(for nervous tension only)*

---

### Shelf Life / Potency After Preparation

- Dried herb: Best within 12 months (airtight, cool, dark)
- Standardized products: Follow manufacturer expiration
- Cold infusion: Refrigerate; use within 24 hours

---

### Herbal Reflections of European Mistletoe

European Mistletoe is the lesson of precision. It does not belong to casual dosing or careless confidence—its power is real, and so are its limits. In the hands of knowledge, it steadies rhythm, calms strain, and invites the body back toward balance.

It teaches that some medicines heal not through force, but through measured correction—where respect becomes part of the remedy.

---

**Herbal Confidence Index:**

*(3/5 green stars — meaningful regulatory potential in supervised settings, but limited by toxicity risk, narrow safe range, and the absolute need for correct preparation.)*

# CISTUS INCANUS

★★★★

### *Cistus incanus*

**Cistus Incanus** is a polyphenol-rich immune-support herb used to strengthen resilience during viral season and soothe irritated respiratory and oral tissues. Best known as "Rock Rose," it is valued for gentle antimicrobial support, antioxidant protection, and steady daily reinforcement—without the harshness of stronger essential-oil herbs.

Taken as tea, it's commonly used for sore throat support, mouth and gum comfort, and general immune steadiness, especially during exposure-heavy periods.

Across Mediterranean regions, Cistus has been used for centuries as tea, wash, and traditional purifier. Modern interest has grown around its unusually high polyphenol content and its role in supporting everyday immune defense. It remains a classic example of a "safe, steady protector" herb—quiet, consistent, and reliable.

---

### Core Herbal Category — Cistus Incanus

**Primary Core: Immune System Support herb** with *(polyphenol-rich antiviral action that strengthens immune defense and inhibits pathogen adhesion)*

**Secondary Cores:** Respiratory Support herb · Digestive Support herb · Liver & Detoxification herb · Skin & Tissue Repair herb

---

### How It Works

Cistus Incanus works primarily through its dense polyphenols, which help reduce oxidative stress and support balanced immune signaling. It is also studied for interfering with pathogen adhesion—making it harder for certain microbes to "grip" onto tissues. In the respiratory and oral pathways, it supports comfort by calming irritated surfaces while reinforcing natural defenses. Overall, it functions as a broad, non-stimulating immune protector that supports resilience through consistent use.

---

### Primary Uses

- Daily immune resilience support (viral season)
- Sore throat and upper-respiratory comfort

- Mouth and gum support (tea as rinse)
- Antioxidant protection during inflammatory stress
- Gentle support for skin irritation when used as wash

---

**Scientific Backing**

Cistus Incanus contains high levels of polyphenols and flavonoids associated with antioxidant activity and immune defense support. Research highlights antimicrobial and antiviral-support potential, reduced oxidative stress, and usefulness in upper-respiratory and oral-health support—especially as a tea-based daily strategy.

---

**Forms Available**

- Dried leaves (tea/infusion)
- Capsules (standardized products)
- Lozenges/sprays (brand-dependent)
- Tinctures/extracts (less common)

---

**How to Use (Dosage & Methods)**

**Tea (Primary Method):**

- 1 Tbsp dried leaf per cup
- Steep 10–15 minutes
- Drink 1–3 cups daily

**Mouth Rinse:**

- Brew strong tea, cool
- Swish 20–30 seconds, spit (1–2× daily)

**Capsules/Extracts:**

- Follow label dosing (commonly 300–600 mg/day)

---

⚠️ **Caution Level:** Safe

- Generally well tolerated
- Very high intake may cause mild stomach discomfort or constipation (astringency)
- May slightly reduce iron absorption—separate from iron supplements if needed
- Pregnancy/Nursing: mild tea typically acceptable; avoid high-dose extracts as a precaution

---

**Gender-Specific Safety**

**Men:** Strong daily immune and oral support; safe for routine use.
**Women:** Helpful for immune resilience and inflammation balance; well tolerated.
**Pregnancy / Nursing:** Mild tea usually okay; avoid concentrated extracts.

---

**Expected Results**

- Throat/oral comfort: 1–3 days
- Immune steadiness: 3–7 days
- Full resilience-building effect: 2–4 weeks of consistent use

**DIY Recipe — Cistus Immune & Throat Tea**

1 Tbsp dried Cistus leaves
1–2 cups hot water
Steep 10–15 minutes, strain. Add honey/lemon if desired.

---

**Same / Similar Results** Elderberry Olive Leaf Echinacea Chamomile Goldenseal *(stronger; shorter-course herb)*

---

**Shelf Life / Potency After Preparation**

Dried leaves: 1–2 years (airtight, cool, dark)
Capsules: 2–3 years (check expiration)
Tincture: 4–6 years

Prepared tea/rinse: 24 hours refrigerated

---

**Herbal Reflections of Cistus Incanus**

Cistus Incanus is the shield you drink. It doesn't announce itself with heat or intensity—it fortifies quietly, strengthening the body's boundary lines day by day. In its steady tea is a kind of discipline: protection built through consistency, not urgency.

Rock Rose reminds us that resilience is not always dramatic. Sometimes the strongest defense is simply the habit of daily reinforcement.

**Herbal Confidence Index:**

*(4/5 green stars — safe, dependable immune protector; excellent for respiratory season, oral support, and antioxidant reinforcement without overstimulation.)*

# MULLEIN LEAF

★★★★★

*Verbascum thapsus*

**Mullein Leaf** is a gentle lung-soothing herb used to calm coughs, ease airway irritation, and support healthy mucus balance. Its demulcent, expectorant nature makes it especially valuable for dry, scratchy throats, lingering bronchial irritation, and congestion that needs softening—not forcing.

Because it supports comfort without harsh stimulation, Mullein is widely favored for sensitive constitutions and long, steady respiratory recovery.

Historically known as the "torch plant," mullein traveled through European and North American traditions as both symbol and medicine—used for lungs, ear support (flower oil), and household respiratory care. Across cultures it earned a reputation as a comfort herb: simple, safe, and deeply restorative.

---

### Core Herbal Category — Mullein Leaf

**Primary Core: Respiratory System Support herb** with *(demulcent, lung-soothing action that calms irritation and supports healthy mucus balance)*

**Secondary Cores:** Immune Support herb · Nervines (Nervous System Support) herb · Liver & Detoxification herb

---

### How It Works

Mullein Leaf works by coating and soothing irritated respiratory tissues, reducing dryness and cough-trigger inflammation. Its gentle expectorant action helps loosen and normalize mucus, making coughs more productive without strain. By easing breathing discomfort, it indirectly reduces nervous-system tension that often accompanies respiratory illness. Overall, it functions as a steady lung-restorative herb that supports clearer, calmer breathing over time.

---

### Primary Uses

- Soothes dry cough and irritated throat
- Helps loosen congestion and stubborn phlegm

- Supports bronchitis recovery and seasonal respiratory stress
- Supports smokers' lung recovery (as tea, not smoke)
- Mullein flower oil traditionally supports ear comfort

---

🧪 **Scientific Backing**

Mullein contains mucilage and saponins associated with soothing, expectorant effects, while flavonoids contribute anti-inflammatory support to respiratory tissues. Traditional use is extensive for cough, bronchial irritation, and lung recovery.

---

💊 **Forms Available**

- Dried leaf (tea/infusion)
- Syrups and respiratory blends
- Tincture
- Mullein flower infused oil (ear-support tradition)

---

📏 **How to Use (Dosage & Methods)**

**Tea/Infusion (Preferred):**

- 1–2 tsp dried leaf per cup
- Steep 10–15 minutes
- Drink 1–3 cups daily as needed
  ✅ **Strain extremely well** (fine hairs can irritate throat)

**Syrup:**

- Follow label or recipe; commonly 1 tsp as needed

**Tincture:**

- 1–2 mL up to 3× daily

⚠️ **Caution Level:** Safe

- Generally very gentle and well tolerated
- Strain tea thoroughly to prevent throat irritation from leaf hairs
- Avoid smoking plant material (can irritate airways)
- If asthma is severe or breathing is compromised, use alongside appropriate medical care

---

**Gender-Specific Safety**

**Men:** Excellent for cough and chest irritation; safe for steady tea use.

**Women:** Supports calm breathing and mucus balance; well tolerated.

**Pregnancy / Nursing:** Generally considered safe as mild tea; avoid high-dose extracts unless advised.

---

**Expected Results**

- Throat/lung soothing: 1–3 doses
- Cough calm + easier breathing: 2–5 days
- Deeper recovery support: 1–2 weeks of consistent use

---

**DIY Recipe — Lung-Soothing Mullein Tea**

1 tsp Mullein Leaf

1 tsp Thyme *(optional for microbial support)*

Steep 10–15 minutes → strain extremely well → sip warm.

---

**Same / Similar Results**

Elecampane

Thyme

Licorice Root

Marshmallow Root

Osha Root

---

**Shelf Life / Potency After Preparation**

Dried leaf: 1–2 years (airtight, cool, dark)

Tincture: 3–5 years

Syrup: 1–2 months refrigerated

Prepared tea: 24 hours refrigerated

---

**Herbal Reflections of Mullein Leaf**

Mullein is comfort made medicinal. It doesn't fight the lungs—it reassures them, softening what is tight, soothing what is raw, and guiding the breath back into ease. Its gift is gentle clearing: the kind of healing that restores without exhausting.

In a world that makes breathing harder than it should be, Mullein remains one of the purest reminders that recovery can be soft, steady, and faithful.

**Herbal Confidence Index:**

*(5/5 green stars — cornerstone lung-soothing herb; exceptionally safe and effective for cough, irritation, and respiratory recovery across a wide range of people.)*

# HAWTHORN BERRY

★★★★★

*Crataegus monogyna*

**Hawthorn Berry** is a classic cardiovascular tonic traditionally used to support heart muscle tone, circulation, and balanced blood pressure. Rich in flavonoids and procyanidins, it nourishes the heart and blood vessels while offering antioxidant protection that supports long-term cardiovascular resilience.

Historically revered across Europe and Asia, Hawthorn has long been associated with protection of both the physical and emotional heart. Today, it remains best known for gently supporting heart rhythm, circulation, and stress-related palpitations without overstimulation.

---

### Core Herbal Category — Hawthorn Berry

**Primary Core: Cardiovascular System Support** herb with (strengthening, regulating action that supports heart muscle tone, vessel integrity, and balanced blood pressure)

**Secondary Cores:** Nervines (Nervous System Support) herb · Immune Support herb · Nutritive & Restorative herb

---

### How It Works

Hawthorn Berry supports the heart by improving coronary and peripheral circulation while gently strengthening myocardial function. Its flavonoids and oligomeric procyanidins enhance vascular tone, support endothelial health, and assist with balanced blood pressure regulation. Antioxidant compounds protect heart and vessel tissues from oxidative stress, while its mild nervine action helps calm emotional tension that can affect heart rhythm and circulation.

---

### Primary Uses

- Heart tone and cardiac performance
- Circulation and microvascular support
- Mild blood pressure balance alongside lifestyle measures
- Stress-related palpitations and anxious heart patterns

• Gentle endurance support for regular walking and activity

---

### Scientific Backing

Hawthorn contains flavonoids and oligomeric procyanidins (OPCs) shown to support coronary blood flow, myocardial efficiency, and vascular elasticity. Clinical research has explored its use in mild heart failure, hypertension, and angina, with improvements noted in exercise tolerance and quality-of-life measures. Hawthorn supports nitric oxide activity and endothelial function while acting as a gentle positive inotrope without stimulant effects.

---

### Forms Available

• Dried berries, leaf, and flower (tea)
• Tincture or liquid extract
• Capsules and standardized tablets

---

### How to Use (Dosage)

**Tea:** 1–2 teaspoons dried herb per 8 oz hot water, steep 10–15 minutes, 1–2× daily
**Tincture:** 1–2 mL, 2–3× daily
**Capsules:** 250–500 mg extract, 2–3× daily
Best used as a long-term tonic: 8–12 weeks or longer for full benefit.

---

### Caution Level: Caution

Monitor use if taking cardiac or blood pressure medications (beta-blockers, calcium-channel blockers, nitrates, digoxin).
May mildly lower blood pressure and enhance cardiac efficiency.
Discontinue 1–2 weeks before surgery due to circulatory effects.
Pregnancy/Nursing: Mild tea only; avoid concentrated extracts unless supervised.

---

### Gender-Specific Safety

**Men:**
Supports endurance, circulation, and heart efficiency. Suitable for long-term use as tea or tincture. Avoid unsupervised use alongside heart medications.
**Women:**
Helpful for stress-related palpitations and emotional tension, particularly during menopause. Safe for daily use; avoid strong extracts if on cardiac medications.
**Pregnancy/Nursing:**

Generally safe as a mild tea. Avoid strong extracts unless guided by a qualified practitioner.

---

**⏳ Expected Results**

- Calmer rhythm or reduced flutter: 1–3 weeks
- Improved circulation and walking comfort: 2–4+ weeks
- Emotional grounding and stress support: 1–2 weeks

---

**🛠 DIY Recipe — Hawthorn-Rose Heart Tonic**

Simmer 1 tablespoon Hawthorn berries in 2 cups water for 20 minutes.
Remove from heat, add 1 teaspoon Hawthorn leaf/flower and 1 teaspoon rose petals.
Cover, steep 10 minutes, strain, and sip 1 cup daily.

---

**🔄 Same / Similar Results**

- Motherwort
- Danshen
- Arjuna
- Grape Seed
- Hibiscus

---

**Shelf Life / Potency After Preparation**

- Dried berries, leaf, or flower: 1–2 years (airtight, cool, dark)
- Tincture: 3–5 years (excellent potency retention)
- Prepared tea: Use within 24 hours if refrigerated

---

**💬 Herbal Reflections of Hawthorn Berry**

Hawthorn reflects the balance of strength and gentleness at the heart's core. With thorn and blossom alike, it teaches protection without rigidity and resilience without force. Its medicine works quietly and steadily, reinforcing both the physical heartbeat and the emotional center, reminding us that endurance is built through harmony and consistency rather than intensity.

---

**⭐ Herbal Confidence Index:** 🌿 🌿 🌿 🌿 🌿

*(5/5 — cornerstone cardiovascular and restorative herb; exceptionally reliable and safe for long-term support of heart strength, circulation, and emotional balance.)*

# TANSY

★★

*Tanacetum vulgare*

**Tansy** is a potent historical antiparasitic and insect-repellent herb known for its strong antimicrobial oils, particularly thujone. While once used internally for cleansing and menstrual regulation, modern herbal practice recognizes its significant toxicity and restricts its use almost entirely to external applications.
Traditionally grown in European monastery and cottage gardens, Tansy symbolized purification and protection. Today, it is best known as a household and environmental deterrent rather than an internal remedy.

---

### 🌿 Core Herbal Category — Tansy

**Primary Core: Immune System Support** herb with (strong antimicrobial and antiparasitic action historically used for purging but associated with significant toxicity)
**Secondary Cores:** Digestive Support herb · Women's Health herb · Skin & Tissue Repair herb

---

### 🌿 How It Works

Tansy's volatile oils disrupt parasites, insects, and pathogenic organisms through strong antimicrobial and neuroactive effects. These same compounds can irritate tissues and overstimulate the nervous and reproductive systems, making internal use unsafe. Modern herbal practice limits Tansy to external and environmental applications where its repellent properties can be used without systemic risk.

---

### 🌱 Primary Uses (Historical / External)

- Insect, lice, and mite deterrent
- Household and storage protection
- Ritual, preservation, and traditional cleansing uses

---

### 🧪 Scientific Backing

Tansy contains thujone-rich essential oils and sesquiterpene lactones with demonstrated insecticidal and antimicrobial activity. While historical use included internal applications, contemporary toxicology recognizes neurological and hepatic risks, supporting external use only and strict avoidance of ingestion.

---

### 💊 Forms Available

- Dried herb (sachets, garlands)
- Hydrosol (external use)
- Essential oil (external only, highly diluted)

---

### 📏 How to Use (External Only)

**Repellent Sachet:** Place dried Tansy with lavender or bay in cloth bags near entryways or wardrobes.

**Household Vinegar:** Steep dried herb in vinegar for 7 days; strain and apply to door frames or baseboards.

⚠️ Internal use is not recommended. Keep all preparations away from children and pets.

---

### ⚠️ Caution Level: 🔴 Supervision Required

🔴 Internal use is strongly discouraged due to thujone toxicity.

🔴 Potential risks include liver damage, neurological symptoms, seizures, and miscarriage.

🔴 External use only; avoid concentrated skin application.

🔴 Absolutely contraindicated during pregnancy and nursing.

---

### 🚹 🚺 Gender-Specific Safety

🔴 **Men:** External use only. Internal use may cause neurological or hepatic harm.

🔴 **Women:** Historically used as an emmenagogue; now recognized as unsafe internally. External aromatic use only.

🔴 **Pregnancy/Nursing:** Absolutely contraindicated in all forms of internal or concentrated use.

---

### ⏳ Expected Results

- Repellent effects: Immediate to several days (refresh as scent fades)

---

### 🛠️ DIY Recipe — Doorway Repellent Garland

Bundle dried Tansy with bay or rosemary and hang above doorways. Replace monthly during insect season.

---

🔄 **Same / Similar Results** ● Neem ● Clove ● Wormwood ● Cedar ● Catnip

---

### Shelf Life / Potency After Preparation

- Dried herb: Up to 2 years (cool, dark storage)
- Hydrosol: 6–12 months refrigerated
- Vinegar preparations: 3–6 months

---

### Herbal Reflections of Tansy

Tansy represents the uncompromising edge of old herbal medicine — powerful, effective, and demanding respect. Once used internally, it now serves as a reminder that discernment is essential in healing. Its modern role as a guardian herb teaches that protection does not always belong inside the body; sometimes it belongs at the threshold.

---

### Herbal Confidence Index:

*(2/5 — historically powerful and externally effective, but internal toxicity limits safe application to environmental and topical use only.)*

# TRIBULUS

★★★★

*Tribulus terrestris*

**Tribulus** is a traditional vitality tonic used to support stamina, libido, and hormonal balance in both men and women. Rather than acting as a stimulant or hormone replacement, it supports natural endocrine signaling and physical resilience, with individual responses varying by dose and extract quality.

Used in Ayurvedic and Chinese traditions, Tribulus has long been valued for restoring strength after illness and supporting urinary and reproductive function. Today, it remains popular in endurance and vitality formulations.

---

### 🌿 Core Herbal Category — Tribulus

**Primary Core: Endocrine & Hormonal Support** herb with (tonifying action that supports healthy androgen signaling without direct hormone replacement)

**Secondary Cores:** Men's Health & Vitality herb · Circulatory & Cardiovascular herb · Urinary & Kidney Support herb

---

### 🌿 How It Works

Tribulus supports endocrine responsiveness related to libido, strength, and recovery, particularly during depletion. Its saponins influence androgen receptor signaling and nitric oxide availability, contributing to vitality, circulation, and urinary tone. It works gradually, supporting long-term resilience rather than short-term stimulation.

---

### 🌱 Primary Uses

- Vitality and exercise recovery
- Libido and reproductive wellness
- Hormonal balance support
- Urinary and prostate tone
- Circulatory endurance support

---

### 🧪 Scientific Backing

Tribulus contains steroidal saponins such as protodioscin, studied for effects on androgen signaling and vascular function. Research outcomes are mixed, but traditional use supports its role as a tonic for physical resilience when paired with proper diet and training.

---

### Forms Available

• Standardized extract capsules or tablets
• Powdered herb
• Alcohol tincture

---

### How to Use (Dosage)

**Capsules:** 500–1,500 mg daily with food (split doses)
**Tincture:** 1–2 mL twice daily
**Powder:** 1 teaspoon daily in smoothies or tonics
Use in cycles: 8–12 weeks on, 2 weeks off.

---

### Caution Level: Caution

Avoid during pregnancy, nursing, or hormone-sensitive conditions.
Monitor if using blood pressure or blood sugar medications.
Discontinue if signs of overstimulation occur (irritability, acne, insomnia).

---

### Gender-Specific Safety

**Men:** Supports libido, endurance, and recovery. Avoid excessive dosing.
**Women:** Supports vitality and hormonal balance; discontinue if androgenic effects appear.
**Pregnancy/Nursing:** Not recommended due to hormonal activity.

---

### Expected Results

• Energy and libido: 2–3 weeks
• Endurance and recovery: 4–6 weeks
• Hormonal balance: 6–8 weeks

---

### DIY Recipe — Tribulus Endurance Cooler

Blend Tribulus powder with hibiscus, water, citrus, and a pinch of sea salt. Sip before activity.

---

### Same / Similar Results

Maca
Ashwagandha
Ginseng

Tongkat Ali

Shilajit

---

**Shelf Life / Potency After Preparation**

Capsules: 2–3 years

Powder: 1–2 years airtight

Tincture: 3–5 years

---

**Herbal Reflections of Tribulus**

Tribulus teaches steady rebuilding rather than quick elevation. It rewards patience, working quietly beneath the surface to restore traction where energy once slipped. Its medicine is not forceful — it is cumulative, strengthening foundations rather than chasing peaks.

---

**Herbal Confidence Index:**

*(4/5 — dependable vitality and endocrine-support herb; effective when used cyclically and responsibly.)*

---

# CHRYSANTHEMUM

★★★★

*Chrysanthemum morifolium*

**Chrysanthemum** is a cooling circulatory herb traditionally used to ease eye strain, head tension, and internal heat. Commonly consumed as a gentle tea, it supports calm blood flow to the head and eyes while offering antioxidant and nervous system support.
Long revered across East Asia, Chrysanthemum symbolizes clarity and balance. Today, it remains best known as a daily cooling tea for visual fatigue, heat, and stress-related tension.

---

### 🌿 Core Herbal Category — Chrysanthemum

**Primary Core: Cardiovascular System Support** herb with (cooling action that supports healthy blood flow to the head and eyes)
**Secondary Cores:** Immune Support herb · Liver & Detoxification herb · Nervines herb

---

### 🌿 How It Works

Chrysanthemum clears excess heat while improving microcirculation to the head and eyes. Its flavonoids calm vascular and inflammatory tension, easing headaches and visual fatigue. It also supports liver function, which influences eye health, and gently settles heat-related nervous agitation.

---

### 🌱 Primary Uses

- Eye strain and visual fatigue
- Tension headaches and head heat
- Cooling cardiovascular support
- Heat and stress relief

---

### 🧪 Scientific Backing

Chrysanthemum contains luteolin, apigenin, and chlorogenic acid, compounds shown to support antioxidant activity, vasorelaxation, and inflammation modulation. Traditional Chinese medicine classifies it as a heat-clearing herb, with modern research supporting its role in microcirculatory and visual comfort.

---

### Forms Available

- Dried flowers
- Tea pearls
- Tincture or syrup
- Powdered herb

---

### How to Use (Dosage)

**Tea:** 1–2 teaspoons dried flowers per 8 oz hot (not boiling) water, steep 8–10 minutes, up to 3× daily
Best paired with hydration and screen breaks.

---

### Caution Level: Caution

Possible sensitivity in those allergic to Asteraceae plants
May mildly lower blood pressure
Use mild tea only during pregnancy; avoid concentrates

---

### Gender-Specific Safety

**Men:** Safe, cooling, and calming; supports eye and head comfort.
**Women:** Helpful for menopausal warmth and eye fatigue.
**Pregnancy/Nursing:** Mild tea acceptable; avoid extracts.

---

### Expected Results

- Head and eye relief: Same day
- Cooling clarity: 3–7 days

---

### DIY Recipe — Chrysanthemum-Goji Eye Tea

Steep Chrysanthemum flowers with Goji berries for 10 minutes; sip warm and eat berries.

---

### Same / Similar Results

Mulberry Leaf
Peppermint
Goji Berry
Schisandra
Elderflower

---

### Shelf Life / Potency After Preparation

- Dried flowers: 12–18 months
- Tincture/syrup: 3–5 years
- Prepared tea: 24 hours refrigerated

---

### Herbal Reflections of Chrysanthemum

Chrysanthemum heals through softness — releasing heat, restoring clarity, and easing tension without depletion. It reminds us that calm circulation and gentle cooling can be among the most restorative forms of medicine.

---

**Herbal Confidence Index:** *(4/5 — safe, cooling, and consistently effective for eye comfort, heat, and tension relief.)*

# *CALAGUALA*

★★★★

*Polypodium leucotomos*

**Calaguala** is a traditional fern remedy used in Central and South American herbalism to support clear skin, calm inflammation, and promote "internal cooling" during heat-driven irritation. It is best known today as an internal skin-support herb that helps the body manage inflammatory stress and maintain healthier tissue resilience over time.
Modern research on standardized *Polypodium leucotomos* extract (PLE) supports its antioxidant and photoprotective activity, making it a bridge between traditional "blood-clearing" practice and contemporary skin science—especially when paired with sensible sun habits and topical barrier care.

---

### 🌿 Core Herbal Category — Calaguala

**Primary Core: Immune System Support** herb with (immune-modulating action that supports a balanced inflammatory response without broadly suppressing immunity)
**Secondary Cores:** Skin & Tissue Repair herb · Liver & Detoxification herb · Musculoskeletal & Pain-Relief herb

---

### 🌿 How It Works

Calaguala helps regulate immune signaling involved in inflammatory flares, supporting calmer skin and tissue responses over time. Its antioxidant compounds reduce oxidative stress and may lessen UV-triggered inflammatory cascades, which can contribute to redness and flare sensitivity. By supporting liver clearance pathways, it may also help the body process inflammatory byproducts that aggravate skin reactivity.

---

### 🌱 Primary Uses

- Adjunct support for inflammatory skin conditions (eczema, psoriasis)
- Internal antioxidant support for UV and environmental stress
- Immune-balancing support during chronic inflammatory tendency
- Skin resilience support alongside topical barrier care

---

### Scientific Backing

Standardized *Polypodium leucotomos* extract (PLE) has been studied for reducing UV-induced erythema and oxidative damage markers in humans. Research also suggests immunomodulatory effects and antioxidant activity that may support inflammatory skin comfort and photoprotection when used as part of a broader skin-health plan.

---

### Forms Available

- Standardized extract capsules/tablets (PLE)
- Traditional decoction (dried rhizome/root)

---

### How to Use (Dosage)

**Capsules:** 240–480 mg/day with meals
**UV-support timing:** 30–60 minutes before sun exposure (label-guided)
**Decoction:** 1 teaspoon cut herb in 2 cups water; simmer 20–25 minutes; take ½–1 cup 1–2× daily
Best paired with hydration, omega-rich foods, and consistent sun-protective habits.

---

### Caution Level: Caution

Immune-modulating: consult a clinician if using immunosuppressants or managing autoimmune disease
Limited pregnancy/lactation data: avoid concentrated extracts unless supervised
Mild digestive upset possible; take with food or reduce dose

---

### Gender-Specific Safety

**Men:** Supports skin resilience and inflammatory balance without known hormonal effects. Use label-guided dosing.
**Women:** Helpful for heat-driven skin flares and inflammatory irritation; best used steadily and moderately.
**Pregnancy/Nursing:** Mild dietary-level use only; avoid concentrated extracts due to limited safety data.

---

### Expected Results

- UV stress support: days to 1–2 weeks
- Skin calm and resilience: 3–6+ weeks

---

### DIY Recipe — Calaguala Skin-Calm Decoction

Simmer 1 teaspoon Calaguala in 2 cups water for 25 minutes.
Cover, cool 10 minutes, strain, and drink ½ cup daily.

---

🔄 **Same / Similar Results**

- 🔘 Burdock
- 🔘 Gotu Kola
- 🔘 Turmeric
- 🔘 Green Tea
- 🔘 Omega-3 (dietary)

---

**Shelf Life / Potency After Preparation**

- Dried herb: Up to 1 year (airtight, cool, dry)
- Capsules/tablets: 2–3 years (per label)
- Prepared decoction: Use within 48 hours refrigerated

---

**Herbal Reflections of Calaguala**

Calaguala works quietly beneath the surface, supporting calmer immune tone and steadier skin responses without force. Its strength is restraint—helping the body return to balance rather than pushing it in one direction. Over time, it becomes a companion for those who need steadiness more than intensity, especially when skin and system are easily triggered by heat, stress, or sun.

**Herbal Confidence Index:** 🌿 🌿 🌿 🌿

*(4/5 — dependable internal skin-support and antioxidant herb; especially useful for inflammatory flares and UV-related stress when used consistently.)*

# DODDER

★★★

*Cuscuta chinensis*

**Dodder** is a classic TCM seed tonic used to support kidney–liver vitality, reproductive strength, and urinary tone during periods of depletion. It is most often used in formulas for fertility support, libido, and recovery after chronic stress, with benefits building gradually through consistent use.
Known in Chinese medicine as *Tu Si Zi*, Dodder has a long history as a "Jing-support" herb—paired with other tonics to nourish core vitality, improve resilience, and support long-term endocrine balance.

---

### 🌿 Core Herbal Category — Dodder

**Primary Core:** Endocrine & Hormonal Support herb with (deep tonic action that supports reproductive vitality and long-term endocrine resilience)
**Secondary Cores:** Urinary & Kidney Support herb · Liver & Detoxification herb · Adaptogen herb

---

### 🌿 How It Works

Dodder supports endocrine and reproductive resilience by nourishing pathways associated with long-term vitality and recovery. Traditionally linked to kidney function and "core reserves," it is used to rebuild stamina, support libido, and promote urinary tone. It also supports the liver's role in hormone metabolism and recovery from stress-related depletion, helping benefits accumulate steadily rather than rapidly.

---

### 🌱 Primary Uses

- Kidney and urinary tone support
- Fertility and libido support (men and women)
- Endocrine resilience during depletion
- Recovery support after prolonged stress or illness
- Traditional support for vision and overall vitality

---

### Scientific Backing

Dodder contains flavonoids, lignans, and quinic-acid derivatives associated with antioxidant and anti-inflammatory activity. Preliminary research suggests potential support for reproductive parameters and endocrine balance, though stronger modern clinical trials are still needed to confirm reliability across diverse populations and products.

---

### Forms Available

- Dried seeds (whole or powdered)
- Capsules/tablets
- TCM combination formulas
- Decoction blends

---

### How to Use (Dosage)

**Powder:** 1–2 g daily
**Capsules:** 400–600 mg, 2× daily
**Decoction:** 1 tablespoon in 2 cups water; simmer 20 minutes; drink ½–1 cup daily
Often blended with Goji, Schisandra, or Licorice in restorative formulas.

---

### Caution Level: Caution

Avoid during pregnancy and nursing due to insufficient safety data and possible uterine effects

Use caution with fertility medications or hormone-sensitive conditions

May cause mild dryness, dizziness, or digestive upset at high doses; use cycles and breaks

Consult a clinician if managing liver/kidney conditions or on related medications

---

### Gender-Specific Safety

**Men:** Supports libido, endurance, and reproductive tone; best used in moderate cycles, especially when targeting fertility.

**Women:** Traditional fertility and vitality support; use moderate dosing and discontinue if overstimulating.

**Pregnancy/Nursing:** Avoid entirely.

---

### Expected Results

- Urinary/sexual vitality: 2–3 weeks
- Energy and stamina: 4–6 weeks
- Fertility/reproductive support: best assessed over months of consistent use

---

### 🛠 DIY Recipe — Dodder Rejuvenation Tonic

Simmer 1 tablespoon Dodder seeds with ½ teaspoon Licorice root in 2 cups water for 20 minutes.

Strain and drink ½ cup in the morning.

---

### 🔄 Same / Similar Results

- Horny Goat Weed
- Ashwagandha
- Maca
- Tribulus
- Shatavari

---

### Shelf Life / Potency After Preparation

- Dried herb: Up to 1 year (airtight, cool, dark)
- Capsules/tablets: 2–3 years (stored properly)
- Prepared decoction: Use within 48 hours refrigerated

---

### 💬 Herbal Reflections of Dodder

Dodder is restoration through steadiness—more nourishing than stimulating. It is best for people rebuilding reserves rather than chasing quick results, and it teaches the long view: vitality grows through patient consistency. When paired wisely in formula, Dodder supports deep resilience—helping the body regain traction after stress, depletion, or long recovery seasons.

---

### ⭐ Herbal Confidence Index: 🌿🌿🌿

*(3/5 — respected traditional reproductive and vitality tonic; moderately effective, but commercial product quality varies and modern clinical confirmation is limited.)*

---

# BARLEY GRASS

★★★★★

*Hordeum vulgare*

**Barley Grass** is a nutrient-dense green food traditionally used to support daily nourishment, antioxidant defense, and gentle detoxification. Rich in chlorophyll, vitamins, minerals, and plant enzymes, it helps replenish depleted diets and support steady energy without stimulant effects.

Popularized through whole-food "green therapy," Barley Grass remains widely used today as an easy daily addition for foundational nutrition, digestive support, and metabolic steadiness—especially when consistency is prioritized over high dosing.

---

### 🌿 Core Herbal Category — Barley Grass

**Primary Core:** Nutritional & Tonic Support herb with (mineral-rich action that rebuilds depleted systems and supports daily cellular nourishment)

**Secondary Cores:** Liver & Detoxification herb · Digestive Support herb · Immune Support herb · Metabolic & Blood Sugar Support herb

---

### 🌿 How It Works

Barley Grass supplies concentrated micronutrients and chlorophyll that support cellular repair and antioxidant protection. Its fiber and plant compounds support digestive regularity and nutrient absorption, while antioxidant enzymes help reduce oxidative stress. This foundational nourishment supports immune resilience and steadier metabolic energy, especially when used consistently in moderate amounts.

---

### 🌱 Primary Uses

- Daily nutritive replenishment and "green" support
- Antioxidant and cellular defense support
- Digestive regularity and gut support
- Gentle liver support and metabolic balance
- Energy support through nourishment (not stimulation)

---

### 🧪 Scientific Backing

Barley Grass is recognized as nutrient-dense, with research noting potential benefits for antioxidant status and supportive effects on lipid and glucose markers in some studies. Compounds such as superoxide dismutase (SOD) contribute to oxidative defense. Outcomes vary by product quality and overall diet.

---

### Forms Available

- Powder
- Freeze-dried capsules
- Fresh juice (where available)

---

### How to Use (Dosage)

**Powder:** 1 teaspoon to 1 tablespoon daily (start low)
**Capsules:** ~500 mg, 1–2× daily (label-guided)
**Fresh juice:** ~1 oz daily, often on an empty stomach

---

### Caution Level: Safe

Generally safe as a food-based supplement in normal dietary amounts.

If celiac/gluten-sensitive: choose certified gluten-free products to avoid cross-contamination.

Start with small doses to reduce bloating or nausea.

Consult a clinician if using anticoagulants or diabetes medications (dietary changes may affect dosing needs).

---

### Gender-Specific Safety

**Men:** Supports energy, recovery, and digestive regularity without hormonal effects.

**Women:** Helpful for nourishment, skin clarity, and steady detox support; suitable for daily use.

**Pregnancy/Nursing:** Generally safe as a food; avoid highly concentrated or unfamiliar products unless clinician-approved.

---

### Expected Results

- Energy steadiness: 3–7 days
- Digestive support: 1–2 weeks
- Immune/metabolic support: 2–4 weeks

---

### DIY Recipe — Daily Green Detox Drink

Mix 1 teaspoon Barley Grass powder with 8 oz water and juice of ½ lemon (optional: 1 teaspoon honey). Drink in the morning.

---

### 🔄 Same / Similar Results

- Wheatgrass
- Spirulina
- Alfalfa
- Chlorella
- Moringa

---

### Shelf Life / Potency After Preparation

- Powder: 1–2 years (sealed, cool, dry)
- Capsules: 2–3 years (airtight, low humidity)
- Fresh juice: Best immediately; within 24 hours refrigerated

---

### Herbal Reflections of Barley Grass

Barley Grass is quiet restoration—simple, steady, and foundational. It doesn't force change; it restores capacity by replenishing what is missing. Its best lesson is consistency: modest daily use that gradually improves the body's ability to repair, digest, and maintain energy. When paired with a balanced diet, it becomes a reliable "baseline" herb that supports resilience from the ground up.

---

### Herbal Confidence Index: 🌿 🌿 🌿 🌿 🌿

*(5/5 — cornerstone nutritive herb; exceptionally safe and consistently helpful for daily replenishment, antioxidant support, and gentle detox foundation.)*

# TAMARIND

★★★★

*Tamarindus indica*

Tamarind's sweet-tart pulp supports digestion, bile flow, and gentle elimination. **Rich in polyphenols, potassium, magnesium, fiber, and organic acids, it eases constipation, reduces post-meal sluggishness, and contributes antioxidants. Beyond the gut, it's used for cholesterol balance, liver support, and fever relief in traditional systems. Historically, Ayurvedic, African, and Southeast Asian lineages relied on Tamarind as food-medicine.** From cooling drinks to spice pastes, it bridged cuisine and care. Its enduring presence across continents reflects a simple truth: palatable remedies encourage steady use—and steady use brings steady results.

---

## Core Herbal Category — Tamarind

**Primary Core: Digestive System Support herb** with (gentle laxative and digestive-regulating action that supports elimination and intestinal comfort)
**Secondary Cores:** Liver & Detoxification herb · Metabolic & Blood Sugar Support herb · Immune Support herb

---

## How It Works

Tamarind works by **stimulating gentle bowel movement and digestive flow**, supporting regular elimination without harsh irritation. Its organic acids help **improve digestion and ease stagnation**, promoting intestinal comfort. This cleansing action supports the **liver's detoxification processes**, aiding waste removal. Tamarind also helps **moderate blood sugar response**, supporting metabolic balance after meals. Overall, it acts as a **mild, food-based digestive herb that restores rhythm, comfort, and metabolic ease**.

---

### *Primary Uses*

- Relieves constipation, gas, and gut inflammation
- Supports liver cleansing & bile production
- Helps regulate cholesterol & blood sugar
- Provides antioxidant cellular protection
- Traditional aid for fever and parasite protocols

## 🧪 Scientific Backing

Soluble fiber aids lipid and glycemic control; polyphenols provide antioxidant and mild antimicrobial actions. Studies support hepatoprotective effects, metabolic regulation, and gentle laxation.

---

## 💊 *Forms Available*

- *Raw pulp or blocks*
- *Dried leaves or bark*
- *Capsules and powdered extracts*
- *Concentrate or syrup*

---

## 📏 How to Use (Dosage)

- *Pulp: 1–2 tsp/day in warm water or food*
- Tea: 1 Tbsp pulp or leaves simmered in 2 cups water for 15 minutes
- *Powder: 500–1,000 mg/day*
- Culinary: Added to stews, tonics, marinades

---

## ⌛ *Expected Results*

- *Digestive ease: 1–3 days*
- *Lipid/liver support: 2–4 weeks*
- *Anti-inflammatory benefits: 3–6 weeks*

## ⚠ Caution Level: ● Safe

Tamarind is generally regarded as a ● **Safe** and food-grade herb when used in normal dietary amounts. Overuse may cause loose stools, mild stomach irritation, or reflux due to natural acidity. Avoid large medicinal doses with blood thinners or diabetic medications, as Tamarind may mildly enhance anticoagulant or blood-sugar-lowering effects.

Safe for children and elders when used as a gentle digestive or culinary spice. Pregnant and breastfeeding women should stick to moderate amounts in food or tea form and avoid concentrated extracts unless advised by a practitioner.

---

## Gender-Specific Safety

- **Men:** Aids digestion, supports healthy cholesterol, and promotes gentle detox without hormonal effects. May assist weight loss goals when paired with movement. Safe for regular use in mild amounts.
- **Women:** Helpful for bloating, fluid retention, and circulation during hormonal shifts. Supports skin clarity through gentle liver detox. Safe in daily culinary or tea doses.
- **Pregnancy / Nursing:** Safe in culinary amounts but avoid concentrated pulp or extract as the mild laxative and uterine-stimulating effects may cause discomfort. Always consult a professional for high-dose use during pregnancy or breastfeeding.

---

## DIY Recipe — Tamarind Cleansing Tonic

- *1 Tbsp tamarind pulp*
- *½ tsp grated fresh ginger*
- *½ tsp honey (optional)*
- 1½ cups warm water
  Steep 10 minutes, strain, sip slowly after meals.

---

## *Same / Similar Results*

- *Triphala — daily detox and bowel tone*
- Dandelion Root — liver and cholesterol support
- Milk Thistle — liver protection and regeneration
- Hawthorn Berry — heart and vascular support
- Turmeric — antioxidant and anti-inflammatory

---

## Shelf Life / Potency After Preparation

- **Pulp or blocks**: Up to 2 years when stored airtight in a cool, dry place

- **Powder or capsules**: 1–2 years sealed and away from light
- **Prepare fresh tonics daily for best potency**

## 🗨 Herbal Reflections of Tamarind

Tamarind is bright balance in a pod — a tart pull that wakes digestion and a soft sweetness that soothes heat and heaviness. It cuts through rich meals, encourages gentle elimination, and leaves the mouth clear rather than coated.

Where Lemon is sharper and Hibiscus more cooling, Tamarind sits in the middle: stimulating without straining, cooling without dampening — a friendly nudge toward ease.

Its lesson is that medicine can feel like a treat. A little sour-sweet sip before meals to prime digestion, or an afternoon tamarind water to steady heat and mind. Tamarind proves that healing often works best when it tastes good enough to become a habit.

---

## ★ Herbal Confidence Index: 🌿🌿🌿🌿

(4/5 green stars — refreshing digestive and cardiovascular-supporting fruit; highly effective for aiding digestion, gentle detoxification, and cholesterol balance, with rich antioxidant content, though its acidity may irritate sensitive stomachs when overused.)

# GINGER ROOT

★★★★★

Zingiber officinale

**Ginger Root** stands as one of the most dependable and time-tested medicinal roots in herbal practice, valued not for a single action but for its ability to restore functional balance where the body has slowed or stalled. **Traditionally used wherever digestion, circulation, and internal warmth required support, ginger works by re-establishing movement—helping food digest properly, energy circulate more freely, and stagnation resolve naturally. Its influence is felt first in the digestive system, but its benefits extend outward, supporting inflammation balance, metabolic activity, and overall physiological resilience.**

Unlike herbs that act narrowly or condition-specifically, Ginger Root serves as a foundational ally, often enhancing the effectiveness of other remedies while remaining reliable on its own. Its warming, aromatic rhizome does not overwhelm the system; rather, it gently stimulates the body's innate capacity to process, eliminate, and adapt. This combination of immediacy, versatility, and long-term safety has secured Ginger Root's place as a cornerstone herb across cultures and generations.

---

## Core Herbal Category — Ginger Root

**Primary Core: Digestive System Support herb** with (warming, carminative action that stimulates digestion, improves motility, and supports efficient elimination)

**Secondary Cores:** Liver & Detoxification herb · Musculoskeletal & Pain-Relief herb · Circulatory & Cardiovascular herb · Metabolic & Blood Sugar Support herb · Immune Support herb

---

## How It Works

Ginger Root works by **warming the digestive system**, stimulating gastric activity and easing gas, bloating, and sluggish elimination. Its pungent compounds help **improve digestive motility and circulation**, supporting smoother nutrient assimilation. This warming action supports the **liver's detoxification role**, aiding metabolic clearance. Ginger also helps **reduce inflammation and stabilize blood sugar response**, especially after meals. Overall, it acts as a **foundational digestive activator that restores warmth, movement, and metabolic efficiency**.

---

## Primary Uses

- Digestive support and motility enhancement
- Relief of nausea, vomiting, and motion sickness
- Gas, bloating, and intestinal discomfort
- Anti-inflammatory support for joints and tissues
- Circulatory stimulation and warming support
- Microbiome balance and gut–immune interaction

---

## Scientific Backing

Modern research confirms ginger's traditional uses, identifying active compounds such as **gingerols**, **shogaols**, and **zingerone**, which demonstrate:

- Pro-motility effects on the gastrointestinal tract
- Anti-nausea action comparable to pharmaceutical agents
- Anti-inflammatory and antioxidant activity
- Supportive effects on metabolic and immune pathways

Clinical studies have validated ginger's effectiveness for nausea (including pregnancy-related nausea), digestive discomfort, and inflammatory conditions.

---

## Forms Available

- *Fresh root (culinary and medicinal)*
- *Dried root powder*
- *Capsules and tablets*
- *Tea and decoction*
- *Tincture*

- *Oil and topical preparations*

## How to Use

Use **fresh or dried ginger root** as a tea, capsule, or food ingredient to support digestion, reduce nausea, and promote healthy gut motility. Typical use includes **½–1 teaspoon fresh root** or **500–1,000 mg dried root**, taken **1–3 times daily** with food or as needed.

## Expected Results

- Digestive comfort may improve within **30–60 minutes**
- *Reduced nausea often felt* ***rapidly***
- Circulatory and warming effects felt within **hours**
- Inflammatory benefits build over **days to weeks**

## Caution Level

**Safe**
Ginger Root is generally safe for most individuals when used in reasonable amounts. Very high doses may cause mild stomach irritation in sensitive individuals. Those on blood-thinning medications should consult a professional before heavy medicinal use.

## Gender-Specific Safety

- ***Men:*** *Safe*
- ***Women:*** *Safe*
- **Pregnancy/Nursing:** Caution
  Low-to-moderate doses are widely used for pregnancy-related nausea; excessive dosing should be avoided unless supervised.

## DIY Preparation (Home Use)

### *Simple Digestive Ginger Tea*

- ½–1 teaspoon fresh grated ginger root or
- *¼–½ teaspoon dried ginger root*
- *1 cup hot water*

***Instructions:***

1. *Add ginger to hot water*
2. *Steep covered for 10–15 minutes*
3. *Strain and drink warm*

✓*Use after meals for bloating, gas, or sluggish digestion*

---

## *Same / Similar Results*

- *Turmeric*
- *Fennel*
- *Peppermint*
- *Chamomile (German)*
- *Cardamom*

### Shelf Life / Potency After Preparation

- **Dried rhizome or powder:** 1–2 years when kept dry and sealed
- **Essential oil:** 2–3 years if stored cool and dark
- Prepared tinctures last 3–5 years when properly made

Store all forms in airtight containers away from heat and light to preserve aromatic compounds.

---

## Herbal Reflections of Ginger Root

Ginger Root is a herb of movement and awakening. Rather than forcing change, it gently reminds the body how to move energy, warmth, and digestion in the direction they were always meant to go. Where stagnation settles—whether in the gut, the joints, or the circulation—ginger brings quiet momentum. Its strength lies not in overpowering symptoms, but in restoring the natural rhythm that allows discomfort to resolve on its own. Unlike milder digestive herbs that soothe passively, Ginger Root participates actively in healing. It warms without excess, stimulates without depletion, and supports elimination without harshness. This balance is what has earned ginger its place across cultures and centuries as both medicine and food. Few herbs are as immediately felt, yet as reliably gentle over time, making Ginger Root a true cornerstone ally for digestive health and whole-body resilience.

### Herbal Confidence Index:

*(5/5 green stars — cornerstone digestive and circulatory herb; highly effective for stimulating digestion, relieving nausea and bloating, enhancing gut motility, and supporting systemic warmth and circulation. Ginger Root is fast-acting, reliable, widely accessible, and historically validated across global medical traditions, making it one of the most trusted and versatile medicinal roots in herbal practice.)*

# ATRACTYLODES

★★★★

*Atractylodes macrocephala*

**Atractylodes (Bai Zhu) is a classic TCM restorative for digestion, energy (Qi), and "dampness." It improves appetite, reduces bloating and loose stools, and enhances nutrient absorption while gently supporting immune tone. By tonifying the spleen/stomach axis, it replaces heaviness with steady, grounded vitality.**

Historically, Bai Zhu anchors many foundational formulas. Paired with ginseng, licorice, or astragalus, it rebuilds after illness and buffers against recurrent depletion. Centuries of clinical use mark it as a reliable builder rather than a quick fix—patient medicine for durable wellness.

---

## Core Herbal Category — Atractylodes

**Primary Core: Digestive System Support herb** with (strengthening, drying action that restores gut tone, improves absorption, and reduces damp digestive weakness)
**Secondary Cores:** Immune Support herb · Metabolic & Blood Sugar Support herb · Urinary & Kidney Support herb · Liver & Detoxification herb

---

## How It Works

Atractylodes works by **strengthening digestive function and improving nutrient assimilation**, especially when digestion is weak or sluggish. Its drying action helps **reduce excess fluid accumulation**, supporting healthy fluid balance and reducing edema. By restoring digestive efficiency, it supports **steady metabolic energy and blood sugar regulation**. This digestive strengthening also enhances **immune resilience**, which depends on proper nutrient uptake. Overall, Atractylodes acts as a **foundational gut-strengthening herb that restores digestion, energy, and internal balance**.

---

### *Primary Uses*

- *Strengthens spleen and stomach Qi*

- Reduces bloating, fatigue, and loose stools
- Improves appetite and nutrient absorption
- *Clears dampness and phlegm*
- *Gently supports immune vitality*

---

## 🧪 Scientific Backing

Atractylodes contains atractylenolides and polysaccharides that show gastroprotective, antimicrobial, immunomodulatory, and anti-fatigue actions. Research supports its ability to enhance digestive motility, maintain mucosal integrity, and modulate immune responses.

---

## 💊 *Forms Available*

- *Dried powdered root*
- *Encapsulated extracts*
- *Traditional decoction blends*
- *Tincture*

---

## 📏 How to Use (Dosage)

- **Decoction:** 1 Tbsp root per 2 cups water; simmer 20 minutes; drink daily
- ***Powder:*** *500–1000 mg, up to 2× daily*
- **Tincture:** 30–60 drops (1–2 mL), up to 3× daily

---

## ⌛ *Expected Results*

- *Digestive relief: 1–3 days*
- *Spleen/stomach tone: 2–4 weeks*
- Energy and immune improvement: 3–6 weeks

---

## ⚠ Caution Level: 🟢 Safe

Atractylodes is considered a 🟢 **safe** tonic herb when used within normal therapeutic dosage.
However:

- Its warming, drying properties may aggravate **yin deficiency** or constitutional dryness.
- Avoid during acute fevers or inflammatory heat states.
- Prolonged high-dose use without balancing herbs can cause digestive dryness, thirst, or overstimulation.

Use in balanced formulas if dryness develops (pair with Licorice, Rehmannia, or moistening herbs).

---

## 🚺🚹 Gender-Specific Safety

- **Men:** Supports digestion, reduces dampness, and strengthens energy without hormonal effects. Safe for daily use; excessive intake may lead to dryness. Excellent post-illness tonic.
- **Women:** Helpful for fatigue, water retention, and sluggish digestion due to hormonal or metabolic imbalances. Traditionally used postpartum to restore strength.
- **Pregnancy / Nursing:** Avoid during early pregnancy due to stimulating digestive nature. May reduce milk flow if used in excess. If needed, use only under professional supervision in later pregnancy or nursing.

---

## 🛠 DIY Recipe — Spleen-Strengthening Tea

- *1 Tbsp Atractylodes root*
- *½ tsp dried Ginger*
- 2 cups water
  Simmer 20 minutes. Sip after meals to support digestive strength.

---

## *Same / Similar Results*

- *Ginseng*
- *Licorice Root*
- *Astragalus*
- *Slippery Elm*
- *Ginger*

---

## 📦 Shelf Life / Potency After Preparation

- **Dried root or powder:** 2+ years when stored airtight and dry
- **Tincture:** 3–5 years when preserved in 40–50% alcohol
- **Decoction:** Refrigerate for 24–48 hours only; discard if cloudiness develops

Store herbs in a cool, dark place to maintain maximum potency and aroma.

---

## 💬 Herbal Reflections of Atractylodes

Atractylodes is the quiet backbone of vitality — a steadfast builder that restores digestive rhythm so energy can pool rather than leak. It moves slowly, drying dampness, tonifying the center, and offering enough strength for the body to restore itself.
Its lesson: **healing is a process of addition, not subtraction.** Meal by meal, cup by cup, this root nourishes the foundation so stamina returns naturally.

---

⭐ **Herbal Confidence Index:** 🌿 🌿 🌿 🌿 🌿
*(5/5 — a foundational Qi tonic and digestive strengthener; exceptionally reliable for dampness resolution, digestive stamina, and steady systemic vitality.)*

# CLOVE BASIL

★★★★

*Ocimum gratissimum*

**Clove Basil**—also known as African Basil or Wild Basil—is a strongly aromatic medicinal basil traditionally used to support immune defense, respiratory comfort, and microbial balance. Rich in eugenol, it offers warming antimicrobial and anti-inflammatory activity that makes it especially useful during acute infections, fevers, and digestive upsets when used with moderation.

Prepared historically as teas, steams, and topical applications across African, Indian, and Caribbean traditions, Clove Basil is best known today for clearing respiratory congestion, supporting digestion, and providing topical protection during short-term challenges rather than daily long-term use.

---

### Core Herbal Category — Clove Basil

**Primary Core: Immune System Support** herb with (aromatic antimicrobial action that supports immune response and respiratory defense)

**Secondary Cores:** Respiratory Support herb · Digestive Support herb · Circulatory & Cardiovascular herb · Skin & Tissue Repair herb

---

### How It Works

Clove Basil delivers volatile aromatic compounds that inhibit microbial growth and support immune activity. Its warming nature helps open respiratory passages and mobilize circulation during congestion or fever. In the digestive tract, it helps reduce microbial imbalance and gas, while topical use supports localized antimicrobial protection when applied appropriately.

---

### Primary Uses

- Immune and antimicrobial support
- Cough, cold, asthma, and chest congestion relief
- Fever and inflammatory support
- Digestive discomfort and microbial imbalance

• Topical cleansing for bites, rashes, and minor wounds

---

### Scientific Backing

Clove Basil contains eugenol, thymol, linalool, and rosmarinic acid—compounds shown to exhibit antimicrobial, antifungal, antiviral, and anti-inflammatory activity. Research supports traditional respiratory, digestive, and topical uses, though potency varies by preparation and dose.

---

### Forms Available

- Fresh or dried leaf
- Tea or infusion
- Tincture or liquid extract
- Essential oil (topical use only, always diluted)

---

### How to Use (Dosage)

**Tea:** 1 teaspoon dried leaf (or 1 tablespoon fresh), steep 5–10 minutes, up to 2× daily
**Steam:** 1 tablespoon herb added to hot water; inhale 10–15 minutes
**Tincture:** ~1 mL (30 drops), 1–2× daily
**Poultice:** Crushed fresh leaves applied topically
Use short-term during acute need.

---

### Caution Level: Caution

May lower blood pressure—monitor if using antihypertensives
Avoid high-dose internal use during pregnancy (eugenol content)
Essential oil is potent—always dilute; external use only
Excessive use may irritate mucous membranes or overstimulate sensitive individuals
Mildly stimulating; not ideal for chronic insomnia

---

### Gender-Specific Safety

**Men:** Supports immune defense, respiratory clarity, and digestive warmth; use concentrated forms sparingly.

**Women:** Helpful for congestion and microbial balance; prefer tea or light tincture.

**Pregnancy/Nursing:** Light culinary or mild tea amounts only; avoid tinctures and essential oil internally.

### Expected Results

- Respiratory relief: 30–60 minutes
- Topical cleansing effects: 1–5 days
- Digestive balance: 1–2 weeks

---

### 🛠 DIY Recipe — Antiseptic Clove Basil Steam

Add 1 tablespoon dried (or a handful fresh) Clove Basil to a bowl of hot water. Cover head with a towel and inhale steam for 10–15 minutes.

---

### 🔄 Same / Similar Results

- Clove
- Thyme
- Holy Basil (Tulsi)
- Oregano
- Eucalyptus

---

### Shelf Life / Potency After Preparation

- Dried leaves: 1–2 years (airtight, dark storage)
- Tincture: 3–5 years
- Essential oil: 2–3 years (cool, dark; dilute before use)
- Prepared tea: Use within 24 hours refrigerated

### 💬 Herbal Reflections of Clove Basil

Clove Basil acts with clarity and purpose—warming, cleansing, and protective without subtlety. It is best called upon when decisive action is needed, reminding us that strong medicine works best with timing, respect, and restraint.

**Herbal Confidence Index:** 🌿 🌿 🌿 🌿

*(4/5 — potent aromatic antimicrobial with strong respiratory and topical benefits; highly effective when used mindfully and in moderation.)*

# OLIVE LEAF

★★★★★

*Olea europaea*

**Olive Leaf** is a well-established immune and cardiovascular support herb traditionally used to help the body manage infections, inflammation, and metabolic stress. Its bitter compound oleuropein provides antioxidant and antimicrobial activity that supports immune balance, vascular resilience, and overall systemic steadiness.

Honored for centuries in Mediterranean and Middle Eastern traditions, Olive Leaf tea was used for fevers, infections, and circulatory complaints. Today, modern research supports these traditional uses, confirming Olive Leaf as a quiet, dependable ally for long-term resilience rather than rapid stimulation.

---

### 🌿 Core Herbal Category — Olive Leaf

**Primary Core: Immune System Support** herb with (antimicrobial and vascular-protective action that supports natural defense and heart–vessel resilience)

**Secondary Cores:** Metabolic Balance herb · Anti-Inflammatory Support herb

---

### 🌿 How It Works

Olive Leaf supports immune defense by inhibiting microbial activity while supplying antioxidant protection to tissues and blood vessels. Its polyphenols help maintain healthy blood pressure, vascular tone, and glucose metabolism, reducing inflammatory stress without overstimulating the system. This steady action makes it well suited for both short-term immune challenges and ongoing foundational support.

---

### 🌱 Primary Uses

- Immune support against viral, bacterial, and fungal stress
- Blood pressure and circulatory balance
- Antioxidant and anti-inflammatory protection
- Cholesterol and metabolic support
- General vitality during seasonal challenges

---

### 🧪 Scientific Backing

Olive Leaf contains oleuropein and related polyphenols shown to support antimicrobial activity, vascular elasticity, oxidative balance, and glucose regulation. Clinical studies support benefits in hypertension, metabolic syndrome, and immune modulation, closely aligning with long-standing traditional use.

---

### Forms Available

- Dried leaf (tea or decoction)
- Standardized extracts or tinctures (15–25% oleuropein)
- Capsules and liquid concentrates

---

### How to Use (Dosage)

**Tea:** 1 tablespoon dried leaf simmered 15 minutes; drink 1–2× daily
**Capsules:** 300–600 mg extract, 1–2× daily
**Tincture:** 1–2 mL up to 2× daily
**Immune cycle:** Use daily for 7–14 days during acute need

---

### Caution Level: Safe

Generally well tolerated
Mild detox symptoms (headache, fatigue, loose stools) may occur initially
Monitor blood pressure and blood sugar if medicated
Maintain adequate hydration

---

### Gender-Specific Safety

**Men:** Excellent support for circulation, cholesterol balance, and immunity; no hormonal concerns.

**Women:** Safe for long-term immune and metabolic stability.

**Pregnancy/Nursing:** Mild tea acceptable; avoid high-potency extracts unless supervised.

---

### Expected Results

- Immune support: 5–7 days
- Circulatory and metabolic effects: 2–3 weeks
- Antioxidant benefits: ongoing with regular use

---

### DIY Recipe — Olive Leaf Immunity Decoction

Simmer 1 tablespoon Olive Leaf in 2 cups water for 15 minutes.
Strain and drink once daily.

---

***Same / Similar Results*** *Garlic* *Oregano* *Elderberry* *Turmeric* *Green Tea*

---

### Shelf Life / Potency After Preparation

- Dried leaves: Up to 2 years
- Capsules/powder: 18–24 months
- Tincture: 4–6 years
- Decoction: Use within 48 hours refrigerated

---

### Herbal Reflections of Olive Leaf

Olive Leaf offers protection through steadiness rather than force. Like the tree itself, it endures—clearing excess, stabilizing fluctuations, and strengthening resilience quietly over time. Its medicine reminds us that lasting health is built through consistency, not urgency.

---

### Herbal Confidence Index:

(5/5 — top-tier antimicrobial and cardiovascular support herb; exceptionally safe, reliable, and effective for long-term systemic resilience.)

# FEVER TREE

★★

*Cinchona officinalis*

**Fever Tree bark** is historically significant as the natural source of quinine, long used to address severe fevers and malaria. Its bitter, alkaloid-rich bark exerts powerful antipyretic and antimicrobial effects, making it effective—but also potentially dangerous—when misused.

Indigenous Andean healers first employed this bark, later introducing it to Europe where it reshaped fever treatment. Today, whole-bark use is largely historical and symbolic, with modern medicine favoring standardized derivatives due to safety concerns.

---

### 🌿 Core Herbal Category — Fever Tree

**Primary Core: Immune System Support** herb with (bitter, heat-clearing action historically used to reduce severe febrile states)

**Secondary Cores:** Liver & Detoxification herb · Digestive Support herb · Circulatory & Cardiovascular herb

---

### 🌿 *How It Works*

*Fever Tree's alkaloids interrupt intense fever patterns and exert antimicrobial effects that historically aided survival during severe infections. Its bitterness stimulates digestion and liver activity, supporting toxin clearance during illness. However, its narrow therapeutic window means these effects are accompanied by significant toxicity risk, limiting safe use to controlled settings.*

---

### 🌱 Primary Uses (Historical / External)

- Historical treatment of malaria and infectious fevers
- Short-term fever reduction under medical supervision
- Circulatory and bitter-digestive stimulation
- External liniments for muscle or joint discomfort

---

### 🧪 Scientific Backing

Cinchona bark contains quinine and related alkaloids with proven antimalarial and antipyretic activity. While historically life-saving, these compounds carry well-documented toxicity risks, leading modern medicine to isolate and strictly dose quinine derivatives rather than use whole bark.

---

### Forms Available

- Dried bark (historical; professional supervision only)
- Tinctures or extracts (controlled, clinical use)
- Quinine-based pharmaceuticals
- Topical liniments or infused oils

---

### How to Use (Dosage)

**Internal use:** Not recommended outside licensed medical supervision.
**Topical use:** Infuse 1 teaspoon powdered bark in 1 cup olive oil for 24 hours; strain and apply to intact skin only. Do not ingest.

---

### Caution Level: ● Supervision Required

● High toxicity risk: nausea, tinnitus, dizziness, vision changes, cardiac irregularities
● Internal use only under licensed medical supervision
● Avoid in pregnancy, nursing, and in heart, liver, or kidney conditions
● Do not combine with blood thinners or cardiac medications
● External use only in diluted form

---

### Gender-Specific Safety

**Men:** Historical fever use acknowledged; internal use requires professional supervision. Diluted external use acceptable.
**Women:** Same restrictions apply; internal use may cause significant side effects.
● **Pregnancy/Nursing:** Absolutely contraindicated due to uterine and fetal risk.

---

### Expected Results

- Fever reduction: 1–2 days (medical supervision only)
- Circulatory support: as fever resolves
- Topical pain relief: hours to 1–2 days

---

### DIY Recipe — External Fever Tree Rub (Topical Use Only)

Infuse 1 teaspoon powdered Fever Tree bark in 1 cup olive oil for 24 hours.
Strain and apply sparingly to intact skin over sore areas. Do not ingest.

---

***Same / Similar Results*** *Andrographis* *Cat's Claw* *Neem* *Elderflower*

Willow Bark

---

**Shelf Life / Potency After Preparation**

Dried bark: 2+ years (cool, dark, airtight)

Tinctures/extracts: 3–5 years

Infused oils: Up to 1 year (cool, dark storage)

---

**Herbal Reflections of Fever Tree**

Fever Tree stands as both triumph and warning—proof of nature's power to save lives when guided, and to harm when mishandled. Its legacy reminds us that strength in medicine must always be balanced by restraint, knowledge, and respect.

---

**Herbal Confidence Index:**

(2/5 — historically vital antimalarial herb; profoundly effective under control, but unsuitable for general internal use due to toxicity.)

# ISATIS

★★★

*Isatis tinctoria / Isatis indigotica*

**Isatis** is a strongly cooling, detoxifying immune herb traditionally used to address acute viral infections, sore throats, swollen glands, and febrile inflammation. In Traditional Chinese Medicine, both the root (Ban Lan Gen) and leaf (Da Qing Ye) are valued for clearing toxic heat while supporting the body's antiviral and antibacterial defenses.

For centuries, Isatis has served as a frontline remedy during epidemics across East Asia. Ban Lan Gen tea was commonly taken at the first sign of illness or during outbreaks as a protective measure. Modern research continues to support its short-term use as a decisive, heat-clearing ally during acute infection rather than a daily tonic.

---

### Core Herbal Category — Isatis

**Primary Core: Immune System Support** herb with (intense antiviral, heat-clearing action that cools toxic heat during acute infection)

**Secondary Cores:** Respiratory Support herb · Liver & Detoxification herb · Musculoskeletal & Pain-Relief herb

---

### *How It Works*

*Isatis works by rapidly clearing pathogenic heat and reducing inflammatory viral load during acute illness. Its cooling compounds help calm immune overactivation while supporting antiviral defense, particularly in the throat and upper respiratory tract. At the same time, it assists the liver in processing inflammatory byproducts. Its role is short-term intervention, not long-term immune tonification.*

---

### Primary Uses

- Viral sore throats, colds, and flu states
- Fever reduction and lymphatic swelling
- Acute respiratory infections
- Liver support during inflammatory overload
- Short-term epidemic or outbreak support

---

🧪 **Scientific Backing**

Isatis contains indigo, indirubin, and tryptanthrin, compounds shown in laboratory and clinical settings to exert antiviral, antibacterial, and anti-inflammatory effects. Studies and TCM clinical use report faster fever and sore-throat resolution when used early in infection.

---

💊 **Forms Available**

- Dried root (Ban Lan Gen)
- Dried leaf (Da Qing Ye)
- Capsules and standardized tinctures

---

📏 **How to Use (Dosage)**

**Decoction:** 1 tsp dried root in 2 cups water, simmer 20 minutes; up to 2× daily
**Tincture:** 30–40 drops, 2× daily at first signs of illness
**Capsules:** 300–600 mg, up to 3× daily
👉 Discontinue once symptoms improve

---

⚠️ **Caution Level:** 🟡 **Caution**

🟡 Safe for short-term use only
🟡 Excessive or prolonged use may cause fatigue, chills, loose stools, or digestive weakness
🟡 Avoid with anemia, chronic fatigue, or weak digestion
🔴 Avoid during pregnancy
🟡 Restore warmth and nourishment after use

---

🚹 🚺 **Gender-Specific Safety**

🟡 **Men:** Effective during acute infection; avoid prolonged use to prevent digestive depletion.

🟡 **Women:** Helpful for short courses during infection or inflammatory flare; limit to 5–10 days.

🔴 **Pregnancy/Nursing:** Avoid entirely due to strong cooling and detoxifying actions.

---

⏳ **Expected Results**

- Throat and fever relief: 24–48 hours
- General symptom improvement: 2–3 days
- Preventive support (short-term): 1–2 weeks

---

🛠️ **DIY Recipe — Immune Defender Decoction**

Simmer 1 tsp Isatis root with ½ tsp Licorice root and 1 tsp Elderflower for 20 minutes.

Strain and sip warm at the first sign of fever or sore throat.

---

***Same / Similar Foundation*** *Andrographis* *Elderberry* *Chinese Skullcap* *Olive Leaf* *Yarrow*

---

**Shelf Life / Potency After Preparation**

- Dried root/leaf: Up to 2 years (airtight, cool, dark)
- Tincture: 3–5 years
- Decoction: Use within 24 hours (refrigerated)

---

**Herbal Reflections of Isatis**

Isatis is a decisive ally, called upon when heat and infection overwhelm the system. It intervenes swiftly, clears excess, and then steps aside—teaching restraint as much as strength. Its medicine lies in knowing when to act and when to withdraw, restoring balance without lingering force.

---

**Herbal Confidence Index:**

(3/5 — reliable antiviral and heat-clearing herb; highly effective for acute infection support, best reserved for short-term or supervised use.)

# PASQUE FLOWER

★★★★★

*Pulsatilla vulgaris*

**Pasque Flower** is a powerful nervine and reproductive-system ally traditionally used for acute nervous agitation, emotional overwhelm, and spasmodic pain associated with PMS and painful menstruation. In carefully controlled micro-doses, it acts as a strong sedative—quieting headaches, nerve tension, uterine cramping, and restlessness rather than serving as a daily calming tonic.

In European folk medicine, Pasque Flower was valued as much for emotional healing as for physical relief. It was used for grief, shock, hysteria, and deep emotional distress, especially during hormonal transitions. While the fresh plant is toxic, traditional tincturing and homeopathic dilution allowed skilled practitioners to transform it into a precise, delicate medicine—one that demands respect and restraint.

---

### Core Herbal Category — Pasque Flower

**Primary Core: Nervous System Support (Nervines)** herb with (strong sedative action that quiets acute nervous agitation and emotional overload)

**Secondary Cores:** Musculoskeletal & Pain-Relief herb · Hormonal & Endocrine Support herb · Immune Support herb

---

### How It Works

Pasque Flower works by strongly reducing nervous system overactivity, producing deep calm during states of acute agitation, spasms, or emotional distress. Its compounds relax nerve-driven tension and smooth spasmodic pain, particularly in the reproductive system. Because it directly affects both the nervous and endocrine systems, its action is intense and short-term. Pasque Flower is not a general tonic and must be used with strict care and professional oversight.

---

### Primary Uses

- Acute anxiety, restlessness, and emotional overload
- PMS, uterine cramps, and spasmodic menstrual pain
- Nervous headaches and tension
- Grief, shock, and hysterical states

• Light insomnia driven by agitation

---

### Scientific Backing

Pasque Flower contains ranunculin and anemonin, compounds associated with sedative, antispasmodic, and antimicrobial activity. Historical pharmacognosy records confirm its use for hysteria, uterine pain, headaches, and nerve agitation. Modern herbal consensus emphasizes that safety depends entirely on dilution and dosing, as the fresh plant is toxic.

---

### Forms Available

Homeopathic tablets or drops

Highly diluted tincture (professional use only)

---

### How to Use (Dosage)

• Tincture (guided use only): 5–15 drops in water, up to 3× daily
• Homeopathic preparations are the safest and most common form
• Dried herb teas are **not recommended**

---

### Caution Level: Supervision Required

Pasque Flower is highly potent and potentially toxic. The fresh plant contains protoanemonin, which can cause severe irritation, nausea, neurological symptoms, or paralysis if misused. Internal use must occur only under qualified professional supervision, in minute doses or homeopathic dilution. Do not self-prepare. Keep away from children and pets.

---

### Gender-Specific Safety

**Men:** Historically used for nerve pain, agitation, and insomnia; internal use only with professional guidance. Even small overdoses may cause nausea or irritation.

**Women:** Occasionally used in very small doses for cramps or emotional distress; self-use strongly discouraged due to narrow safety margin.

**Pregnancy / Nursing: Strictly contraindicated.** Uterine-stimulating and toxic potential makes all internal use unsafe.

---

### Expected Results

• Emotional calming: within hours
• Menstrual or spasm relief: 1–3 days
• Nervous system settling: 1–2 weeks (guided use)

---

### DIY Recipe — PMS Calming Tonic (Professional guidance required)

10 drops Pasque Flower tincture
20 drops Lemon Balm tincture
1 tsp warm water
Stir gently and sip before rest.

---

### 🔄 Same / Similar Results

- Motherwort
- Lemon Balm
- Chamomile
- Cramp Bark
- Valerian

---

### Shelf Life / Potency After Preparation

- Dried aerial parts: 1–2 years (potency declines after ~18 months)
- Diluted tincture: 4–6 years (most stable form)
- Tea / infusion: **Not recommended**
- Fresh plant: Use immediately only by experienced herbalists

---

### Herbal Reflections of Pasque Flower

Pasque Flower is a medicine of tenderness and restraint—capable of easing profound emotional and physical distress when used with care. It teaches balance through precision: too much harms, but the right dose restores calm and composure. Its lesson is one of respect, reminding us that the most powerful medicines demand the greatest humility.

---

### Herbal Confidence Index: 🌿 🌿

(2/5 green stars — potent nervine and antispasmodic herb; historically valuable but restricted to micro-doses or professional supervision due to toxicity.)

# *HEARTSEASE*

★★★★

*Viola tricolor*

**Heartsease** is a gentle skin-, lung-, and nervous-supporting herb traditionally used for eczema, acne, coughs, and grief-related stress. Its mild anti-inflammatory and demulcent actions make it especially useful for chronic rashes, respiratory irritation, and sensitive constitutions. Prepared as teas, washes, or poultices, it offers steady relief without strain. In European tradition, Heartsease was regarded as both a physical and emotional remedy. Its name reflects its long use for easing grief and nervous tension, while healers valued it for clearing the lungs, soothing inflamed skin, and gently purifying the blood. Small yet resilient, it became known as a quiet but dependable restorative.

---

### 🌿 Core Herbal Category — Heartsease

**Primary Core: Lymphatic & Skin Support** herb with (demulcent and gentle astringent action that soothes irritated surface tissues)

**Secondary Cores:** Anti-Inflammatory Support herb · Lymphatic Support herb · Nervous System Support herb

---

### 🌿 How It Works

Heartsease soothes inflamed skin and sensitive tissues through its demulcent compounds while gently toning with mild astringency. It supports lymphatic movement, helping clear inflammatory byproducts that contribute to rashes. Its light nervine action calms stress that often aggravates skin conditions. Through consistent, gentle use, it restores balance without drying or overstimulation.

---

### 🌱 Primary Uses

- Eczema, acne, and chronic rashes
- Coughs, phlegm, and bronchial irritation
- Gentle cardiovascular and circulatory support
- Emotional calm during grief or nervousness
- Blood- and lymph-cleansing support

---

### 🔬 Scientific Backing

Research on Viola tricolor supports its traditional use as a skin-clearing, anti-inflammatory, and mild diuretic herb. It contains flavonoids, saponins, and salicylate derivatives shown to reduce skin irritation and support eczema, acne, and psoriasis. Studies also note antioxidant and expectorant properties, explaining its value in coughs and bronchial congestion.

---

### 💊 Forms Available

- Dried herb
- Extracts and tinctures
- Skin washes, salves, and poultices

---

### 📏 How to Use (Dosage)

- Tea: 1–2 tsp dried herb, steep 10 minutes, up to 3× daily
- Tincture: 1–2 mL (30–40 drops), 2–3× daily
- Topical: Use cooled tea or poultice on irritated skin

---

### ⚠️ Caution Level: 🟢 Safe

Generally well tolerated.

- Avoid internal use if allergic to salicylates or aspirin
- Large doses may cause mild stomach irritation
- Patch-test topical applications on sensitive skin

Safe for children and seniors.

---

### 👨 👩 Gender-Specific Safety

🟢 **Men:** Supports skin clarity, circulation, and mild respiratory issues; non-hormonal.

🟢 **Women:** Helpful for hormonal breakouts, PMS-related skin changes, and emotional balance.

🟢 **Pregnancy / Nursing:** Generally safe in tea or food-level amounts; avoid prolonged high-dose extracts.

---

### ⏳ Expected Results

- Respiratory relief: 1–3 days
- Skin clarity: 5–7 days
- Emotional calm: ~1 week

---

### 🛠️ DIY Recipes

**Heart-Centered Skin Wash**
1 Tbsp Heartsease + 1 tsp Calendula
Steep in 1 cup hot water, cool, strain, and apply gently.

**Heartsease Comfort Tea**
1 tsp Heartsease + ½ tsp Lemon Balm
Steep 10 minutes; sip for skin, nerves, and emotional ease.

---

**🔄 Same / Similar Results**

- Calendula
- Red Clover
- Sweet Violet
- Chamomile
- Skullcap

---

**Shelf Life / Potency After Preparation**

- Dried herb: 1–2 years (airtight, cool, dark)
- Tincture: 3–5 years
- Washes / salves: 6–12 months depending on base

---

**Herbal Reflections of Heartsease**

Heartsease offers quiet resilience—softening inflamed skin, easing troubled breath, and gently lifting grief. It bridges outer and inner healing, reminding us that restoration often arrives patiently and without force.

**Herbal Confidence Index:** 🌿 🌿 🌿 🌿
(4/5 green stars — gentle, reliable skin and lymphatic herb; exceptionally safe and effective for inflammatory skin conditions and emotional soothing.)

# LABRADOR TEA

★★

*Rhododendron groenlandicum*

**Labrador Tea** is a warming northern herb traditionally used for respiratory irritation, mild digestive upset, and nervous tension. Indigenous peoples of North America prepared it as a light tea to ease coughs, sinus congestion, nausea, and fatigue during illness or harsh seasonal conditions. Its aromatic compounds offer short-term soothing and anti-inflammatory support.

Among Arctic and boreal cultures, Labrador Tea carried both medicinal and ceremonial significance. Valued as a calming lung tea and a survival herb during scarcity, it was respected for its strength and used sparingly. This tradition reflects its narrow but meaningful therapeutic window.

---

### Core Herbal Category — Labrador Tea

**Primary Core: Respiratory System Support** herb with (astringent, aromatic action that tones inflamed mucous membranes and eases airway irritation)

**Secondary Cores:** Nervous System Support herb · Digestive Support herb · Immune Support herb

---

### How It Works

Labrador Tea tones irritated respiratory tissues, helping reduce inflammation and excessive secretions. Its aromatic constituents calm nervous tension that can aggravate breathing and digestion. In very small doses, it soothes mild nausea and spasms. Its action is short-term and situational, making it unsuitable as a daily tonic.

---

### Primary Uses

- Coughs, colds, and chest congestion
- Sinus pressure and restricted breathing
- Mild nausea and digestive discomfort
- Nervous tension and seasonal fatigue
- Antioxidant and immune support

---

### Scientific Backing

Labrador Tea contains ledol, arbutin, and quercetin—compounds with antimicrobial and anti-inflammatory activity. Research supports its traditional respiratory and digestive uses. However, ledol contributes to potential neuro- and hepatotoxic effects when used in excess or concentrated form.

---

### 💊 Forms Available

- Dried leaves (tea)
- Low-concentration tincture
- Essential oil — **external use only**

---

### 📏 How to Use (Dosage)

- **Light tea:** 1 tsp dried leaves, steep ≤10 minutes; **max 1 cup daily for up to 3 days**
- **Tincture:** 20–30 drops in water, 1× daily (short-term only)
- **Steam:** Small amount added to hot water for sinus relief

Only use **Rhododendron groenlandicum** — other "wild teas" may be toxic.

---

### ⚠️ Caution Level: ● Supervision Required

High doses or prolonged use may cause nausea, dizziness, liver strain, or neurological effects. Avoid internal use during pregnancy, nursing, liver disease, or in children. Never ingest essential oil. Use only occasionally, in low doses, and with care.

---

### 🚹 🚺 Gender-Specific Safety

● **Men:** May ease bronchial congestion or winter fatigue when used sparingly; avoid repeated use.

● **Women:** Can calm sinus pressure or anxiety in small doses; not for long-term use.

● **Pregnancy / Nursing: Contraindicated.** Avoid completely.

---

### ⏳ Expected Results

- Respiratory easing: 1–2 days
- Digestive or nausea relief: within hours
- Nervous relaxation: 30–60 minutes
- Sinus clearing: immediate with steam

---

### 🛠️ DIY — Northern Lung Tea (Short-Term Use)

1 tsp Labrador Tea
1 tsp Mullein
½ tsp Thyme
Steep 10 minutes. Limit to **1 cup daily for no more than 3 days**.

---

### 🔄 Same / Similar Results

- Mullein
- Thyme
- Lemon Balm
- Yarrow
- Chamomile

---

### Shelf Life / Potency After Preparation

- Dried leaves: 1–2 years (airtight, cool, dark)
- Tincture: ~3 years
- Prepared tea: Use within 24 hours

Do not store or reuse strong infusions.

---

### Herbal Reflections of Labrador Tea

Labrador Tea reflects the discipline of the North—strong medicine that demands restraint. It offers clarity and warmth when needed, but teaches that power must be bounded by respect. Its lesson is simple: healing is strongest when limits are honored.

---

### Herbal Confidence Index: 🌿 🌿

(2/5 green stars — effective respiratory and digestive aid with narrow safety margins; best reserved for short-term, guided use.)

# ROSEMARY

★★★★★

*Rosmarinus officinalis*

**Rosemary** is a classic stimulant for the brain, circulation, and digestion. Traditionally used to sharpen memory, uplift mood, and reduce inflammation, its aromatic oils enhance mental clarity while supporting cardiovascular and digestive function. It has long been massaged into the scalp for hair growth and inhaled for focus and alertness.
Across the Mediterranean, Rosemary symbolized remembrance, vitality, and protection. Used in food, ritual, and medicine, it bridged daily nourishment with therapeutic power. Modern research now confirms its antioxidant, antimicrobial, and circulation-enhancing effects, validating centuries of traditional use.

---

### Core Herbal Category — Rosemary

**Primary Core: Cardiovascular System Support** herb with (stimulating action that enhances cerebral and peripheral blood flow, improving clarity and vitality)
**Secondary Cores:** Nervous System Support herb · Digestive Support herb · Immune Support herb

---

### How It Works

Rosemary stimulates circulation, especially to the brain, improving oxygen delivery and cognitive performance. Its aromatic compounds activate and tone the nervous system without sedation. Digestively, it stimulates gastric function and relieves sluggishness. Antioxidant constituents protect tissues from oxidative stress, supporting immune and cardiovascular resilience.

---

### Primary Uses

- Memory, focus, and mental clarity
- Scalp circulation and hair support
- Inflammation, stiffness, and muscle tension
- Bloating and sluggish digestion
- Circulatory and energy support
- Antimicrobial respiratory and skin aid

---

### Scientific Backing

Rosemary contains carnosic acid, rosmarinic acid, cineole, and camphor—compounds shown to be antioxidant, neuroprotective, anti-inflammatory, and antimicrobial. Clinical studies confirm improved cognition, alertness, mood, circulation, and topical benefits for scalp and skin health.

---

### Forms Available

- Fresh or dried herb (culinary, tea)
- Essential oil (aromatherapy, topical)
- Tinctures and capsules

---

### How to Use (Dosage)

- **Tea:** 1 tsp dried herb, steep 10–12 minutes
- **Infused oil:** Apply to scalp or sore muscles
- **Aromatherapy:** Diffuse or inhale gently
- **Bath:** 2 Tbsp dried herb or 5 diluted oil drops

---

### Caution Level: Caution

Generally safe in food and tea amounts. Use care with concentrated extracts.

- Avoid high doses during pregnancy
- May raise blood pressure in sensitive individuals
- Always dilute essential oil
- Avoid internal essential-oil use

---

### Gender-Specific Safety

**Men:** Supports circulation, focus, stamina, and hair health; safe long-term in food or tea form.

**Women:** Enhances mood, digestion, circulation, and scalp health; safe in moderate use.

**Pregnancy / Nursing:** Safe in small food or tea amounts; avoid concentrated internal products.

---

### Expected Results

- Mental clarity: 15–30 minutes
- Digestive comfort: 30–45 minutes
- Circulatory or joint support: 1–2 weeks
- Hair/scalp improvement: 2–4 weeks

---

🛠 **DIY — Rosemary Clarity Oil**

1 cup Rosemary

1½ cups olive or jojoba oil

Infuse gently or in sunlight 3–4 weeks. Strain and apply to scalp or muscles.

---

🔄 **Same / Similar Results**

- Peppermint
- Ginkgo
- Gotu Kola
- Thyme
- Lavender

---

**Shelf Life / Potency After Preparation**

- Dried herb: 1–2 years
- Essential oil: 3–4 years
- Infused oil: ~12 months
- Tea: Best within 24 hours

---

💬 **Herbal Reflections of Rosemary**

Rosemary awakens remembrance—not only of memory, but of purpose. It clears stagnation, sharpens thought, and restores motion where dullness lingers. Its lesson is renewal through awareness: when circulation flows, life follows.

---

⭐ **Herbal Confidence Index:** 🌿 🌿 🌿 🌿 🌿

(5/5 green stars — cornerstone circulatory and cognitive herb; exceptionally reliable, safe, and validated across cultures and science.)

# THYME

★★★★★

*Thymus vulgaris*

**Thyme** is a compact yet formidable antimicrobial and lung-supportive herb used to clear mucus, soothe sore throats, and calm spasmodic coughs. Rich in thymol and carvacrol, it provides broad-spectrum protection against bacteria, fungi, and viruses while easing digestive gas and gently steadying the nerves. Prepared as tea, steam, syrup, or diluted oil, Thyme is a first-line ally for colds, bronchitis, and seasonal infections.
From ancient Egypt and Greece to modern kitchens, Thyme has been used for purification, protection, and resilience—burned during plagues and infused to fortify the sick. Its name traces to thumos (spirit or courage), reflecting its tonic lift to weary bodies. A pantry staple with clinical relevance, Thyme bridges daily nourishment and dependable medicine.

---

### 🌿 Core Herbal Category — Thyme

**Primary Core: Respiratory System Support** herb with (aromatic antimicrobial and expectorant action that clears infection and supports airway function)
**Secondary Cores:** Immune Support herb · Digestive Support herb · Circulatory & Cardiovascular herb

---

### 🌿 How It Works

Thyme delivers potent aromatics that inhibit respiratory pathogens while loosening and clearing mucus. Its expectorant action supports productive cough and open airways. Concurrently, it stimulates immune response during infection and acts as a carminative in the gut, easing gas and microbial imbalance. Overall, Thyme is a rapid, warming respiratory herb that restores clarity and defense.

---

### 🌱 Primary Uses

- Clears mucus; soothes sore throats
- Eases coughs, bronchitis, chest congestion
- Supports immune response during illness
- Relieves bloating and digestive discomfort
- Broad antimicrobial support
- Mildly calming to nerves

---

### Scientific Backing

Contains thymol, carvacrol, rosmarinic acid, and flavonoids with validated antimicrobial, antiviral, and antioxidant activity. Clinical studies show Thyme syrups reduce cough and bronchitis symptoms; laboratory data confirm strong antibacterial and antifungal potency.

---

### Forms Available

- Dried herb · Fresh sprigs
- Essential oil
- Syrups, tinctures, capsules

---

### How to Use (Dosage)

- **Tea:** 1 tsp dried herb (or 2–3 fresh sprigs), steep 10–15 min
- **Steam:** Handful in hot water; inhale 5–10 min
- **Chest rub:** Essential oil diluted (1–2 drops per 1 tsp carrier)
- **Gargle:** Cooled tea as throat rinse

---

### Expected Results

- Cough relief: 20–30 minutes
- Digestive ease: 30–60 minutes
- Immune/antimicrobial support: 1–3 days

---

### Caution Level: Caution

- Always dilute essential oil; **no internal EO use**
- Avoid large doses during pregnancy
- Use mild teas only for children under 5
- Watch for mint-family sensitivities
- Avoid concentrated extracts with seizure or blood-pressure medications

---

### Gender-Specific Safety

**Men:** Excellent for sinus congestion, sore throats, digestion; safe in food, tea, steam. Avoid internal EO.

**Women:** Helpful for colds and sinus pressure; supports digestion and circulation. Safe in culinary/tea/topical use.

**Pregnancy / Nursing:** Safe in culinary amounts and mild tea. Avoid concentrated extracts and internal EO; diluted external use is typically safe.

---

### DIY — Thyme Cough Syrup

Simmer 2 Tbsp dried Thyme in 1 cup water for 15 minutes. Strain, cool, add ½ cup raw

honey.
Take 1 tsp every 2–3 hours as needed.

---

**🔄 Same / Similar Results**

- Oregano
- Eucalyptus
- Sage
- Peppermint
- Mullein

---

**Shelf Life / Potency After Preparation**

- Dried herb: 1–2 years (airtight, cool, dark)
- Essential oil: 2–4 years
- Syrup: Up to 2 months refrigerated
- Tea: Same day (24 hrs refrigerated)

---

**Herbal Reflections of Thyme**

Thyme restores movement—loosening phlegm, brightening digestion, and firming boundaries when the chest feels heavy. A humble kitchen leaf that becomes clinic-grade medicine, it reminds us that courage and clarity often arrive in small forms.

---

**Herbal Confidence Index:** 🌿 🌿 🌿 🌿 🌿

(5/5 green stars — cornerstone antimicrobial and respiratory herb; exceptionally reliable, safe, and well-validated across cultures.)

# ST. JOHN'S WORT

★★★★★

*Hypericum perforatum*

**St. John's Wort** is a classic nervine for mild–moderate depression, anxious tension, and nerve irritation. It supports emotional steadiness, sleep quality, and stress resilience while offering notable analgesic and anti-inflammatory effects. Its infused oil is especially valued for nerve pain, sciatica, burns, and sun-irritated skin.

Long regarded as a "sun herb" in European folk medicine, St. John's Wort symbolizes the restoration of light during emotional darkness. Modern research confirms its effectiveness for mild–moderate depression and nerve pain. However, its strong interaction profile requires informed and responsible use.

---

### Core Herbal Category — St. John's Wort

**Primary Core: Nervous System Support (Nervines)** herb with (uplifting, mood-stabilizing action that supports emotional balance and nerve resilience)

**Secondary Cores:** Musculoskeletal & Pain-Relief herb · Liver & Detoxification herb · Immune Support herb · Skin & Tissue Repair herb

---

### How It Works

St. John's Wort supports neurotransmitter balance, helping stabilize mood and reduce mild to moderate depressive states. It calms nerve irritation, eases neuralgia, and supports nerve recovery. Topically, it promotes tissue repair and reduces inflammation. Systemically, it offers antiviral and immune support during stress-related depletion. Overall, it functions as a nerve-restorative herb for mood, pain, and recovery.

---

### Primary Uses

- Supports mild–moderate depression and nervous exhaustion
- Reduces anxiety and stress-related sleep disturbance
- Soothes nerve pain and neuralgia
- Anti-inflammatory and mild analgesic
- Topical healing for burns, bruises, and wounds

---

### Scientific Backing

Key compounds include hypericin and hyperforin, which influence serotonin, dopamine, and norepinephrine pathways. Clinical trials show comparable effectiveness to some antidepressants in mild–moderate cases. Strong evidence confirms significant drug–herb interactions via CYP450 induction.

---

### Forms Available

- Dried herb (tea or capsules)
- Standardized extracts
- Infused oil (topical)
- Homeopathic preparations

---

### How to Use (Dosage)

- **Tea:** 1–2 tsp dried herb, steep 10–15 min
- **Tincture:** 30–60 drops, 2–3× daily
- **Capsules:** 300 mg standardized extract, 1–3× daily
- **Infused oil:** External use for nerve pain or skin repair

---

### Expected Results

- Mood support: 7–14 days
- Improved sleep and calm: ~1 week
- Nerve pain relief (topical): 15–30 minutes
- Wound soothing: 2–4 days

---

### Caution Level: Caution

- **Major drug interactions** (SSRIs, MAOIs, birth control, anticoagulants, immunosuppressants, HIV meds)
- May reduce effectiveness of hormonal therapies
- Photosensitivity possible
- Avoid in bipolar spectrum without supervision

---

### Gender-Specific Safety

**Men:** Useful for low mood and nerve pain; monitor medication interactions and sun sensitivity.

**Women:** Supports mood and menopausal anxiety; may reduce birth-control effectiveness.

**Pregnancy / Nursing:** Avoid unless under qualified supervision.

---

### Same / Similar Foundation

Lemon Balm

- Ashwagandha
- Passionflower
- Rhodiola
- Valerian

---

**Shelf Life / Potency**

- Dried herb: 1–2 years (dark, airtight)
- Infused oil: ~1 year
- Tincture: 4–5 years
- Extracts: 2–3 years (check label)

---

**Herbal Reflections of St. John's Wort**

St. John's Wort restores light where emotional fatigue has settled, gently repairing the nervous system while lifting the spirit. Its medicine is steady rather than abrupt, asking for patience and respect. It teaches that illumination heals best when paired with discernment.

---

**Herbal Confidence Index:**

(4/5 — highly effective and well-studied; loses one star due to significant drug interactions.)

---

# HIBISCUS

★★★★★

Hibiscus sabdariffa

**Hibiscus** is a cooling circulatory tonic that supports healthy blood pressure, liver clearance, and cholesterol balance. Rich in anthocyanins and vitamin C, it helps reduce oxidative stress, cool excess metabolic heat, and promote gentle detoxification while refreshing the body.

Used worldwide as both medicine and celebration, hibiscus tea has earned strong clinical support for cardiometabolic health. It stands out as one of the rare herbs that is both therapeutically effective and suitable for daily enjoyment, bridging traditional use with modern validation.

---

### 🌿 Core Herbal Category — Hibiscus

**Primary Core: Cardiovascular System Support** herb with (cooling, vasodilatory action that supports healthy blood pressure and vascular tone)

**Secondary Cores:** Digestive Support herb · Liver & Detoxification herb · Skin & Tissue Repair herb · Women's Health herb

---

### 🌿 How It Works

Hibiscus works by gently relaxing blood vessels and cooling the circulatory system, supporting balanced blood pressure and smoother blood flow. Its antioxidant-rich compounds protect cardiovascular and liver tissues from oxidative damage while easing inflammation and metabolic heat. Mild diuretic action supports fluid balance, and liver support enhances detoxification efficiency. Overall, Hibiscus restores circulatory calm and systemic clarity without stimulation.

---

### 🌱 Primary Uses

- Supports healthy blood pressure and circulation
- Promotes liver and cardiovascular health
- Reduces inflammation and oxidative stress
- Supports cholesterol balance
- Assists metabolic and weight-management goals
- Refreshes and hydrates during heat or fatigue

---

### Scientific Backing

Hibiscus contains anthocyanins, polyphenols, and organic acids responsible for its cardiovascular and antioxidant effects. Clinical studies confirm reductions in systolic and diastolic blood pressure, LDL cholesterol, and oxidative stress with regular use. Research also supports liver protection, metabolic balance, and anti-inflammatory activity, validating its long-standing traditional use.

---

### Forms Available

- Dried petals (tea or cold infusion)
- Powder or capsules
- Liquid extract / tincture
- Beverage blends and concentrates

---

### How to Use (Dosage)

- **Tea:** 1–2 tsp dried petals, steep 10–15 minutes (hot or cold)
- **Cold Brew:** Steep overnight for smoother extraction
- **Capsules/Powder:** Follow product label guidance
- **Tincture:** As directed by practitioner or product instructions

---

### Caution Level: Caution

- May mildly lower blood pressure — monitor if using antihypertensives
- Avoid high-dose extracts during pregnancy
- Review use if taking diuretics or hypotensive medications
- Generally very safe when used as tea

---

### Gender-Specific Safety

**Men:** Supports blood pressure, cholesterol balance, and liver health without hormonal effects. Safe for regular tea use.

**Women:** Helpful for fluid balance, circulation, skin clarity, and heat-related fatigue. Supports women's cardiovascular wellness.

**Pregnancy / Nursing:** Mild tea is generally acceptable; avoid concentrated extracts or medicinal dosing without guidance.

---

### Expected Results

- Cooling hydration and refreshment: immediate
- Circulatory and blood pressure support: 1–2 weeks
- Skin tone and vitality: 2–4 weeks
- Metabolic and systemic balance: ongoing with regular use

---

### 🛠 DIY Recipe — Hibiscus Heart-Cooling Tonic

1 tbsp Hibiscus petals
½ tsp Cinnamon
1 slice fresh Ginger
Steep 10–15 minutes. Enjoy warm or iced to support circulation and digestion.

---

### 🔄 Same / Similar Foundation

- Hawthorn
- Dandelion Leaf
- Green Tea
- Lemon Balm
- Schisandra

---

### Shelf Life / Potency After Preparation

- Dried petals: 1–2 years (airtight, away from light and heat)
- Powder/capsules: Up to 2 years (check label)
- Tincture: 4–5 years (alcohol-based)
- Prepared tea: Refrigerate and use within 48–72 hours

Fading color or aroma indicates reduced potency.

---

### Herbal Reflections of Hibiscus

Hibiscus is the color of circulation restored — cooling the blood, lifting stagnation, and renewing vitality with grace. Its medicine refreshes rather than forces, offering clarity where heat and heaviness once lingered. Both tonic and celebration, Hibiscus reminds us that healing can be beautiful, flavorful, and sustaining.

---

### Herbal Confidence Index: 🌿🌿🌿🌿🌿

(5/5 — cornerstone circulatory and antioxidant herb; exceptionally safe and effective in tea form for long-term cardiovascular, liver, and metabolic support.)

# BUTCHER'S BROOM

★★★★

*Ruscus aculeatus*

**Butcher's Broom** is a structural circulatory tonic that tones veins, reduces swelling, and improves lower-body circulation. It is especially valued for varicose veins, hemorrhoids, and heavy, fatigued legs. Its ruscogenins strengthen vascular walls while easing inflammation and fluid retention.
Historically used throughout the Mediterranean, this resilient shrub moved from sweeping butcher stalls to sweeping stagnation from the body. Modern research confirms its effectiveness in chronic venous insufficiency, particularly when paired with vitamin C or citrus bioflavonoids. Its action is gradual, steady, and deeply supportive.

---

### 🌿 Core Herbal Category — Butcher's Broom

**Primary Core: Cardiovascular System Support** herb with (venotonic, vessel-tightening action that strengthens veins and improves venous return)
**Secondary Cores:** Musculoskeletal & Pain-Relief herb · Urinary & Kidney Support herb · Immune Support herb

### 🌿 How It Works

Butcher's Broom tightens and strengthens venous walls, improving blood return from the legs and reducing pooling. This venotonic action decreases swelling and inflammation while supporting comfort and mobility. Improved circulation also assists lymphatic drainage and fluid balance. Overall, it functions as a targeted structural circulatory herb for venous congestion and lower-body heaviness.

---

### 🌱 Primary Uses

- Varicose veins and hemorrhoids
- Leg swelling, heaviness, and fatigue
- Chronic venous insufficiency
- Mild fluid retention and lymphatic congestion
- Circulatory support for prolonged standing or sitting

---

### 🔬 Scientific Backing

Butcher's Broom contains ruscogenins — steroidal saponins shown to tighten vein walls, improve microcirculation, and reduce edema. Clinical studies demonstrate reduced pain and swelling in chronic venous insufficiency (CVI), with enhanced benefits when combined with vitamin C or hesperidin. Its mild diuretic action supports fluid balance without electrolyte depletion.

---

### 💊 How to Use (Dosage)

- **Capsules/Tablets:** 300–500 mg daily
- **Tincture:** 2–4 mL, twice daily
- **Topical:** Creams or compresses for veins or hemorrhoids
- **Decoction:** 1 tsp dried root, simmered 10–15 min (less common)

---

### ⏳ Expected Results

- Hemorrhoid relief: 2–4 days
- Reduced leg swelling/heaviness: 5–7 days
- Improved vein tone and appearance: 4–6 weeks

---

### ⚠️ Caution Level: 🟡 Caution

Generally safe when used as directed.

- Avoid during pregnancy and breastfeeding
- May interact with anticoagulants, antihypertensives, or diuretics
- Seek guidance with cardiovascular or blood-pressure conditions

---

### 🚹 🚺 Gender-Specific Safety

🔵 **Men:** Supports vein tone, circulation, and prostate comfort; useful for occupational leg fatigue.

🟣 **Women:** Beneficial for menstrual-related swelling, varicose veins, and circulatory sluggishness.

🟡 **Pregnancy / Nursing:** Avoid high-dose internal use; mild topical use is generally acceptable with guidance.

---

### 🛠️ DIY Recipe — Vein Support Topical Blend

1 tbsp Butcher's Broom tincture
1 tbsp Witch Hazel extract
2 tbsp Aloe Vera gel
Mix and apply to affected areas 1–2× daily.

---

### 🔄 Same / Similar Foundation

🟢 Horse Chestnut

- Gotu Kola
- Witch Hazel
- Yarrow
- Hawthorn

---

**Shelf Life / Potency**

- Capsules/Tablets: 2–3 years
- Tincture: 4–5 years
- Dried root: 2 years
- Topicals: 12–18 months

Replace if aroma, color, or texture degrades.

---

**Herbal Reflections of Butcher's Broom**

Butcher's Broom is the quiet sentinel of circulation — firm, grounded, and structural. It restores ease where heaviness once ruled and strengthens the channels through which vitality flows. Its medicine teaches that stability and support are active forces, reshaping how the body stands, moves, and endures.

**Herbal Confidence Index:**

(4/5 — dependable venous tonic with excellent clinical backing; requires caution with medications and pregnancy.)

# CAMU CAMU

★★★★★

*Myrciaria dubia*

**Camu Camu** is an exceptionally concentrated, food-based source of vitamin C that strengthens immunity, supports collagen formation, and delivers powerful antioxidant protection. Even small daily amounts help fortify resistance to colds and flu, enhance skin and joint repair, and counter oxidative stress from modern life.

Traditionally used by Indigenous Amazonian cultures long before its rise as a modern "superfruit," Camu Camu reflects whole-plant nutrition at its best. Its vitamin C arrives with natural synergists—flavonoids, ellagic acid, and amino acids—enhancing absorption and broadening benefits. Bright, sour, and remarkably efficient, it offers high impact in modest doses.

---

### Core Herbal Category — Camu Camu

**Primary Core: Immune System Support** herb with (exceptionally high antioxidant and vitamin-C–rich action that strengthens immune resilience and tissue protection)

**Secondary Cores:** Skin & Tissue Repair herb · Nervines (Nervous System Support) herb · Metabolic & Blood Sugar Support herb

---

### How It Works

Camu Camu works by supplying concentrated vitamin C and antioxidant compounds that reinforce immune defenses and neutralize oxidative stress. This activity supports collagen synthesis and tissue repair, benefiting skin, joints, and connective tissue. By lowering inflammatory burden, it indirectly supports mood stability and nervous system resilience. Its dense micronutrient profile also enhances metabolic efficiency and recovery. Overall, Camu Camu functions as a potent nutritive immune herb that restores resilience through nourishment rather than stimulation.

---

### Primary Uses

- Rapid immune reinforcement
- Collagen support (skin, joints, connective tissue)
- Antioxidant protection from oxidative stress
- Supports mood and serotonin pathways

• Enhances energy, stamina, and recovery

---

**Scientific Backing**

Camu Camu contains 30–60× more vitamin C than oranges and is rich in anthocyanins, flavonoids, and ellagic acid. Clinical studies show reductions in C-reactive protein (CRP), improved liver markers, increased antioxidant capacity, and potential neuroprotective and mood-supportive effects linked to serotonin modulation.

---

**Forms Available**

- Freeze-dried powder (most potent and common)
- Capsules or tablets
- Tincture or liquid extract
- Rarely, dried whole fruit

---

**How to Use (Dosage)**

- **Powder:** ¼–½ tsp daily in water, juice, or smoothies (start low due to potency)
- **Capsules:** 500–1,500 mg daily, divided if sensitive
- **Tincture:** 1–2 mL, 1–2× daily

Best taken earlier in the day to support energy and immunity.

---

**Caution Level: Safe**

- Very high doses may cause mild digestive upset
- Those with kidney stone history should moderate intake
- May enhance effects of blood thinners or anti-inflammatories
- Pregnant or nursing individuals should use food-level amounts only

---

**Gender-Specific Safety**

**Men:** Excellent for immunity, collagen repair, oxidative stress recovery, and energy. No hormonal concerns.

**Women:** Supports skin radiance, mood resilience, immune balance, and daily vitality. Very well tolerated.

**Pregnancy / Nursing:** Safe in dietary amounts; avoid high-dose powders or extracts.

---

**Expected Results**

- Immune reinforcement: 1–3 days
- Improved skin tone and joint comfort: 1–2 weeks
- Enhanced energy, mood, and resilience: 2–3 weeks

---

🛠️ **DIY Recipe — Immunity Power Shot**
½ tsp Camu Camu powder
Juice of 1 orange
Pinch of cayenne (optional)
Mix and drink once daily for immune and liver support.

---

🔄 **Same / Similar Foundation**

- Amla
- Acerola
- Rosehip
- Baobab
- Goji

---

**Shelf Life / Potency After Preparation**

- Powder: 1–2 years (airtight, cool, dry)
- Capsules: 2–3 years
- Tincture: 4–5 years

Potency declines with heat, light, and humidity.

💬 **Herbal Reflections of Camu Camu**

Camu Camu carries the brightness of stored sunlight—clean, immediate, and deeply nourishing. Rather than forcing the body, it rebuilds resilience quietly, strengthening tissues and defenses through steady nourishment. Its lesson is simple: true vitality grows from consistency, not excess.

---

⭐ ***Herbal Confidence Index:*** 🌿 🌿 🌿 🌿 🌿

*(5/5 — cornerstone whole-food vitamin C source; exceptionally safe, efficient, and reliable for immune, antioxidant, and collagen support.)*

# CARAWAY SEED

★★★★

*Carum carvi*

**Caraway Seed** is a classic digestive herb valued for its warming, aromatic ability to ease gas, bloating, and intestinal cramping. Used for centuries across Europe and the Middle East, these small crescent-shaped seeds stimulate digestion, calm spasms, and help the body process heavy or sluggish meals with greater ease.
Beyond the kitchen, Caraway Seed has long been trusted as a gentle balancer of the gut. Frequently paired with fennel, anise, or chamomile, it supports digestive rhythm while offering mild antimicrobial and antioxidant benefits. Safe, familiar, and dependable, it remains a daily digestive ally across cultures.

---

## 🌿 Core Herbal Category — Caraway Seed

**Primary Core: Digestive System Support** herb with (aromatic carminative and antispasmodic action that relieves gas, cramping, and digestive tension)
**Secondary Cores:** Women's Health herb · Immune Support herb · Metabolic & Blood Sugar Support herb

---

## 🌿 How It Works

Caraway Seed works by relaxing smooth muscle in the digestive tract, easing spasms, bloating, and trapped gas. Its aromatic oils stimulate digestive secretions, improving breakdown and assimilation of food. This carminative action calms irritation and restores digestive rhythm. It also helps relieve cramp-related pelvic and intestinal tension, particularly after meals.

---

## 🌱 Primary Uses

- Relieves gas, bloating, and indigestion
- Reduces intestinal spasms and cramping
- Stimulates appetite and sluggish digestion
- Supports infant colic (carefully dosed)
- Traditionally supports lactation

---

## 🧪 Scientific Backing

Caraway Seed contains carvone and limonene, essential oils shown to relax intestinal muscle and reduce gas formation. Clinical trials demonstrate that Caraway combined with

Peppermint significantly improves symptoms of IBS and functional dyspepsia. Additional studies support antimicrobial, antioxidant, and anti-inflammatory activity beneficial to gut balance.

---

**Forms Available**

- Whole or lightly crushed seeds
- Capsules
- Tincture or extract
- Essential oil (topical only, diluted)

---

**How to Use (Dosage)**

- **Tea:** 1 tsp lightly crushed seeds, steep 10 minutes after meals
- **Chew:** ¼–½ tsp seeds after eating for gas
- **Capsules:** 300–600 mg as directed
- **Topical oil:** Diluted massage over abdomen for cramps

---

**Caution Level: Caution**

- Avoid internal use of concentrated essential oil
- Use cautiously in severe liver disease
- Monitor infants carefully when used for colic
- Generally very safe in food and tea amounts

---

**Gender-Specific Safety**

**Men:** Excellent digestive support with no hormonal effects. Safe for daily culinary or tea use.

**Women:** Supports digestion, reduces menstrual bloating, and traditionally supports lactation.

**Pregnancy / Nursing:** Safe in food or tea amounts; avoid essential oil and strong extracts.

---

**Expected Results**

- Relief from gas and bloating: ~30 minutes
- Improved digestive balance: 1–2 weeks
- Lactation support (when applicable): several days

---

**DIY Recipe — Soothing Digestive Tea**

1 tsp Caraway Seed
½ tsp Fennel Seed

1 cup hot water
Steep covered 10–15 minutes. Drink after meals.

---

**Same / Similar Foundation**

- Fennel Seed
- Anise
- Chamomile
- Dill Seed
- Ginger

---

**Shelf Life / Potency After Preparation**

- Whole seeds: 2–3 years (airtight, cool, dark)
- Crushed seeds: 6–12 months
- Tincture: 3–5 years
- Prepared tea: Use within 24 hours

---

**Herbal Reflections of Caraway Seed**

Caraway Seed is quiet reassurance for the gut — steady, warming, and dependable. Its medicine works gently yet persistently, restoring comfort where digestion falters. It reminds us that some of the most effective remedies are those trusted long enough to become tradition.

---

**Herbal Confidence Index:**

(4/5 — foundational digestive carminative; safe, effective, and time-tested for daily gastrointestinal support.)

# CHAGA

★★★★★

*Inonotus obliquus*

**Chaga Mushroom** is among the most potent natural antioxidants known, valued for strengthening immune resilience, protecting cellular DNA, and reducing chronic inflammation. Rich in polyphenols, beta-glucans, and melanin, it supports long-term balance in conditions shaped by oxidative stress, immune depletion, and environmental burden.

Unlike fast-acting herbs aimed at immediate symptoms, Chaga works slowly and cumulatively—building endurance, restoring inner reserves, and protecting tissues over time. For centuries, it has been consumed as a daily tea across Siberia and Northern Europe, where it was revered as a life-extending tonic. Modern science now confirms what tradition long observed: Chaga is a deep restorative, not a stimulant—strengthening the body from the inside out.

---

## Core Herbal Category — Chaga

**Primary Core: Immune System Support** herb with (antioxidant-rich, immune-modulating action that strengthens defense while reducing inflammatory stress)

**Secondary Cores:** Adaptogen herb · Liver & Detoxification herb · Nutritive & Restorative herb

---

## How It Works

Chaga works by modulating immune activity rather than forcing stimulation, helping strengthen defense responses while calming chronic inflammatory signaling. Its dense antioxidant compounds reduce oxidative damage and protect tissues over time, easing long-term cellular stress. This immune-balancing effect supports liver detoxification and metabolic clarity. Chaga's action is gradual but profound—supporting recovery, resilience, and longevity through steady restoration.

---

## Primary Uses

- Strengthens immune resilience
- Protects DNA and cellular integrity
- Powerful antioxidant defense
- Reduces systemic inflammation
- Supports blood sugar and chronic-condition balance

---

### Scientific Backing

Chaga contains polyphenols, melanin, beta-glucans, and triterpenes responsible for its exceptional antioxidant capacity. Research demonstrates strong free-radical scavenging activity, DNA-protective effects, improved inflammatory markers, and early evidence of blood-sugar regulation. Human trials remain limited but consistently promising for immune modulation.

---

### Forms Available

- Dried chunks or powder
- Dual-extract tinctures (water + alcohol)
- Capsules and standardized supplements

---

### How to Use (Dosage)

- **Decoction/Tea:** 1–2 tsp chopped or powdered Chaga, simmer 30–60 minutes; drink 1–2 cups daily
- **Dual-extract tincture:** 20–40 drops in water, 1–3× daily
- **Capsules/Powders:** Typically 500–1,000 mg daily

Best used consistently for several weeks for immune or antioxidant support.

---

### Caution Level: Caution

- Contains mild anticoagulant compounds — use caution with blood thinners
- Long-term heavy use may stress kidneys (oxalate content)
- Avoid during pregnancy or nursing unless supervised
- Take periodic breaks if used daily for extended periods

---

### Gender-Specific Safety

**Men:** Supports endurance, immunity, and recovery from physical stress. Non-hormonal and safe in moderate daily use.

**Women:** Helps reduce fatigue, improve immune balance, and support skin and tissue repair. Useful during post-illness recovery.

**Pregnancy / Nursing:** Limited data — avoid concentrated extracts; mild tea only with professional guidance.

---

### Expected Results

- Improved energy: several days
- Immune reinforcement: 1–2 weeks
- Deep antioxidant protection: 3–4 weeks of consistent use

---

🛠 **DIY Recipe — Chaga Vitality Tea**
2 tsp dried Chaga chunks
3 cups water
Optional: cinnamon stick, ginger, or orange peel
Simmer gently for 1 hour. Strain and enjoy warm.
(Chunks may be reused 2–3 times.)

---

🔄 **Same / Similar Foundation**
- Reishi
- Turkey Tail
- Shiitake
- Maitake
- Cordyceps

---

**Shelf Life / Potency After Preparation**
• Dried chunks/powder: 2–3 years (airtight, cool, dark)
• Dual-extract tincture: 4–6 years
• Prepared tea/decoction: Use within 48–72 hours refrigerated
• Double extract: 5+ years (highest stability)

---

💬 **Herbal Reflections of Chaga Mushroom**
Chaga is a teacher of endurance. Forged in cold and scarcity, it restores strength through patience rather than force. Its medicine unfolds quietly—fortifying immunity, calming inflammation, and rebuilding reserves where chronic stress has taken its toll. To drink Chaga is to drink resilience itself: slow, steady, and enduring.

---

⭐ **Herbal Confidence Index:** 🌿 🌿 🌿 🌿 🌿
(5/5 — cornerstone immune and longevity mushroom; exceptionally effective for immune balance, inflammation reduction, and long-term resilience when used consistently.)

# GALANGAL ROOT

★★★★

*Alpinia officinarum*

**Galangal Root** is a bold, warming digestive and circulatory herb long valued in Southeast Asian and Ayurvedic traditions. Often compared to ginger but sharper and more invigorating, it stimulates digestion, enhances circulation, and restores warmth to sluggish systems.

Traditionally used for indigestion, joint discomfort, respiratory congestion, and low vitality, galangal's antimicrobial and antioxidant qualities make it especially useful during cold, damp, or stagnant conditions. Where heaviness and inertia dominate, galangal acts as a spark—reviving movement, clarity, and digestive fire.

---

### 🌿 Core Herbal Category — Galangal Root

**Primary Core: Digestive System Support** herb with (warming, aromatic action that stimulates digestion and improves circulatory movement)

**Secondary Cores:** Circulatory & Cardiovascular herb · Respiratory Support herb · Musculoskeletal & Pain-Relief herb

---

### 🌿 How It Works

Galangal Root works by warming and activating digestive function, increasing appetite, secretion, and motility. Its aromatic compounds enhance circulation, supporting the movement of blood and energy throughout the body. This warming action helps open the respiratory system during cold congestion and reduces inflammatory tension in joints and muscles. Overall, galangal restores momentum where cold and stagnation have slowed the system.

---

### 🌱 Primary Uses

- Eases indigestion, bloating, and nausea
- Reduces joint and muscle stiffness
- Relieves coughs and cold congestion
- Boosts circulation and vitality
- Provides antimicrobial digestive support

---

### 🧪 Scientific Backing

Galangal contains galangin, alpinin, kaempferol, and aromatic essential oils with demonstrated antioxidant, antimicrobial, and anti-inflammatory activity. Research highlights activity against bacteria and fungi linked to digestive imbalance, circulation-enhancing effects, and early evidence of lipid-modulating and cardioprotective action—supporting its long traditional use.

---

### Forms Available

- Fresh rhizome
- Dried slices or powder
- Tincture or capsules

---

### How to Use (Dosage)

- **Tea/Decoction:** 1–2 tsp fresh or dried root, simmer 10–15 minutes, 1–2× daily
- **Capsules:** 400–600 mg, up to 2× daily
- **Powder:** ¼–½ tsp added to food or tea
- **Tincture:** 15–30 drops, up to 3× daily

Use with food if sensitive to warming herbs.

---

### Caution Level: Caution

- Avoid high doses during pregnancy (warming/stimulating)
- May irritate sensitive stomachs
- Use caution with blood thinners or blood-pressure medications
- Best used periodically rather than continuously

---

### Gender-Specific Safety

**Men:** Supports digestion, circulation, and energy without hormonal effects. Excessive use may increase heat.

**Women:** Helpful for cold-type fatigue and digestive sluggishness; avoid overuse during heat-dominant states.

**Pregnancy / Nursing:** Culinary amounts only. Avoid tinctures, capsules, and strong teas.

---

### Expected Results

- Digestive relief: within hours
- Cold and respiratory support: 1–3 days
- Anti-inflammatory benefits: 1–2 weeks

---

### DIY Recipe — Galangal Digestive Tonic

1 tsp grated fresh galangal
1 tsp honey
Pour hot water over ingredients and steep 10 minutes.
Sip after meals to support digestion and warmth.

---

### 🔄 Same / Similar Foundation

- Ginger
- Turmeric
- Licorice Root
- Black Pepper
- Cinnamon

---

### Shelf Life / Potency After Preparation

- Fresh root: 2–3 weeks refrigerated
- Dried slices/powder: 1–2 years
- Tincture: 4–6 years
- Prepared tea: Use within 24–48 hours

---

### Herbal Reflections of Galangal Root

Galangal is purposeful fire—direct, clarifying, and invigorating. It lifts digestion out of stagnation and restores movement where heaviness lingers. Used wisely, its heat is not harsh but awakening, reminding the body how to move, digest, and circulate with confidence.

---

### Herbal Confidence Index: 🌿 🌿 🌿 🌿

(4/5 — powerful warming digestive and circulatory tonic; fast-acting and reliable, best suited for moderate, periodic use.)

# *GERMAN CHAMOMILE*

★★★★★

*Matricaria chamomilla*

**German Chamomile**—often simply called "Chamomile"—is one of the world's most beloved calming herbs, treasured for its gentle ability to ease nervous tension, support sleep, and settle digestive upset. In traditional European medicine it has been a go-to ally for insomnia, anxiety, colic, and "nervous stomach." Its pleasant apple-like aroma makes it equally loved as a bedtime tea and as a daily comfort herb.

Beyond emotional calm, chamomile is a versatile healer. It eases cramps, quiets spasms, reduces skin inflammation, and supports tissue repair. Though its flowers appear delicate, chamomile's anti-inflammatory chemistry can be surprisingly strong—especially in properly prepared infusions, topical compresses, and diluted oil applications.

---

### Core Herbal Category — German Chamomile

**Primary Core: Nervous System Support (Nervines)** herb with (gentle calming, antispasmodic action that settles anxiety while soothing the digestive tract)

**Secondary Cores:** Digestive Support herb · Anti-Inflammatory Support herb · Women's Health herb · Skin & Tissue Repair herb

---

### How It Works

German Chamomile works by calming nervous-system overactivity while relaxing smooth muscle spasms in the gut and uterus. Its flavonoids (notably apigenin) support relaxation and sleep quality, while its aromatic constituents ease digestive tension, gas, and cramping. Topically, chamomile reduces inflammatory irritation and supports tissue comfort. Overall, it functions as a gentle, wide-use soother—nervous system first, digestion closely behind.

---

### Primary Uses

- Calms anxiety and supports restful sleep
- Relieves indigestion, gas, and bloating
- Soothes menstrual cramps and PMS tension
- Reduces topical irritation and inflammation
- Gentle support for children's colic (properly diluted/mild)

---

### Scientific Backing

Chamomile contains apigenin, bisabolol, and chamazulene, supporting sedative, antispasmodic, and anti-inflammatory effects. Studies align well with traditional use for mild anxiety/sleep support, digestive discomfort (including IBS-type tension), infant colic relief, and improved skin comfort/wound soothing when used topically.

---

### Forms Available

- Dried flowers (tea)
- Tincture
- Capsules/syrups
- Salves/compresses
- Essential oil (topical/aromatic; diluted)

---

### How to Use (Dosage)

- **Tea:** 1–2 tsp dried flowers, steep 10–15 minutes, up to 3× daily
- **Tincture:** 30–60 drops in water, up to 3× daily
- **Compress:** Apply cooled tea to irritated skin
- **Essential oil:** External/aromatic use only; dilute heavily

For sleep: drink tea 30–60 minutes before bedtime.

---

### Caution Level: Safe

Generally safe for most people in tea, tincture, or topical form.

- Use caution with **Asteraceae** allergies (ragweed family)
- Excess may cause drowsiness or mild stomach upset
- May **enhance sedatives**; use caution with blood thinners
- Pregnancy: mild tea is commonly used; avoid high-dose extracts early in pregnancy unless guided

---

### Gender-Specific Safety (GS)

**Men:** Safe; excellent for stress, digestion, and sleep support.

**Women:** Safe; traditional cramp and PMS support; useful during hormonal tension.

**Pregnancy / Nursing:** Mild tea is generally well tolerated; avoid concentrated tinctures/extracts unless guided.

---

### Expected Results

- Relaxation/sleep support: 30–60 minutes
- Digestive relief: within 1 hour
- Skin soothing: 2–4 days of consistent topical use

🛠 **DIY Recipe — Chamomile Bedtime Tea**

1 tsp Chamomile
½ tsp Lemon Balm
¼ tsp Lavender
Steep 10 minutes. Sip warm before bed.

---

🔄 **Same / Similar Foundation**

🟢 Lemon Balm
⚪ Passionflower
🟣 Valerian Root
🟡 Fennel Seed
🟣 Lavender

⏳ **Shelf Life / Potency After Preparation**

• Dried flowers: 1–2 years (airtight, dark, cool)
• Tincture: 4–6 years
• Essential oil: 2–3 years (cool, dark, amber glass)
• Prepared tea: use within 24 hours refrigerated
• Compress: use within 24–48 hours refrigerated

---

💬 **Herbal Reflections of German Chamomile**

Chamomile is quiet protection—soft enough for the tender, strong enough for the inflamed. It calms the mind without dulling it, and settles the stomach without forcing it. In a world that runs too fast, chamomile teaches the body to unclench, breathe, and return to peace—one warm cup at a time.

⭐ **Herbal Confidence Index:** 🌿 🌿 🌿 🌿 🌿

(5/5 — cornerstone calming and digestive herb; exceptionally safe, widely effective, and universally usable for sleep, anxiety tension, gut spasms, and gentle inflammation support.)

# FIGWORT

★★★★

*Scrophularia nodosa*

**Figwort** is a deep-cleansing lymph and skin herb valued for reducing chronic inflammation, clearing stubborn eruptions, and helping swollen glands move toward relief. Traditionally called a "blood purifier," it supports circulation and elimination—especially when sluggish lymph flow contributes to eczema, acne, psoriasis-type flare patterns, or long-standing inflammatory congestion.

Used across European and Chinese traditions, figwort became known for clearing "heat" and swelling from the body. Its action is not flashy—it works steadily, gradually opening blocked pathways and helping the body release what has been stored too long.

---

### Core Herbal Category — Figwort

**Primary Core: Lymphatic & Skin Support herb** with (lymphatic-clearing action that supports immune drainage and reduces chronic inflammatory congestion)

**Secondary Cores:** Skin & Tissue Repair herb · Liver & Detoxification herb · Urinary & Kidney Support herb

---

### How It Works

Figwort supports lymphatic movement, helping the body clear inflammatory byproducts that can surface through the skin. This drainage action reduces congestion in glands and tissues while supporting liver and kidney elimination. Over time, its cooling alterative nature helps restore clearer skin tone and calmer inflammatory patterns.

---

### Primary Uses

- Supports lymphatic drainage and detoxification
- Helps chronic skin eruptions (eczema/acne-type patterns)
- Reduces glandular swelling and inflammatory congestion
- Promotes circulation and "stagnation clearing"
- Supports gentle liver and kidney activity

---

### Scientific Backing

Figwort contains iridoids, saponins, and flavonoids associated with anti-inflammatory, antimicrobial, and mild diuretic effects. Research and traditional systems both support its role in chronic inflammatory skin patterns and swelling/"heat" congestion, especially when lymph movement is sluggish.

---

### 🏷 Forms Available

- Dried root/herb
- Tincture extract
- Decoction blends

---

### 📏 How to Use (Dosage)

- **Tincture:** 30–60 drops (1–2 mL) in water, 2× daily
- **Decoction:** 1 tsp dried root, simmer 10–15 minutes; 1–2× daily
- **Poultice:** softened root applied to swollen glands/irritated skin

Best used in cycles (1–3 weeks), then break.

---

### ⚠ Caution Level: ● Caution

- High doses may loosen stools
- Avoid during pregnancy/nursing
- Use caution with diuretics or heart medications
- Moderate dosing is preferred during cleansing protocols

---

### 🚹 🚺 Gender-Specific Safety (GS)

● **Men:** Useful for chronic skin/lymph congestion; use in short cycles, not prolonged high-dose.

● **Women:** Helpful for lymph stagnation and inflammatory skin patterns; avoid during pregnancy; caution with prescriptions.

● **Pregnancy / Nursing:** Avoid.

---

### ⏳ Expected Results

- Reduced swelling/tender glands: 2–4 days
- Skin calming/clarity: 5–10 days
- Improved lymph flow/detox: 1–2 weeks

---

### 🛠 DIY Recipe — Lymph-Clearing Tea (Cycle Use)

1 tsp Figwort root
1 tsp Cleavers
1 tsp Red Clover
Simmer 15 minutes in 3 cups water. Drink 1 cup, 1–2× daily for up to 10–14 days.

---

### Same / Similar Foundation

- Cleavers
- Burdock Root
- Red Clover
- Oregon Grape Root
- Dandelion

---

### Shelf Life / Potency After Preparation

- Dried root: 1–2 years (dark, dry, airtight)
- Tincture: 4–6 years
- Decoction: 24–48 hours refrigerated
- Poultice: prepare fresh; discard after use

---

### Herbal Reflections of Figwort

Figwort is the quiet mover—entering the hidden pockets of stagnation and helping the body release what it has carried too long. Its medicine is slow honesty: steady drainage, steady clearing, steady return to flow. For chronic skin flare patterns and swollen, sluggish pathways, figwort offers patient renewal.

---

### Herbal Confidence Index: 🌿 🌿 🌿 🌿

(4/5 — reliable lymph/skin cleansing herb with strong historical use; best used in cycles due to its cleansing intensity and medication/pregnancy cautions.)

---

# CORYDALIS

★★★★

*Corydalis yanhusuo*

**Corydalis** (Yan Hu Suo) is a respected Chinese pain-relief herb used for cramps, injury pain, nerve tension, and "stagnation" patterns that create stubborn discomfort. It is valued for helping ease pain while also encouraging relaxation and sleep—especially when pain and emotional tension are interlocked.

Its alkaloids influence pain signaling and circulation dynamics, making Corydalis a powerful but respectful ally—best used in short cycles rather than daily long-term.

---

### Core Herbal Category — Corydalis

**Primary Core: Anti-Inflammatory & Pain Support** herb with (analgesic, circulation-moving action that relieves pain by improving blood flow and calming nerve signaling)

**Secondary Cores:** Nervines (Nervous System Support) herb · Circulatory & Cardiovascular herb · Women's Health herb

---

### How It Works

Corydalis helps reduce pain through two main pathways: calming pain signaling in the nervous system and improving circulation where stagnation contributes to pressure and inflammation. This dual action makes it useful for cramps, injury pain, nerve-driven discomfort, and tension that disrupts sleep. It is potent and best used cyclically—short-term support, then a break.

---

### Primary Uses

- Eases nerve, joint, and musculoskeletal pain
- Relieves menstrual cramps and abdominal spasm
- Supports sleep when pain or tension is present
- Moves "blood stasis" patterns (circulatory stagnation)
- Supports recovery from injuries and inflammation

---

### Scientific Backing

Corydalis contains several alkaloids (including dehydrocorybulbine and related compounds) studied for analgesic, sedative, and anti-inflammatory effects. Research supports pain-relief activity without the same dependency profile as opioids, along with circulation-moving and antispasmodic benefits consistent with traditional use.

### Forms Available
- Capsules/standardized extract
- Dried root (decoction)
- Tincture extract

---

### How to Use (Dosage)
- **Tincture:** 30–60 drops in water, up to 3× daily
- **Capsules:** 500–1,000 mg standardized extract, 1–2× daily
- **Decoction:** 1 tsp dried root simmered 15–20 minutes

⚠ Best used in 2–3 week cycles with short breaks.

---

### ⚠ Caution Level: Caution
- Avoid combining with sedatives, sleep aids, or alcohol
- Do not use during pregnancy or breastfeeding
- May cause dizziness/drowsiness
- Not recommended for continuous long-term daily use

---

### Gender-Specific Safety (GS)
**Men:** Useful for pain and tension; may increase drowsiness or lower BP in sensitive users—avoid mixing with sedatives/alcohol.

**Women:** Helpful for cramp pain and tension patterns; use cyclically, not daily long-term.

**Pregnancy / Nursing:** Avoid.

---

### Expected Results
- Pain relief: 30–60 minutes
- Cramp reduction: 1–2 uses
- Sleep/emotional calm: 2–5 days of consistent use

---

### DIY Recipe — Corydalis Sleep-Pain Blend (Tincture)
1 part Corydalis
1 part California Poppy
1 part Skullcap
Steep 4 weeks in high-proof alcohol. Strain. Use in small, cautious doses as needed.

---

### Same / Similar Foundation
California Poppy

- Valerian Root
- Turmeric
- Passionflower
- Skullcap

---

**Shelf Life / Potency After Preparation**

- Dried root: 2–3 years (airtight, cool, dark)
- Capsules: 1–2 years (check label)
- Tincture: 4–6 years
- Decoction: use within 24 hours refrigerated

---

**Herbal Reflections of Corydalis**

Corydalis is relief with quiet intelligence—softening pain without erasing awareness, restoring movement where tightness and stagnation have taken hold. It teaches that healing often begins when the body can finally unclench. Used with respect, it brings comfort back into the nervous system and rest back into the night.

---

**Herbal Confidence Index:**

(4/5 — strong, reliable analgesic and antispasmodic herb; highly effective for pain patterns rooted in stagnation and tension, but potent enough to require cyclical, careful use.)

# ELDER LEAF

★★★

*Sambucus nigra folium*

**Elder Leaf** is the lesser-known counterpart to elderflower and elderberry, and it is **stronger, sharper, and more caution-requiring** in its traditional use. Historically, herbalists relied on the **properly prepared leaves** mainly for **external applications**—helping calm hot swelling, soothe bruises, ease sprains, and support wound-area cleanliness. In older folk practice, small, carefully prepared decoctions were sometimes used internally to support fever and congestion, but **modern herbalism generally treats internal leaf use as non-routine** because the leaf contains cyanogenic compounds that can cause nausea and toxicity if misused.
Elder Leaf has held an important place in European folk medicine—respected as both "protector" and "purger." In rural tradition, the elder tree was viewed as sacred, and the leaves were used for protection in both practical and symbolic ways. Today, the leaf is best understood as a **topical helper with boundaries**: useful, but not casual.

---

### 🌿 Core Herbal Category — Elder Leaf

**Primary Core: Lymphatic & Skin Support** herb with (topical anti-inflammatory and cleansing action that helps reduce swelling and supports tissue comfort)
**Secondary Cores:** Musculoskeletal & Pain-Relief herb · Lymphatic Support herb · Immune Support herb

---

### 🌿 How It Works

Elder Leaf works mainly through **external action**: calming inflamed, swollen tissues and supporting local cleansing where irritation or bruising is present. Traditional poultice and wash use may help reduce heat, tightness, and discomfort by supporting fluid movement and easing local inflammatory congestion. While elder's family is known for antiviral activity (especially berry/flower), the **leaf is not a primary internal immune tonic** in modern practice due to toxicity risk. Overall, Elder Leaf is best treated as a **short-term, topical support herb**—not a daily internal remedy.

---

### 🌱 Primary Uses

- Helps reduce swelling and heat (topical)
- Supports comfort in bruises, sprains, and sore joints (topical)
- Traditional wash/poultice support for irritated skin (intact skin preferred)

• Supports local fluid movement (congestion-type swelling)

---

### Scientific Backing

Most modern Sambucus research focuses on **elderberry and elderflower**, which show antiviral and anti-inflammatory activity. Elder Leaf contains **cyanogenic glycosides** (e.g., sambunigrin) that can release cyanide under certain conditions—explaining why raw or improperly prepared leaf can be toxic. Folk evidence supports external use in poultices, salves, and washes; internal use is now generally reserved for trained practitioners and is **not** standard household practice.

---

### Forms Available

Infused oils / salves (topical)

Prepared poultices (boiled leaves)

Dried leaf (for external use)

Internal decoctions (rare; professional guidance only)

---

### How to Use (Dosage)

• **Salve / infused oil:** apply to bruised or sore areas 1–2× daily (avoid eyes/mucous membranes)

• **Poultice:** use **boiled** leaves (never raw), cool, apply 10–20 minutes

• **Wash:** strained, cooled leaf decoction used externally as a rinse

⚠ **Internal use is not recommended** in this system without qualified supervision.

---

### ⚠ Caution Level: Supervision Required

• **Do not take Elder Leaf internally** in routine home practice

• Never use raw leaf preparations

• Avoid use on deep/open wounds unless professionally guided (irritation risk)

• Do not confuse leaf with **elderflower/elderberry**, which are the commonly used safer parts

---

### Gender-Specific Safety (GS)

**Men:** Topical use only; helpful for swelling/soreness. Avoid internal leaf use.

**Women:** Topical use only; avoid internal leaf use.

**Pregnancy / Nursing:** Avoid (internal and topical) due to limited safety data and toxicity concerns—use elderflower or elderberry instead when appropriate.

---

### Expected Results

• Swelling/bruise comfort: 12–24 hours

- Joint soreness ease (topical): 1–3 days
- Skin comfort: ~3–7 days (depending on cause)

---

🛠 **DIY Recipe — Elder Leaf Comfort Salve (Topical)**

1 cup **boiled** elder leaves (well strained and dried of excess water)
1 cup olive oil
¼ cup beeswax
Infuse leaves in oil on very low heat ~2 hours, strain thoroughly, combine with beeswax, pour into jars.

⚠ **Topical use only.**

---

🔄 **Same / Similar Foundation**

● Calendula — skin repair + gentle antimicrobial support
● Plantain Leaf — irritation + skin comfort
● Arnica (topical) — bruises + soreness (intact skin only)
● St. John's Wort oil — nerve pain + bruising comfort
● Comfrey (topical) — tissue comfort (use with care; not on infected wounds)

---

**Shelf Life / Potency After Preparation**

- Dried leaf (external): 1–2 years (airtight, cool, dark)
- Infused oil: ~12 months (cool/dark; refrigerate if preferred)
- Salve: 1–2 years (sealed, cool, dark)
- Fresh poultice: use immediately; discard after use

💬 **Herbal Reflections of Elder Leaf**

Elder Leaf is the elder tree's stern side—protective, cleansing, and unafraid of boundaries. It reminds the herbalist that some medicines are not meant for casual use: they serve best when prepared carefully, applied wisely, and then set down. Elder Leaf teaches respect—the kind that keeps healing safe.

---

⭐ **Herbal Confidence Index:** 🌿 🌿 🌿 (3/5 green stars)

Reasoning: Historically valued for topical swelling and bruising support, but **limited modern internal safety** and the presence of cyanogenic compounds keep it from higher status. Best used **externally** and sparingly.

# CARDAMOM

★★★★★

*Elettaria cardamomum*

**Cardamom**, often honored as the "Queen of Spices," is a fragrant, warming seed treasured for both its flavor and its healing power. Beyond its wide use in kitchens, this spice has long been valued in Ayurvedic and Chinese medicine for easing digestion, supporting clear breathing, and uplifting the spirit. Its aromatic seeds are known to calm bloating, freshen the breath, ease nausea, and restore balance when the body feels sluggish or heavy after rich meals. Whether taken as a tea, chewed whole, or blended into herbal formulas, cardamom acts as a gentle stimulant that comforts the stomach while soothing the mind. This dual action makes it a trusted daily ally for harmony in body and spirit.

Historically, Cardamom has carried prestige not only as a medicine but as a symbol of luxury and refinement. Native to the lush forests of India and Sri Lanka, it was traded along spice routes into the Middle East and Europe, where it became prized in both cuisine and healing traditions. Ancient temples used cardamom in incense for its uplifting aroma, while healers employed it in tonics for digestion, colds, and melancholy. Its reputation as both a sacred spice and a household remedy shows its remarkable versatility — bridging food, ritual, and medicine. Today, cardamom remains a universal herb that connects centuries of tradition, offering comfort, clarity, and resilience across cultures.

---

### Core Herbal Category — Cardamom

**Primary Core: Digestive System Support herb** with (aromatic carminative action that relieves gas, warms digestion, and restores digestive rhythm)

**Secondary Cores:** Respiratory Support herb · Circulatory & Cardiovascular herb · Musculoskeletal & Pain-Relief herb

---

### How It Works

Cardamom works by stimulating digestive secretions and relaxing intestinal spasms, easing gas, bloating, and heaviness. Its warming aromatic oils help restore digestive movement, especially when digestion is cold or sluggish. This warming action extends to the respiratory system, helping open airways and ease congestion. By gently improving circulation, it supports heat movement and reduces stagnant tension. Overall, Cardamom acts as a refined warming digestive herb that restores comfort, flow, and vitality.

---

### Primary Uses

- Relieves gas, bloating, indigestion
- Eases nausea (including mild morning sickness)

• Clears mucus and supports lung comfort
• Freshens breath and supports oral wellness
• Uplifts mood and eases fatigue

---

### Scientific Backing

Cardamom's essential oils — including 1,8-cineole, limonene, and terpinyl acetate — are associated with:
• Carminative digestive relief
• Antispasmodic action for cramping and bloating
• Antimicrobial effects (especially oral and respiratory)
• Antioxidant and mild anti-inflammatory support
Clinical findings support improvements in dyspepsia/indigestion, nausea patterns, and breath/oral microbial balance. Early research also suggests potential support for blood pressure and metabolic balance, though more human trials are needed.

---

### How to Use (Dosage)

• **Tea:** Steep 1–2 lightly crushed pods in hot water for 10 minutes
• **Powder:** ¼–½ tsp in warm milk, tea, or meals
• **Tincture:** 20–30 drops, up to 3× daily

---

### Forms Available

Whole pods (green or black)
Powder
Essential oil (aromatherapy or diluted topical use only)

---

### Expected Results

• Nausea relief: 15–30 minutes
• Digestive improvement: 30–60 minutes
• Respiratory clearing: 1–3 days

---

### Caution Level: Safe

Cardamom is exceptionally safe for daily use in tea or culinary amounts. Mild cautions:
• Concentrated extracts may trigger warmth/heartburn in sensitive people
• Use moderation if prone to gallbladder irritation or reflux
• Avoid medicinal-strength tinctures during pregnancy unless guided

---

### Gender-Specific Safety (GS)

**Men:** Safe — excellent for digestion, circulation, breath freshness, and post-meal relief. No hormonal concerns.

**Women:** Safe — helpful for bloating, nausea, and menstrual digestive discomfort. Uplifts mood and relaxes tension.

**Pregnancy/Nursing:** Safe as culinary spice or mild tea. Avoid medicinal-strength dosing or strong tinctures unless professionally guided.

---

### 🔄 Same / Similar Results

🟢 Ginger — nausea + digestion
🟡 Clove — warming + antimicrobial
🟢 Fennel — bloating + breath freshening
🟢 Peppermint — nausea + clarity
🟤 Cinnamon — warming digestion

---

### 🛠 DIY Recipe — Soothing Cardamom Milk

- 1 cup warm milk (dairy or plant-based)
- ½ tsp cardamom powder
- ¼ tsp cinnamon
- Honey to taste

Drink after meals or before bed for comfort, digestion, and calm.

---

### 📦 Shelf Life / Potency After Preparation

- Whole pods: 2–3 years (airtight, cool, dark)
- Powder: 1–2 years (best within 12 months)
- Infused oils: ~1 year (refrigerated)
- Essential oil: 3–5 years (dark glass, cool storage)

---

### 💬 Herbal Reflections of Cardamom

Cardamom is the gentle harmonizer — a fragrant, elegant herb that soothes the stomach while uplifting the mind. It clears heaviness, refreshes the breath, and restores balance after rich meals or stressful days. Unlike harsher digestive stimulants, Cardamom works with grace: warming yet soft, correcting without force. It blends effortlessly with Ginger, Fennel, and Cinnamon, forming a cornerstone of aromatic healing traditions across cultures.

---

🌟 **Herbal Confidence Index:** 🌿 🌿 🌿 🌿 🌿 (5/5 green stars)

Reasoning: Cornerstone digestive and aromatic tonic — exceptionally safe, effective, and time-honored for calming the stomach, easing nausea, refreshing the breath, and gently uplifting the mind.

# FO-TI (*He Shou Wu*)

★★★★

*Polygonum multiflorum*

**Fo-Ti**, also known in Traditional Chinese Medicine as He Shou Wu, is one of the most legendary herbs of vitality and longevity. Revered for centuries, it has been celebrated as a restorative tonic said to nourish the blood, strengthen kidney and liver energy, and support deep reserves. Its folklore stems from the tale of "Black-haired Mr. He," an elderly man said to have regained youthful vigor and hair vitality after taking the root daily. In TCM tradition, Fo-Ti became synonymous with graceful aging and the rebuilding of foundational strength.

Modern herbalists recognize Fo-Ti as both a powerful restorative and a herb of caution. In its **properly prepared (cured)** form, Fo-Ti is valued for supporting stamina, fertility, hair strength, and long-term resilience. However, **raw/unprocessed Fo-Ti has a documented history of liver stress in some users**, and should not be taken. This dual nature — deep promise and real risk — makes Fo-Ti an herb that must be used with precision, sourcing, and respect.

---

### Core Herbal Category — Fo-Ti (He Shou Wu)

**Primary Core: Nutritional & Tonic Support** herb with (deep blood- and essence-nourishing action that supports long-term vitality, liver function, and kidney resilience)

**Secondary Cores:** Hormonal & Endocrine Support herb · Skin & Tissue Repair herb · Immune Support herb

---

### How It Works

Fo-Ti works by nourishing blood and foundational reserves, supporting long-term vitality and resilience rather than quick stimulation. Its compounds support liver and kidney function—systems traditionally associated with aging strength and hair vitality in TCM. This deeper nourishment may support skin and tissue restoration in deficiency patterns and strengthen recovery capacity during stress or aging. Overall, it functions as a slow, rebuilding tonic best used consistently and conservatively.

---

### Primary Uses

- Supports hair vitality and early graying patterns (traditional use)
- Nourishes foundational vitality and stamina
- Supports liver and kidney resilience (TCM foundation)
- Gentle support for bowel regularity (varies by form)
- Supports aging-related depletion and recovery

---

### Scientific Backing

Fo-Ti contains stilbene glycosides, phospholipids, anthraquinones, and antioxidant compounds. Research suggests potential antioxidant and anti-inflammatory effects, lipid support, and neuroprotective activity in early models.

⚠ **Important:** Documented cases of liver stress and hepatotoxicity have been associated with Fo-Ti—especially raw/unprocessed forms and high dosing—reinforcing the necessity of **prepared/cured root only** and conservative use.

---

### How to Use (Dosage) (Prepared/Cured Root Only)

- **Prepared root capsules/powder:** 1–2 g daily (low, steady tonic range)
- **Tea/decoction:** 1–2 tsp prepared root simmered 20–30 minutes
- **Tincture:** 30–60 drops, up to 3× daily

Best used in small, consistent tonic amounts — not high doses.

---

### Forms Available

- Prepared (cured) root slices or powder (**Zhi He Shou Wu**)
- Standardized tinctures/extracts (reputable sourcing strongly recommended)
- Raw root (**Sheng He Shou Wu**) — not recommended

---

### Expected Results

- Bowel regularity support (if it occurs): 24–72 hours
- Increased stamina and vitality: 1–2 weeks
- Hair/nail support: 1–2 months (slow-building)

---

### ⚠ Caution Level: Caution

- Never take raw/unprocessed Fo-Ti (risk of liver toxicity)
- Use prepared/cured root only
- Avoid with active liver disease or unexplained elevated liver enzymes
- Avoid during pregnancy or breastfeeding
- Use caution with medications processed through the liver

**Requirement:** Products must clearly state **Prepared/Cured Root (Zhi He Shou Wu)**

---

### Gender-Specific Safety (GS)

**Men:** Helpful for stamina and hair vitality; prepared form only. Keep dose conservative and avoid long-term unsupervised high dosing.

**Women:** Traditionally used to nourish blood and vitality; prepared form only. Use extra caution with liver-active medications.

**Pregnancy/Nursing:** Avoid — choose safer nutritives such as Nettle Leaf or Red Raspberry Leaf.

---

### Same / Similar Results

🟢 Ashwagandha — vitality + adrenal resilience
🟢 Nettle Leaf/Root — nourishment + hair support
🟢 Panax Ginseng — endurance + longevity support
🟡 Rehmannia — kidney/blood tonic support
🟢 Saw Palmetto — male hair/hormone support patterns

---

🛠 **DIY Recipe — Hair Vitality Tea (Prepared Root Only)**
• 1 tsp **cured** Fo-Ti root
• 1 tsp nettle leaf
Simmer gently for 20 minutes. Strain and sip daily to support hair nourishment and deeper vitality.

---

📦 **Shelf Life / Potency After Preparation**
• Prepared root slices: 3–5 years (cool, dark, sealed)
• Powder: 2–3 years (airtight, away from heat/humidity)
• Tincture: 4–6 years
• Raw root: ❌ Not recommended for use

---

💬 **Herbal Reflections of Fo-Ti**
Fo-Ti is an herb of paradox: a profound restorer of life force that also requires discipline and respect. In Chinese lore it symbolizes a return to youth—renewed stamina, deeper reserves, and hair vitality restored over time. Energetically, it feels like deep nourishing water that slowly refills the system from the inside outward. Yet Fo-Ti also teaches a hard truth: longevity is not a shortcut. When prepared properly and used conservatively, it can be a steady ally for long-term rebuilding.

---

🌟 **Herbal Confidence Index:** 🌿 🌿 🌿 🌿 (4/5 green stars)
Reasoning: Deep restorative longevity herb revered for nourishing blood and reserves, supporting vitality and hair strength. Loses one star due to liver-risk history and the strict requirement for prepared form, conservative dosing, and reputable sourcing.

# RED RASPBERRY LEAF

★★★★★

*Rubus idaeus*

**Red Raspberry Leaf is one of the most celebrated herbs in Western herbalism, treasured especially for women's reproductive health.** Known as the "herb of midwives," it is rich in minerals (iron, magnesium, calcium, potassium) and the compound fragarine, which tones uterine muscles and supports smoother cycles, fertility, and childbirth.

**Beyond reproduction, Red Raspberry Leaf also offers digestive, immune, and nutritive benefits.** Its mild astringency makes it a gentle remedy for diarrhea or tissue weakness, while its rich nutrient profile strengthens the body as a daily tonic.

For centuries, Red Raspberry has been treasured across Europe and North America as a woman's ally and household healer. **Midwives of the 16th and 17th centuries relied on its leaves to strengthen the womb and ease childbirth, while Native American herbalists brewed it as a restorative tonic for fevers, wounds, and digestive calm.** In Victorian England, it became a symbol of gentle strength — a tea of resilience and renewal passed down from mother to daughter.

---

## *Core Herbal Category — Red Raspberry Leaf*

**Primary Core: Reproductive & Women's Health Support herb** with (uterine-toning, mineral-rich action that strengthens reproductive tissues and supports hormonal balance)

**Secondary Cores:** Digestive Support herb · Nutritive & Restorative herb · Immune Support herb

---

## *How It Works*

Red Raspberry Leaf works by **toning and strengthening uterine and pelvic tissues**, supporting reproductive resilience without overstimulation. Its high mineral content helps **nourish depleted systems**, especially during menstruation, pregnancy, and recovery. The herb's gentle astringency supports **digestive tone and nutrient absorption**. This nutritive support contributes to **steady hormonal rhythm and vitality**. Overall, Red Raspberry Leaf acts as a **deeply nourishing reproductive tonic that restores strength, balance, and endurance**.

---

## *Primary Uses*

- Tones and nourishes the uterus
- Eases menstrual cramps and hormonal shifts
- Supports fertility and pregnancy balance

• Helps prepare the body for childbirth (late-pregnancy use)
• Provides gentle digestive support
• Serves as a daily mineral-rich nutritive tonic

---

## Scientific Backing

Research highlights **fragarine**, tannins, and ellagic acid as key compounds contributing to:
• Uterine toning and smoother muscular coordination
• Menstrual and pregnancy support
• Astringent digestive action
• Immune and cardiovascular benefits
Mineral density (iron, magnesium, potassium, antioxidants) validates its role as a safe daily nutritive herb.

---

## How to Use (Dosage)

• **Tea:** 1 tbsp dried leaves; steep 10–15 minutes; 1–3 cups daily
• **Capsules:** 300–500 mg, 1–3× daily
• **Infused oil:** Topical toning or massage applications

---

## Expected Results

• Menstrual comfort: **1–2 days**
• Pregnancy/uterine tone: **1–3 weeks**
• General vitality + nutrient renewal: **within 1 week**

---

## Caution Level: Safe / Mild Caution

• Safe for most users
• Mild uterine-toning activity — use professional guidance during **first trimester**
• Avoid high-dose extracts early in pregnancy
• Appropriate during **second and third trimesters** in moderate tea amounts

---

## Gender-Specific Safety (GS)

**Men:** Safe — Supports digestive tone, oral/gum health, and overall vitality. No hormonal concerns.
**Women:** Safe — One of the most respected herbs for uterus, cycles, hormones, and pregnancy preparation.
**Pregnancy / Nursing:** Caution — Safe in moderate tea amounts during the 2nd & 3rd

trimesters; avoid strong extracts or very early use. Supports postpartum recovery and lactation.

## Forms Available

- Dried leaves
- Capsules or tincture
- Infused oil

---

## Same / Similar Results

- Nettle Leaf — mineral-rich vitality
- Chamomile — digestive + nervous balance
- Lemon Balm — mood + gentle circulation
- Alfalfa — nutrient tonic
- Dong Quai — deeper hormonal support

## DIY Recipe — Raspberry Leaf Renewal Tea

1 tbsp dried raspberry leaves
1 cup boiling water
Steep 10–15 minutes. Drink warm, up to 3× daily for reproductive tone and nourishment.

---

## Shelf Life / Potency After Preparation

- **Dried leaves:** 1–2 years (airtight, away from light)
- **Tincture:** 3–5 years
- **Prepared tea:** Refrigerate; use within 24 hours
- **Infused oil:** 6–12 months (refrigerated)

## Herbal Reflections of Red Raspberry Leaf

Red Raspberry Leaf represents gentle strength—supporting cycles, fertility, pregnancy, and feminine renewal. Its minerals fortify, its tannins tighten and protect, and its fragarine helps the womb remember its natural rhythm.

A companion herb for women across generations, it nourishes from within, offering steadiness rather than stimulation.

---

## Herbal Confidence Index:

*(5/5 green stars — a cornerstone herb for reproductive vitality, uterine tone, menstrual harmony, fertility, and pregnancy support. One of the safest and most dependable daily herbs for long-term nourishment and childbearing strength.)*

# YOHIMBE

★★½

Pausinystalia johimbe

**Yohimbe, derived from the bark of a West African tree, is a powerful stimulant long recognized for its effects on circulation, stamina, and intimacy. Its key alkaloid, yohimbine, acts directly on the nervous system to increase blood flow, heighten sexual response, and energize the body.** Herbalists and researchers alike **consider Yohimbe both potent and risky** — a herb that can bring noticeable results but requires careful, professional guidance.
**Historically, Yohimbe was revered in traditional African medicine as a sacred aphrodisiac, courage enhancer, and stamina tonic.** Tribal healers valued it for its ability to strengthen vitality and confidence in body and spirit. Later, **it gained worldwide recognition for improving erectile function and inspiring modern pharmaceutical interest.** Its legacy, however, remains dual-edged: a symbol of both potency and caution.

---

## *Core Herbal Category — Yohimbe*

**Primary Core: Cardiovascular System Support herb** with (strong vascular-stimulating action that increases blood flow and nervous system activation)
**Secondary Cores:** Nervines (Nervous System Support) herb · Men's Health & Vitality herb · Metabolic & Blood Sugar Support herb

---

## *How It Works*

Yohimbe works by **stimulating adrenergic receptors**, increasing blood flow and heightening nervous system activity. This vascular activation enhances **circulation to peripheral tissues**, contributing to libido and performance effects. Its stimulant action also **elevates energy and alertness**, influencing mood and responsiveness. Because it strongly activates the nervous and cardiovascular systems, its effects are **fast and pronounced**. Overall, Yohimbe functions as a **potent, short-term circulatory stimulant rather than a restorative tonic**.

---

## *Primary Uses*

- Supports erectile dysfunction and sexual performance
- Enhances libido and circulation
- Increases stimulation, alertness, and short-term energy

• Explored for athletic performance and fat mobilization

---

## 🔬 Scientific Backing

Research confirms that **yohimbine** is a strong vasodilator and adrenergic stimulant that increases sexual response by enhancing neural and circulatory function. Prescription forms exist for erectile dysfunction, demonstrating documented physiological effects.

Studies on weight loss and athletic performance show mixed results — and side effects increase sharply with dosage. Yohimbe's clinical usefulness lies in **precise, low-dose, supervised applications**, not casual use.

---

## 💊 How to Use (Dosage)

(Professional supervision strongly recommended)

• **Tea/Decoction:** 1 tsp dried bark simmered 10–15 minutes; **max 1 cup daily**
• **Capsules/Tablets:** Follow standardized extract guidelines only under expert direction
• **Tincture:** Rarely recommended; use only with clinical guidance

---

## ⏳ Expected Results

• Libido/erectile support: **2–5 days**
• Nervous-system stimulation: **within hours**
• Energy/fatigue boost: **variable; short-term only**

---

## ⚠️ Caution Level: 🔴 Supervision Required

• Contains **yohimbine**, a powerful stimulant affecting blood pressure, heart rate, and mood
• May cause rapid heartbeat, hypertension, anxiety, agitation, dizziness, nausea
• **Never combine with:**
– Antidepressants (SSRIs, MAOIs)
– Caffeine or stimulant herbs
– Blood pressure medication
– Erectile dysfunction drugs (Viagra, Cialis, etc.)
• Avoid with heart disease, hypertension, kidney issues, anxiety disorders, or PTSD
• Pregnant or breastfeeding individuals should strictly **avoid**
• Commercial Yohimbe products vary widely in potency; some are unsafe or adulterated
• **Not a tonic** — use only short-term, in ritual or supervised therapeutic contexts

---

## Gender-Specific Safety (GS)

**Men:** Supervision Required — Effective for circulation and libido but easily causes overstimulation and cardiovascular strain. Use only under professional guidance; avoid all stimulants or ED drugs.
**Women:** Supervision Required — Strong nervous-system activation may trigger anxiety, insomnia, or mood agitation. Not recommended during hormonal therapy.
**Pregnancy/Nursing:** Avoid — Unsafe at all stages. Risks include blood pressure changes and neurovascular stress.

---

## Forms Available

- Dried bark (decoction)
- Capsules/tablets (standardized extract only — safer, but still supervised)

---

## Same / Similar Results

- Muira Puama — libido + nervous stimulation
- Ginseng — stamina + circulation
- Horny Goat Weed — sexual vitality + stimulant
- Maca Root — hormone balance + energy
- Damiana — aphrodisiac + calming nerve support

---

## DIY Recipe — Yohimbe Infusion

1 tsp dried Yohimbe bark
1½ cups water
Simmer 10–15 minutes.
**Do not exceed 1 cup per day** and only use under professional supervision.

---

## Shelf Life / Potency After Preparation

- **Dried bark:** 2–3 years (cool, dark, airtight)
- **Capsules/tablets:** 1–2 years (follow label dates)
- **Prepared decoction:** Refrigerate; use within **24 hours**

---

## Herbal Reflections of Yohimbe

Yohimbe is a force — bold, hot, and commanding. It energizes, sharpens, and intensifies, but rarely does so gently. Unlike Maca or Ginseng, which build vitality over time, Yohimbe strikes quickly and can overwhelm sensitive systems.

It teaches that potency requires boundaries. Used respectfully and with guidance, it can awaken vitality and passion. Used casually, it becomes chaotic and hazardous. Yohimbe belongs to the category of ritualistic, precision herbs — one that demands respect more than enthusiasm.

---

## Herbal Confidence Index: ½

(2.5/5 red stars — potent but unpredictable stimulant and aphrodisiac; capable of enhancing circulation and libido, yet burdened with high safety risks including hypertension, nervous agitation, and cardiovascular strain. Effective only within a narrow therapeutic window and under expert supervision. Not suitable as a daily or tonic herb.)

# YERBA MANSA

★★★★

*Anemopsis californica*

**Yerba Mansa**, a medicinal treasure of the American Southwest, has been valued by Native American tribes and Hispanic healers for its ability to calm inflammation, clear infection, and soothe irritated tissues. Its peppery-spicy root has earned a reputation as a natural cleanser and tonic, particularly for the respiratory, urinary, and digestive systems. Often referred to as a "calming cleanser," Yerba Mansa helps dry damp congestion, ease chronic sinus issues, and restore balance in mucous membranes and joints. Whether prepared as a tea or applied topically, this desert healer addresses both acute irritation and lingering inflammatory states with steady, grounding action.

---

### Core Herbal Category — Yerba Mansa

**Primary Core: Respiratory System Support** herb with (astringent antimicrobial action that tones mucous membranes, reduces excessive secretions, and supports resolution of damp inflammatory states)

**Secondary Cores:** Respiratory Support · Urinary & Kidney Support · Digestive Support · Skin & Tissue Repair

---

### How It Works

Yerba Mansa works by tightening and toning mucous membranes while discouraging microbial overgrowth, making it especially effective for damp, inflamed tissue states. Its astringent properties help reduce excessive secretions and swelling in the respiratory and urinary tracts. At the same time, its mild circulatory stimulation supports tissue repair and immune response. Overall, Yerba Mansa functions as a mucosal-toning immune herb that restores tissue integrity where chronic irritation or infection has taken hold.

---

### Primary Uses

- Supports resistance to bacterial & fungal overgrowth (internal and topical)
- Eases sinus, throat, and lung congestion
- Calms inflammation in the digestive and urinary tracts
- Supports wound healing, gum irritation, and oral health
- Helps regulate dampness and lingering inflammatory patterns

---

### Scientific Backing

Yerba Mansa contains volatile oils (including piperitone derivatives) and tannins with demonstrated antimicrobial, antifungal, and astringent activity. Research and ethnobotanical evidence support its traditional use for oral infections, sinus inflammation, urinary irritation, and digestive imbalance. Its dual action — drying excess moisture while supporting circulation — aligns closely with Indigenous and Hispanic clinical traditions.

---

### How to Use (Dosage)

- **Tea/Decoction:** 1 tsp dried root simmered 15–20 minutes; 1–2× daily
- **Tincture:** 20–40 drops in water, up to 3× daily
- **Topical:** Poultice or infused oil for wounds, fungal areas, or gum irritation

---

### Expected Results

- Sinus & respiratory relief: 1–2 days
- Digestive & urinary comfort: 3–5 days
- Skin and wound support: within 1 week

---

### Caution Level: Safe / Mild Caution

- Generally safe when used in moderate doses
- Excessive use may cause dryness or mild digestive irritation
- Not suited for very dry constitutions
- Avoid during pregnancy due to astringent and mildly stimulating effects

---

### Gender-Specific Safety (GS)

**Men:** Caution — Supports urinary, sinus, and digestive health. Avoid prolonged high doses if prone to dryness or dehydration.

**Women:** Caution — Helpful for chronic congestion and mucosal imbalance. Excessive use may overly dry tissues.

**Pregnancy/Nursing:** Avoid — Not recommended due to mucosal-tightening and stimulating properties. Choose gentler alternatives such as Marshmallow, Calendula, or Chamomile.

---

### Forms Available

Dried root

Tincture

Topical infused oil / salve

---

### Same / Similar Results

🔘 Goldenseal — mucous membrane tonic + antimicrobial
🔘 Echinacea — immune activation and infection defense
🔘 Oregon Grape Root — antimicrobial + liver/skin support
🔘 Myrrh — oral and wound antiseptic
🔘 Calendula — gentle tissue repair

---

🛠 **DIY Recipe — Cleansing Yerba Mansa Steam**
1 tbsp chopped Yerba Mansa root
4 cups hot water
Inhale steam for 5–10 minutes under a towel for sinus congestion and damp irritation.

---

**Shelf Life / Potency After Preparation**
• Dried root: 2 years
• Tincture: 4–6 years
• Infused oil: 6–12 months (refrigerated)
• Prepared decoction: Refrigerate; use within 48 hours

---

🌙 **Herbal Reflections of Yerba Mansa**
Yerba Mansa restores balance by clearing stagnation rather than overpowering it. Thriving in harsh environments, it teaches that healing often comes from correcting terrain — drying what is excessive, calming what is inflamed, and strengthening what has been irritated too long.

---

⭐ **Herbal Confidence Index:** 🌿 🌿 🌿 🌿
(4/5 — a dependable Southwestern immune and mucosal tonic with strong antimicrobial and tissue-balancing action; highly effective when used appropriately, though excessive use may cause dryness.)

# WHITE PEONY

★★★★★

*Paeonia lactiflora*

**White Peony**, known in Traditional Chinese Medicine as Bai Shao, is one of the most balancing tonic herbs for women's health. Cherished for its ability to calm the liver, nourish the blood, and harmonize hormones, it is widely used in fertility, menstrual, and menopausal formulas. Gentle yet powerful, White Peony reduces cramping, cools irritation, eases mood swings, and restores emotional steadiness without sedation.
For over a thousand years, White Peony has held an honored place in classical Chinese medicine texts, appearing in formulas alongside Dong Quai and Licorice Root to strengthen women's vitality and promote harmony. Its reputation as both an elegant ornamental flower and trusted medicinal root symbolizes endurance, grace, and feminine resilience.

---

### 🌿 Core Herbal Category — White Peony

**Primary Core: Endocrine & Hormonal Support** herb with (blood-nourishing, liver-calming action that harmonizes hormonal rhythm and eases tension-driven imbalance)
**Secondary Cores:** Women's Health · Nervous System Support · Digestive Support · Musculoskeletal & Pain Relief

---

### 🌿 How It Works

White Peony works by nourishing the blood while calming excessive liver-driven tension, allowing hormonal rhythm and muscle tone to normalize. This harmonizing action reduces menstrual cramping, muscle tightness, and irritability linked to imbalance. By softening nervous reactivity, it promotes emotional steadiness without sedation and gently supports digestion. Overall, White Peony functions as a restorative tonic that brings balance across hormones, mood, and muscular systems.

---

### 🌱 Primary Uses

- Reduces PMS, cramps, and menstrual irregularity
- Supports fertility and menopausal transition
- Nourishes blood and calms liver tension (TCM)
- Eases muscle spasms and stress-related irritability
- Promotes emotional steadiness and hormonal balance

---

### Scientific Backing

White Peony contains paeoniflorin, a compound shown to have antispasmodic, anti-inflammatory, and neuro-calming effects. Clinical and traditional evidence supports its use for dysmenorrhea, PMS, mood instability, and hormonal imbalance. In TCM, it is classified as a yin-nourishing, blood-tonifying herb used to cool liver heat and stabilize reproductive function.

---

### How to Use (Dosage)

- **Decoction:** 1 tbsp dried root simmered 15–20 minutes; 1–2 cups daily
- **Capsules:** 300–600 mg extract, 1–2× daily
- **Tincture:** 2–4 mL daily (commonly used in formulas)

---

### Expected Results

- PMS & cramp relief: 1–2 days
- Emotional steadiness: 1–2 weeks
- Hormonal balance: 1–2 cycles
- Blood nourishment: gradual, cumulative improvement

---

### Caution Level: Safe / Mild Caution

- Generally well tolerated
- Avoid high doses in early pregnancy
- May potentiate anticoagulant medications
- Excessive long-term dosing may cause mild digestive upset

---

### Gender-Specific Safety (GS)

**Men:** Safe — Calms liver tension and muscular tightness without hormonal disruption.

**Women:** Caution — Premier reproductive tonic; avoid excessive dosing.

**Pregnancy/Nursing:** Avoid — Not recommended due to uterine-modulating effects.

---

### Forms Available

- Dried root
- Capsules / extracts
- Tincture
- Often included in classic formulas

---

### Same / Similar Results

- Dong Quai — blood and menstrual support
- Vitex — cycle regulation

🟣 Black Cohosh — menopausal transition support
🟣 Shatavari — fertility tonic
🟡 Licorice Root — adrenal and liver harmony

---

### 🛠 DIY Recipe — White Peony Harmony Tea

1 tbsp dried root
2 cups water
Simmer gently 15–20 minutes; drink daily as a reproductive tonic.

---

### Shelf Life / Potency After Preparation

- Dried root: 2–3 years
- Capsules/powder: 1–2 years
- Tincture: 5–7 years
- Decoction: Refrigerate; use within 48–72 hours

---

### 🌙 Herbal Reflections of White Peony

White Peony teaches balance through gentleness. It does not force the body into change — it helps the body remember its rhythm. Where tension, overwork, or emotional strain has tightened the system, White Peony softens and restores.
Compared with Dong Quai, which moves and builds blood more actively, White Peony is calmer and more harmonizing — especially helpful when cramps, irritability, and stress are tied to liver tension. Compared with Black Cohosh, which is often used for stronger menopausal shifts, White Peony tends to be steadier and more nourishing over time.
Its unique gift is grace: strengthening without agitation, calming without dullness, and supporting women's vitality without pushing the body past its limits.

---

### 🌟 Herbal Confidence Index: 🌿 🌿 🌿 🌿 🌿

(5/5 — a cornerstone hormonal harmonizer with exceptional safety and depth; highly reliable for menstrual, fertility, and menopausal balance.)

# WORMWOOD

★★★

*Artemisia absinthium*

**Wormwood** is a sharply bitter herb long valued for stimulating digestion, activating bile flow, and disrupting parasitic overgrowth. Its volatile oils — particularly thujone — account for both its medicinal strength and strict safety limits. Used correctly, it revives sluggish digestion and supports short-term cleansing; misused, it becomes neurotoxic.

---

### 🌿 Core Herbal Category — Wormwood

**Primary Core: Digestive System Support** herb with (intensely stimulating action that activates digestion and disrupts parasitic overgrowth)

**Secondary Cores:** Liver & Gallbladder Support · Immune Support · Metabolic Support

---

### 🌿 How It Works

Wormwood works by powerfully stimulating digestive secretions, increasing stomach acid and bile flow. Its bitter compounds create an inhospitable environment for parasites and certain microbes while activating liver and gallbladder function. This intensity breaks severe stagnation but strictly limits duration of use. Wormwood is corrective — never tonic.

---

### 🌱 Primary Uses

- Short-term parasite cleansing
- Appetite stimulation
- Bile and digestive activation
- Liver and gallbladder support
- Relief of severe digestive stagnation

---

### 🧪 Scientific Backing

Thujone-rich volatile oils account for Wormwood's antiparasitic and digestive effects. Research confirms increased bile secretion and enhanced digestive enzyme activity. Thujone is neurotoxic in excess, requiring strict dosage control and professional supervision.

---

### How to Use (Dosage)

- **Tea:** 1 tsp dried herb steeped 5–7 minutes; once daily

⚠ **Maximum duration:** 7–10 days only

- **Formulas:** Commonly combined with Black Walnut and Cloves
- **Extracts:** Professional supervision only

---

### Expected Results

- Digestive stimulation: 30–60 minutes
- Parasite response: 24–48 hours
- Appetite improvement: 1–3 days

---

### ⚠ Caution Level: ● Supervision Required

**PRECAUTION:** Wormwood contains thujone. Misuse may cause neurological, hepatic, or cardiovascular harm. Never combine with alcohol or other thujone-containing herbs. Avoid entirely if pregnant/nursing or if you have a seizure disorder.

---

### Gender-Specific Safety (GS)

**Men:** ● Supervision Required — Short-term use only.

**Women:** ● Supervision Required — Uterine-stimulating potential.

**Pregnancy/Nursing:** ● Avoid — Unsafe.

---

### Forms Available

● Dried herb

● Capsules (cleanse formulas)

● Tincture (professional use)

---

### Same / Similar Results

● Black Walnut Hull — antiparasitic

● Cloves — antiparasitic synergy

● Oregano Oil — antimicrobial support

● Barberry — bile stimulant

● Mugwort — bitter digestive stimulant

---

### DIY Recipe — Wormwood Cleanse Tea

1 tsp dried Wormwood

Steep 5–7 minutes

Drink once daily for no more than 7 days

⚠ Best used as part of a supervised parasite protocol.

---

### Shelf Life / Potency After Preparation

- Dried herb: 2 years
- Capsules/powders: 1–2 years
- Tincture: 5–7 years
- Tea: Refrigerate; use within 24–48 hours

---

### Herbal Reflections of Wormwood

Wormwood is the strict teacher of herbalism — powerful, effective, and unforgiving of casual use. It clears what is stubborn: heavy stagnation, sluggish digestion, and parasitic burden. But it teaches an equally important lesson: strength without boundaries becomes harm.

Compared with Gentian or Dandelion bitters, Wormwood is far more intense and far less suited for general digestive support. Compared with Mugwort, it is sharper and more neurologically risky due to thujone. Wormwood has a place, but that place is narrow: short-term, corrective, supervised.

Its deeper value is precision. When used properly, it can be transformative. When used carelessly, it becomes a warning written into the plant itself.

---

### Herbal Confidence Index:

(3/5 — highly effective but narrow-margin antiparasitic and digestive bitter; valuable only for brief, supervised use, never a daily tonic.)

---

# RUE

★★★

*Ruta graveolens*

**Rue** — the ancient "Herb of Grace" — is a sharp, bitter, commanding plant historically used for cramps, circulation, and protective cleansing. Its essential oils and alkaloids make it potent and also hazardous, with a narrow safety margin that limits modern medicinal use. Today, Rue is primarily respected as an external herb, ritual plant, or homeopathic preparation rather than a routine internal remedy.

---

### 🌿 Core Herbal Category — Rue

**Primary Core:** Cardiovascular System Support herb with (strong activating action that stimulates smooth muscle and pelvic circulation)
**Secondary Cores:** Women's Health · Digestive Support · Immune Support

---

### 🌿 How It Works

Rue works by strongly stimulating circulation and smooth muscle activity, especially in the pelvic region. This may reduce certain spasmodic tensions, but it also introduces significant risk — including uterine stimulation and systemic toxicity. Its bitter compounds can activate digestive secretions, and its volatile oils can irritate tissues. Rue is non-tonic and unsuitable for routine internal use.

---

### 🌱 Primary Uses

- External use for sore muscles, bruises, and localized inflammation
- Historical use for cramps and digestive stagnation (⚠ not appropriate for casual internal use)
- Traditional protective/clearing uses in folk practice

---

### 🧪 Scientific Backing

Rue contains rutin and strong volatile oils associated with circulation effects and antimicrobial activity. These same constituents can irritate the stomach and nervous system. Fresh Rue can cause blistering, photosensitive dermatitis, and inflammatory skin reactions. Modern practice generally restricts Rue to external use or homeopathic preparations.

---

### 💊 How to Use (Dosage)

**Internal use:** ● Not recommended except under medical supervision.

**External:**

- Infused oil or diluted salve for sore muscles/joints (patch test first)
- Wear gloves when handling fresh plant material

**Homeopathic:** Follow labeled directions only.

---

### ⏳ Expected Results

- Topical comfort: 30–60 minutes
- Internal effects: variable and unsafe without supervision

---

### ⚠ Caution Level: ● Supervision Required

**PRECAUTION:** Rue is a high-risk herb with abortifacient history and documented toxicity. Avoid internal use. Avoid fresh handling without protection. Avoid if sensitive to sunlight or prone to skin reactions. Never use during pregnancy or while nursing.

---

### Gender-Specific Safety (GS)

**Men:** ● Supervision Required — Prefer external use only; internal use risks toxicity.

**Women:** ● Supervision Required — Strong uterine stimulation risk; internal use is unsafe.

**Pregnancy/Nursing:** ● Avoid — Unsafe in all forms.

---

### 💊 Forms Available

● Dried herb (external use only)

● Infused oil (topical use)

● Homeopathic preparations

---

### 🔄 Same / Similar Results

● Chamomile — cramps + nervous relaxation

● Lavender — topical comfort + calm

● Mugwort — uterine/digestive stimulant (caution)

● Wormwood — bitter digestive (supervised)

● Arnica (topical) — bruising and soreness support

---

### 🛠 DIY Recipe — Rue Joint & Nerve Oil (External Only)

1 small handful dried Rue

1 cup olive oil
Infuse 2 weeks in a cool, dark place. Strain and apply sparingly.
⚠ Avoid sunlight on treated skin; discontinue if irritation occurs.

---

### Shelf Life / Potency After Preparation

• Dried herb: 1–2 years
• Infused oil: up to 1 year (refrigeration preferred)
• Homeopathic: follow labeled expiration

---

### Herbal Reflections of Rue

Rue is the boundary herb — sharp, protective, and uncompromising. Historically, it was used to "clear the room" in both body and spirit, and that symbolism still fits: Rue pushes, stimulates, and provokes change.

But Rue also carries a sobering truth about herbal medicine: not every traditional remedy belongs in casual modern use. Compared with Chamomile, which soothes cramps safely, Rue is forceful and risky. Compared with Mugwort, it is more likely to irritate the nervous system and provoke uterine response. Its modern role is narrow — best respected as an external or ceremonial plant, approached with caution and skill.

Rue's lesson is reverence: potency must always be matched with restraint.

---

### Herbal Confidence Index: 🌿 🌿

(2/5 — historically important and physiologically active, but too hazardous for general internal use; best reserved for external, limited applications and respectful handling.)

# HORSETAIL

★★★★

*Equisetum arvense*

**Horsetail** is a mineral-rich restorative herb valued for strengthening bones, joints, hair, nails, and connective tissue. Its naturally high silica content supports structural integrity and long-term tissue repair, while its mild diuretic action assists urinary elimination and gentle cleansing. Herbal traditions have long relied on Horsetail as a slow-building ally for rebuilding what has been worn down by age, injury, or stress.
Often used both internally and topically, Horsetail supports wound healing, joint comfort, and urinary tone. Its effects are gradual rather than dramatic, making it best suited for steady, cyclical use rather than short bursts.

---

### Core Herbal Category — Horsetail

**Primary Core: Nutritional & Tonic Support herb** with (silica-rich, remineralizing action that strengthens connective tissue and structural integrity)
**Secondary Cores:** Urinary & Kidney Support · Skin & Tissue Repair · Musculoskeletal Support

---

### How It Works

Horsetail supplies bioavailable silica and trace minerals that support collagen formation and connective tissue repair. This strengthens bones, joints, skin, hair, and nails over time. Its gentle diuretic effect promotes urinary elimination without electrolyte depletion, supporting bladder tone and tissue cleansing. Together, these actions make Horsetail a slow, structural rebuilder rather than a fast-acting stimulant.

---

### Primary Uses

- Strengthens bones, hair, nails, and skin
- Supports joint and connective tissue repair
- Aids wound healing and tissue recovery
- Relieves mild urinary irritation and fluid retention

---

### Scientific Backing

Horsetail's silica content has been linked to collagen support, connective tissue repair, and wound healing. Studies also confirm mild diuretic effects without significant potassium loss. **Only Equisetum arvense** is used medicinally; other species may contain higher thiaminase or unwanted compounds.

---

### How to Use (Dosage)

- **Decoction:** 1–2 tsp dried herb simmered 10–15 minutes; 1–2× daily
- **Capsules/Powder:** 300–500 mg, 1–2× daily with food
- **Topical:** Strong decoction as compress or rinse

---

### Expected Results

- Urinary support: 1–3 days
- Skin/wound recovery (topical): several days
- Hair and nail strength: 3–6 weeks
- Bone and joint support: 8–12 weeks

---

### Caution Level: Caution

- Contains thiaminase — avoid long-term continuous daily use
- Avoid with kidney disease or strong diuretics
- Use verified E. arvense only
- Pregnancy/Nursing: light use only unless supervised

---

### Gender-Specific Safety (GS)

**Men:** Safe — Supports structural and urinary health with moderate cyclic use.

**Women:** Safe — Helpful for connective tissue and post-menopausal bone support.

**Pregnancy/Nursing:** Mild Caution — Avoid high-dose or prolonged use.

---

### Forms Available

Dried herb (decoction)

Capsules / powder

Tincture

Topical compresses / salves

---

***Same / Similar Results*** *Nettle Leaf · Oatstraw · Bamboo Leaf · Gotu Kola · Comfrey (topical)*

---

### DIY Recipe — Horsetail Mineral Decoction

Simmer 1–2 tsp dried Horsetail in 1 cup water for 10–15 minutes.
Strain and use as tea or cooled for compresses.

### Shelf Life / Potency After Preparation

- Dried herb: 1–2 years
- Capsules/powder: 18–24 months
- Tincture: 5+ years
- Decoction: refrigerate; use within 24–48 hours

### Herbal Reflections of Horsetail

Horsetail rebuilds quietly. Its medicine restores strength through nourishment rather than force, reminding us that resilience returns when structure is patiently supported.

### Herbal Confidence Index:

(4/5 — a dependable structural and urinary restorative; most effective when used in sensible cycles.)

# GUAVA LEAF

★★★★

*Psidium guajava folium*

**Guava Leaf** is a stabilizing herbal remedy used worldwide for digestive distress, blood sugar balance, and microbial defense. Rich in tannins and flavonoids, it helps calm diarrhea, strengthen intestinal tissue, and support metabolic steadiness. Unlike harsher astringents, Guava Leaf balances rather than shocks the system.
Traditionally brewed as a daily tea across tropical regions, Guava Leaf remains valued for its reliability in digestive and metabolic care, as well as its supportive role in skin and oral health.

---

### 🌿 Core Herbal Category — Guava Leaf

**Primary Core: Digestive System Support** herb with (regulating, antioxidant action that supports steadier glucose response)
**Secondary Cores:** Digestive Support · Immune Support · Skin & Tissue Repair · Respiratory Support

---

### 🌿 How It Works

Guava Leaf helps regulate post-meal glucose response while its astringent tannins strengthen and protect the intestinal lining. This reduces excessive fluid loss and discourages microbial overgrowth during digestive upset. Antioxidant compounds further support immune function and tissue protection.

---

### 🌱 Primary Uses

- Supports blood sugar balance
- Calms diarrhea and digestive irritation
- Supports antimicrobial defense
- Assists cough and cold recovery
- Supports skin and wound care (topical)

---

### 💉 Scientific Backing

Guava Leaf contains quercetin, tannins, and flavonoids shown to reduce post-meal glucose spikes, shorten infectious diarrhea duration, and provide antimicrobial activity.

---

### How to Use (Dosage)

- **Tea:** 3–5 leaves (or 1 tbsp crushed), simmer 10–15 minutes; 1–2 cups daily
- **Capsules:** 300–500 mg, 1–2× daily
- **Topical:** Strong tea as wash or rinse

---

### Expected Results

- Digestive relief: 1–2 days
- Blood sugar support: 1–2 weeks
- Skin support: 5–10 days

---

### Caution Level: Safe

- High doses may cause constipation
- Monitor if prone to low blood sugar or using diabetes medication

---

### Gender-Specific Safety (GS)

**Men:** Safe — Supports digestion and metabolic stability.

**Women:** Safe — Helpful for digestion and microbial balance.

**Pregnancy/Nursing:** Caution — Mild tea acceptable; avoid concentrates.

---

### Forms Available

Dried/fresh leaves

Capsules / powder

Tincture

---

### Same / Similar Results

Bay Leaf · Blackberry Leaf · Chamomile · Goldenseal

---

### DIY Recipe — Guava Leaf Digestive Tea

Simmer 5–6 leaves in 2 cups water for 15 minutes.

Strain and drink warm for short-term digestive support.

---

### Shelf Life / Potency After Preparation

- Dried leaves: 1–2 years
- Capsules/powder: up to 2 years
- Tincture: 4–5 years
- Prepared tea: refrigerate; use within 24–48 hours

🌙 **Herbal Reflections of Guava Leaf**

Guava Leaf restores calm through steadiness. Its strength lies in regulation — guiding digestion, sugar balance, and immune tone back toward equilibrium without disruption.

---

⭐ **Herbal Confidence Index:** 🌿 🌿 🌿 🌿

(4/5 — a reliable digestive and metabolic stabilizer with broad traditional and scientific support.)

---

# GRAPEFRUIT SEED

★★★

*Citrus × paradisi semen*

**Grapefruit Seed** is most commonly used as Grapefruit Seed Extract (GSE), a modern botanical product valued for its strong antimicrobial properties. It is frequently employed in short-term protocols for yeast, bacterial, and fungal imbalance. While effective, it requires careful sourcing and disciplined use.

---

### Core Herbal Category — Grapefruit Seed

**Primary Core: Immune System Support** herb with (targeted antimicrobial action against bacteria and fungi)

**Secondary Cores:** Digestive Support · Respiratory Support · Skin & Tissue Repair

---

### How It Works

Grapefruit Seed Extract disrupts microbial growth, helping reduce bacterial and fungal overgrowth in the digestive and oral environment. Its concentrated nature makes it effective for short-term cleansing, but unsuitable for continuous daily use.

---

### Primary Uses

- Candida and yeast overgrowth
- Bacterial and fungal infections
- Digestive imbalance
- Oral and skin hygiene support

---

### Scientific Backing

Studies confirm antimicrobial activity against Candida, E. coli, and Staphylococcus. Commercial variability is a known limitation, making reputable sourcing essential.

---

### How to Use (Dosage)

- **Liquid extract:** 5–10 drops diluted in water, 1–2× daily
- **Capsules/Tablets:** Follow label; short-term use only
- **Topical:** Dilute before skin application

---

### Expected Results

- Digestive/immune support: 1–3 days
- Microbial balance: 5–10 days

---

### Caution Level: Caution

- May interact with many medications (statins, BP meds, antidepressants)
- Always dilute; avoid long-term use
- Pregnancy/Nursing: avoid concentrated extracts

---

### Gender-Specific Safety (GS)

**Men:** Safe — Short-term use only; monitor medication interactions.

**Women:** Safe — Avoid if using hormonal or anticoagulant medications.

**Pregnancy/Nursing:** Caution — Food-level exposure only.

---

### Forms Available

Liquid extract

Capsules/tablets

Topical preparations

---

**Same / Similar Results** Olive Leaf · Oregano Oil · Garlic · Black Walnut Hull · Neem

---

### DIY Recipe — Antifungal Skin Spray

Dilute 10 drops extract in 1 cup distilled water.
Apply to affected areas once or twice daily.

---

### Shelf Life / Potency After Preparation

- Liquid extract: 3–5 years
- Capsules/tablets: 2–3 years
- Diluted spray: refrigerate; use within 30 days

---

### Herbal Reflections of Grapefruit Seed

Grapefruit Seed teaches precision. It acts quickly and decisively, but only when used with restraint. Its value lies in correction, not maintenance.

---

**Herbal Confidence Index:** ½ (3.5/5 — a potent modern antimicrobial; effective short-term, limited by sourcing and interaction concerns.)

# GREEN TEA

★★★★★

*Camellia sinensis (folium viride)*

**Green Tea** is one of the world's most respected daily herbs, valued for antioxidant protection, metabolic support, and clear, steady mental energy. Its catechins (especially EGCG) help defend cells from oxidative stress and support cardiovascular wellness. At the same time, its natural caffeine paired with L-theanine creates a focused alertness that is typically smoother than coffee.

Historically used for centuries in China and Japan, Green Tea has served as both daily nourishment and mindful ritual. Its long use in culture and traditional health systems reflects its rare combination of safety, effectiveness, and practicality.

---

### 🌿 Core Herbal Category — Green Tea

**Primary Core: Cardiovascular System Support** herb with (antioxidant-rich, gently stimulating action that supports energy metabolism and cellular resilience)

**Secondary Cores:** Circulatory & Cardiovascular Support · Nervous System Support · Immune Support

---

### 🌿 How It Works

Green Tea provides catechins that reduce oxidative stress and support healthier metabolic signaling. Mild caffeine increases alertness, while L-theanine helps smooth nervous system stimulation for calmer focus. Together, these actions support metabolic efficiency, cardiovascular tone, and balanced immune response over time. It functions best as a steady daily supportive herb rather than a "quick fix."

---

### 🌱 Primary Uses

- Antioxidant and cellular protection
- Cardiovascular support
- Calm alertness and focus
- Metabolic and weight-supportive routines
- Supports healthier post-meal glucose response

---

### 🧪 Scientific Backing

Research supports Green Tea catechins (including EGCG) for antioxidant activity, lipid and vascular support, and mild metabolic enhancement. Studies also support the caffeine + L-theanine pairing for improved attention and calmer concentration compared with caffeine alone.

---

### How to Use (Dosage)

- **Tea:** 1 tsp loose leaf (or 1 bag) per 8 oz water; steep 2–4 minutes; 1–3 cups daily
- **Matcha:** 1/2–1 tsp, 1–2× daily
- **Capsules/Extracts:** typically 200–400 mg/day catechins (follow label)
- **Topical:** cooled brewed tea as compress for mild soothing support

---

### Expected Results

- Calm alertness: within 30–60 minutes
- Metabolic/cardiovascular support: 3–6 weeks of daily use
- Topical soothing effects: 7–10 days

---

### Caution Level: Safe / Mild Caution

- Excess intake may cause insomnia, jitteriness, or stomach irritation
- Tannins can reduce iron absorption — avoid around iron-rich meals if iron-deficient
- Concentrated extracts may irritate the stomach (especially on an empty stomach)
- May interact with warfarin and certain stimulant-sensitive conditions
- Pregnancy: avoid high-dose extracts; keep caffeine modest

---

### Gender-Specific Safety (GS)

**Men:** Safe — Supports metabolism, circulation, and steady energy; reduce if caffeine-sensitive.

**Women:** Safe — Supports focus and metabolic balance; reduce around insomnia-prone hormonal phases if needed.

**Pregnancy/Nursing:** Caution — 1–2 lightly brewed cups daily; avoid concentrated extracts and high caffeine.

---

### Forms Available

Loose leaf / tea bags

Matcha powder

Standardized extracts / capsules

Ready-to-drink teas (quality varies)

---

### Same / Similar Results

Matcha · White Tea · Tulsi (Holy Basil) · Ginkgo Biloba · Yerba Mate

### 🛠 DIY Recipe — Green Tea Skin Tonic (Simple)

Brew 1 cup Green Tea, cool completely, and use as a gentle facial rinse or compress.

---

### Shelf Life / Potency After Preparation

- Dried leaves: 1–2 years (airtight, cool, dark)
- Matcha: 6–12 months (kept cool; refrigerate if needed)
- Extracts: 4–6 years (per label storage)
- Brewed tea: refrigerate; use within 24 hours
- Topical preparations: best within 24–48 hours refrigerated

---

### Herbal Reflections of Green Tea

Green Tea offers clarity without force. It lifts attention while keeping the nervous system steadier, making it a daily ally for focus, longevity, and metabolic balance. Its lesson is simple: consistent small support often outperforms intense short bursts.

---

### Herbal Confidence Index: 🌿 🌿 🌿 🌿 🌿

(5/5 — a cornerstone antioxidant and longevity herb with extensive research support for metabolic, cardiovascular, and cognitive benefits; exceptionally practical and safe when used moderately.)

---

# SHEPHERD'S PURSE

★★★★

*Capsella bursa-pastoris*

**Shepherd's Purse** is a classic short-term hemostatic herb used to help reduce excessive bleeding and support capillary tone. Traditionally, it has been used for heavy menstrual flow, minor wound bleeding, and nosebleeds. Its role is corrective and situational — best used when bleeding is active rather than as a daily tonic.
Historically, it was used in field medicine and midwifery when immediate bleeding control was needed. That legacy continues today in careful, targeted herbal practice.

---

### Core Herbal Category — Shepherd's Purse

**Primary Core: Cardiovascular System Support** herb with (hemostatic action that supports vessel tone and helps control acute bleeding)
**Secondary Cores:** Women's Health · Musculoskeletal Support · Immune Support

---

### How It Works

Shepherd's Purse supports constriction of small vessels and improves capillary integrity, helping reduce excessive bleeding. This can be useful for heavy menstrual flow and minor external bleeding when used short-term. It may also support tissue calm by reducing inflammatory irritation associated with vascular leakage. It is a targeted bleeding-control herb, not a daily wellness tonic.

---

### Primary Uses

- Supports reduction of heavy menstrual bleeding (short-term)
- Helps with minor nosebleeds and small cuts (topical)
- Supports capillary tone and circulatory steadiness
- Supports mild urinary irritation (supportive use)

---

### Scientific Backing

Shepherd's Purse contains flavonoids and vessel-toning compounds traditionally associated with hemostatic effects. Historical and clinical herbal use supports its role in reducing excessive bleeding, with the key safety note that it may influence uterine tone.

---

### How to Use (Dosage)

- **Tincture:** 1–2 mL up to 3× daily during acute need (short-term)
- **Tea:** 1–2 tsp steeped 10 minutes; 1–2× daily for 2–3 days
- **Topical:** cooled tea or diluted tincture applied to minor bleeding

---

### ⏳ Expected Results

- Minor topical bleeding: minutes to hours
- Heavy menstrual flow support: 1–3 days
- Urinary irritation support: 2–4 days

⚠ **Caution Level:** ● Caution

- Avoid during pregnancy (uterine influence)
- Postpartum use only with professional guidance
- Avoid prolonged continuous internal use
- Use caution with anticoagulants or clotting disorders

---

### Gender-Specific Safety (GS)

**Men:** ● Safe — Short-term topical or internal use only; not for long-term daily use.

**Women:** ● Caution — Useful for heavy flow short-term; avoid pregnancy; not a daily tonic.

**Pregnancy/Nursing:** ● Avoid — Pregnancy: avoid; Nursing/postpartum: supervised use only.

---

### Forms Available

● Dried herb (tea/compress)

● Tincture / liquid extract

---

### Same / Similar Results

● Yarrow · ● Red Raspberry Leaf · ● Lady's Mantle · ● Witch Hazel · ● Agrimony

---

### DIY Recipe — Short-Term Flow Support Tea

Steep 1 tsp Shepherd's Purse + 1 tsp Red Raspberry Leaf for 10 minutes.
Use short-term during heavy flow (not during pregnancy).

---

### Shelf Life / Potency After Preparation

- Dried herb: 1–2 years
- Tincture: 4–6 years
- Prepared tea: refrigerate; use within 24 hours
- Compress: best within 24–48 hours

---

🌙 **Herbal Reflections of Shepherd's Purse**

Shepherd's Purse is a "steadying" herb — useful when the body is losing too much too fast. It reminds us that some medicines are meant for moments, not seasons: precise, short-term support that restores order when balance slips.

---

⭐ **Herbal Confidence Index:** 🌿 🌿 🌿 🌿

(4/5 — dependable short-term bleeding support with a long traditional track record; best used briefly and thoughtfully.)

# JUJUBE

★★★★★

*Ziziphus jujuba*

**Jujube** (Chinese Red Date) is a nourishing fruit-herb used to calm the nervous system, support sleep, and restore gentle vitality. In Traditional Chinese Medicine, it is valued for "building and harmonizing" — supporting digestion and emotional steadiness while helping the body recover from stress and fatigue. Its sweet, supportive nature makes it well suited for long-term use.

For thousands of years, Jujube has also been used as a harmonizer in formulas, helping moderate stronger herbs while providing steady nourishment.

---

### Core Herbal Category — Jujube

**Primary Core: Nervous System Support (Nervines)** herb with (calming, nourishing action that supports sleep quality and steadies emotional tone)

**Secondary Cores:** Digestive Support · Immune Support · Nutritive & Restorative Support

---

### How It Works

Jujube nourishes and calms the nervous system, reducing restlessness and supporting more restorative sleep. Its gentle sugars, minerals, and phytochemicals support steady mood and stress resilience without harsh sedation. By supporting digestion and comfort, it indirectly improves sleep quality and energy restoration. Over time, it functions as a replenishing nervine-tonic that supports calm vitality.

---

### Primary Uses

- Supports restful sleep and calmer nights
- Reduces mild anxiety and emotional tension
- Supports digestion and gentle energy restoration
- Supports immune resilience and antioxidant protection
- Helps recovery from stress-related fatigue

---

### Scientific Backing

Jujube contains saponins, triterpenoids, and flavonoids studied for calming, sleep-supportive, and neuroprotective effects. Research supports improvements in sleep quality and stress modulation, aligning with its long-standing traditional use as a spirit-calming, restorative tonic.

---

### How to Use (Dosage)

- **Dried fruits:** 2–6 daily, or add 5–8 fruits to tea blends
- **Decoction:** simmer 5–6 fruits in 2 cups water for 10–15 minutes; 1–2× daily
- **Tincture:** 2–4 mL up to 2× daily
- **Powder/Extract:** 1–2 g daily (follow label)

---

### Expected Results

- Sleep and calmer nights: 3–7 days
- Mood steadiness: 1–2 weeks
- Vitality restoration: 2–4 weeks

---

### Caution Level: Safe / Mild Caution

- Very safe for long-term use
- Naturally sweet — moderate portions if diabetic/insulin-resistant
- Large doses may increase drowsiness or digestive heaviness
- May enhance sedatives in sensitive individuals

---

### Gender-Specific Safety (GS)

**Men:** Safe — Supports sleep, digestion, and stress recovery.

**Women:** Safe — Supports mood steadiness, sleep, and gentle nourishment.

**Pregnancy/Nursing:** Safe — Food-level and tea use are traditionally common; keep amounts moderate.

---

### Forms Available

Fresh or dried fruits

Teas/decoctions

Syrups/tonics

Capsules/powder/extract

Tincture

---

### Same / Similar Results

Goji Berry · Licorice Root · Schisandra · Ashwagandha · Passionflower

---

### DIY Recipe — Jujube Sleep Tea (Simple)

Simmer 5–6 dried Jujubes in 2 cups water for 15 minutes.
Strain and sip warm in the evening.

### Shelf Life / Potency After Preparation

• Dried fruit: 1–2 years
• Powder/extract: 1–2 years
• Syrups/tonics: 6–12 months refrigerated
• Tincture: 4–6 years
• Decoction/tea: refrigerate; use within 24–48 hours

---

### Herbal Reflections of Jujube

Jujube heals by replenishing. It doesn't force calm — it feeds it. Its medicine is the steady rebuilding that happens when the body feels safe, nourished, and supported long enough to rest deeply again.

---

### Herbal Confidence Index:

(5/5 — exceptionally safe, nourishing, and effective for sleep support, stress recovery, and gentle vitality; ideal for long-term use.)

# NIGHTSHADE

★★

*Atropa belladonna*

**Nightshade is one of the most infamous and controversial herbs in the history of medicine. Known for its potent alkaloids — atropine, scopolamine, and hyoscyamine — it demonstrates both strong medicinal effects and extreme toxicity. In small, controlled doses, these alkaloids have been used for muscle relaxation, pain relief, and motion sickness, but the margin between therapeutic and fatal is dangerously narrow.**

**Historically, Nightshade carried a shadowy reputation.** In medieval Europe, it was tied to apothecaries, ritual practices, and even witchcraft. Its dramatic effects on the nervous system made it both revered and feared. Today, only isolated compounds are used in regulated pharmaceuticals, while the herb itself is avoided in modern herbalism due to the extreme risk of poisoning.

---

## *Core Herbal Category — Nightshade*

**Primary Core:** **Nervous System Support (Nervines)** **(Nervous System Support) herb** with (powerful anticholinergic, sedative action that suppresses nerve signaling and muscle spasm)
**Secondary Cores:** Musculoskeletal & Pain-Relief herb · Immune Support herb · Metabolic & Blood Sugar Support herb

---

## *How It Works*

Nightshade works by **blocking acetylcholine signaling**, profoundly reducing nerve transmission and muscle activity. This suppression produces **strong sedation, spasm relief, and pain dampening**, but also carries significant risk. By inhibiting autonomic nervous system activity, it can **lower fever and reduce severe inflammatory reactions**. These effects are **dose-critical and unpredictable**, separating therapeutic from toxic response. Overall, Nightshade functions as a **high-risk, non-tonic nervous system suppressant reserved for controlled medical contexts only**.

---

### Primary Uses (Historical & Pharmaceutical Context Only)

- Pain relief and muscle relaxation (historic European medicine)
- Motion sickness and anesthesia (via modern pharmaceutical alkaloids)
- Nervous system sedation under strict medical control

• Ceremonial and ritual use in ancient European folk practices

⚠ **Not used in modern herbalism. Self-use of whole herb is dangerous and prohibited.**

---

## 🧪 Scientific Backing

Nightshade contains the tropane alkaloids atropine, hyoscyamine, and scopolamine. These compounds block acetylcholine at muscarinic receptors, causing:

• Pupil dilation
• Muscle relaxation
• Reduced secretions
• Decreased gastrointestinal activity
• Sedative and hallucinogenic effects

Atropine and scopolamine remain indispensable in regulated medicine today, used in ophthalmology, cardiac care, and motion-sickness patches.

However, the whole plant is dangerously unpredictable. Alkaloid concentration varies with soil, light, and plant age, making unregulated ingestion extremely unsafe.

---

## 🧪 How to Use (Medical Context Only)

🚫 **There are NO safe dosages for home or herbal use.**

All uses of Nightshade must occur under licensed medical supervision using pharmaceutical preparations, not whole-plant extracts.

*Examples include:*

• **Atropine (Rx):** eye exams, cardiac uses • **Scopolamine patch (Rx):** motion sickness • **Hyoscyamine (Rx):** severe digestive spasm

⚠ The whole herb — tincture, tea, powder, smoke, or salve — is **unsafe** and not used in modern herbal practice.

---

## 💊 Forms Available (Restricted / Medical)

⚪ Prescription pharmaceutical alkaloids only

🚫 Whole-plant tinctures, teas, or powders are prohibited and unsafe for internal use

🚫 Home preparations do not exist in safe form

---

## ⚠ Caution Level: ⚫ Supervision Required

### Nightshade is one of the most toxic herbs known. Risks include:

• Hallucinations, delirium, agitation
• **Severe dry mouth & pupil dilation**
• Rapid heartbeat, arrhythmia
• **Paralysis and respiratory failure**
• Permanent neurological damage

• **Coma or death**
***Even touching the plant can irritate sensitive skin.**
****Never harvest, prepare, or ingest wild Nightshade.**

---

## 🚹 🚺 Gender-Specific Safety (GS)

**Men:** 🔴 Supervision Required — Internal use of whole herb unsafe. Pharmaceutical alkaloids only under medical direction.
**Women:** 🔴 Supervision Required — Avoid all herbal forms; strong cardiovascular and neurological effects.
**Pregnancy / Nursing:** 🔴 Avoid — Contraindicated in all forms. May cause uterine stimulation, neurological disturbance, and fetal toxicity.

---

## ⌛ Expected Results (Medical Derivatives Only)

• Pain/spasm relief: **30–60 minutes**
• Motion sickness relief (scopolamine patch): **1–2 hours**
⚠️ 🔴 **Unsupervised ingestion leads to unpredictable, dangerous, or fatal outcomes.**

---

## 🔄 Same / Similar Results (Safe Alternatives)

🟢 Skullcap — nerve relaxation and sleep support
🟢 Passionflower — gentle calm, anxiety support
🟢 California Poppy — mild pain and nervous tension
🟢 Valerian Root — sleep and muscle relaxation
🟢 Lemon Balm — nervous system soothing

## 🧴 Shelf Life / Potency After Preparation

• Pharmaceutical atropine/scopolamine: per pharmacy labeling
• Whole-plant products: 🚫 Not used — unsafe, improper, and prohibited

---

## 🛠 *DIY Preparations*

🚫 **None.**
There are **no** safe home preparations of Nightshade.

## 🌙 Herbal Reflections of Nightshade

Nightshade is the shadow-teacher of the herbal world — a reminder that great potency carries equally great responsibility. Revered and feared across history, it shaped medicine by revealing how narrow the line between healing and harm can be.

Its presence whispers a quiet truth: nature offers gifts of immense power, but wisdom demands discernment. Nightshade does not invite use; it invites respect. It teaches humility to the healer, caution to the curious, and reverence for the unseen edges of herbal medicine.

---

## ★ Herbal Confidence Index: 🌿 🌿 (2/5 green stars)

(Powerful but unsafe as an herbal remedy; primarily useful only through modern, controlled pharmaceutical derivatives.)

# WHITE OAK BARK

★★★★

*Quercus alba cortex*

**White Oak Bark has been prized for centuries as one of nature's most dependable astringents.** Rich in **tannins, it excels at tightening tissues, reducing inflammation, and halting excess discharges** such as diarrhea, bleeding gums, or varicose vein seepage. Herbalists continue to turn to White Oak Bark for gum care, wound healing, and soothing irritated skin, where its steady, contracting action restores integrity and strength.

**Its legacy in folk and medical traditions spans both Europe and North America.** Colonists and herbalists relied on it for oral health, wounds, and skin irritations, while Native American traditions also employed it for its reliable firming action. Symbolically, White Oak Bark became associated with **resilience and grounded strength,** sealing and reinforcing tissues much like the mighty oak tree itself. Its place in herbal medicine is a testament to both its practicality and its enduring reliability.

---

## *Core Herbal Category — White Oak Bark*

**Primary Core: Lymphatic & Skin Support herb** with (strong astringent, tissue-tightening action that firms lax tissue and reduces excessive discharge or bleeding)
**Secondary Cores:** Digestive Support herb · Immune Support herb · Musculoskeletal & Pain-Relief herb

---

## *How It Works*

White Oak Bark works by **binding proteins in tissues**, causing them to contract and tighten, which reduces bleeding, seepage, and inflammation. This astringent action helps **restore integrity to weakened skin and mucous membranes**, both externally and internally. In the digestive tract, it **firms intestinal tissue**, helping control diarrhea and irritation. Its antimicrobial and anti-inflammatory properties support **tissue protection during injury or infection**. Overall, White Oak Bark functions as a **powerful structural-support herb for acute tissue laxity and excessive discharge**, not long-term daily use.

---

## *Primary Uses*

- Astringent for wounds, bleeding gums, hemorrhoids, and varicose veins
- Tones tissues of the digestive and urinary systems
- Reduces inflammation in mouth, throat, and skin
- Helps stop diarrhea and restore intestinal balance
- Strengthens weakened or sagging tissues

---

## Scientific Backing

White Oak Bark contains up to 15–20% tannins, including catechins, ellagic acid, gallic acid, and quercetin — compounds known for strong astringent, antimicrobial, antioxidant, and anti-inflammatory activity.

Research supports its ability to:

- tighten and contract connective tissue
- reduce microbial load
- protect mucous membranes
- reduce irritation and swelling
- encourage wound recovery

Traditional use for gums, ulcers, skin eruptions, diarrhea, and hemorrhoids aligns well with modern understanding of its tannin-mediated effects.

---

## How to Use (Dosage & Methods)

**Decoction (Tea):**

- 1 tsp bark per cup of water
- Simmer 10–15 minutes
- Drink up to 2× daily for short-term needs (1–2 weeks max)

***Tincture:***

- *2–4 mL, up to 2× daily*

**External Use:** • Apply cooled decoction or diluted tincture as a compress, gargle, mouth rinse, sitz bath, or topical wash. • Excellent for gums, wounds, hemorrhoids, rashes, or oozing skin irritation.

---

## *Forms Available*

- Dried bark (whole or powdered)
- Tinctures and extracts
- Topical washes, compresses, soaks, rinses

---

## ⚠ Caution Level: Caution

- Safe for short-term use; avoid high-dose or long-term internal use due to tannin content.
- May cause nausea or stomach irritation if taken on an empty stomach.

• Avoid with chronic constipation or dryness-prone digestion.
• Use in cycles of 1–2 weeks followed by a break.
• During pregnancy: reserve primarily for diluted topical use, as internal strong astringents may reduce nutrient absorption.

---

## 🚹 🚺 Gender-Specific Safety (GS)

**Men:** 🟢 Safe. Beneficial for gum care, hemorrhoids, wounds, or skin inflammation. Internal use should be short-term, as prolonged use may cause mild constipation.
**Women:** 🟢 Safe. Useful as a soothing wash, sitz bath, or rinse for vaginal irritation or postpartum toning. Limit internal use to short-term cycles.
**Pregnancy / Nursing:** 🟡 Caution — Topical use is generally safe (rinses, washes, compresses). Avoid strong internal preparations unless advised, as high astringency can interfere with nutrient uptake or cause digestive tightening.

---

## ⏳ *Expected Results*

• Inflammation relief & tissue tightening: **2–3 days**
• Gum or wound improvement: **3–5 days**
• Digestive strengthening & diarrhea relief: **3–7 days**

---

## 🔄 *Same / Similar Results*

🟢 Witch Hazel Bark — skin + veins
🟢 Yarrow — wound repair + circulation
🟢 Plantain Leaf — external soothing
🟢 Bayberry Root Bark — mucosal astringent
🟢 Slippery Elm — mucosal restoration

---

## 🧴 Shelf Life / Potency After Preparation

• Dried bark: **2–3 years** (airtight, dry, cool)
• Tincture: **4–6 years**
• Decoction (tea): refrigerate; best within **24 hours**
• Topical wash/soak: **24–48 hours** if refrigerated
• Powder: **1–2 years**, but potency slightly decreases after 12 months

---

## 🛠 DIY Recipe — White Oak Bark Healing Wash

1 tbsp dried White Oak Bark
2 cups water

Simmer 15 minutes, cool, strain.
Use as a gargle, compress, sitz bath, wound rinse, or mouthwash to tone and soothe irritated tissues.

---

## 🌙 Herbal Reflections of White Oak Bark

White Oak Bark is the architect of resilience — the tree that lends its strength to whatever leans upon it. It teaches the medicine of boundaries: the ability to restore form, reinforce integrity, and reclaim structure where life has loosened it.
Its action is steady, grounded, and clarifying.
Where tissues sag, seep, or lose tone, White Oak gathers them back into strength.
Where irritation scatters the body's order, it restores coherence with calm authority.
It reminds us that healing sometimes begins with firmness — with the quiet re-establishment of strength where the body has grown weary or weak.

## ★ Herbal Confidence Index: 🌿🌿🌿🌿

(4/5 green stars — dependable traditional astringent and tissue strengthener; excellent for wounds, gums, hemorrhoids, diarrhea, and inflammation when used properly. Powerful externally, effective internally when used short-term with awareness.)

# YUCCA ROOT

★★★★

*Yucca filamentosa / Yucca glauca*

**Yucca Root is a hardy desert plant valued for its cleansing and anti-inflammatory powers.** Rich in **saponins, antioxidants, and detoxifying compounds, it helps the body reduce oxidative stress, ease joint pain, and support healthy digestion.** Often taken as decoctions, tinctures, or capsules, Yucca Root works gradually to relieve stiffness, improve mobility, and cleanse sluggish systems weighed down by inflammation or toxic buildup.

**Native American tribes revered Yucca as both a medicine and a survival plant.** It was used for **arthritis, rheumatism, and digestive stagnation,** while its fibrous leaves provided material for rope, mats, and baskets. The plant's dual value — practical and medicinal — made it a cornerstone of desert living. Today, Yucca Root continues to be recognized as a time-honored ally in addressing chronic inflammatory and degenerative conditions, embodying the resilience of the harsh landscapes it grows in.

---

## *Core Herbal Category — Yucca Root*

**Primary Core: Anti-Inflammatory & Pain Support herb** with (anti-inflammatory, saponin-rich action that reduces joint irritation and supports connective-tissue comfort)
**Secondary Cores:** Digestive Support herb · Liver & Detoxification herb · Skin & Tissue Repair herb

---

## *How It Works*

Yucca Root works by **reducing inflammatory compounds**, particularly those that aggravate joints and connective tissue. Its natural saponins help **bind and escort inflammatory byproducts out of the body**, easing stiffness and discomfort. This cleansing action supports **digestive comfort and detoxification**, especially where inflammation contributes to irritation. By lowering systemic inflammatory burden, it aids **joint mobility and tissue resilience**. Overall, Yucca Root functions as a **joint-supportive herb that calms inflammation while supporting internal cleansing**.

---

## Primary Uses

- Relieves arthritis, rheumatism, and joint stiffness
- Supports detoxification and colon cleansing
- Helps regulate cholesterol and systemic inflammation
- Soothes minor skin irritations (topical)
- Reduces oxidative stress and tissue irritation

---

## Scientific Backing

Yucca Root contains steroidal saponins, polyphenols, resveratrol-like antioxidants, and anti-inflammatory compounds that:

- reduce joint and connective tissue inflammation
- assist in cholesterol balance
- enhance digestive cleansing
- provide antimicrobial and antioxidant protection

Studies suggest benefits for osteoarthritis, inflammatory pain, and metabolic support. Its saponins may assist in breaking down waste buildup in the colon, contributing to improved nutrient absorption and reduced inflammatory load.

---

## How to Use (Dosage & Methods)

**Decoction:**

- 1 tsp dried root in 2 cups water
- Simmer 20–30 minutes
- Drink ½–1 cup daily for 2–3 weeks, then pause 1 week

**Capsules / Tinctures:**

- As directed on label (commonly 300–500 mg capsules or 1–2 mL tincture, 1–2× daily)

**Topical:**

- Diluted extract or tea applied to inflamed skin, rashes, or irritated joints

**Timing:**

- Morning or early afternoon is best to avoid stimulating nighttime detox effects.

---

## Forms Available

- Dried root slices (for decoction)
- Capsules and tinctures
- Topical extracts and salves

## ⚠ Caution Level: Caution

- Safe in moderate, short-term use.
- Excess intake may irritate stomach or intestines due to saponins.
- Can cause mild nausea or loose stools in sensitive individuals.

• Not advised with gallbladder obstruction, active ulcers, or chronic digestive weakness.
• Avoid during pregnancy or breastfeeding unless supervised.
• Long-term or high-dose use may stress the liver or kidneys — use in cycles of **2–3 weeks on, 1 week off**.

---

## 🚹 🚺 Gender-Specific Safety (GS)

**Men:** 🟡 Caution — Supports joint health, inflammation reduction, and detoxification. May cause digestive looseness or dehydration if overused. Avoid if prone to very low blood pressure.
**Women:** 🟡 Caution — Useful for arthritis, gout, and inflammatory conditions. Limit to short-term or guided protocols to prevent liver strain.
**Pregnancy / Nursing:** 🔴 Avoid — No confirmed safety data; possible uterine or hormonal effects. Choose safer anti-inflammatories (Turmeric, Ginger, Boswellia).

---

## ⏳ *Expected Results*

• Joint relief: **1–2 weeks**
• Digestive detox & cleansing: **2–4 weeks**
• Topical relief: **1–3 applications**

---

## 🔄 *Same / Similar Results*

🟢 Devil's Claw — joint inflammation
🟢 Turmeric — systemic anti-inflammatory
🟢 Boswellia — arthritis & connective tissue support
🟢 Ginger — circulation + gut support
🟢 Nettle — mineral-rich anti-inflammatory

## 🧴 Shelf Life / Potency After Preparation

• Dried root: **2–3 years** airtight
• Powder: **1–2 years**
• Tincture: **4–6 years**
• Decoction: **Use within 24–48 hours**, refrigerated
• Topical extract: **1–2 years**

---

## 🛠 DIY Recipe — Joint Relief Decoction

1 tsp Yucca Root
2 cups water
Simmer 25 minutes, strain, and drink ½–1 cup daily during 2–3 week cycles.

## 🗨 Herbal Reflections of Yucca Root

Yucca Root embodies the endurance of the desert — a plant that thrives where life is harsh and passes that resilience to those who use it. Its medicine is steady and cleansing, easing stiff joints, inflamed tissues, and systems weighed down by stagnation. Yucca does not offer quick fixes; instead, it restores in cycles, sweeping away what burdens the body while rekindling mobility and ease.

Energetically, Yucca offers survival wisdom: strength earned through patience, healing born from persistent renewal. Its presence teaches that even in the harshest internal landscapes, regeneration is possible. The journey may be gradual, but it is deeply grounding — the kind of healing that lasts because it arises from within.

## ★ Herbal Confidence Index: 🌿🌿🌿🌿

(4/5 green stars — valuable anti-inflammatory and cleansing herb long used for arthritis, gout, joint pain, and systemic stagnation. Effective when used in moderation or cycles; avoid excessive intake to protect digestive and liver health.)

# FALSE UNICORN ROOT

★★★★

*Chamaelirium luteum*

**False Unicorn Root** is a deeply respected reproductive tonic in traditional North American herbal medicine, prized for its ability to strengthen, balance, and restore vitality within the female reproductive system. Despite its name, it is neither related to unicorns nor particularly mythical — its reputation was earned through centuries of consistent use by Indigenous healers and early herbal practitioners.

This herb is best known for its role in addressing weakness, depletion, and imbalance rather than acute symptoms. False Unicorn Root does not force hormonal changes; instead, it nourishes and stabilizes the underlying systems that support menstrual regularity, uterine tone, and reproductive resilience. It has historically been used when the body shows signs of exhaustion, infertility related to weakness, or repeated reproductive stress.

Gentle yet profound, False Unicorn Root is especially valued in long-term constitutional support, helping restore equilibrium where vitality has been gradually diminished rather than suddenly lost.

---

## 🌿 Core Herbal Category — False Unicorn Root

**Primary Core: Reproductive & Women's Health Support** (tonic that strengthens uterine tone and hormonal balance)
**Secondary Cores:** Endocrine Support · Nervous System Support · Digestive Support

---

### 🌿 How It Works

False Unicorn Root works by nourishing and stabilizing the endocrine and reproductive systems. Rather than acting as a stimulant or suppressor, it improves tissue tone, enhances regulatory balance, and supports communication between the ovaries, uterus, and hormonal signaling centers. Its bitter and tonic properties also gently support digestion and nutrient assimilation, indirectly strengthening reproductive vitality.

---

### 🌿 Primary Uses

- Supports uterine tone and reproductive strength
- Aids menstrual regularity associated with weakness or depletion

• Supports fertility when linked to constitutional deficiency
• Helps restore vitality after repeated reproductive stress
• Provides gentle endocrine system support

---

### 🌿 Scientific Backing

False Unicorn Root contains steroidal saponins and bitter compounds associated with tonic and adaptogenic actions. While modern clinical studies are limited, extensive historical use and contemporary herbal practice support its role as a restorative reproductive tonic, particularly in conditions involving weakness, imbalance, or chronic reproductive strain.

---

### 🌿 How to Use (Dosage)

• Tincture: 0.5–1 mL once daily (often used long-term)
• Decoction: Rarely used due to bitterness; small doses only
• Capsules: Follow product guidelines; commonly used in tonic protocols

---

### 🌿 Shelf Life

• Dried root (properly stored): 2–3 years
• Tincture: 4–5 years
• Capsules: Follow manufacturer expiration

---

### 🌿 Potency After Preparation 👍 👍

• Tincture: Stable potency throughout shelf life
• Capsules: Consistent with proper storage

---

### ● Caution Level: Caution

Traditionally used in small, consistent doses. Avoid during pregnancy. Use caution in individuals with hormone-sensitive conditions unless guided by a qualified practitioner.

---

### 🌿 Gender-Specific Safety (GS)

● **Women:** Beneficial — especially for reproductive strength and balance
● **Men:** Generally safe — tonic support only
● **Pregnancy:** Avoid
● Nursing: Caution — professional guidance recommended

---

### 🌿 Expected Results

• Improved reproductive tone: 2–4 weeks
• Hormonal stabilization: 1–3 months
• Constitutional strengthening: gradual with continued use

---

### 🌿 Same / Similar Results

Vitex · Red Raspberry Leaf · Blue Cohosh · Dong Quai · Shatavari

---

### 🌿 Herbal Reflections of False Unicorn Root

False Unicorn Root teaches the value of quiet restoration. It does not rush the body or demand immediate change; instead, it rebuilds strength patiently and deliberately. In its steady support lies the reminder that true balance is restored not through force, but through nourishment and time.

---

🌿 Herbal Confidence Index

★★★★☆
(4/5 — highly valued for long-term reproductive support; best used with intention and respect.)

# RED ROOT

★★★★

Ceanothus americanus

**Red Root** is a deep lymphatic and splenic tonic valued for its ability to reduce congestion, restore healthy lymph flow, and support the body's natural filtration systems. Traditionally used when glands are swollen, tissues feel dense or stagnant, or recovery from chronic illness is slow, Red Root works quietly but profoundly to bring movement where the body has become congested.

Long respected in North American herbal medicine, Red Root has been relied upon in cases involving chronic inflammation, fibrotic tissue, and compromised immune drainage. It is not a fast-acting herb, but a restorative one — best suited for long-standing imbalances where strength and circulation must be rebuilt rather than forced.

---

## Core Herbal Category — Red Root

**Primary Core: Lymphatic & Skin Support** (deep lymph and spleen tonic that restores circulation and reduces tissue congestion)
Secondary Cores: Immune Support · Circulatory Support · Anti-inflammatory

---

### How It Works

Red Root works by toning lymphatic vessels and supporting the spleen's role in filtering blood and lymph. Its astringent and alterative properties help shrink swollen tissues, reduce excess fluid accumulation, and improve circulation through congested lymph channels. Over time, this enhanced drainage supports immune efficiency, reduces inflammatory load, and helps the body resolve chronic stagnation.

---

### Primary Uses

- Reduces swollen lymph nodes and glandular congestion
- Supports spleen health and lymph filtration
- Assists recovery from chronic infections or inflammation
- Helps resolve cysts, fibrotic tissue, and lymph stagnation
- Supports immune resilience in long-term conditions

---

### 🌿 Scientific Backing

Red Root contains tannins and alkaloids that contribute to its astringent, anti-inflammatory, and circulatory-supportive actions. While modern clinical studies are limited, traditional use and contemporary herbal practice consistently recognize its effectiveness in lymphatic and splenic support, particularly in chronic conditions involving tissue congestion.

---

### 🌿 How to Use (Dosage)

- Decoction: 1 tsp dried root per cup of water; simmer 15–20 minutes; 1–2× daily
- Tincture: 1–2 mL up to 2× daily
- Capsules: Follow product guidelines; typically used in longer-term protocols

---

### 🌿 Shelf Life

- Dried root (properly stored): 2–3 years
- Tincture: 4–5 years
- Decoction: Best used within 24 hours (refrigerate if needed)

---

### 🌿 Potency After Preparation 👍👍

- Decoction: strongest within the first 12–24 hours
- Tincture: stable potency throughout shelf life

---

### 🟡 Caution Level: Caution

Generally safe when used appropriately. Avoid high doses in cases of acute infection or during pregnancy unless guided by a qualified practitioner. Long-term use should be monitored.

---

### 🌿 Gender-Specific Safety (GS)

🟢 Men: Safe — supports lymph circulation and immune recovery

🟢 Women: Safe — beneficial for glandular and inflammatory conditions

🟡 Pregnancy/Nursing: Caution — avoid unless professionally supervised

---

### 🌿 Expected Results

- Reduction in lymph swelling: 1–3 weeks
- Improved circulation and tissue tone: 3–6 weeks
- Immune resilience: gradual with continued use

### 🌿 Same / Similar Results

🟢 Cleavers · 🟣 Red Clover · 🟡 Yellow Dock · 🟤 Burdock Root · 🌸 Poke Root

---

### 🌿 Herbal Reflections of Red Root

Red Root teaches patience and persistence. It does not rush the body, nor does it overwhelm it. Instead, it restores quiet movement — reminding us that healing often begins when what has been stuck is finally allowed to flow again.

---

### 🌿 Herbal Confidence Index

⭐⭐⭐⭐☆
(4/5 — deeply effective for lymphatic and splenic support; especially valuable in chronic congestion and immune stagnation.)

# PRICKLY ASH BARK

★★★★

Zanthoxylum americanum

**Prickly Ash Bark** is one of the great warming restoratives of North American herbal medicine — a tree revered not for subtlety, but for its ability to awaken what has gone cold, stagnant, or unresponsive. Long used by Indigenous healers and early American herbalists, it earned the name "the warming tree" for its profound effect on circulation, nerve activity, and vital flow throughout the body.

This is an herb turned to when tissues lack warmth, when digestion feels weak or unmotivated, and when pain or stiffness is rooted not in inflammation alone, but in poor blood movement and nerve stagnation. Prickly Ash does not numb discomfort or suppress symptoms; instead, it restores movement — bringing blood, sensation, and metabolic energy back to areas that have grown sluggish or deprived.

Traditionally employed for cold extremities, rheumatic conditions, nerve weakness, and digestive insufficiency, Prickly Ash Bark is especially valued in constitutional states marked by chill, fatigue, and diminished vitality. Its action is stimulating but purposeful, reminding the body how to circulate, respond, and reengage with its own strength rather than forcing relief from the outside.

---

## Core Herbal Category — Prickly Ash Bark

**Primary Core: Cardiovascular System Support** (warming stimulant that improves peripheral blood flow and nerve responsiveness)
**Secondary Cores:** Nervous System Support · Digestive Support · Musculoskeletal Support

---

### How It Works

Prickly Ash Bark works by stimulating peripheral circulation and activating sensory nerve pathways. Its pungent alkaloids increase blood flow to cold or under-perfused tissues, improving oxygen delivery and metabolic exchange. By enhancing circulation, it indirectly strengthens digestion, reduces rheumatic stiffness, and restores nerve signaling in areas affected by stagnation or constitutional cold.

---

### 🌿 Primary Uses

• Improves circulation to cold hands, feet, and extremities
• Supports nerve responsiveness and sensation
• Eases rheumatic and joint discomfort linked to poor blood flow
• Strengthens digestion weakened by circulatory insufficiency
• Supports vitality in cold, depleted, or stagnant conditions

---

### 🌿 Scientific Backing

Prickly Ash Bark contains alkaloids and pungent compounds that stimulate circulation and nerve activity. While modern clinical research is limited, traditional use and contemporary herbal practice consistently support its role as a circulatory, digestive, and nervous system stimulant, particularly in conditions marked by coldness, poor perfusion, and sluggish response.

---

### 🌿 How to Use (Dosage)

• Decoction: ½–1 tsp dried bark per cup of water; simmer 15–20 minutes; 1× daily
• Tincture: 0.5–1 mL up to 2× daily
• Capsules: Follow product guidelines; typically used short- to moderate-term

---

### 🌿 Shelf Life

• Dried bark (properly stored): 2–3 years
• Tincture: 4–5 years
• Decoction: Best used within 24 hours (refrigerate if needed)

### 🌿 Potency After Preparation 👍 👍

• Decoction: strongest within the first 12–24 hours
• Tincture: stable potency throughout shelf life

---

### ● Caution Level: Caution

A warming, stimulating herb. Avoid excessive use in heat conditions, active inflammation, or high fever. Use cautiously in individuals with sensitive digestion. Not recommended during pregnancy unless guided by a qualified practitioner.

---

### 🌿 Gender-Specific Safety (GS)

● **Men: Safe** — supports circulation, joint comfort, and vitality
● **Women: Safe** — beneficial for cold-related discomfort and nerve stagnation
● **Pregnancy/Nursing: Caution** — avoid unless professionally supervised

---

### Expected Results

• Increased warmth and circulation: within days to 1 week
• Reduced stiffness and nerve discomfort: 1–3 weeks
• Digestive strengthening: gradual with continued use

---

### Same / Similar Results

Cayenne · Ginger Root · Ginkgo Biloba · Hawthorn Berry · Black Pepper

---

### Herbal Reflections of Prickly Ash Bark

Prickly Ash Bark reminds us that healing often begins with movement. It stirs what has gone cold, awakens what has fallen quiet, and encourages the body to reclaim its natural circulation. In its warmth is the lesson that flow is life — and where circulation returns, strength soon follows.

---

## Herbal Confidence Index

★★★★☆ (4/5 stars — highly effective for circulatory and nerve stagnation; best used with intention and moderation.)

# ECLIPTA ALBA

★★★★★

*Eclipta prostrata / Eclipta alba*

**Eclipta Alba**—known in Ayurveda as **Bhringraj, the "King of Hair"**—is a deeply restorative herb prized for its ability to regenerate hair, strengthen the liver, and calm inflammatory stress throughout the body. While widely celebrated for preventing premature graying and supporting hair regrowth, its true power lies beneath the surface: protecting liver tissue, stabilizing the nervous system, and replenishing depleted reserves. Used for centuries in Ayurveda and Traditional Chinese Medicine, Eclipta Alba was often paired with Amla, Brahmi, or Gotu Kola to support longevity, memory, and youthful vitality. Its dual action—beautifying outward appearance while restoring internal balance—has earned it a reputation as an herb of renewal, resilience, and steady regeneration rather than quick cosmetic effect.

---

### Core Herbal Category — Eclipta Alba

**Primary Core: Liver & Detoxification Support** herb with (cooling, hepatoprotective action that supports liver regeneration and toxin clearance)
**Secondary Cores:** Skin & Tissue Repair · Immune Support · Nutritive & Restorative

---

### How It Works

Eclipta Alba supports liver health by protecting hepatocytes and encouraging efficient detoxification pathways. Its cooling, anti-inflammatory nature helps reduce oxidative stress and metabolic burden on the liver. As liver balance improves, downstream effects appear in the skin, scalp, and hair follicles, where nourishment and circulation gradually return. By replenishing foundational reserves, Eclipta supports steady hair vitality, calmer nervous tone, and long-term tissue resilience.

---

### Primary Uses

- Supports hair regrowth and scalp vitality
- Protects and regenerates liver tissue
- Calms inflammatory stress
- Supports nervous-system balance and resilience

---

### Scientific Backing

Eclipta Alba contains **wedelolactone, ecliptine, and flavonoids** shown to:

- Protect liver cells
- Reduce systemic inflammation
- Stimulate dormant hair follicles
- Support antioxidant defenses

Animal and early human studies support both hepatoprotective and hair-restorative effects, aligning with its long-standing traditional use.

---

### How to Use (Dosage & Methods)

- **Tea:** 1–2 tsp dried herb, steep 10 minutes; drink 1–2× daily
- **Capsules:** 500–1000 mg daily
- **Tincture:** 1–2 mL up to 2× daily
- **Hair Oil:** Massage infused oil into scalp 2–3× weekly

---

### Forms Available

- Dried herb (tea)
- Tincture
- Capsules / powdered extract
- Hair oils / topical preparations

---

### Caution Level: Safe / Mild Caution

- Very safe for daily use
- High doses may cause mild digestive looseness
- Avoid combining with multiple strong liver detoxifiers
- Consult if using liver medications or blood thinners

---

### Gender-Specific Safety (GS)

**Men:** Safe — Supports hair, liver strength, clarity, and restorative tone

**Women:** Safe — Excellent for hair vitality, hormonal calm, and stress balance

**Pregnancy / Nursing:** Caution — Mild tea acceptable; avoid concentrated extracts

---

### Expected Results

- Scalp nourishment & hair strength: 4–6 weeks
- Liver support & inflammatory calming: 2–3 weeks
- Nervous-system steadiness: 2–4 weeks

---

### Same / Similar Results

Amla · Gotu Kola · Milk Thistle · Bacopa

---

### Shelf Life / Potency After Preparation

- Dried herb: 1–2 years
- Powder/capsules: ~2 years
- Tincture: 5–7 years
- Hair oil: 6–12 months

---

### Herbal Reflections of Eclipta Alba

Eclipta Alba restores beauty by restoring balance. Its work is slow, cooling, and deeply nourishing—reminding us that true vitality emerges from internal harmony rather than force. Few herbs unite cosmetic benefit with systemic healing so completely.

---

### Herbal Confidence Index:

(5/5 — premier restorative tonic for liver health, hair vitality, and calm resilience; exceptionally safe and deeply nourishing when used consistently.)

# COWSLIP

★★★★

*(Primula veris)*

**Cowslip** is a gentle meadow herb long valued for calming the nervous system while easing respiratory tension. Traditionally used for restlessness, mild insomnia, headaches, and congestive coughs, it bridges nervous and respiratory support with a soft, reassuring touch rather than sedation.

Folklore across Europe associated Cowslip with emotional lightness during times of gloom, earning it a place in home remedies for melancholy, nervous fatigue, and winter coughs. Its action remains mild but dependable—ideal for those needing comfort rather than force.

---

### 🌿 Core Herbal Category — Cowslip

**Primary Core: Respiratory System Support herb** with (expectorant, anti-inflammatory action that loosens mucus and soothes irritated airways)

**Secondary Cores:** Nervines · Musculoskeletal & Pain Relief · Immune Support

---

### 🌿 How It Works

Cowslip gently thins and loosens mucus, supporting easier clearance from the lungs. Its anti-inflammatory compounds calm airway irritation while mild nervine activity helps settle tension that accompanies illness or fatigue. Relief of congestion often reduces associated headaches and restlessness, supporting more comfortable breathing and rest.

---

### 🌱 Primary Uses

- Promotes restful sleep and relaxation
- Relieves tension headaches
- Eases mild coughs and respiratory congestion

---

### 🧪 Scientific Backing

Cowslip contains **flavonoids, saponins, and salicylates** that provide:

- Gentle expectorant action
- Mild sedative and calming effects
- Anti-inflammatory support

Traditional and modern herbal use supports its role in nervous and respiratory comfort.

---

### 💊 How to Use (Dosage & Methods)

• **Tea:** 1–2 tsp dried flowers, steep 10 minutes; up to 3× daily
• **Tincture:** 1–2 mL up to 3× daily
• **Capsules:** 300–500 mg daily

---

### 💊 Forms Available

• Dried flowers
• Tincture
• Syrup
• Capsules

---

### ⚠ Caution Level: ● Caution

• Generally safe in moderate doses
• Possible sensitivity in those allergic to primrose or aspirin-like compounds
• Avoid during pregnancy or breastfeeding due to limited data
• Use caution with blood-thinning medications

---

### Gender-Specific Safety (GS)

**Men:** ● Safe — Helpful for tension headaches and evening relaxation
**Women:** ● Safe — Supports nervous calm and sleep during stress or transition
**Pregnancy / Nursing:** ● Caution — Light tea only; avoid frequent or concentrated use

---

### ⏳ Expected Results

• Nervous calming: often within first cup
• Cough relief: 2–3 doses
• Sleep support: 2–4 days

---

### 🔄 Same / Similar Results

● Chamomile · ● Lemon Balm · ● Skullcap · ● Valerian · ● Passionflower

---

### Shelf Life / Potency After Preparation

• Dried flowers: 1–2 years
• Tincture: 3–5 years
• Syrup: 6–12 months refrigerated
• Tea: best within 12 hours

---

### 🌙 Herbal Reflections of Cowslip

Cowslip teaches the medicine of softness. It doesn't overpower tension—it dissolves it gently, inviting rest to arrive naturally. Its quiet reassurance is often exactly what frayed nerves and tired lungs need.

---

**Herbal Confidence Index:**
(4/5 — gentle, reliable nervine and respiratory ally for sleep, tension, and mild congestion.)

---

# DEVIL'S CLUB

★★★★

*(Oplopanax horridus)*

**Devil's Club** is one of the most respected and guarded medicinal plants of the Pacific Northwest. Armed with spines and ecological sensitivity, it has long been used by Indigenous peoples for deep immune weakness, lung infections, inflammatory pain, and metabolic imbalance—always with restraint and respect.

Revered as both medicine and protector, Devil's Club is not a casual herb. Its power lies in restoring strength where systems are exhausted, but improper handling or dosing carries real risk. Modern herbalism recognizes its value as a **specialist adaptogenic and immune-modulating herb**, not a household tonic.

---

### Core Herbal Category — Devil's Club

**Primary Core: Adaptogens** herb with (strengthening principles that support respiratory resilience and stress recovery)

**Secondary Cores:** Immune Support · Metabolic Balance · Anti-Inflammatory Support

---

### How It Works

Devil's Club supports adaptive stress response by modulating immune and inflammatory pathways. Bitter compounds strengthen respiratory tissues and improve resilience during chronic infection or fatigue. Metabolically, it assists cellular response to glucose while calming joint inflammation through non-stimulatory pathways. Its effects build slowly and require disciplined, guided use.

---

### Primary Uses

- Strengthens lungs during infection
- Supports immune recovery after exhaustion
- Eases inflammatory joint pain
- Assists blood sugar balance (guided use only)

---

### Scientific Backing

Contains **polyynes, lignans, saponins, and aromatic compounds** with:

- Anti-inflammatory activity
- Antimicrobial effects

• Early evidence for blood-sugar modulation
Traditional use is extensive; modern research is ongoing.

---

### 💊 How to Use (Medical–Herbal Context Only)

• **Decoction:** 1 tsp properly dried root bark, simmer 20–25 minutes
• **Tincture:** Practitioner-guided dosing only
• **Topical salve:** For joint inflammation
⚠ Fresh plant material is unsafe.

---

### 💊 Forms Available

• Dried root bark
• Tincture (professional preparation)
• Salves

---

### ⚠ Caution Level: ● Supervision Required

• Raw inner bark & berries are toxic
• Spines cause skin injury
• Not for pregnancy or nursing
• May amplify antidiabetic medications
• Do not self-harvest; ecosystem is fragile
• Requires skilled preparation and dosing

---

### Gender-Specific Safety (GS)

**Men:** ● Caution — Use only with guidance
**Women:** ● Caution — Strong endocrine effects; guided use only
**Pregnancy / Nursing:** ● Avoid

---

### ⏳ Expected Results

• Respiratory support: 3–5 days
• Joint inflammation relief: 1–2 weeks
• Metabolic effects: long-term, supervised use

---

### 🔄 Same / Similar Results

● Astragalus · ● Reishi · ● Elecampane · ● Licorice · ● Burdock

---

### Shelf Life / Potency After Preparation

• Dried root bark: 2–3 years
• Tincture: 4–6 years

- Salve: ~1 year
- Decoction: 48 hours refrigerated

---

🌙 **Herbal Reflections of Devil's Club**

Devil's Club teaches boundaries. It offers strength only to those who approach with patience and respect. Its medicine is not gentle—but it is honest, restoring resilience where lesser tonics fall short.

---

⭐ **Herbal Confidence Index:** 🌿🌿🌿✨

(3.5/5 — powerful specialist herb requiring guidance; effective but not for casual use.)

# GRAVEL ROOT

★★★★

*(Eupatorium purpureum)*

**Gravel Root** is a classic North American urinary-tract herb traditionally used for **kidney "gravel," urinary irritation, and sluggish flow**. Herbalists valued it as a targeted diuretic that supports elimination while calming heat and discomfort in the urinary passages. It also appears in old formulas for **uric-acid burden** (gout-type patterns), swelling, and rheumatic discomfort.

The name "Joe-Pye Weed" is linked to a Native healer remembered in oral tradition for helping communities during fevers and urinary complaints. Gravel Root became a household remedy in early American herbalism—used carefully and usually short-term—especially when hydration, diet, and rest weren't enough to restore comfortable urinary function.

---

### 🌿 Core Herbal Category — Gravel Root

**Primary Core: Kidney & Urinary Support** herb with (diuretic, soothing principles that support urine flow and urinary-tract comfort)

**Secondary Cores:** Anti-Inflammatory Support · Fluid Balance Support

---

### 🌿 How It Works

Gravel Root increases gentle urine flow, which supports flushing of the urinary tract and may help discourage small mineral buildup from lingering. It also contains constituents that calm irritated tissues, easing burning, pressure, or urinary spasm. By supporting fluid movement and reducing inflammatory irritation, Gravel Root helps restore clearer, more comfortable urinary function over short, focused use.

---

### 🌱 Primary Uses

- Supports urine flow and reduces retention
- Soothes burning or irritated urination
- Supports kidney/bladder "gravel" discomfort (traditional use)
- Supports uric-acid clearance patterns (gout-type support)
- Helps reduce swelling related to fluid stagnation

---

### 🧪 Scientific Backing

Traditional literature and ethnobotanical records describe Gravel Root as a diuretic and urinary-soothing herb. Reported constituents include flavonoids and sesquiterpene lactones; however, modern clinical trial data is limited. Its best-supported use remains **short-term urinary support** in traditional practice.

---

### 💊 How to Use (Dosage & Methods)

- **Decoction:** 1 tsp dried root simmered 15–20 minutes; 1 cup daily
- **Tincture:** 1–2 mL up to 3× daily

**Duration:** short-term only (commonly 7–21 days)

---

### 💊 Forms Available

- Dried root (decoction)
- Tincture / liquid extract

---

### ⚠ Caution Level: ● Caution

- Use short-term; avoid prolonged continuous use
- Avoid if pregnant or nursing
- Avoid with liver disease or significant kidney disease
- Use only from reputable sources; discontinue if nausea or unusual fatigue occurs
- Do not combine long-term with other herbs known to contain pyrrolizidine alkaloids (PA-risk category)

---

### Gender-Specific Safety (GS)

**Men:** ● Safe (short-term) — Useful for urinary flow and uric-acid burden patterns; avoid prolonged use

**Women:** ● Safe (short-term) — Helpful for urinary irritation; avoid prolonged use; not for pregnancy

**Pregnancy / Nursing:** ● Avoid — choose safer urinary soothers (Corn Silk, Marshmallow Root)

---

### ⏳ Expected Results

- Urinary comfort: 3–7 days
- Improved flow/pressure: 1–2 weeks
- Uric-acid pattern support: 2–4 weeks (with lifestyle support)

---

### 🔄 Same / Similar Results

● Marshmallow Root · ● Corn Silk · ● Celery Seed · ● Hydrangea Root · ● Parsley (short-term) · ● Juniper Berry

🛠 **DIY Recipe — Urinary Comfort Decoction**

1 tsp Gravel Root + 1 tsp Marshmallow Root
Simmer in 2 cups water for 20 minutes; strain.
Sip 1 cup daily for up to 7–10 days.

---

🕯 **Shelf Life / Potency After Preparation**

- Dried root: 1–2 years
- Tincture: 3–5 years
- Decoction: 48 hours refrigerated

---

🌙 **Herbal Reflections of Gravel Root**

Gravel Root is the steady "flow-restorer"—not flashy, but practical. Its gift is helping the body move what has grown stuck: pressure, heat, grit, and heaviness in the urinary pathway. It teaches a quiet lesson in wellness: when hydration, rhythm, and elimination return, comfort often returns with them.

---

⭐ **Herbal Confidence Index:** 🌿🌿🌿🌿

(4/5 — strong traditional urinary ally for short-term support; reliable when used responsibly and not treated as a daily tonic.)

# GROUND IVY

★★★★

*(Glechoma hederacea)*

**Ground Ivy** is a modest mint-family plant traditionally used to **clear sinus and bronchial congestion**, soothe irritated tissues, and support sluggish digestion. Older European traditions also used it during "heavy-headed" colds—when mucus, pressure, and fatigue settled into the face and chest.
Historically called "Alehoof," it was used in brewing and as a household herb for coughs, ear discomfort, and spring cleansing. While modern clinical research is limited, its long folk use centers on **aromatic clearing, mild antimicrobial support, and steady drainage** rather than strong stimulation.

---

### Core Herbal Category — Ground Ivy

**Primary Core: Respiratory System Support** herb with (aromatic expectorant principles that loosen mucus and ease sinus/bronchial congestion)
**Secondary Cores:** Lymphatic Support · Digestive Support

---

### How It Works

Ground Ivy's volatile oils gently loosen and move mucus, supporting easier drainage from sinuses and upper airways. Mild astringent and anti-inflammatory constituents help calm irritated tissues. By supporting lymphatic movement and digestive comfort during colds or allergies, it helps the system "clear the backlog" that can keep congestion stuck.

---

### Primary Uses

- Eases sinus pressure and thick mucus
- Supports cough relief and easier breathing
- Supports lymphatic drainage during congestion
- Calms bloating or sluggish digestion (especially during illness)
- Traditional support for ear and head-pressure discomfort

---

### Scientific Backing

Ground Ivy contains flavonoids and aromatic compounds associated with anti-inflammatory and mild antimicrobial activity in laboratory research. Clinical trials are limited, but traditional European use consistently emphasizes respiratory drainage and tissue calming.

---

### How to Use (Dosage & Methods)

- **Tea:** 1 tsp dried herb per cup; steep 10–15 minutes; 1–2× daily for 7–10 days
- **Topical poultice:** fresh herb (optional) for localized soothing (avoid broken skin)

---

### Forms Available

- Dried herb (tea)
- Fresh herb (topical preparations)

---

### Caution Level: Caution

- Avoid high-dose or long-term use (may irritate stomach/kidneys in sensitive people)
- Avoid during pregnancy
- Use caution with significant kidney disease
- Source carefully; avoid misidentified mint-family look-alikes

---

### Gender-Specific Safety (GS)

**Men:** Safe (short-term) — best as light tea during congestion

**Women:** Safe (short-term) — discontinue if irritation occurs; avoid during pregnancy

**Pregnancy / Nursing:** Avoid in pregnancy; Caution while nursing (light, brief use only)

---

### Expected Results

- Sinus drainage: 24–48 hours
- Digestive calming: same day
- Congested cough relief: 2–3 days

---

### Same / Similar Results

Thyme · Mullein · Eyebright · Horseradish (strong) · Elecampane

---

### DIY Recipe — Sinus & Chest Tea

1 tsp Ground Ivy + 1 tsp Mullein

Steep 15 minutes; drink 1 cup daily for up to 7 days.

---

### Shelf Life / Potency After Preparation

- Dried herb: 1–2 years
- Tea: 24 hours refrigerated
- Infused oil: ~1 year

---

**Herbal Reflections of Ground Ivy**

Ground Ivy is a quiet path-clearer. It doesn't overwhelm congestion—it patiently loosens what's stuck and encourages the body to drain and breathe again. Its lesson is humble: steady relief often comes from gentle persistence, not force.

---

**Herbal Confidence Index:**

(4/5 — dependable for sinus and mucus clearing when used short-term; mild but effective in the right lane.)

# YELLOW JASMINE

★★

*Gelsemium sempervirens*

**Yellow Jasmine** is a striking southern vine with a long history as a **dangerous medicinal plant**. Its alkaloids act strongly on the nervous system and were once used—under medical supervision—for severe neuralgia, tremor, and spasm. The line between "effect" and poisoning is extremely narrow, and the plant is considered unsafe for home herbal use. In modern practice, Yellow Jasmine is treated as an educational example of high-risk botanical medicine. Contemporary clinical use centers on regulated medicine and highly diluted homeopathic preparations under qualified supervision—not whole-plant herbal dosing.

---

### 🌿 Core Herbal Category — Yellow Jasmine

**Primary Core: Nervous System Support (Nervines)** herb with (strong depressant, antispasmodic action that suppresses nerve signaling)

**Secondary Cores:** Spasm-Relief Support · Pain-Relief Support

**Important Note:** Restricted, high-toxicity plant—whole-herb use is not appropriate in modern herbal practice.

---

### 🌿 How It Works

Yellow Jasmine contains alkaloids that depress central nervous system signaling and can relax severe spasm or neural overactivity. That same mechanism can rapidly progress into dangerous weakness, slowed breathing, and respiratory failure. Because its dosing margin is unreliable and the plant varies in potency, it is not suitable for non-clinical use.

---

### 🌱 Primary Uses (Historical / Restricted Context Only)

- Severe neuralgia and spasmodic pain (historic)
- Tremor and intense nervous agitation (historic)
- Sedation in controlled settings (historic)

⚠️ Not recommended for modern home herbal use.

---

### 🧪 Scientific Backing

Documented alkaloids (including gelsemine-related compounds) show strong CNS depressant effects. Toxicity is well-established, with risk of respiratory suppression, paralysis, and death. Plant potency varies widely—making whole-herb use unsafe.

---

**How to Use (Medical Context Only)**

**No safe home dosage.**

Use is restricted to regulated medicine or qualified clinical/homeopathic supervision.

---

**Forms Available**

- Regulated clinical/homeopathic preparations only

Whole-plant teas, tinctures, powders, or DIY extracts are unsafe.

---

**Caution Level:** Supervision Required

- High poisoning risk; dosing errors can be fatal
- Avoid all self-harvesting and self-administration
- Contraindicated in pregnancy/nursing and in heart/lung/neurologic disorders

---

**Gender-Specific Safety (GS)**

**Men:** Avoid — not appropriate for self-use

**Women:** Avoid — not appropriate for self-use

**Pregnancy / Nursing:** Avoid — strictly contraindicated

---

**Expected Results (Restricted Context Only)**

- Sedation/spasm reduction: hours (unreliable)

Toxic reactions may occur rapidly and unpredictably.

---

**Same / Similar Results (Safe Alternatives)**

Skullcap · Passionflower · Valerian · California Poppy · Lemon Balm

---

**DIY Recipe**

None. No safe DIY preparations exist.

---

**Shelf Life / Potency After Preparation**

- Clinical/homeopathic products: follow labeled expiration

Whole-plant storage for medicinal use is not appropriate.

---

**Herbal Reflections of Yellow Jasmine**

Yellow Jasmine is a "boundary plant"—beautiful, powerful, and not meant for casual use.

Its primary value today is educational: a reminder that wisdom in herbalism includes knowing when not to use a plant, and choosing safer nervines that support the same goals without risking life.

---

⭐ **Herbal Confidence Index:** 🌿 🌿
(2/5 — historically significant but unsafe as an herbal remedy; best replaced by safer alternatives.)

# Willow Bark

★★★★

*Salix alba* (also *Salix nigra, Salix purpurea*)

**Willow Bark** is a classic pain-and-fever herb and the historical botanical inspiration behind aspirin. Traditionally used for headaches, body aches, back pain, and inflammatory joint discomfort, it tends to act **more gradually** than standard NSAIDs. When used correctly, it can support comfort and mobility without "forcing" the body—though it still carries the same salicylate cautions as aspirin.

Across Europe, Asia, and North America, Willow Bark became a practical remedy for cold-and-fever aches and overuse pain. In modern herbalism, it remains a respected option for short-term inflammatory discomfort, especially when a steadier, slower onset is acceptable.

---

### 🌿 Core Herbal Category — Willow Bark

**Primary Core: Anti-Inflammatory & Pain Support** herb with (salicylate-based anti-inflammatory action that eases pain and fever signaling)

**Secondary Cores:** Immune Support · Circulatory Support · Digestive Support

---

### 🌿 How It Works

Willow Bark provides natural salicylates (notably salicin) that the body converts into salicylic acid derivatives, helping reduce inflammatory prostaglandin activity. This lowers pain and fever signals and can ease swelling over time. Because conversion is gradual, effects can feel slower but longer-lasting than rapid-acting pain relievers. Willow also contains supportive polyphenols that contribute to tissue-calming effects.

---

### 🌱 Primary Uses

- Back pain and overuse aches
- Osteoarthritis discomfort
- Headaches and body aches
- Fever and flu-like aches
- Joint stiffness and inflammatory pain patterns

---

### 🔬 Scientific Backing

Willow Bark contains salicin plus flavonoids and polyphenols associated with analgesic and anti-inflammatory effects. Clinical evidence supports benefit for certain pain conditions (including low back pain and osteoarthritis) in standardized preparations. Safety and tolerability depend on dose, source quality, and salicylate sensitivity.

---

### How to Use (Dosage & Methods)

- **Decoction:** 1–2 tsp dried bark simmered 20–30 minutes; 1/2–1 cup up to 2× daily
- **Capsules:** follow label directions (standardized products vary)
- **Tincture:** follow label; use short-term

---

### Forms Available

- Dried bark (decoction)
- Powder/capsules (standardized products vary)
- Tincture

---

### Caution Level: Caution

- Avoid if allergic to aspirin/salicylates
- Avoid with bleeding disorders, active ulcers, or anticoagulant therapy unless medically guided
- Avoid combining with high-dose NSAIDs or multiple blood-thinning agents
- Avoid in children/teens with viral illness (Reye's syndrome risk applies to salicylates)
- Pregnancy: avoid routine internal use unless supervised

---

### Gender-Specific Safety (GS)

**Men:** Safe (when appropriate) — short-term pain/fever support; avoid with blood thinners/ulcers/salicylate sensitivity

**Women:** Safe (when appropriate) — helpful for aches; avoid if heavy bleeding tendency or anticoagulants

**Pregnancy / Nursing:** Caution — avoid concentrated/internal use unless professionally guided; choose safer pain supports when possible

---

### Expected Results

- Pain relief: often 1–3 days
- Inflammation reduction: builds over 5–10 days
- Best results: short, consistent use rather than chronic daily dosing

---

### Same / Similar Results

Meadowsweet · Turmeric · Boswellia · Devil's Claw · Ginger ·

---

**🛠 DIY Recipe — Traditional Willow Decoction**

Simmer 1–2 tsp Willow Bark in 2 cups water for 20–30 minutes.
Strain; drink 1/2–1 cup up to 2× daily for short-term aches.

---

**Shelf Life / Potency After Preparation**

- Dried bark: 2–3 years (airtight, cool, dry)
- Decoction: 24 hours refrigerated
- Tincture: 3–5 years

---

**Herbal Reflections of Willow Bark**

Willow Bark teaches patience. It doesn't silence pain instantly; it steadily reduces the inflammatory "noise" beneath it. In a world that wants immediate numbing, Willow reminds us that relief can be built—quietly, consistently, and with respect for the body's pace.

---

**Herbal Confidence Index:** 🌿 🌿 🌿 🌿

(4/5 — reliable traditional pain-and-fever herb with solid historic use and modern support; loses a point for salicylate sensitivity and medication-interaction limits.)

# WILD YAM

★★★★★

*Dioscorea villosa*

**Wild Yam** is a classic comfort root used for **cramping, spasms, and pelvic or digestive tension**. It's often marketed as "natural progesterone," but the key compound (diosgenin) **does not convert into human hormones inside the body**—its value is better understood as antispasmodic support that helps muscles release tight, painful patterns.
Historically used by Native American healers and early American herbalists, Wild Yam became a trusted ally for menstrual cramps, menopausal transition discomfort, and intestinal spasm. In modern use, it remains a steady choice for people who need **relaxation of smooth muscle** without heavy sedation.

---

### 🌿 Core Herbal Category — Wild Yam

**Primary Core: Reproductive & Women's Health Support herb** with (antispasmodic action that eases uterine and pelvic tension)
**Secondary Cores:** Digestive Support · Musculoskeletal & Pain-Relief · Hormonal & Endocrine Support (indirect rhythm support—not a hormone replacement)

---

### 🌿 How It Works

Wild Yam relaxes smooth muscle in the uterus and digestive tract, helping reduce cramping and spasmodic pain. Its steroidal saponins contribute to tissue-calming, antispasmodic effects and may support endocrine "rhythm" indirectly by lowering stress-tension patterns that worsen symptoms. Its primary strength is **comfort and release**, not forcing hormonal change.

---

### 🌱 Primary Uses

- Menstrual cramps and PMS tension
- Pelvic tightness and spasm discomfort
- Menopause transition discomfort (tension/irritability patterns)
- Intestinal cramping, gas-related spasm
- Muscular spasm and rheumatic tightness (supportive)

---

### 🧪 Scientific Backing

Wild Yam contains diosgenin and related saponins associated with antispasmodic and anti-inflammatory activity. Evidence and clinical commentary consistently clarify that diosgenin converts to hormones only through laboratory processing, not human metabolism. Traditional use supports its role as a cramp-relieving comfort herb.

---

### 💊 How to Use (Dosage & Methods)

- **Decoction:** 1–2 tsp dried root simmered 20 minutes; 1–2× daily as needed
- **Tincture:** 1–2 mL up to 3× daily
- **Capsules:** 500–1000 mg daily (follow label)
- **Topical creams:** comfort support only; not "hormone replacement"

---

### 💊 Forms Available

- Dried root (decoction)
- Tincture
- Capsules
- Creams/salves (comfort support)

---

### ⚠ Caution Level: 🟢 Safe / 🟡 Caution

- Generally well tolerated; may cause mild nausea if taken on an empty stomach
- Use caution with hormone-sensitive conditions (medical guidance recommended)
- Pregnancy: avoid routine use unless professionally guided due to uterine/smooth muscle effects
- Nursing: use mild forms only unless guided

---

### 🚹 🚺 Gender-Specific Safety (GS)

**Men:** 🟢 Safe — may ease muscle tension/spasm; no direct hormone conversion in the body

**Women:** 🟢 Safe — excellent for cramp patterns and pelvic tension; clarify it is not direct progesterone

**Pregnancy / Nursing:** 🟡 Caution — avoid during pregnancy unless guided; nursing: mild tea may be acceptable, avoid strong extracts unless guided

---

### ⏳ Expected Results

- Cramp/spasm relief: often 1–3 days
- Menopause transition comfort: 2–4 weeks
- Digestive spasm calming: 1–3 days

---

### Same / Similar Results

Cramp Bark · Black Cohosh · Dong Quai · Vitex · Ginger

---

### DIY Recipe — Wild Yam Comfort Tea

Simmer 1 tsp dried Wild Yam root in 1½ cups water for 20 minutes, covered. Strain; drink warm during menstrual or digestive cramping.

---

### Shelf Life / Potency After Preparation

- Dried root: 1–2 years
- Decoction: 24–48 hours refrigerated
- Tincture: 4–6 years
- Capsules/creams: follow label dating

---

### Herbal Reflections of Wild Yam

Wild Yam is a quiet negotiator—helping the body release what it has been gripping too tightly. Its gift is honest comfort: it doesn't promise hormone miracles; it eases tension, softens spasm, and restores a more livable rhythm. Healing, here, comes through relaxation and steadiness.

---

### Herbal Confidence Index:

(5/5 — exceptional antispasmodic comfort herb for pelvic and digestive cramp patterns with strong traditional reliability; safest when its true role is understood.)

# WILD INDIGO

★★★

*Baptisia tinctoria*

**Wild Indigo** is a **high-potency, short-term immune herb** historically used for swollen glands, severe sore throat patterns, and septic-type infection states. Eclectic physicians and traditional herbalists used it in controlled dosing when the body seemed overwhelmed—especially with thick inflammation, lymph stagnation, and spreading infection.
Today, Wild Indigo is best understood as a **crisis-level herb**, not a daily immune tonic. It is commonly used in modern practice as a small-dose tincture ingredient in acute formulas, often combined with gentler immune and lymph herbs.

---

### 🌿 Core Herbal Category — Wild Indigo

**Primary Core: Immune System Support** herb with (powerful, short-term immune-stimulating action used in acute infectious states)
**Secondary Cores:** Lymphatic Support · Circulatory Support · Digestive Support

---

### 🌿 How It Works

Wild Indigo strongly stimulates immune activity and lymphatic movement, helping the body respond to acute infection patterns. Its intensity can support rapid "turning" of swollen gland and throat patterns, but it can also irritate digestion and overstimulate sensitive systems. For that reason, it is used **briefly, in low doses**, and typically as part of a combined formula rather than as a stand-alone tonic.

---

### 🌱 Primary Uses (Short-Term / Acute)

• Swollen glands and lymph congestion during infection
• Severe sore throat patterns (formula use)
• Acute infection states needing strong immune escalation (guided use)
• Topical diluted rinses for gum or wound support (careful dilution)

---

### 🧪 Scientific Backing

Wild Indigo contains alkaloid and isoflavone constituents associated with antimicrobial and immune-modulating actions. Historic Eclectic use is well documented for septic states and glandular swelling. Modern clinical data is limited; its strongest support remains traditional/clinical herbal practice emphasizing low-dose, short-term use.

---

### How to Use (Dosage & Methods)

• **Tincture (preferred):** 5–20 drops, 2–3× daily during acute needs, up to 5 days
• **Tea/decoction:** generally avoided; if used, extremely low-dose and short-term only
• **Topical rinse:** very dilute infusion for gums/skin (do not use concentrated preparations)

---

### Forms Available

• Tincture (most common)
• Dried root (specialist use)
• Diluted topical rinse preparations

---

### Caution Level: Supervision Required

• Not for casual use, high dosing, or long-term use
• Avoid in pregnancy/nursing
• Avoid with autoimmune disease or significant inflammatory disorders unless medically guided
• May cause nausea, dizziness, or GI upset—stop if adverse effects occur
• Safer acute alternatives often include Echinacea and other gentler immune herbs

---

### Gender-Specific Safety (GS)

**Men:** Caution — only short-term, measured dosing; avoid with autoimmune/liver concerns

**Women:** Caution — short-term, guided use only; avoid with autoimmune/liver concerns

**Pregnancy / Nursing:** Avoid

---

### Expected Results

• Swollen gland/throat turning: 24–72 hours
• Acute immune escalation effects: 1–3 days
• Topical support: 1–2 applications

---

### Same / Similar Results

Echinacea · Goldenseal (short-term) · Red Root · Cleavers · Oregon Grape Root

---

### 🛠️ DIY Recipe

🚫 Not recommended. This is a specialist herb; home blending is not appropriate without guidance.

---

### 🧍🧍 Shelf Life / Potency After Preparation

- Dried root: ~2 years
- Tincture: 4–6 years
- Diluted topical rinse: 24 hours refrigerated

---

### 🌙 Herbal Reflections of Wild Indigo

Wild Indigo is the "emergency lever," not the daily routine. It steps forward when infection patterns look heavy and fast-moving—but its lesson is restraint. Used briefly and wisely, it can be a decisive ally. Used casually, it becomes unnecessary risk. Its power is real, and so is its boundary.

---

### ⭐ Herbal Confidence Index: 🌿 🌿 🌿

(3/5 — highly effective in its narrow lane as a short-term crisis herb; rated lower only because it requires careful dosing and is not suited for routine use.)

# WINTERGREEN

★★★½

*Gaultheria procumbens*

**Wintergreen** is a low-growing North American evergreen best known for its minty aroma and bright red berries. Its key compound, **methyl salicylate**, is intensely pain-relieving and anti-inflammatory—**but also highly toxic if misused**. For that reason, Wintergreen's best and safest role in modern herbal practice is **diluted topical use** (balms/liniments) for muscle and joint soreness.

In Native American traditions it was used carefully for pain, fever, and congestion. In later Western practice it became a familiar external remedy for rheumatism and strain. Today, Wintergreen remains effective—but it must be handled with strict respect for dosage, age restrictions, and salicylate risks.

---

### 🌿 Core Herbal Category — Wintergreen

**Primary Core: Anti-Inflammatory & Pain Support** herb with (strong salicylate-based action used primarily for topical pain relief)

**Secondary Cores:** Circulatory Support · Respiratory Support (aromatic/steam only) · Skin & Tissue Repair (external only)

---

### 🌿 How It Works

Wintergreen's methyl salicylate penetrates tissues and reduces local inflammatory signaling, which helps dull pain and relax tight muscles when used **topically in very low dilution**. It also creates a warming sensation by increasing local circulation. Because methyl salicylate can absorb through skin and behave like a high-dose salicylate, safety depends on **small amounts, proper dilution, limited surface area**, and avoiding heat/occlusion.

---

### 🌱 Primary Uses (Topical / Aromatic)

- Muscle aches, sprains, and overuse soreness (topical)
- Arthritic and rheumatic joint discomfort (topical)
- Tension-type aches from tight muscles (topical)
- Occasional steam inhalation for congestion (aromatic only; not internal)

---

### 🔬 Scientific Backing

Wintergreen oil is a well-known source of methyl salicylate, a strong topical analgesic used in many liniments. Research supports its localized pain-relief effects while also documenting serious toxicity risk if ingested or used undiluted/excessively on skin. It must be treated as a **high-risk salicylate source**.

---

### How to Use (Dosage & Methods)

- **Topical dilution: 0.5–1%** for most adults (higher is unnecessary and increases risk)
- Apply to **small areas only**, 1–2× daily
- **Steam inhalation:** if used, aromatic only (no ingestion); keep exposure brief and ventilated
- **Internal use:** 🚫 **Unsafe — do not ingest**

---

### Forms Available

- Essential oil (external only; **must be diluted**)
- Infused oils, balms, liniments (preferred)
- Dried leaves (rare; traditional use only—**not recommended internally**)

---

### ⚠ Caution Level: ● Supervision Required

**Do NOT ingest.** Even small internal amounts can be toxic or fatal.

Avoid entirely if: salicylate/aspirin allergy, blood thinners, bleeding disorders, active ulcers, kidney disease, aspirin-exacerbated asthma.

**Never** apply undiluted, to large areas, to broken skin, or under heat/occlusion (heating pads, tight wraps).

**Children/teens:** avoid due to salicylate toxicity risk (and viral-illness salicylate concerns).

Toxicity signs: ringing ears, nausea/vomiting, confusion, rapid breathing—seek urgent medical care.

**PRECAUTION:** Wintergreen is effective but has strong potential for harm. Safer options include **Peppermint (diluted), Arnica (external), Ginger, Turmeric**.

---

### Gender-Specific Safety (GS)

**Men:** ● Caution — topical diluted use only; avoid with anticoagulants/daily aspirin; stop if irritation or salicylate symptoms occur

**Women:** ● Caution — topical diluted use only; avoid with salicylate sensitivity or heavy bleeding tendency; use sparingly

**Pregnancy / Nursing:** ● Avoid — methyl salicylate can absorb systemically; avoid all topical/internal use

---

### ⏳ Expected Results (Topical Use)

- Relief of soreness/tightness: 15–60 minutes
- Stiffness easing: 1–3 days with careful use
- Ongoing support: short-term cycles only (avoid daily long-term use)

---

### 🔄 Same / Similar Results (Safer Options)

⚪ Peppermint (diluted) · ⚪ Arnica (external) · ⚪ Ginger · ⚪ Turmeric · ⚪ White Willow Bark (internal—only if appropriate)

---

### 🛠 DIY Recipe — Safer Micro-Dilution Muscle Oil

Add **1 drop** Wintergreen essential oil to **2 teaspoons** carrier oil (about ~0.5%). Massage into a **small area** 1× daily as needed. Patch test first.

🚫 Do not use on broken skin or under heat.

---

### Shelf Life / Potency After Preparation

- Essential oil: 3–5 years (sealed, cool, dark)
- Balms/infused oils: 1–2 years (shorter if oils go rancid)
- Dried leaves: ~1 year (aroma fades)

---

### 🌙 Herbal Reflections of Wintergreen

Wintergreen is a lesson in potency and restraint. It can bring fast, targeted relief—yet it demands boundaries that many herbs do not. Used with precision, it serves the body well; used casually, it becomes a risk. In The Herbal Resurrection system, Wintergreen is best honored as **a carefully diluted external specialist**, not a general household herb.

---

### ⭐ Herbal Confidence Index: 🌿 🌿 🌿 ½

(3.5/5 — very effective for topical pain relief, but scored lower for narrow safety margins and serious toxicity risk if misused.)

# WESTERN RED CEDAR

★★½

*Thuja plicata*

**Western Red Cedar** is a powerful aromatic evergreen deeply respected by Indigenous peoples of the Pacific Northwest. Traditionally called the "Tree of Life," it has been used for **external cleansing, respiratory steaming, and ceremonial purification**, especially during seasonal illness and environmental heaviness. Its resinous aroma can support a sense of clearer breathing and a cleaner environment.
However, Western Red Cedar contains **thujone-rich oils** that can be neurotoxic if misused. In The Herbal Resurrection system, it is best treated as an **external/steam/ritual herb**, not a routine internal remedy.

---

### Core Herbal Category — Western Red Cedar

**Primary Core: Respiratory System Support** herb with (aromatic antimicrobial action used externally and in steam/ceremonial use)
**Secondary Cores:** Immune Support · Skin & Tissue Repair (external) · Circulatory Support (warming aromatic influence)

---

### How It Works

Western Red Cedar's volatile compounds can inhibit some microbes in the environment and on the skin when used in diluted external preparations. In steam or aromatic use, its resinous scent may help open the feeling of the airways and reduce "stale" congestion sensation—without requiring ingestion. Because internal use increases toxicity risk, its safest benefits come through **external contact (diluted)**, **steam (brief, ventilated)**, and **ceremonial cleansing practices**.

---

### Primary Uses (External / Steam / Ritual)

- Steam support for congestion (brief, ventilated)
- External cleansing for minor fungal/skin concerns (diluted wash)
- Environmental purification/ceremonial use (with ventilation)
- Supportive immune-season ritual ally (non-ingested)

---

### Scientific Backing

Cedar species contain essential oils and tannins with demonstrated antimicrobial and antifungal activity in laboratory settings. Safety literature also warns that thujone-containing oils can be harmful if ingested or used excessively. This supports a **restricted external/steam-only** approach.

---

### 🩹 How to Use (Dosage & Methods)

- **Steam:** a small handful of leaves in hot water; inhale 5–8 minutes with good ventilation
- **Topical wash:** mild decoction applied to skin (avoid broken skin); discontinue if irritation
- **Essential oil:** external only; very dilute (many products are too strong—use extreme caution)
- **Internal use:** 🚫 not recommended in this system due to thujone risk

---

### 🩹 Forms Available

- Fresh/dried leaves (steam, wash)
- Salves/washes (external)
- Essential oil (external only; caution)

---

### ⚠️ Caution Level: ● Supervision Required

- Avoid internal ingestion and concentrated oils
- Avoid in pregnancy/nursing
- Avoid with epilepsy/seizure history, kidney disease, or thujone-sensitive conditions
- Avoid combining with other thujone-heavy herbs (e.g., Wormwood)
- When burned ceremonially: ventilate well; avoid heavy smoke exposure

**PRECAUTION:** Western Red Cedar is effective but can cause harm if misused. Safer respiratory aromatic options include **Pine, Spruce, mild Thyme steam** (when appropriate).

---

### 🚹 🚺 Gender-Specific Safety (GS)

**Men:** ● Caution — use external/steam only; avoid if seizure/kidney issues; stop if dizziness/nausea

**Women:** ● Caution — external/steam only; avoid strong oils; stop if irritation or nausea

**Pregnancy / Nursing:** ● Avoid — thujone concerns and safety uncertainty

---

### ⏳ Expected Results

- Steam respiratory ease: often same day (1–2 steams)
- Skin/fungal improvement: 1–2 weeks (consistent gentle external use)
- Ritual clarity/grounding: immediate (non-medical)

---

### 🔄 Same / Similar Results

🟢 Pine Needles · 🟢 Spruce Tips · 🟣 Juniper (external/aromatic) · 🔵 Eucalyptus (external/aromatic)

---

### 🛠️ DIY Recipe — Cedar Steam for Congestion (External Use Only)

Add a small handful of cedar leaves to a bowl of hot water.
Steam 5–8 minutes with good ventilation.
Stop if headache, dizziness, or irritation occurs.

---

### 🧍 🧍 Shelf Life / Potency After Preparation

- Dried leaves: 1–2 years (airtight, dark)
- Decoction/wash: 24–48 hours refrigerated
- Essential oil: 3–5 years sealed, cool, dark

---

### 🌙 Herbal Reflections of Western Red Cedar

Western Red Cedar is protection medicine—best approached through scent, steam, and respectful external use rather than ingestion. It teaches that some plants heal by **presence** and **boundary**, offering clearing and steadiness when used correctly. In The Herbal Resurrection system, Cedar is honored as a strong ally with a narrow lane: **external and ceremonial, not casual internal use.**

---

### ⭐ Herbal Confidence Index: 🌿 🌿 ½

(2.5/5 — meaningful external and ceremonial ally with antimicrobial value, but scored lower due to thujone-related safety limits and restricted internal suitability.)

# JUNIPER BERRY

★★★★

*Juniperus communis*

**Juniper Berry** is a warming, aromatic herb long valued as a **urinary and digestive tonic**, prized for its ability to stimulate kidney function, ease fluid retention, and support digestive warmth. Traditionally used for sluggish digestion, bloating, and urinary discomfort, it is valued for its **brisk, penetrating action**.
Historically burned as a purifying incense and distilled into gin across Europe, Juniper Berry has also been associated with protection and cleansing—yet its practical strengths are clear: **urinary stimulation, digestive warmth, and antimicrobial support**.

---

**Core Herbal Category — Juniper Berry** (Juniperus communis)
**Primary Core: Kidney & Urinary Support** herb with (warming, diuretic volatile-oil principles that stimulate kidney filtration and support fluid balance)
**Secondary Cores:** Digestive Support · Antimicrobial Support · Circulatory Warmth

---

### How It Works

Juniper Berry stimulates kidney filtration through its volatile oil content, particularly terpinen-4-ol, encouraging healthy fluid elimination and easing water retention. Its warming, carminative action supports sluggish digestion, easing gas and bloating. Antimicrobial compounds help discourage unwanted microbial overgrowth within the urinary tract. The result is a brisk, penetrating herb that stimulates elimination pathways without depleting the system.

---

### Primary Uses

- Supports healthy urinary flow and mild fluid retention
- Eases bloating, gas, and sluggish digestion
- Provides antimicrobial support for occasional urinary discomfort
- Warms cold, damp constitutions
- Traditionally used for joint stiffness (topical/warming use)

---

### Scientific Backing

Juniper Berry contains volatile oils (including alpha-pinene and terpinen-4-ol) along with flavonoids, historically associated with diuretic, carminative, and antimicrobial activity.

Traditional European herbalism consistently describes its warming, stimulating action on the kidneys and digestive tract.

---

### 💊 How to Use (Dosage & Methods)

- **Tea/infusion:** ½–1 tsp crushed berries per cup; steep 10 minutes; up to 2× daily
- **Tincture:** 1–2 mL, up to 2× daily
- **Culinary:** crushed berries in savory dishes and marinades
- **Capsules/powder:** follow label dosing

---

### 💊 Forms Available

- Dried berries (tea/culinary)
- Tincture or liquid extract
- Essential oil (external use only)
- Capsules or powder

---

### ⚠️ Caution Level: 🟡 Caution

- Avoid prolonged or high-dose internal use
- Not recommended with kidney disease or inflammation
- Avoid during pregnancy (traditional uterine-stimulant use)
- Essential oil for external use only, well diluted

---

### 🚹 🚺 Gender-Specific Safety (GS)

**Men:** 🟢 Safe — supportive for urinary flow, digestion, and joint warmth

**Women:** 🟡 Caution — supportive in moderate use; avoid concentrated forms with kidney sensitivity

**Pregnancy / Nursing:** 🔴 Avoid — traditional uterine-stimulant action; insufficient safety data

---

### ⏳ Expected Results

- Digestive warmth and gas relief: within hours
- Urinary flow support: 1–3 days
- Fluid retention relief: several days of consistent use

---

### 🔄 Same / Similar Results

🟢 Corn Silk · 🟢 Uva Ursi · 🟢 Gravel Root · 🟢 Parsley

---

### 🛠️ DIY Recipe — Juniper Berry Digestive Tea

Crush ½–1 tsp dried juniper berries and steep in 1 cup hot water for 8–10 minutes.

Strain and sip after meals for digestive warmth and urinary support.

---

### 🕯 🕯 Shelf Life / Potency After Preparation

- Dried berries: 2–3 years (airtight, cool, dark)
- Tincture: 4–5 years
- Essential oil: 2–3 years (cool, dark storage)
- Prepared tea: use within 24 hours

---

### 🌙 Herbal Reflections of Juniper Berry

Juniper Berry carries the resinous strength of the evergreen forest—warming, penetrating, and quietly protective. It moves what has stagnated, clearing dampness from the body just as it has long been burned to clear stagnant air from a room. Its medicine is brisk and purposeful, reminding the body how to release what no longer serves it.

---

### ⭐ Herbal Confidence Index: 🌿 🌿 🌿 🌿

(4/5 — a reliable, time-tested urinary and digestive stimulant, valued across centuries of European herbal tradition; best used short-term and with respect for its warming intensity.)

# VERBENA

★★★½

*Verbena officinalis*

**Verbena (Vervain)** is a classic European nervine known for easing stress patterns that "sit in the body"—tight shoulders and neck, tension headaches, shallow sleep, and stress-linked digestive cramping. It calms without dulling the mind, helping the nervous system unwind while keeping clarity intact. Many herbalists also use Verbena as a gentle bitter-tonic that supports the liver and digestion during periods of emotional overload.
Historically revered across Egyptian, Roman, Druidic, and early Christian traditions, Verbena bridged ritual and remedy. In modern practice, its value remains practical: it releases tension, supports sleep quality, and helps the body recover from the strain of prolonged stress.

---

### 🌿 Core Herbal Category — Verbena

**Primary Core: Nervous System Support (Nervines)** herb with (tension-releasing, calming principles that relax a strained nervous system without heavy sedation)
**Secondary Cores:** Digestive Support · Liver & Detoxification Support · Musculoskeletal & Pain-Relief Support (tension headaches)

---

### 🌿 How It Works

Verbena works by gently lowering nervous-system overactivity and relaxing stress-driven muscle guarding—especially in the neck, shoulders, jaw, and upper back. Its bitter constituents help normalize digestive function when anxiety disrupts appetite, motility, or comfort. By supporting healthy bile flow and liver processing, it can assist the body's recovery during "stuck" stress patterns that feel both emotional and physical. Overall, Verbena functions as a clarifying nervine: it softens tension, steadies mood, and supports smoother digestion and sleep.

---

### 🌱 Primary Uses

- Stress and mild anxiety with muscular tension
- Tension headaches and tight neck/shoulders
- Stress-related indigestion, cramping, or appetite disruption
- Restless sleep from an overactive mind/body
- Gentle support in "stagnation" patterns (stress + digestive heaviness)

---

## Scientific Backing

**Verbena** contains iridoid glycosides (including verbenalin), flavonoids, and mild bitters associated with calming, anti-inflammatory, and digestive-support effects. Traditional European use strongly supports its role for tension, headaches, nervous digestion, and sleep quality. Evidence is best described as **supportive and traditional**, with modern studies suggesting mild analgesic and neuro-calming activity rather than strong sedative force.

---

## How to Use (Dosage & Methods)

**Tea (infusion):** 1 tsp dried herb per cup; steep 8–10 minutes; up to 2–3× daily, or 1 cup in the evening
**Tincture:** 1–2 mL up to 2–3× daily
**Capsules/Tablets:** 300–600 mg/day (follow label)
**Bath/Compress:** add strong tea to a bath or cloth compress for relaxation

---

## Forms Available

- Dried herb (tea/infusion)
- Tincture/extract
- Capsules/tablets
- Fresh herb (compresses/baths)

---

## Caution Level: Caution

Generally safe in normal amounts, but use with awareness:
- **Pregnancy:** avoid concentrated preparations (traditional uterine-tone cautions)
- **Low blood pressure:** may feel too relaxing for some
- **Sedatives/alcohol:** can add to drowsiness in sensitive individuals
- Excess bitterness may cause mild nausea—take with a small snack if needed

---

## Gender-Specific Safety (GS)

**Men:** Safe — helpful for tension headaches, stress digestion, and tight muscles; use caution only if very low blood pressure or strong sedatives

**Women:** Safe — excellent for emotional overload, PMS-related tension, and nervous digestion; avoid very high doses during heavy menstrual flow if it feels overly relaxing

**Pregnancy / Nursing:** Caution — avoid concentrated tinctures/extracts during pregnancy; if used at all, keep to mild tea only under professional guidance; avoid strong dosing while nursing if infant shows drowsiness or digestive upset

---

### ⏳ Expected Results

- Nervous calming and tension softening: 1–2 doses
- Tension headache relief: 1–3 days (pattern-dependent)
- Sleep quality improvement: ~1 week
- Stress-digestion resilience: 2–3 weeks

---

### 🔄 Same / Similar Results

🟢 Lemon Balm · 🟢 Chamomile · 🟢 Skullcap · 🟢 Passionflower · 🟢 Holy Basil

---

### 🛠️ DIY Recipe — Verbena Rest & Renewal Tea

1 tsp Verbena
1 tsp Chamomile
1 tsp Lemon Balm
Steep 10 minutes covered. Sip slowly in the evening to unwind.

---

### 🧴 Shelf Life / Potency After Preparation

- Dried herb: 1–2 years (cool, dry, airtight)
- Tincture: 3–5 years
- Capsules/tablets: 1–2 years (per manufacturer)
- Fresh preparations: use immediately

Potency loss signs: fading aroma, weak bitterness, dull color

### 🌙 Herbal Reflections of Verbena

Verbena is the herb for the person who has been "holding it together" for too long. It loosens the hidden knots—emotional, muscular, and digestive—without taking away clarity. Its medicine is not a heavy sedation; it is a steady unwinding. In The Herbal Resurrection system, Verbena stands as a calm rebalancer: helping the body release tension, settle the stomach, and return to natural rest.

---

### ⭐ Herbal Confidence Index: 🌿🌿🌿½

(3.5/5 — reliable for tension patterns, nervous digestion, and headache-prone stress. Not a powerhouse sedative, but an excellent harmonizer when used consistently and appropriately.)

# VELVET BEAN

★★★★

(*Mucuna pruriens*)

**Velvet Bean** is a dopamine-supportive adaptogen best known for its natural **L-DOPA**, which can improve motivation, mood, libido, focus, and stress resilience when used in **small, cycled doses**. It is one of the most "chemical-impact" herbs in the book—excellent for the right person at the right time, but not an everyday casual tonic for everyone. In Ayurveda (Kapikacchu), it is used to rebuild vitality during nervous exhaustion and depleted drive, often paired with grounding routines (sleep, protein, sunlight, steady meals).

---

### Core Herbal Category — Velvet Bean

**Primary Core:** Nervous System Support (Nervines) herb with (dopaminergic, mood-lifting principles that support motivation, focus, and neurological resilience)
**Secondary Cores:** Adaptogen · Men's Health & Vitality · Hormonal & Endocrine Support

---

### How It Works

Velvet Bean works by providing **L-DOPA**, a direct precursor to dopamine, which can raise dopamine availability and improve drive, mood tone, and neurological signaling. This support may reduce stress-fatigue patterns linked to low motivation, low libido, and mental "flatness." Because dopamine influences sleep-wake rhythm and endocrine signaling, Velvet Bean can also improve recovery and vitality—but it can overstimulate sensitive systems if dosed too high or used without cycling. Overall, Velvet Bean functions as a **targeted neuro-restorative** best used with precision, breaks, and medication awareness.

---

### Primary Uses

- Low motivation / low drive / stress-related "flatness"
- Libido and vitality support (especially for depletion patterns)
- Nervous fatigue and stress recovery (cycled)
- Focus support when dopamine tone is low (not a stimulant substitute)

---

### Scientific Backing

Velvet Bean is naturally rich in **L-DOPA**, plus antioxidants and supportive phytochemicals. Research supports:

- dopaminergic activity (mood/motivation support)
- potential adjunctive support in Parkinsonian conditions (medical supervision)
- antioxidant and neuroprotective effects
- support for male fertility parameters in some studies

Because it directly impacts neurotransmitter pathways, it should be treated as **highly active** rather than "gentle."

---

### How to Use (Dosage & Methods)

**Powder:** ¼–½ tsp daily in smoothie/tea (start low; increase only if calm and well tolerated)

**Capsules:** 250–500 mg once daily (often best in short cycles)

**Standardized extracts:** follow label; start low

**Cycling options:**

- 5 days on / 2 days off **OR**
- 3–6 weeks on / 1–2 weeks off

**Timing:** morning or early afternoon (avoid close to bedtime if it makes you alert)

---

### Forms Available

- Powder
- Capsules
- Tincture (less common; practitioner-guided)
- Standardized extracts

---

### Caution Level: Caution — Use With Guidance

Avoid or use only with professional guidance if taking:

- antidepressants (SSRIs/SNRIs/MAOIs)
- antipsychotics
- Parkinson's meds (levodopa/carbidopa, etc.)
- ADHD stimulants
- blood pressure or blood sugar medications

Use caution with: anxiety/insomnia tendencies, glaucoma, diabetes, heart rhythm concerns, bipolar-spectrum mood instability. Start small; stop if agitation, rapid heartbeat, nausea, insomnia, irritability, or headaches appear.

---

### Gender-Specific Safety (GS)

**Men:** Caution — strong benefits for drive/libido and depleted motivation, but dose must stay modest and cycled; avoid with dopamine-altering meds.

**Women:** ⚪ Caution — can lift mood and motivation, but may worsen anxiety/insomnia if pushed; avoid with antidepressants, thyroid meds, or hormonal therapies unless supervised.
**Pregnancy / Nursing:** ⚫ Avoid — dopaminergic action may affect prolactin and pregnancy/nursing physiology; not appropriate.

---

### ⏳ Expected Results

- Mood/drive shift: 2–4 days (often subtle at first)
- Focus/energy steadier: 1 week
- Libido/vitality improvement: 2–3 weeks (with cycling)
- Longer-term nervous tone: 1–2 months **only if** cycled properly and well tolerated

---

### 🔄 Same / Similar Results

⚪ Rhodiola — motivation + stress resilience
⚫ Ashwagandha — calm vitality + recovery
⚪ Maca — endurance + libido
⚪ Damiana — mood + sensual balance
⚫ Ginkgo — focus + circulation (non-dopaminergic)

### 🛠 DIY Recipe — Dopamine-Support Morning Elixir

¼ tsp Velvet Bean powder
1 tsp raw cacao
Warm almond milk
Drizzle of honey
Blend and sip in the morning. (Avoid near bedtime.)

---

### 🧴 Shelf Life / Potency After Preparation

- Powder: 1–2 years (airtight, cool, moisture-free)
- Capsules: 1–2 years (manufacturer-dependent)
- Tincture: 3–5 years
- Extracts: 2–3 years

Potency loss signs: clumping, stale odor, softened capsules, dull bitter-sweet scent.

---

### 🌙 Herbal Reflections of Velvet Bean

Velvet Bean returns the spark—but it teaches restraint. It is a precision herb: enough to brighten the inner engine, not so much that it turns into restlessness or edge. Its lesson is that motivation is not merely willpower; sometimes it is chemistry, nourishment, and recovery aligning again. Used thoughtfully, Velvet Bean helps life regain color and forward motion. Used carelessly, it becomes too sharp a flame. The wisdom is in dosage, timing, and the humility to cycle.

🌟 ***Herbal Confidence Index:*** *🌿 🌿 🌿 🌿 4/5 — exceptional for the right "low-dopamine depletion" pattern and vitality recovery, but its neurotransmitter strength demands cycling, medication awareness, and respect. High benefit, higher responsibility.)*

# TURMERIC

★★★★★

(*Curcuma longa*)

**Turmeric** is one of the world's most respected anti-inflammatory roots, valued for its ability to calm pain, cool systemic inflammation, and support long-term resilience. Its curcuminoids act broadly yet gently—supporting joints, digestion, cardiovascular health, immune balance, and cognitive clarity without suppressing natural healing processes. As both food and medicine, Turmeric is unusually suited for **daily, lifelong use**.
Used for thousands of years in Ayurveda and Traditional Chinese Medicine, Turmeric has served as a blood purifier, digestive ally, and longevity tonic. In modern herbalism it bridges kitchen and clinic, offering steady, cumulative benefits rather than sharp or stimulating effects.

---

### 🌿 Core Herbal Category — Turmeric

**Primary Core: Anti-Inflammatory & Pain Support** herb with (curcuminoid-driven modulation of inflammatory signaling that reduces pain and tissue irritation)
**Secondary Cores:** Digestive Support · Liver & Gallbladder Support · Cardiovascular Support · Immune Support

---

### 🌿 How It Works

Turmeric works by moderating overactive inflammatory pathways through its curcuminoids, particularly curcumin. This reduces swelling and discomfort while allowing tissue repair to proceed naturally. Turmeric also stimulates bile flow, improving digestion and liver detoxification, and its antioxidant activity protects blood vessels and cells from oxidative stress. Taken consistently, Turmeric restores comfort and balance rather than producing short-term suppression.

---

### 🌱 Primary Uses

- Joint pain, arthritis, and inflammatory stiffness
- Digestive sluggishness and liver congestion
- Cardiovascular and metabolic inflammation
- Immune modulation and oxidative stress protection
- Long-term preventive wellness

---

### Scientific Backing

Curcumin is one of the most researched natural compounds in modern science. Studies show modulation of **NF-κB, COX-2, and TNF-α**, with documented benefits for joint pain, metabolic markers, liver enzymes, gut inflammation, immune regulation, and cognitive resilience. Absorption is enhanced when taken with fats or black pepper (piperine).

---

### How to Use (Dosage & Methods)

**Powder/Capsules:** 500–1,000 mg daily with food and fat
**Tea / Golden Milk:** 1 tsp powder simmered 8–10 minutes
**Extracts:** follow label or practitioner guidance
Consistency matters more than high dosing.

---

### Forms Available

- Fresh or dried root
- Powder
- Capsules/Tablets (standardized curcumin)
- Teas
- Tinctures / extracts

---

### Caution Level: Caution

Generally very safe.

- Use caution with **high-dose supplements** if on blood thinners
- Avoid high doses with gallstones or bile duct obstruction
- Excessive intake may cause warmth or loose stools in sensitive individuals

---

### Gender-Specific Safety (GS)

**Men:** Safe — excellent daily joint, liver, and cardiovascular support
**Women:** Safe — supports hormonal liver balance and inflammation
**Pregnancy / Nursing:** Caution — food-level use is acceptable; avoid high-dose curcumin supplements

---

### Expected Results

- Joint comfort: 4–7 days
- Digestive and liver tone: 1–2 weeks
- Systemic inflammation reduction: 2–3 weeks

---

### Same / Similar Results

Ginger · Boswellia · Devil's Claw · White Willow · Cayenne · Feverfew

---

**Shelf Life / Potency After Preparation**

• Powder: 2–3 years
• Fresh root: 1–2 weeks refrigerated (6 months frozen)
• Capsules: 1–2 years
• Tincture: 3–5 years

Potency loss signs: fading color, weak aroma, clumping.

---

**Herbal Reflections of Turmeric**

Turmeric is slow medicine with deep reach. It does not force change—it **restores flow**. Through warmth, patience, and nourishment, it brings the body back toward balance. Its power lies not in immediacy, but in reliability. Taken daily, it quietly rebuilds comfort and resilience across systems.

---

**Herbal Confidence Index:**

(5/5 — a cornerstone herb: safe, versatile, deeply researched, and ideal for lifelong support.)

# HARITAKI

★★★★★

*Terminalia chebula*

**Haritaki** is revered in Ayurveda as the **"King of Medicines"**, valued for its rare ability to cleanse, tone, and restore digestion without dependency. Rather than forcing elimination, it teaches the digestive system to work properly again—balancing constipation, sluggish digestion, and toxin accumulation over time.

Beyond digestion, Haritaki is considered a rejuvenative herb of clarity and longevity. Traditional systems hold that when elimination is balanced, the entire system benefits—from energy and cognition to immunity and metabolic harmony.

---

### 🌿 Core Herbal Category — Haritaki

**Primary Core: Digestive System Support herb** with (regulating, bowel-toning action that restores natural elimination rhythm)

**Secondary Cores:** Liver & Detoxification · Metabolic Support · Nutritive & Restorative Support

---

### 🌿 How It Works

Haritaki gently stimulates peristalsis while toning intestinal tissue, improving elimination without laxative dependence. It supports liver detoxification, reduces internal stagnation, and improves nutrient absorption. Over time, it strengthens digestive intelligence—helping the gut respond appropriately rather than reactively.

---

### 🌱 Primary Uses

- Constipation or irregular elimination
- Sluggish digestion and bloating
- Gentle detoxification and metabolic balance
- Gut repair and nutrient assimilation
- Longevity and internal cleansing support

---

### 🔬 Scientific & Traditional Insight

Haritaki contains **chebulinic and chebulagic acids**, tannins, and polyphenols with antioxidant, antimicrobial, and gut-toning activity. Traditional use emphasizes **non-habit-**

**forming bowel regulation** and long-term digestive repair rather than short-term evacuation.

---

### How to Use (Dosage & Methods)

**Powder:** ½ tsp once daily with warm water (often at night)
**Capsules:** 500–1,000 mg daily
**Decoction:** ½–1 tsp simmered 10 minutes
Low, consistent dosing is preferred.

---

### Forms Available

- Powder
- Capsules/Tablets
- Decoction (tea)
- Classical formulas (e.g., Triphala)

---

### Caution Level: Generally Safe

- Avoid high doses during pregnancy
- Reduce dose if stools become too loose
- Excessive use may cause dehydration

---

### Gender-Specific Safety (GS)

**Men:** Safe — supports digestion and metabolic balance
**Women:** Safe — reduce dose during menstruation if sensitivity occurs
**Pregnancy / Nursing:** Caution — use only under professional guidance

---

### Expected Results

- 3–7 days: improved regularity, less bloating
- 2–3 weeks: cleaner digestion, lighter energy
- 1–2 months: improved gut tone and metabolic clarity

---

### Same / Similar Results

Triphala · Psyllium Husk · Amla · Senna (short-term only)

---

### DIY — Haritaki Night Tonic

½ tsp Haritaki powder
1 cup warm water
Drink before bed to encourage gentle morning elimination.

---

### 🌙 Herbal Reflections of Haritaki

Haritaki restores intelligence to digestion. Where harsh laxatives exhaust the bowel, Haritaki rebuilds it. Its gift is patience—cleansing without force, repair without depletion. This is why it stands at the foundation of many formulas: when elimination works, everything else follows.

---

### ⭐ Herbal Confidence Index: 🌿 🌿 🌿 🌿 🌿

(5/5 — foundational, intelligent, and restorative. One of the safest and most effective long-term digestive allies.)

# TEA TREE

★★★★

*Melaleuca alternifolia*

**Tea Tree** is a potent Australian antiseptic renowned for its broad-spectrum antimicrobial action. Distilled from the leaves, its essential oil demonstrates antibacterial, antifungal, and antiviral activity and is widely used for acne, fungal skin and nail infections, dandruff, lice, and cold sores. Traditional Aboriginal use included crushed leaves applied to wounds and inhaled vapors for respiratory hygiene.
Modern herbal practice values Tea Tree for **rapid external sanitation** when properly diluted. It is **for external use only** and must be diluted (typically ≤5%) to avoid irritation. In steam inhalation, a single drop may assist sinus clearance; in shampoos and washes it supports scalp and skin hygiene when used with restraint and patch testing.

---

### Core Herbal Category — Tea Tree

**Primary Core: Lymphatic & Skin Support** herb with (powerful antimicrobial action that protects skin from bacterial and fungal overgrowth)
**Secondary Cores:** Immune Support · Respiratory Support · Musculoskeletal & Pain-Relief

---

### How It Works

Tea Tree acts through volatile antimicrobial compounds that inhibit bacteria, fungi, and certain viruses when applied externally. Its penetrating nature allows it to reach deeper skin layers, supporting wound hygiene and faster resolution of irritation. Aromatically, diluted vapor exposure may support respiratory hygiene by reducing microbial load. Tea Tree functions as a **topical antimicrobial specialist**, not an internal remedy.

---

### Primary Uses

- Acne and bacterial skin irritation
- Athlete's foot and fungal skin issues
- Nail fungus (persistent use required)
- Minor cuts, scrapes, and wound hygiene
- Dandruff and scalp irritation
- Lice support (proper dilution only)
- Steam inhalation for sinus congestion
- Household disinfectant applications

---

### Scientific Backing

Tea Tree oil contains terpinen-4-ol, γ-terpinene, and α-terpineol. Research confirms strong antibacterial and antifungal activity, reduction of acne lesions, inhibition of Candida, Staphylococcus, and dermatophytes, and support for scalp health via suppression of Malassezia. Tea Tree is among the most studied essential oils for topical antimicrobial control.

---

### Forms Available

- Essential oil
- Infused creams and lotions
- Shampoos and cleansers
- Spray-on hygiene blends

---

### How to Use

- **Topical:** Dilute to 1–5% in carrier oil; apply 1–3× daily
- **Steam:** 1 drop in hot water (eyes closed)
- **Scalp:** 2–3 drops added to shampoo
- **Household:** 10–20 drops in natural cleaners

---

### Expected Results

- Acne: 2–7 days
- Dandruff/scalp irritation: 3–5 uses
- Athlete's foot/fungal skin issues: 1–2 weeks
- Nail fungus: 4–8+ weeks

---

### Caution Level: Moderate — External Use Only

- **Never ingest** (risk of neurological toxicity)
- Always dilute before skin use
- Avoid eyes, ears, mucous membranes
- Patch test if sensitive or asthmatic
- Do not use on infants under 6 months
- Avoid use on pets (especially cats)

---

### Gender-Specific Safety — Tea Tree

**Men:** Safe externally when diluted; avoid undiluted use on broken skin

**Women:** Safe externally; may be drying—use soothing carriers

**Pregnancy/Nursing:** External use only; avoid heavy inhalation or undiluted oil

---

**Same / Similar Results** *Oregano Oil · Thyme Oil · Eucalyptus · Neem · Calendula*

---

**Shelf Life & Potency**

- Essential oil: 2–3 years (sealed, dark)
- Diluted oils: 6–12 months
- Creams/shampoos: As labeled

---

**DIY — Acne Spot Treatment**

1 drop Tea Tree + 1 tsp aloe gel or jojoba oil. Apply once daily.

---

**Herbal Reflections of Tea Tree**

Tea Tree is the swift cleanser—decisive, protective, and boundary-setting. It clears invasion without negotiation and reminds us that power must be paired with restraint. When respected, it restores clarity; when misused, it warns quickly. Its wisdom is precision.

**Herbal Confidence Index:** (4/5)

---

# *SWEDISH BITTERS*

★★★★

*Traditional Herbal Formula (multi-herb compound, not a single botanical species)*

**Swedish Bitters** is a classic multi-herb digestive tonic built around the power of bitterness. Bitter herbs stimulate bile flow, liver function, appetite, and peristalsis, easing gas, bloating, and sluggish elimination. Traditionally, it has also been used externally for bruises, bites, and skin irritation.

Rooted in formulas attributed to Paracelsus and revived by Maria Treben, Swedish Bitters reflects Europe's bitters tradition: **taste bitterness → awaken digestion**. While formulas vary, bitterness remains the unifying therapeutic driver.

---

### 🌿 Core Herbal Category — Swedish Bitters

**Primary Core: Digestive System Support** herb with (classic bitter action that stimulates digestion, bile flow, and elimination)

**Secondary Cores:** Liver & Detoxification · Metabolic Support · Skin & Tissue Repair

---

### 🌿 How It Works

Swedish Bitters activates bitter receptors that trigger digestive secretions and bile release, improving fat digestion and metabolic clearance. This stimulation restores digestive rhythm and supports liver detox pathways. Used externally, it assists tissue cleansing and protection. It functions as a **digestive wake-up formula**, not a daily beverage.

---

### 🌱 Primary Uses

- Sluggish digestion, gas, bloating
- Appetite and bile stimulation
- Liver and metabolic support
- Topical support for bruises and bites
- Diluted oral rinse for gum hygiene (spit only)

---

### 📊 Scientific Backing

Though not standardized, Swedish Bitters' actions are supported by research on its components: Gentian and Angelica stimulate gastric secretion; Aloe and Rhubarb influence bowel tone; Myrrh provides antimicrobial support. Pharmacology recognizes bitters as digestive secretagogues with mild laxative effects.

---

### Forms Available

- Alcohol tinctures
- Glycerites
- Topical creams
- DIY dried herb blends

---

### How to Use

- **Internal:** 1 tsp diluted in water, up to 3× daily before meals
- **Topical:** Apply diluted on cloth to affected areas
- **Oral rinse:** Dilute, swish, spit (do not swallow)

---

### Expected Results

- Gas/bloating relief: 20–30 minutes
- Digestive improvement: 1–3 days
- Topical response: 2–5 days

---

### Caution Level: Caution

- Contains alcohol and strong bitters
- Avoid with pregnancy, ulcers, GERD, reflux
- Overuse may cause cramping or loose stools
- Always dilute

---

### Gender-Specific Safety — Swedish Bitters

**Men:** Use diluted; avoid with ulcers or reflux

**Women:** Avoid high doses if cramp-prone

**Pregnancy/Nursing:** Avoid

---

### Same / Similar Results

Gentian · Dandelion Root · Artichoke Leaf · Milk Thistle · Wormwood

---

### Shelf Life

- Alcohol tincture: 3–5 years
- Glycerite: 1–2 years
- Dried blend: 1–2 years

---

### Herbal Reflections of Swedish Bitters

Swedish Bitters restores rhythm through discipline. It reminds digestion how to wake, secrete, and move—not by force, but by bitter intelligence. It teaches that discomfort, in small doses, can be medicine.

🌼 **Herbal Confidence Index:** 🌿 🌿 🌿 🌿 (4/5)

---

# *SUMAC*

★★★★

*Rhus coriaria*

**Sumac's** ruby berries offer food-grade medicine—cooling, astringent, and antioxidant. Used as spice or tea, Sumac tones tissues, soothes sore throats and diarrhea, supports urinary cleansing, and contributes antioxidant and glycemic balance. Its bright tang reflects vitamin-C-rich polyphenols.

Mediterranean and Indigenous traditions valued Sumac as nourishment and remedy. **Correct identification is essential**: culinary Sumac (Rhus coriaria) is safe; poison sumac is a different, toxic species.

---

### 🌿 Core Herbal Category — Sumac

**Primary Core: Lymphatic & Skin Support** herb with (cooling astringent and antioxidant action that tones tissue and reduces irritation)

**Secondary Cores:** Immune Support · Urinary & Kidney Support · Digestive Support · Circulatory Support

---

### 🌿 How It Works

Sumac gently tightens tissues, reducing excess discharge and soothing irritated membranes. Its antioxidants neutralize inflammatory stress, supporting immune and vascular integrity. Cooling astringency calms digestion and supports urinary tone without stimulation.

---

### 🌱 Primary Uses

- Sore throat, diarrhea, digestive upset
- Urinary and mucosal toning
- Antioxidant and metabolic support
- Immune and vascular strengthening

---

### 📊 Scientific Backing

Rich in polyphenols, flavonoids, tannins, and vitamin C. Studies show antioxidant, antimicrobial, anti-inflammatory activity and potential blood sugar and cholesterol benefits. Traditional use supports mucosal and tissue integrity.

---

### Forms Available

- Powdered berries
- Whole dried berries
- Capsules or tincture

---

### How to Use

- Powder: ½–1 tsp daily in food or water
- Tea: Steep 10 min or cold-infuse 30–60 min
- Tincture: 20–30 drops, 1–3× daily

---

### Expected Results

- Throat/digestive relief: 1–2 uses
- Urinary toning: 3–5 days
- Antioxidant support: 2–3 weeks

---

### Caution Level: Safe / Mild Astringent

- Avoid excessive use if constipated
- Use culinary-grade Rhus coriaria only
- Avoid if allergic to Anacardiaceae family

---

### Gender-Specific Safety — Sumac

**Men:** Safe; monitor if hypoglycemic

**Women:** Safe; avoid excess dryness

**Pregnancy/Nursing:** Food-level use only

---

***Same / Similar Results*** *Hibiscus · Elderberry · Cranberry · Raspberry Leaf · Goldenrod*

---

### Herbal Reflections of Sumac

Sumac offers clarity through cooling strength. It restores tone without force, refreshing tissues fatigued by heat, irritation, or excess. Neither aggressive nor passive, its medicine steadies where inflammation has loosened structure and gently tightens where resilience has thinned. Sumac teaches that recovery does not always require intensity—sometimes balance itself is the cure.

🌟 **Herbal Confidence Index:**
🌿 🌿 🌿 🌿 ½ (4.5/5 — A safe, food-grade, antioxidant-rich herb with broad daily usefulness. Exceptionally reliable for cooling, tissue toning, and gentle systemic support. While not highly aggressive, its consistency, safety, and versatility make it a standout long-term ally.)

# SPIKENARD

★★★★

*Nardostachys jatamansi*

**Spikenard** is a deeply grounding nervine and sacred aromatic native to the Himalayan regions. Closely related to Valerian, it quiets anxiety, restores nervous exhaustion, supports restful sleep, and calms emotional agitation without dulling awareness. Traditionally used for trauma, grief, and spiritual centering, Spikenard bridges emotional regulation with physical relaxation, offering steadiness where the nervous system has been overworked. Across Ayurvedic, Unani, and biblical traditions, Spikenard held a dual role as both medicine and sacred anointing oil. Modern herbalism continues this lineage, using Spikenard primarily at night for insomnia, PTSD-related tension, and stress overload, as well as topically in diluted oils for deep somatic release. It is not a stimulant herb; its strength lies in **descent**—bringing the body gently out of overdrive and back into rest.

---

### Core Herbal Category — Spikenard

**Primary Core: Nervous System Support (Nervines)** herb with (deeply calming, sedative action that quiets overstimulation and grounds emotional tension)

**Secondary Cores:** Hormonal & Endocrine Support herb · Digestive Support herb · Immune Support herb

---

### *How It Works*

Spikenard works by calming excessive nervous-system signaling and supporting parasympathetic activation. Its aromatic compounds help reduce anxiety, restlessness, and emotional agitation, preparing the body for deeper rest and sleep. This nervous-system calming indirectly supports hormonal and adrenal balance by reducing chronic stress load. Used aromatically or gently internally (traditional practice), Spikenard promotes emotional grounding and recovery from prolonged nervous exhaustion. Overall, it functions as a **deep-settling nervine** that restores calm, rest, and internal stability.

---

### *Primary Uses*

- Anxiety, insomnia, PTSD, emotional overload
- Nervous exhaustion and chronic stress
- Topical support for inflammation and fungal skin concerns

## 🧪 Scientific Backing

- Clinical research shows Nardostachys jatamansi preparations significantly lowered blood pressure in essential hypertension over four weeks.
- Preclinical studies confirm CNS-depressant, anxiolytic, and adaptogenic activity.
- Demonstrates antioxidant, neuroprotective, and mood-regulating properties.
- Aligns strongly with traditional use for insomnia, agitation, and nervous tension.

---

## *Forms Available*

- Essential oil (always diluted)
- Powder or capsules
- Light tea or decoction (less common)

---

## *How to Use*

**Powder:** 250–500 mg nightly
**Essential oil:** 1–3 drops diluted in 1 tbsp carrier oil; apply to temples, neck, or feet
**Tea:** ½ tsp root simmered 10 minutes; once daily (optional)

---

## *Expected Results*

Nervous-system calming: 30–60 minutes
Sleep improvement: several nights
Emotional grounding: 1–3 weeks

---

## ⚠ Caution Level: Generally Safe / Gentle Sedative

- May cause mild drowsiness at higher doses
- Avoid during pregnancy and breastfeeding (limited safety data)
- Use caution with sedatives, antidepressants, or sleep medications
- Essential oil must be diluted (≤2%)
- Patch-test topical use due to rare skin sensitivity

---

## Gender-Specific Safety — Spikenard

**Men — Safe:**
Supports stress recovery, sleep, and emotional grounding. Start low if using alongside sedatives.

**Women — Safe:**
Helpful for insomnia, adrenal strain, and emotional tension. Avoid stacking with multiple calming herbs at night.

**Pregnancy / Nursing — Caution:**
Avoid essential oil and strong internal use. Light aromatic diffusion may be acceptable only if no dizziness or nausea occurs.

---

## *Same / Similar Results*

Valerian · Ashwagandha · Chamomile · Holy Basil · Passionflower

---

## Shelf Life & Potency After Preparation

- Dried root: 2 years
- Powder/capsules: 1 year
- Essential oil: 3–5 years
- Tea/decoction: Use within 24 hours

---

## DIY Recipe — Spikenard Relaxation Oil

2 drops Spikenard essential oil
1 tbsp almond or jojoba oil
Massage into temples, feet, or back of neck before bed.

---

## Herbal Reflections of Spikenard

Spikenard speaks the language of stillness—earthy, ancient, and steady. It guides the nervous system into an exhale, easing the tension that accumulates from prolonged stress and emotional burden. Once used to anoint and consecrate, it continues to offer sanctuary for the overwhelmed.

Spikenard teaches the body how to soften again, reminding us that true restoration begins not with force, but with surrender into quiet.

**Herbal Confidence Index:** ½

(4.5/5 — a profoundly calming and restorative nervine with exceptional grounding strength. Reliable and effective when used respectfully.)

# SPEEDWELL

★★★★

*Veronica officinalis*

**Speedwell is a gentle, restoring tonic for lungs, gut, and skin.** Once hailed as a "cure-all," it offers **mild expectorant, astringent, and anti-inflammatory** support for **coughs, sore throats, indigestion/ulcers,** and **irritated skin** (as washes/soaks). Suitable for **children, elders,** and sensitive constitutions.

**Historically prized in European herbals,** Speedwell teas steadied **mucous membranes** and eased **convalescence.** Modern herbalists keep it for **steady, subtle repair** when stronger herbs feel too pushy—an everyday comforter that helps tissues knit back to calm.

---

## Core Herbal Category — Speedwell

**Primary Core: Respiratory System Support herb** with (soothing, mucilage-assisted action that calms irritated airways and supports healthy mucus balance)

**Secondary Cores:** Digestive Support herb · Skin & Tissue Repair herb · Nervines (Nervous System Support) herb

---

## How It Works

Speedwell works by **soothing irritated mucous membranes**, helping calm coughs and respiratory irritation. Its gentle compounds support **balanced mucus production**, making breathing more comfortable. In the digestive tract, it **eases mild irritation and supports gentle digestion**, which often reflects in respiratory comfort. Applied externally or taken internally, it aids **skin repair and calming of minor inflammation**. Overall, Speedwell functions as a **mild, supportive respiratory herb that restores comfort and tissue calm without stimulation**.

---

## Primary Uses

- Coughs, sore throat, mild bronchitis
- Indigestion, bloating, ulcers
- Topical wash for wounds, rashes, irritation
- Gentle immune and mucosal support

---

## Scientific Backing

Modern analysis strongly validates Speedwell's traditional uses:

- Contains **iridoid glycosides** (aucubin, catalpol) proven to reduce inflammation and stabilize mucous membranes
- Shows **antioxidant + antimicrobial** action (Mocan et al., 2015)
- Demonstrated **mast-cell inhibition** and anti-inflammatory properties (Gründemann et al., 2013)
- Review articles confirm **hepatoprotective, diuretic, and wound-healing** action (Salehi et al., 2019)
- Topical extract shown to **stimulate collagen regeneration** and skin repair (Lee et al., 2015)

Together these findings reveal an herb that is soft but highly reliable for respiratory, digestive, and skin recovery.

---

## Forms Available

- Dried herb (tea/infusion)
- Powdered herb
- Topical washes / compresses

---

## How to Use

**Tea:** 1–2 tsp dried herb per cup, steep 10–15 min; 2–3× daily
**Tincture:** 2–4 mL, up to 3× daily
**Topical:** Apply cooled tea to skin with clean cloth

---

## Expected Results

Respiratory relief: **1–2 days**
Digestive ease: **2–4 doses**
Skin support: **2–3 days**
Gentle calming: **30–60 minutes**

---

## ⚠ Caution Level: Safe / Mild-Acting

Speedwell is considered extremely gentle.

- Very rare side effects
- Avoid during pregnancy/nursing due to limited safety data
- Possible mild digestive looseness if overused
- Start small for those sensitive to Plantaginaceae plants

Suitable for long-term use in moderate amounts.

---

## Gender-Specific Safety — Speedwell

**Men — Safe:**
Supports mucous membranes, digestion, and respiratory ease. No known medication conflicts at normal doses. Very gentle on digestion and nerves.

**Women — Safe:**
Excellent for throat, lung, skin, and digestive irritation. Safe for long-term tea use. Mildly cooling and soothing during menstrual inflammation.

**Pregnancy/Nursing — Mild Caution:**
Traditionally considered quite safe, but modern data is limited. Use only light tea amounts. Avoid tinctures and high-dose preparations.

---

## Same / Similar Results

- Plantain Leaf — mucosal soother
- Chamomile — gentle anti-inflammatory
- Mullein — respiratory support
- Skullcap — mild nervine
- Sweet Violet — lymph + throat relief

---

## Shelf Life & Potency After Preparation

- **Dried Herb:** 1 year (airtight, away from light)
- **Powder:** 6–9 months
- **Tincture:** 4–5 years
- **Prepared Tea:** Use within 24 hours (refrigerated)

- **Topical Wash:** Use within 24 hours

Potency slowly declines after 9–12 months in dried form.

---

## DIY Recipe – Speedwell Lung Tea

- 1 tsp Speedwell
- 1 tsp Mullein
- ½ tsp Thyme
  Steep 10–12 minutes. Sip warm for gentle respiratory clearing.

## Herbal Reflections of Speedwell

Speedwell carries the quiet humility of the meadow. Its small blue blossoms hold a deep healing intelligence — subtle, persistent, and precise. Once honored as "All-Heal," it tended wounds, cleared phlegm, and soothed digestion without force.
Energetically, it teaches the art of modest restoration. Speedwell never pushes; it invites. It reminds us that healing often begins with softness — the quiet easing of tension and the slow return of comfort.

## Herbal Confidence Index: 🌿🌿🌿🌿 **4/5 —** A soft but

trustworthy ally for respiratory, digestive, and skin repair, safe for long-term daily use and effective without overwhelming the system. It's reliable, gentle, and ideal for sensitive users

# SOURSOP

★★★★

*Annona muricata*

**Soursop (also known as Graviola or Guanábana)** is a tropical tree whose leaves are widely used for nervous-system calming, immune support, and metabolic balance. Traditional systems throughout the Caribbean, Latin America, Africa, and Asia rely on Soursop leaf tea for anxiety, insomnia, fever, hypertension, digestive upset, and parasitic imbalance. While the fruit is nutritive, the **leaf** carries the primary medicinal value. Modern interest focuses on leaf acetogenins, alkaloids, and polyphenols that demonstrate antioxidant, anti-inflammatory, and immune-modulating activity. Though laboratory studies have explored cytotoxic effects, **human clinical evidence remains limited**, and Soursop should therefore be viewed as being **supportive** and **not curative at this stage**. In traditional use, it is valued most for its gentle nervine sedation—helping restless minds and tense bodies descend into calm.

---

### Core Herbal Category — Soursop

**Primary Core: Nervous System Support (Nervines)** herb with (calming action that eases emotional tension and supports relaxed nervous-system tone)

**Secondary Cores:** Immune Support herb · Digestive Support herb · Circulatory & Cardiovascular herb

---

### *How It Works*

Soursop works by gently calming nervous-system activity and supporting parasympathetic balance. Its compounds reduce emotional agitation, promote relaxation, and support sleep readiness. By soothing digestive irritation and systemic inflammation, it indirectly eases stress responses that affect mood and blood pressure. Overall, Soursop functions as a **gentle calming nervine** that supports emotional ease, digestive comfort, and whole-body balance.

---

### *Primary Uses*

- Nervous tension, anxiety, restlessness

- Insomnia and nighttime overactivity
- Fever and immune imbalance
- Mild hypertension support
- Digestive upset and parasitic concerns
- Liver heat and inflammation

---

## Scientific Backing

**Acetogenins:**
- Show antioxidant and immune-modulating activity
- Demonstrate cytotoxic effects in lab studies (not clinical treatment)

**Alkaloids & Polyphenols:**
- Support anti-inflammatory pathways
- Contribute to nervous-system calming

**Traditional & Observational Use:**
- Widely used for sleep, anxiety, fever, parasites, and blood pressure balance

⚠ No high-quality human trials support cancer treatment claims.

---

## *Forms Available*

- Dried leaves (tea / decoction)
- Powdered leaf
- Tincture or extract
- Fresh fruit (nutritional only)

---

## *How to Use*

**Tea:** 1–2 tsp dried leaf, steep 10–15 minutes; 1–2× daily
**Decoction:** Simmer 5–7 leaves for 10 minutes (stronger nighttime use)
**Tincture:** 1–2 mL up to 2× daily
Best taken 1–2 hours before bedtime for calming effects.

---

## *Expected Results*

Relaxation: 30–90 minutes
Sleep improvement: 1–3 nights
Digestive comfort: 2–3 uses
Blood-pressure calming: several days of consistent use

---

### ⚠ Caution Level: ▨ Caution

- Avoid high doses or long-term heavy use
- May cause nausea or neurological overstimulation if overused
- Avoid during pregnancy and breastfeeding
- Use caution with neurological conditions
- May lower blood pressure—monitor with antihypertensive medications

Moderate tea-level use is generally safe for most adults.

---

### Gender-Specific Safety — Soursop

● **Men — Safe in Moderate Use:**
Supports stress reduction and cardiovascular ease. Avoid excess with BP medication.

● **Women — Safe in Moderate Use:**
Helpful for insomnia and nervous tension. Begin with tea-level dosing.

● **Pregnancy / Nursing — Avoid:**
Insufficient safety data; avoid all internal use.

---

### *Same / Similar Results*

● Passionflower · ● Lemon Balm · ● Chamomile · ● Blue Vervain · ● Linden Flower

---

### Shelf Life & Potency After Preparation

- Dried leaf: 1 year
- Powder: 6–9 months
- Tincture: 4–5 years
- Prepared tea: Use within 24 hours

---

### DIY Recipe — Soursop Night Calm Tea

5–7 dried Soursop leaves
Simmer gently 10 minutes, rest 5 minutes covered
Drink warm 1 hour before bed.

---

### Herbal Reflections of Soursop

Soursop carries the medicine of quiet strength. It slows what races, softens what clenches, and steadies the nervous system when life becomes overwhelming. Brewed nightly in many cultures, it offers comfort rather than force—helping the body remember its natural rhythm of rest.

Soursop teaches restraint and balance, reminding us that some of the most effective medicine works gently, over time, and with respect.

🌟 **Herbal Confidence Index:** 🌿 🌿 🌿 🌿

(4/5 — a dependable calming and immune-supporting herb with long traditional use. Effective for stress and sleep when used moderately, with necessary safety boundaries.)

# SOAPWORT

★★★★

*Saponaria officinalis*

**Soapwort (Saponaria officinalis) is a classic "plant soap" rich in natural saponins that gently lather for fabric and skin cleansing while offering low-dose expectorant and mild hepatic support.** Herbalists use carefully prepared teas and washes to **loosen bronchial phlegm** and **calm irritated, acne-prone or eczematous skin**, favoring it when a **delicate, non-stripping cleanser** is needed; conservative dosing and brief courses help prevent GI upset in sensitive users. **Historically, Soapwort was the washer's ally—its Latin name comes from *sapo* (soap), and its old nickname "Bouncing Bet" nods to the laundress.** Medieval **fullers** and dyers steeped the roots to scour **fine wool and silk**, planting it near washhouses and monastery gardens; along trade routes it naturalized across Europe and North America, often marking old homesteads with pale pink blooms. Even today, **textile conservators** may choose a very dilute Soapwort decoction to clean fragile tapestries because it is gentler than modern detergents—an enduring reminder that a humble roadside herb helped keep both **cloth and skin** clean for centuries.

---

## Core Herbal Category — Soapwort

**Primary Core: Respiratory System Support herb** with (saponin-driven expectorant and cleansing action that loosens mucus and aids airway clearance)
**Secondary Cores:** Skin & Tissue Repair herb · Liver & Detoxification herb · Digestive Support herb

---

## How It Works

Soapwort works through **natural saponins** that reduce surface tension, helping **thin and mobilize thick mucus** for easier expectoration. This cleansing effect supports **respiratory comfort** during congestion. Externally, its mild surfactant action assists **skin cleansing and tissue support**. Internally, when used cautiously and traditionally, it can **stimulate gentle detox pathways**, though sensitivity varies. Overall, Soapwort functions as a **cleansing, mucus-mobilizing herb best used with restraint and clear purpose**.

---

## Primary Uses

- Clears bronchial phlegm
- Supports liver detox pathways
- Soothes irritated or acne-prone skin
- Traditional natural shampoo/cleanser

---

## Scientific Backing

Soapwort contains natural **saponins**, which:
- Create foaming/cleansing action
- Act as **mild expectorants**, helping clear mucus
- Support gentle **liver stimulation** at very low doses
- Offer mild **antimicrobial** benefits externally

Early pharmacology supports its topical use and careful internal use in small, controlled amounts.

---

## Forms Available

- Dried herb or root (cut/powder)
- Infused liquids, washes, shampoos
- Included in natural cleansers and textile-care formulas

---

## How to Use

**Internal Tea:**
- ½–1 tsp dried root in 1 cup water
- Simmer 10 minutes
- *Max 1 cup/day; short-term only*

**Topical Wash:**
- 2 tbsp dried root
- Simmer in 2 cups water
- Strain, cool, and apply to skin

**Fabric/Foaming Cleanser:**
- Simmer root until gentle foam forms
- Use for delicate fabrics or as a mild skin wash

---

## Expected Results

**Respiratory relief:** 1–2 days
**Skin soothing:** 3–5 applications

**Light hepatic "reset":** with brief, consistent use

## ⚠ Caution Level: ● Supervision Required

Soapwort's saponins can irritate the stomach and red blood cells if used improperly.

- Internal use must be minimal and supervised
- Too much may cause nausea, vomiting, or diarrhea
- Avoid with ulcers, gastritis, IBS flare, or GI inflammation
- Avoid during pregnancy or breastfeeding
- External washes and cleansers are generally safe and well tolerated

PRECAUTION ●: Soapwort is considered to be very effective in the herbal community for gentle cleansing and phlegm relief, but it is also known to have a strong potential for harm if misused internally. Readers are advised to explore safer long-term alternatives such as Calendula, Burdock Root, or Plantain Leaf.

## Gender-Specific Safety — Soapwort

### Men — Caution:

Useful for phlegm, skin cleansing, and mild detox support. Internal use should remain low-dose and brief. Avoid if prone to stomach irritation or gallbladder issues.

### Women — Caution:

Helpful for gentle cleansing and soothing inflamed skin. Internal amounts must remain small; avoid during heavy menstrual GI sensitivity. Topical use is safe.

### Pregnancy / Nursing — Avoid:

Due to potential GI irritation and limited safety data, avoid all internal use. External mild washes are safe for most but avoid large areas of application.

## Same / Similar Results

- Calendula — skin repair
- Chamomile — soothing anti-inflammatory
- Burdock Root — skin & detox support
- Plantain Leaf — topical healing
- Licorice Root — mucosal soother

## Shelf Life & Potency After Preparation

**Dried Root/Herb:** 1 year (airtight, dark container)
**Powdered Herb:** 6–8 months
**Tincture/Extract:** 3–5 years
**Topical Wash:** Use within 48 hours (refrigerated)
**Prepared Cleanser:** Best within 48 hours
Potency declines after 10–12 months in dried form.

---

## DIY Recipe — Soapwort Skin-Soothing Wash

1 tbsp dried Soapwort root
2 cups water
Simmer 15 minutes → strain → cool
Use as a facial or body wash for gentle cleansing.

---

## Herbal Reflections of Soapwort

Soapwort's gift is clean clarity — lifting residue from skin, breath, and even fabric without stripping what is healthy. It cleans through gentleness, not force. The herb teaches that purification can be soft, rhythmic, and respectful to the tissues it touches.
Energetically, Soapwort represents simplicity and ritual care. Where heaviness accumulates, it restores openness and breath, reminding us that cleansing is both physical and symbolic: a clearing of space, inside and out.

---

## Herbal Confidence Index: 🌿 🌿 🌿 (3/5)

A valued traditional cleansing herb with unique saponin chemistry. Excellent externally and helpful for clearing phlegm, but internal use remains limited by safety considerations requiring practitioner supervision.

# SNOWBERRY

★★

*Symphoricarpos albus*

**Snowberry (Symphoricarpos albus) is an ornamental North American shrub with striking white, waxy berries and a very narrow medicinal window.** Traditional use kept it **external-only**—cooled washes and poultices for **burns, rashes, sores, and warts,** with rare, highly diluted folk eyewashes—valued for a **cooling, drying, mildly cleansing** touch.
**Because its tissues contain saponins and bitter constituents, internal use is unsafe.** Modern herbalism limits Snowberry to **cautious, topical applications** only, acknowledging its **cleansing/astringent** action while emphasizing the **toxicity risk if ingested**—best treated as a historical, external aid rather than a home remedy.

---

## Core Herbal Category — Snowberry

*(Symphoricarpos albus)*

**Primary Core: Lymphatic & Skin Support herb** with (gentle astringent principles that help tone and repair minor surface wounds)
**Secondary Cores:** Antimicrobial Support **herb** · Anti-Inflammatory Support **herb**
**Important Note:** This herb is intended for **external use only** in traditional skin and wound applications.

---

## How It Works

Snowberry works by providing mild natural astringent action that helps tighten and protect damaged skin.
Its antimicrobial compounds assist the body in resisting minor infections in surface tissues.
The herb calms local inflammation and swelling in small wounds or irritations.
These actions help create a cleaner environment for natural skin repair.

---

## Primary Uses (External Only)

- Poultices for burns, sores, warts, rashes
- Cooled decoctions for mild skin irritation
- Traditional eye washes (historical use only; extremely diluted; not recommended today)
- Cleansing topical applications due to natural saponins

## 🧪 Scientific Backing

Snowberry contains saponins, tannins, and bitter alkaloids that:
• Provide mild antimicrobial and astringent actions
• Help tighten and dry irritated tissues
• Create a natural cleansing foam effect
However:
🚫 **Internal use causes GI irritation and toxicity** — nausea, vomiting, dizziness, diarrhea
🚫 **No modern clinical trials support internal medicinal use**
Therefore, modern herbalism limits Snowberry to **external-only, cautious use.**

---

## 🧴 Forms Available

● Bark or Leaves (decoctions, washes, poultices)
● Fresh or dried berries (topical only — never internal)
● Rare presence in niche natural skin products

---

## 🌡️ How to Use (External Only)

**Skin Wash:**
Boil bark/berries 15 minutes → cool fully → apply with cloth
**Poultice:**
Mash fresh berries/leaves → apply to affected area → remove after 10–15 minutes
🚫 **Do NOT ingest the berries, roots, or leaves.**

---

## ⏱️ Expected Results

• Skin cooling/drying: **24–48 hours**
• Minor irritation relief: **2–3 applications**
• Traditional support: **historical, not clinically verified**

---

## ⚠️ Caution Level: ● Supervision Required

Snowberry has a **narrow therapeutic window**:
• Berries are **mildly poisonous**
• Internal use can cause nausea, vomiting, diarrhea, dizziness
• Avoid during pregnancy, nursing, or with children

• Keep away from pets (especially dogs & livestock)
Safe only for **external, diluted use.**

---

## 🚹 🚺 Gender-Specific Safety — Snowberry

⚪ **Men — Caution (External Only):**
Safe as a diluted skin wash or poultice. Never internal. Avoid broken skin or open wounds.
⚪ **Women — Caution (External Only):**
May soothe mild rashes or irritations, but sensitive skin may react to saponins. Patch-test is recommended.
🔴 **Pregnancy / Nursing — Avoid:**
Due to toxicity risk and lack of safety data, avoid entirely during pregnancy or breastfeeding.

---

## 🌿 Same / Similar Results

🟢 Plantain Leaf — gentle skin repair
🟢 Yarrow — wound cleansing & astringent
🟡 Witch Hazel — tissue toner & anti-inflammatory
🟡 Goldenseal — antimicrobial astringent
🔴 Poke Root — powerful but toxic; historical external-only use

---

## 🧪 Shelf Life & Potency After Preparation

Dried Bark/Leaves: **1–2 years** (airtight, dark, cool)
Fresh Berries (topical only): **Use immediately**
Prepared Decoction/Wash: **24 hours refrigerated**
Potency declines rapidly after preparation due to saponin breakdown.

---

## 📜 DIY Recipe — Snowberry Skin Wash (External Only)

• 1 small handful bark + leaves
• Simmer in 2 cups water for 15 minutes
• Cool completely
• Apply with clean cloth
🚫 **Do NOT ingest under any circumstances**

---

## 💭 Herbal Reflections of Snowberry

Snowberry stands at the threshold between medicine and caution. Its luminous berries catch the eye, yet its chemistry warns the hand. Where it helps, it does so softly—cooling heat, drying irritation, steadying troubled skin—inviting careful, respectful use.

Energetically, Snowberry teaches discernment. It reminds us that healing plants are powerful allies, not harmless ornaments, and that wisdom lies in knowing when to use a remedy—and when to simply admire it. Snowberry offers a lesson in restraint: not every gift in nature is meant for the cup; some are meant only for the surface, the skin, and the story.

### ⭐ Herbal Confidence Index: 🌿 🌿

(2/5 — useful mild external skin-support herb with reliable astringent and antimicrobial action; appropriate for minor wounds and irritations but limited to topical use due to narrow potency and safety range.)

# SKUNK CABBAGE

★★★

*Symplocarpus foetidus*

**Skunk Cabbage (Symplocarpus foetidus) is a potent, once-pharmacopeial wetland herb historically used as an antispasmodic and expectorant.** Properly dried root was given in **minute doses** for asthma, bronchitis, spasmodic coughs, and nervous agitation, while poultices eased swelling and joint pain—use reserved for trained hands due to its strength.
**Its power comes with a tight safety margin and notable cautions.** The **fresh plant is irritant/toxic** (calcium oxalate), and even dried root demands practitioner guidance; safer modern allies (e.g., mullein, thyme, elecampane) now fill its role. Historically notable, it can **generate heat to bloom through snow,** a reminder of its force—best regarded today as a teacher from the past rather than a home remedy.

---

## Core Herbal Category — Skunk Cabbage

*(Symplocarpus foetidus)*

**Primary Core: Nervous System Support (Nervines) herb** with (antispasmodic principles that help relax severe cough-spasm and muscle tension)
**Secondary Cores:** Respiratory Support **herb** · Antimicrobial Support **herb** (topical)
**Important Note:** This herb is used historically in small professional preparations and occasionally as a topical poultice.

---

## How It Works

Skunk Cabbage works by calming intense nervous-system and muscle spasm through resinous bioactive compounds.
These antispasmodic principles help relax cough-spasm signaling in irritated lungs.
The herb supports easier breathing by reducing over-tightened respiratory muscles.
Topically, it has been used in poultices to soothe localized pain and tension.
Because of strong odor and potency, it requires modest, careful external or expert-guided use.

---

# Primary Uses (Historical / Restricted)

- Eases bronchospasm, wheezing, thick mucus
- Antispasmodic for tremors, convulsions

Calms agitation and nervous distress

Poultices for swelling, painful joints

Modern herbalism no longer recommends internal home use.

---

## Scientific Backing

Research and pharmacognosy confirm the presence of:

- **Calcium oxalate crystals** — irritant/toxic unless fully dried
- **Volatile oils & alkaloids** — antispasmodic, expectorant effects
- **Acrid resins** — explain strong mucous-moving action

Drying reduces some irritant components, but **toxicity and unpredictable potency remain major concerns**, limiting its role to supervised use only.

---

## Forms Available

Dried root (rare; practitioner-only)

Tincture from dried root

Dried root for external poultices

(Fresh plant is never used internally.)

---

## How to Use (Under Supervision Only)

**Tincture:** 5–10 drops in water, 2–3× daily (dried root only)

**Tea:** ½ tsp dried root, steep 15 minutes (professional guidance required)

**Poultice:** Crushed dried root applied to swollen joints

🚫 **Never use the fresh plant internally.**

---

## Expected Results

- Respiratory easing: **~30 minutes**
- Nervous system relief: **several days with micro-dosing**
- Swelling reduction (external): **2–3 applications**

Results vary due to unpredictable potency.

---

## ⚠ Caution Level: Supervision Required

Skunk Cabbage must be handled with *extreme respect*:

- Fresh plant is **toxic** — causes severe burning & irritation
- Improper dosing → nausea, vomiting, respiratory irritation
- Never use during pregnancy, nursing, or for children
- Not recommended internally for modern home herbalism

• Can interact with sedatives, respiratory medications, or antispasmodics
Only dried root should ever be used—and only with expert guidance.

---

## 🚹 🚺 Gender-Specific Safety — Skunk Cabbage

**Men — Caution:**
Safe *only* for carefully supervised micro-doses of dried root for historical respiratory indications. Avoid if using sedatives, asthma medication, or blood pressure drugs.

**Women — Caution:**
Not recommended except under strict practitioner guidance due to toxicity, irritant compounds, and unpredictable potency. External-only poultices tolerated.

● **Pregnancy / Nursing — Avoid:**
Never use during pregnancy or breastfeeding. The plant's chemistry poses toxicity risks and uterine irritation potential.

---

## 🌿 Same / Similar Results (Much Safer)

● Chamomile — gentle antispasmodic
● Valerian — stronger nervine & muscle relaxant
● Lobelia — potent respiratory relaxant (still requires caution)
● Wild Lettuce — calming, antispasmodic
● Poke Root — strong but toxic; historical comparison only

---

## Shelf Life & Potency After Preparation

Dried Root: **2–3 years** (airtight, away from light/moisture)
Tincture: **5 years**
Poultice Material: **Use within 24 hours of preparation**
Potency remains strong for years—another reason internal use should be supervised.

---

## 🛠 DIY Recipe — Skunk Cabbage Tincture (Dried Root Only)

1 part dried root
5 parts 60% alcohol
Steep 3–4 weeks → strain → store in dark glass
Dose: **5–10 drops diluted**, under professional direction
🚫 Never tincture the *fresh* plant.

## 💭 Herbal Reflections of Skunk Cabbage

Skunk Cabbage is a winter miracle—one of the few plants capable of generating heat strong enough to melt snow and erupt into bloom while the world still sleeps. That same raw power is mirrored in its medicine: forceful, penetrating, and uncompromising. It breaks through stagnation, spasm, and congestion with an energy that demands respect.
Yet it is not an herb for everyday hands. Its lesson is restraint. Strength without wisdom becomes harm; strength in the right measure becomes healing. Skunk Cabbage reminds us that the strongest medicines in nature are often the ones we approach slowly, reverently, or not at all—teachers more than tonics, guardians more than remedies.

## 🌟 Herbal Confidence Index: 🌿🌿🌿☆☆ (3 / 5)

**Potent Traditional Antispasmodic & Respiratory Herb**
Historically respected for severe spasmodic cough, asthma-like conditions, and muscular tension when properly dried and prepared. Effectiveness is real but narrow, with significant irritation and toxicity risk if misused or used fresh. One star deducted for harshness and preparation sensitivity, and another for limited suitability outside experienced or supervised use.

# HOUTTUYNIA

★★★

*Houttuynia cordata*

**Houttuynia** is a daytime-friendly respiratory and mucosal ally used widely across East and Southeast Asia**. Its aromatic volatiles help open the upper airways, soothe post-nasal drip, reduce lingering throat tickle, and support gum, urinary, and immune comfort.** Traditionally enjoyed as a tea, steam, or fresh culinary herb, Houttuynia clears without heaviness—making it ideal for workdays, travel, and seasonal transitions.

Best used in **steady, light doses**, its action is clarifying rather than sedating. Over several days of consistent use, it gently dries dampness, freshens the sinus–throat corridor, eases low-grade congestion, and encourages mucosal resilience.

---

## Core Herbal Category — Houttuynia

**Primary Core: Respiratory System Support herb** with (cooling, mucosal-balancing action that clears heat and supports healthy airway secretions)

**Secondary Cores:** Immune Support herb · Urinary & Kidney Support herb · Digestive Support herb

---

## How It Works

Houttuynia works by **cooling inflamed mucous membranes** and helping regulate excessive or stagnant secretions in the respiratory tract. Its antimicrobial compounds assist the body in **reducing pathogenic load** while preserving tissue integrity. This cooling action extends to the urinary system, where it **soothes irritation and supports cleansing flow**. As a food-grade medicinal plant, it gently supports digestion and elimination. Overall, Houttuynia functions as a **cooling, infection-responsive herb that restores mucosal balance across respiratory and urinary systems**.

---

## Primary Uses

- Sinus comfort, post-nasal drip, throat tickle
- Mild antimicrobial + immune support
- Gentle urinary soothing
- Gum/mouth mucosal maintenance

- Culinary herb for broths & salads

---

## Scientific Backing

Research supports several of its traditional actions:
- **Volatiles (houttuynin)** → antimicrobial, mucosal-clearing
- **Flavonoids (quercetin-type)** → antioxidant & anti-inflammatory
- Preclinical studies show support for **upper-respiratory recovery**, **immune modulation**, and gentle **antibacterial/antiviral effects**
- Traditional use aligns with findings on mucosal hydration and mild expectorant action

While promising, clinical human data remains limited, and results depend on species identity and preparation.

---

## Forms Available

- Loose-leaf tea (fresh or dried)
- Steam inhalation (fresh or dried leaf)
- Tincture or extract
- Capsules (usually blends—verify species)
- Culinary fresh leaf (soups, salads, stir-fries)

## How to Use / Dosage

**Tea:** 1 tsp leaf per cup, steep 10–12 min; 2–3× daily during flares
**Steam:** 1 tsp leaf in hot water; inhale 3–5 min, then drink the infusion
**Caps / Tincture:** follow manufacturer label; confirm *Houttuynia cordata*
**Culinary:** add small amounts to broths or salads (strong flavor)

---

## Expected Results

- Throat/nasal comfort: **1–3 days**
- Sinus clarity / reduced drip: **3–7 days**
- Lingering mucosal support: **1–2 weeks** steady use

---

## Caution Level: Caution

Houttuynia is generally safe short-term but requires mindful use:
- May cause mild digestive upset or loose stools in sensitive users
- Rare skin or respiratory allergies reported
- Avoid high-dose or long-term use without guidance
- Those with **kidney or liver conditions** should use with practitioner oversight

- **Avoid during pregnancy and breastfeeding** due to limited safety data
- Ensure correct species—look-alike plants may not be edible

---

## Gender-Specific Safety — Houttuynia

**Men — Safe:**
Excellent for sinus clarity, mucosal balance, mild infection support, and urinary ease. Generally non-sedating and compatible with daytime activities. Minimal interactions at tea doses.

**Women — Caution:**
Safe in moderate, short-term doses; however, stronger extracts may cause digestive sensitivity or headaches. Women with kidney issues, autoimmune flares, or allergies should start with small amounts. Avoid if sensitive to strong aromatic herbs.

**Pregnancy / Nursing — Avoid:**
Insufficient data. Avoid internal use during pregnancy or breastfeeding, especially tinctures or high-dose preparations. Culinary micro-amounts in food are generally avoided unless cleared by a professional.

---

## Same / Similar Results

- Thyme — respiratory antimicrobial
- Cistus (Rockrose) — immune + mucosal support
- Pelargonium (Umcka) — sinus & throat health
- Licorice Root — throat + mucosal soothing
- Sage — antimicrobial gargle & steam ally

---

## Shelf Life & Potency After Preparation

Dried Leaf: **1 year** (sealed, away from heat/light)
Fresh Leaf (culinary): **3–5 days refrigerated**
Tincture/Extract: **4–5 years**
Capsules: **2 years**
Prepared Tea: **Use within 24 hours** (refrigerated)
Steam Infusion: **Use immediately**
Potency declines noticeably after 9–12 months in dried leaf form.

---

## DIY Recipe — Houttuynia–Thyme Steam & Sip

1 tsp Houttuynia leaf
½ tsp Thyme

Pour 12 oz steaming water.
Tent with a towel → inhale 3–5 minutes.
Then sip the warm infusion for throat and sinus support.
Use up to **2× daily** during respiratory flare-ups.

---

## 💭 Herbal Reflections of Houttuynia

Houttuynia is a quiet defender—sharp in scent, humble in form, yet unwavering in its clarifying power. It cuts through the fog of damp congestion and helps the body reclaim freshness where heaviness lingers.
Energetically, it is the herb of hidden renewal. Growing in shaded riverbanks and overlooked corners, it reminds us that clarity often emerges from the simplest rituals: a warm cup, a steady breath, a moment of pause. Houttuynia's medicine begins with awakening and ends with relief—subtle, cleansing, and honest.

---

## 🌟 Herbal Confidence Index: 🌿 🌿 🌿 (3/5)**A solid, dependable respiratory ally**—best for mild infections, sinus drip, and general mucosal clarification.

# CANARY SEED

★★★

*(Phalaris canariensis)*

**Canary Seed (silica-free, human-grade) is a protein- and enzyme-rich grain used to support metabolic, renal, and glycemic balance.** Traditional and modern use highlights **gentle diuresis, kidney tone, cholesterol balance, and blood sugar regulation**, with its natural lipase and clean protein profile making it a quiet ally for daily metabolic hygiene. Unlike ordinary birdseed, **only silica-free seed prepared for human consumption** is appropriate, reflecting a shift from feed to functional food.

**Its appeal lies in food-like nourishment rather than drug-like force.** Prepared as a light **"milk"** or added as **flour/powder**, it pairs well with steady diet and movement to support **detox pathways and pancreas function** while easing fluid stagnation. Results come from consistency: small servings woven into routine — always **using verified human-grade, silica-free seed** for safety and effectiveness.

---

## Core Herbal Category — Canary Seed

**Primary Core: Endocrine & Hormonal Support herb** with (enzyme-modulating, nutritive action that supports glycemic balance and lipid regulation)

**Secondary Cores:** Urinary & Kidney Support herb · Nutritive & Restorative herb · Liver & Detoxification herb

---

## How It Works

Canary Seed works by **supporting enzymes involved in carbohydrate and fat metabolism**, helping moderate blood sugar response and lipid balance. Its mild diuretic influence supports **renal cleansing and fluid balance**. As a nutrient-dense, food-grade herb, it provides **gentle nourishment** that aids metabolic resilience over time. This combined action supports **detox pathways and metabolic efficiency** without stimulation. Overall, Canary Seed functions as a **soft, nutritive metabolic-support herb suited for steady, long-term use**.

---

## Primary Uses

- Kidney and bladder support; mild diuretic cleansing

- Gentle detox and liver/lipid balance
- Blood sugar and insulin support
- Adjunct in weight-management routines

---

## Scientific Backing

• Human-grade Canary Seed contains **lipase enzymes**, amino acids (including tryptophan), and high-quality proteins
• Early studies show potential benefits for **blood glucose control**, **cholesterol reduction**, and **anti-inflammatory action**
• Demonstrates **diuretic** activity supportive of kidney tone
• Evidence is promising but still **emerging**, with quality and processing purity being critical

---

## Forms Available

- Silica-free Canary Seed milk (homemade or commercial)
- Ground flour or powder for smoothies
- Capsules/powders (available in select markets)

---

## How to Use / Dosage

**Milk:** 1 cup on an empty stomach daily
**Powder:** 1–2 tbsp in smoothies or porridge
**Capsules:** follow manufacturer guidance
**Note:** Always confirm **hull-less, silica-free** seed.

---

## Expected Results

• Renal/diuretic effect: **2–4 days**
• Blood sugar support: **1–2 weeks**
• Lipid & metabolic improvements: **3–4 weeks** steady use

---

## Caution Level: Caution

• Only consume **human-grade, silica-free** Canary Seed
• Older hairy varieties contain silica fibers unsafe for humans
• May cause mild digestive looseness in sensitive users
• Verify gluten-free processing if intolerant
• Limited safety data → avoid during **pregnancy or breastfeeding**
• Long-term use should be balanced with adequate protein and hydration

## 🚹 🚺 Gender-Specific Safety — Canary Seed

**Men — Generally Safe:**
Supports metabolism, renal flow, and glycemic stability. Safe as a food-like daily beverage. Watch for mild diuretic effects.

**Women — Caution:**
Often well tolerated, though some women may experience digestive sensitivity when first using the milk. Those with iron deficiency or low blood pressure should monitor effects due to Canary Seed's mild diuretic nature.

**Pregnancy / Nursing — Avoid:**
No clinical safety data. Avoid internal use during pregnancy or breastfeeding. Choose proven nutritive allies like oats or chia instead.

---

## Same / Similar Results

- Dandelion Root — renal/liver support
- Milk Thistle — liver & detox pathways
- Nettle Seed — kidney and metabolic vitality
- Fenugreek — glycemic support
- Chia Seeds — gentle metabolism & gut support

---

## Shelf Life & Potency After Preparation

Whole Seed (silica-free): **1 year** (airtight, cool, dry)
Seed Flour/Powder: **6–8 months**
Commercial Milk: as dated on packaging
Homemade Milk: **3–4 days refrigerated**
Capsules: **1–2 years**
Potency declines after 9–12 months in whole seed form.

---

## DIY Recipe — Canary Seed Milk (Detox & Energy)

- Soak **5 tbsp** silica-free Canary Seed overnight
- Blend with **1½ cups** fresh water
- Strain through nut-milk bag
- Drink **1 cup** on an empty stomach

Light, smooth, cleansing, and ideal for daily metabolic tone.

---

## 💭 Herbal Reflections of Canary Seed

Canary Seed's story is one of rediscovery—an everyday grain transformed into a metabolic ally. Its enzyme-rich profile acts like a gentle broom for the kidneys and bloodstream, steadying metabolic rhythms with quiet persistence.

Energetically, it represents **humble nourishment** rather than force. Its medicine is subtle but dependable, reminding us that daily routines often hold more healing than dramatic interventions. In this way, Canary Seed teaches that transformation can come from the simplest cup, taken with intention.

---

## ⭐ Herbal Confidence Index: 🌿 🌿 🌿 (3/5)

A rising nutritive with promising metabolic and glycemic benefits. Safe when using **modern silica-free varieties**, gentle on digestion, and supportive for daily detox—but limited research and quality-control challenges keep it in the moderate range.

# MAGNOLIA

★★★★

*Magnolia officinalis*

**Magnolia (Hou Po)** is an evening-friendly bark for the mind–gut axis, easing restless thoughts, chest tightness, and the sensation of "pressure under the ribs" when stress stalls digestion. Its aromatic lignans—honokiol and magnolol—create a calm, grounded state without next-day fog, helping the body unwind while preserving mental clarity. Magnolia's warm, moving nature supports GI motility, relieves gas and bloating, loosens stress-related chest tightness, and assists sleep onset in tense, wired states.

Historically, Magnolia bark anchors classical East Asian formulas for stress-induced stagnation such as "plum-pit qi." Recorded since Han-dynasty texts, it appears in long-standing preparations alongside Citrus peel and Pinellia, valued for its ability to move stuck energy, dry dampness, and settle the middle. This medicinal bark—distinct from ornamental magnolias—remains a practical remedy for modern stress-digestive patterns and heavy evenings.

---

### Core Herbal Category — Magnolia

**Primary Core: Nervous System Support (Nervines)** herb with *(anxiolytic, calming action that settles nervous tension and supports mind–gut communication)*

**Secondary Cores:** Digestive Support herb · Respiratory Support herb · Hormonal & Endocrine Support herb

---

### How It Works

Magnolia works by quieting overstimulated nervous signaling, reducing anxiety-driven tension that disrupts digestion and sleep. Its active compounds promote parasympathetic activation, improving gut motility and easing stress-related digestive stagnation. This calming effect also relaxes chest tightness and phlegm-associated tension. Overall, Magnolia functions as a bridge herb for the mind–gut axis, restoring calm, flow, and coordinated digestive rhythm.

---

### Primary Uses

- Supports sleep onset and evening unwinding
- Eases anxious tension with chest or shoulder tightness
- Relieves gas, bloating, and stress-stalled digestion
- Supports breathing when stress triggers chest constriction
- Calms worry loops and emotional overactivation

---

### Scientific Backing

Magnolia bark contains honokiol and magnolol, compounds shown to:
• Modulate GABA-A receptors for calming without heavy sedation
• Relax smooth muscle, supporting GI motility and gas relief
• Reduce oxidative and neuro-inflammatory stress
• Support anxiety reduction and sleep onset
Preclinical and early clinical data strongly align with traditional use.

---

**Forms Available**

Standardized extract capsules/tablets

Tincture

Decoction (simmered bark)

Traditional combination formulas

---

**How to Use / Dosage**
• Capsules: per label (commonly 200–500 mg extract, evening)
• Tincture: 0.5–1 mL, 45–60 minutes before bed
• Decoction: Simmer bark 10–15 minutes; sip warm
• Pairing: Passionflower (racing thoughts), Lemon Balm (stress digestion), small Valerian dose for difficult nights

---

**Expected Results**
Evening relaxation: first nights–1 week
Sleep onset improvement: 1–2 weeks
Digestive ease after stress or heavy meals: days–2 weeks
Chest/throat pressure relief: gradual over days

---

**Caution Level: Caution**
• May cause drowsiness, dizziness, or nausea at higher doses
• Can enhance sedatives or sleep medications
• Avoid before driving or operating machinery
• Monitor if prone to low blood pressure
• Avoid during pregnancy or breastfeeding

---

**Gender-Specific Safety — Magnolia**

**Men — Safe / Helpful:**
Supports stress digestion, sleep onset, and chest tension when used in evening doses.

**Women — Mild Caution:**
Helpful for emotional stress and digestive stagnation; start low if using sedatives or prone to dizziness.

**Pregnancy / Nursing — Avoid:**
Insufficient safety data; gentler herbs preferred.

---

### Same / Similar Results

- Passionflower — mental quieting
- Lemon Balm — mood + digestion
- Valerian — stronger sedative
- Jatamansi — deep calming nervine
- Chamomile — gentle unwind

---

### Shelf Life & Potency After Preparation

Dried Bark: 1–2 years
Powder: 6–9 months
Decoction: 24 hours refrigerated
Tincture: 4–6 years
Capsules/Extracts: 2–3 years

---

### DIY Recipe — Simple Evening Magnolia Blend

• 0.5–1 mL Magnolia tincture
• Optional: 0.5 mL Passionflower or Lemon Balm
Take 45–60 minutes before bed; reduce dose if morning feels heavy.

---

### Herbal Reflections of Magnolia

Magnolia is the dimming-lights herb—softening the chest, easing the belly, and quieting the mind without collapse. It unties the subtle knots between thought and digestion, allowing rest to arrive naturally.

Energetically, Magnolia teaches alignment rather than force: breath loosens, pressure lifts, and calm returns. A steady evening ally, it turns tension into exhale and worry into gentle unwinding.

---

### Herbal Confidence Index: (4 / 5)

A time-honored, reliable herb for sleep onset, stress-driven digestive stagnation, and mind–gut tension. Loses one star for sedative strength and interaction potential, requiring mindful dosing.

# BLUEBERRY

★★★★★

*Vaccinium corymbosum*

**Blueberry** (Vaccinium spp.) is a food-grade cornerstone herb for long-term brain, eye, heart, and vascular health. Rich in anthocyanins and flavonoids, it protects capillaries, supports retinal tissue, enhances cognitive clarity, and promotes vascular elasticity and healthy blood pressure. With regular intake, Blueberry also aids glycemic balance, insulin sensitivity, and gut-microbiome diversity—making it one of the most reliable daily botanicals for longevity and metabolic resilience. Traditionally, Indigenous peoples of the Northeastern woodlands gathered wild lowbush blueberries for nourishment and medicine, drying them for winter use and brewing leaf teas for urinary and blood-sugar support. In the early 20th century, botanical cultivation carried this wild food into modern orchards, preserving a lineage of nourishment that remains as relevant today as ever.

---

### Core Herbal Category — Blueberry

**Primary Core: Cardiovascular System Support** herb with *(anthocyanin-rich antioxidant action that protects blood vessels and supports long-term vascular integrity)*

**Secondary Cores:** Nervines (Nervous System Support) herb · Skin & Tissue Repair herb · Metabolic & Blood Sugar Support herb · Digestive Support herb

---

### How It Works

Blueberry works by supplying concentrated anthocyanins that strengthen capillary walls and reduce oxidative stress within blood vessels. This vascular protection supports healthy circulation, memory, and eye tissue resilience. Its antioxidant activity moderates inflammatory signaling, contributing to metabolic balance and cardiovascular stability. As a gentle food-medicine, Blueberry also nourishes beneficial gut bacteria, supporting digestion and systemic immune tone. Overall, it functions as a longevity-supportive antioxidant herb that protects vessels while steadily nourishing brain, eye, and metabolic health.

---

### Primary Uses

- Supports memory, cognition, and mental clarity
- Protects vision and retinal microcirculation
- Strengthens heart, vessels, and capillaries
- Reduces oxidative stress and inflammation
- Supports blood-sugar balance and insulin sensitivity
- Promotes gut health and digestive regularity

---

### Scientific Backing

Blueberry is one of the most extensively researched medicinal fruits. Its anthocyanins, flavonoids, and polyphenols have been shown to:

- Improve memory and executive function
- Protect retinal photoreceptors and microvasculature
- Reduce arterial stiffness and support healthy blood pressure
- Enhance insulin sensitivity and glucose regulation
- Strengthen capillaries and reduce vascular oxidative damage
- Support gut-microbiome diversity and lower inflammatory markers

---

### Forms Available

Fresh or frozen berries

Dried berries

Blueberry leaf (tea)

Juice or concentrate

Powder (smoothies or capsules)

---

### How to Use / Dosage

- Berries: ¾–1 cup daily (fresh or frozen)
- Powder: 1–2 tsp daily
- Leaf Tea: 1 tsp leaf per cup, steep 10–12 min, 1–2× daily
- Concentrate: Follow label directions

Daily intake supports cumulative, long-term benefits.

---

### Expected Results

Cognitive clarity: 1–2 weeks

Eye support: 3–4 weeks

Antioxidant/vascular effects: within days–1 week

Metabolic support: 2–4+ weeks of steady use

---

### Caution Level: Safe

Blueberry is exceptionally safe as both food and medicine.

Use mild caution if:

- Taking blood thinners (very large extract doses)
- Managing low blood sugar (concentrates may enhance effects)
- Sensitive to salicylates (rare)

Fresh and frozen berries are safe for all ages and suitable for long-term daily use.

---

### Gender-Specific Safety — Blueberry

**Men — Safe:**

Supports cardiovascular protection, cognition, metabolism, and energy with no known conflicts at food-level doses.

**Women — Safe:**
Supports vascular tone, memory, eye health, and inflammatory balance; especially helpful during midlife transitions.

**Pregnancy / Nursing — Safe:**
One of the safest nutritive botanicals. Prefer whole berries; use extracts moderately.

---

**Same / Similar Results** Bilberry — vision and circulation support Goji Berry — eye and immune vitality Ginkgo — cognitive circulation support Grape Seed Extract — vascular protection Elderberry — immune antioxidant support

---

### Shelf Life & Potency After Preparation

Fresh/Frozen Berries: best within months (freezing preserves nutrients)
Dried Berries: 1 year
Leaf Tea: 1–2 years
Powder: 6–12 months (airtight, light-proof)
Juice Concentrate: per manufacturer instructions

---

### DIY Recipe — Daily Blueberry Brain Tonic

- 1 cup blueberries
- 1 tsp ground flaxseed
- ½ cup almond milk
- Dash cinnamon

Blend and enjoy for antioxidant, cognitive, and vascular support.

---

### Herbal Reflections of Blueberry

Blueberry is nature's quiet guardian of vitality—sweet, steady, and deeply restorative. Its gentle flavor conceals profound strength, protecting vision, sharpening the mind, and fortifying the heart through daily nourishment rather than force.

Energetically, Blueberry teaches endurance through care. It cools inflammation, feeds resilience, and reminds us that true longevity is built through small, faithful rituals repeated over time.

**Herbal Confidence Index:** **(5 / 5)**

A cornerstone longevity herb with unmatched safety, broad-spectrum nourishment, and exceptional support for brain, eye, vascular, and metabolic health. One of the finest daily herbs for graceful aging and lifelong vitality.

# BLACK CARDAMOM

★★★★

*Amomum subulatum*

**Black Cardamom** (Amomum subulatum) is a smoky, warming spice-herb long valued across the Himalayan region for clearing cold-damp stagnation in the lungs and digestion. Smoke-dried pods develop resinous, camphor-eucalyptol aromatics that help open the chest, stimulate sluggish digestion, and restore circulation in cold, heavy conditions. Known as *badi elaichi*, it traveled through Tibet, Bhutan, and North India, while related species shaped Chinese and Southeast Asian broths—linking breath, warmth, and nourishment.

Medicinally, Black Cardamom is a **strategic mover rather than a daily tonic**. It excels at breaking up thick phlegm, easing gas and bloating, and warming chilled digestive and respiratory systems. Compared with green cardamom's lighter lift, Black Cardamom works deeper and hotter, best used sparingly in stews, broths, or short warming decoctions to restore flow without excess heat.

---

### Core Herbal Category — Black Cardamom

**Primary Core: Respiratory System Support** herb with *(warming, aromatic decongestant action that clears dampness and eases airway obstruction)*

**Secondary Cores:** Digestive Support herb · Circulatory & Cardiovascular herb · Immune Support herb

---

### How It Works

Black Cardamom works through warming aromatic compounds that loosen congestion and dry excess dampness in the respiratory tract, supporting clearer breathing and reduced chest tightness. In digestion, it stimulates digestive fire, improving motility and easing gas and bloating. Its volatile oils provide mild antimicrobial support, while circulatory warming improves tissue perfusion. Overall, it functions as a warming decongestant that restores movement and clarity in cold, stagnant conditions.

---

### Primary Uses

- Stimulates sluggish digestion; reduces gas and bloating
- Breaks up chest congestion and thick phlegm
- Warms cold digestive and respiratory conditions
- Supports circulation in damp, heavy climates
- Assists breathing when mucus is dense or persistent

---

### Scientific Backing

Black Cardamom contains cineole, terpenes, flavonoids, and aromatic volatile oils shown to:

- Act as carminatives, reducing gas and bloating
- Support expectoration and clearance of thick mucus
- Provide antimicrobial activity in respiratory and digestive contexts
- Relax smooth muscle, aiding motility
- Stimulate circulation and digestive heat

Smoke-drying contributes unique resinous compounds linked to its lung-opening effects.

---

### Forms Available

- Whole dried pods
- Ground spice
- Decoction ingredient
- Tinctures or respiratory blends

---

### How to Use / Dosage

- **Culinary:** Crack 1–2 pods into soups, stews, or broths
- **Decoction:** 1 crushed pod with ginger or thyme; simmer 10–15 minutes
- **Tincture:** Short courses only, per label instructions

Use sparingly; this is a warming stimulant, not a daily tonic.

---

### Expected Results

Digestive relief: 30–60 minutes
Respiratory clearing: 1–3 days
Warming circulatory support: 1–2 weeks

---

### Caution Level: Caution

- May aggravate GERD, ulcers, or gastritis
- Large doses can cause heartburn, dryness, or throat irritation
- Avoid medicinal doses during pregnancy (culinary use is fine)
- Use cautiously with hypertension or strong stimulants
- Always source high-quality, unadulterated pods

Best used intentionally and in moderation.

---

### Gender-Specific Safety — Black Cardamom

**Men — Safe (Moderate Use):**

Supports digestion, circulation, and respiratory clearing; avoid excess if prone to reflux.

**Women — Caution:**

Helpful for cold digestion and mucus stagnation; avoid high doses if prone to heat or dryness.

**Pregnancy / Nursing — Mild Caution:**

Culinary amounts are safe; avoid medicinal dosing.

---

### 🌿 Same / Similar Results

- Ginger — warming digestion & lung support
- Elecampane — expectorant decongestant
- Thyme — antimicrobial lung tonic
- Clove — aromatic digestive stimulant
- Mullein — soothing expectorant

---

### Shelf Life & Potency After Preparation

Whole Pods: up to 2 years
Ground Powder: 6–9 months
Decoction: 24 hours refrigerated
Tincture: 4–5 years

---

### DIY Recipe — Simple Warming Lung Tea

• 1 crushed Black Cardamom pod
• 1 tsp ginger
• Simmer in 2 cups water for 15 minutes
Strain and sip warm once or twice daily during cold, damp congestion.

---

### Herbal Reflections of Black Cardamom

Black Cardamom is the apothecary's hearth fire—smoky, grounding, and purposeful. It dispels cold heaviness from lungs and belly, thinning stubborn phlegm and rekindling digestive warmth. Energetically, it teaches restraint. Used with intention, it restores flow and breath; used carelessly, it overwhelms. Black Cardamom reminds us that heat is medicine only when guided.

---

### Herbal Confidence Index: 🌿 🌿 🌿 🌿 (4 / 5)

A reliable warming digestive and respiratory herb, highly effective for cold-damp stagnation and mucus. Loses one star for heat intensity and the need for mindful, moderate use.

# Purslane

★★★★★

*Portulaca oleracea*

**PURSLANE** is one of the most nutrient-dense edible herbs in the world—cooling, succulent, and rich in plant-based omega-3 fatty acids, magnesium, potassium, antioxidants, and gentle mucilage. For centuries, it has been gathered across the Mediterranean, Middle East, Africa, Asia, and Indigenous North America as both food and medicine.

Its crisp leaves cool internal heat, soothe irritated tissues, support hydration, and provide rare omega-3 nourishment for the heart, joints, skin, and brain. Traditional systems valued Purslane for calming inflammation, easing digestive irritation, and restoring vitality during heat or depletion. Today, it remains a quiet, food-grade restorative that strengthens health through steady nourishment rather than force.

---

## Core Herbal Category — Purslane

**Primary Core: Nutritional & Tonic Support** herb (omega-3–rich, mineral-dense nourishment that calms low-grade inflammation)

**Secondary Cores:** Circulatory & Cardiovascular · Skin & Tissue Repair · Digestive Support · Metabolic Support

---

### How It Works

Purslane delivers bioavailable omega-3 fatty acids, antioxidants, and trace minerals that nourish cells and reduce inflammatory stress. Its cooling, demulcent nature soothes digestive irritation, supports skin hydration, and promotes vascular and metabolic balance. Overall, it functions as a gentle, food-grade restorative that rebalances multiple systems.

---

### Primary Uses

- Supports heart and vascular health
- Improves skin hydration and tissue repair
- Cools inflammatory joint and tissue discomfort
- Supports digestion and regularity

---

### Scientific Backing

Purslane is among the richest known plant sources of alpha-linolenic acid (ALA) omega-3s and contains flavonoids and polysaccharides shown to reduce inflammatory stress, support cardiometabolic balance, and protect skin and vascular tissues. Nutritional research supports its role as a functional food for metabolic and cardiovascular support.

---

### Forms Available

🟢 Fresh leaves (food)
🟢 Dried leaf or powder
🟢 Juice or smoothie ingredient
🟢 Capsules

---

📏 **How to Use / Dosage**
- Fresh leaves: ½–1 cup daily in meals
- Powder: 1–2 teaspoons daily
- Juice/smoothies: up to ½ cup blended with greens
- Topical: crushed fresh leaves applied to irritated skin

---

⏱ **Expected Results**
Digestive comfort: 2–7 days
Skin hydration & calming: 1–2 weeks
Cardiometabolic tone: 3–6 weeks with regular use

---

⚠ **Caution Level:** 🟢 *Generally Safe*
Extremely safe as food and herb.
Use mild caution with kidney stone history or gout due to natural oxalates.
Avoid harvesting from treated or polluted areas.

---

**Gender-Specific Safety — Purslane**
🟢 **Men:** Safe — supports cardiovascular and metabolic health.
🟢 **Women:** Safe — cooling and hydrating; helpful during heat or inflammation.
🟡 **Pregnancy / Nursing:** Safe as food; avoid concentrated powders or extracts.

---

🌿 **Same / Similar Results**
🟢 Spinach · 🟢 Watercress · 🟢 Gotu Kola

**Shelf Life / Potency After Preparation**
Fresh: 3–5 days refrigerated
Dried leaf: up to 1 year
Powder: 6–9 months

💬 **Herbal Reflections — Purslane**
Purslane is the people's tonic—humble, cooling, and deeply generous. It restores vitality through simplicity, reminding us that some of the strongest medicines arrive quietly, through daily nourishment.

⭐ **Herbal Confidence Index:** 🌿 🌿 🌿 🌿 🌿 *(5 / 5) A cornerstone nutritive herb — exceptionally safe, accessible, reliable, and historically validated.*

# BETEL LEAF

★★★

*Piper betle*

**Betel Leaf** is a warming, aromatic leaf traditionally used for oral hygiene, digestion, and respiratory clearing. Rich in phenolic compounds, it freshens breath, tones gums, stimulates digestion, eases gas and bloating, and helps break up upper-airway phlegm. Light infusions or occasional chewing provide a clean, clarifying lift without jitter.

Culturally revered across South and Southeast Asia, Betel Leaf is distinct from harmful betel-quid practices that add areca nut or tobacco. Used on its own, it remains a respected ritual and medicinal ally in Ayurveda and Unani traditions.

---

### Core Herbal Category — Betel Leaf

**Primary Core: Digestive System Support herb** with *(warming, aromatic carminative action that stimulates digestion and relieves gas and stagnation)*

**Secondary Cores:** Respiratory Support herb · Nervines herb · Skin & Tissue Repair herb

---

### How It Works

Betel Leaf stimulates digestive secretions and motility, relieving bloating and heaviness. Its warming aromatics help loosen respiratory congestion while gently stimulating mental clarity and digestive–nervous coordination. Used orally, it supports gum health and microbial balance. Overall, it functions as a warming, aromatic mover that restores flow and comfort.

---

### Primary Uses

- Natural breath freshener and oral cleanser
- Digestive stimulant for gas and stagnation
- Breaks up upper-airway phlegm
- Mild antimicrobial and anti-inflammatory support
- Headache relief (traditional poultice)

---

### Scientific Backing

Betel Leaf contains chavicol, eugenol, and allylpyrocatechol, shown to:

- Reduce oral bacteria
- Stimulate gut motility
- Provide antimicrobial and expectorant effects
- Offer antioxidant and anti-inflammatory activity

Preliminary research suggests possible metabolic benefits; further human trials are needed.

---

### Forms Available
Fresh leaves
Leaf tea or juice
Topical poultices

### How to Use / Dosage
- Tea: 1–2 fresh leaves per cup, steep 10 minutes
- Chewed leaf: after meals for oral cleansing
- Poultice: warmed, bruised leaf applied externally

---

### Expected Results
Digestive relief: 30–60 minutes
Oral cleansing: immediate
Respiratory clearing: 2–4 days

---

### Caution Level: Caution
- Use moderately; naturally stimulating
- **Never** combine with areca nut or tobacco
- Excess may cause mouth irritation, palpitations, or nausea
- Avoid during pregnancy and breastfeeding

---

### Gender-Specific Safety — Betel Leaf
**Men — Safe (Occasional Use):** Helpful for digestion and oral hygiene; avoid chronic use.
**Women — Caution:** Limit if prone to reflux or stimulant sensitivity.
**Pregnancy / Nursing — Avoid:** Not recommended due to stimulating compounds.

---

### Same / Similar Results
Peppermint · Fennel · Ginger · Thyme · Clove

---

### Shelf Life & Potency
Fresh leaves: 5–7 days refrigerated
Dried leaf: 1–2 years
Tea/Infusion: 24 hours
Tincture: 4–5 years

### Herbal Reflections of Betel Leaf
Betel Leaf is a ritual cleanser—warming, aromatic, and precise. It clears the mouth, wakes the gut, and lifts respiratory damp with restraint. Used respectfully and without harmful additives, it teaches that small, intentional doses can restore flow without excess.

---

**Herbal Confidence Index:** **(3 / 5)** A traditional aromatic digestive and respiratory stimulant. Effective in moderation but limited by safety concerns and cultural misuse when combined with areca nut or tobacco.

# BALSAM FIR

★★★★

*Abies balsamea*

**Balsam Fir** is the woodland healer — an evergreen rich with resin, aroma, and clarity. Its needles and sap carry gentle expectorant, antimicrobial, and muscle-soothing qualities long valued in northern herbal traditions. Whether used as steam for congested lungs, a resin salve for sore joints, or an uplifting aromatic, Balsam Fir brings the clean breath of the forest into the body and space. Indigenous healers used its resin for wounds and lung support, while early apothecaries prized "Canada balsam" for purity and clarity. Today, its familiar winter scent and warming topical action make it a steady ally for breathing ease, muscular comfort, and seasonal resilience.

---

## Core Herbal Category — Balsam Fir

**Primary Core: Respiratory System Support herb** with (aromatic, resinous action that opens airways and supports lung clarity)
**Secondary Cores:** Musculoskeletal & Pain-Relief herb · Immune Support herb · Nervines (Nervous System Support) herb

---

## How It Works

Balsam Fir works through volatile resins and essential oils that loosen congestion and promote clearer breathing when inhaled or diffused. These compounds stimulate local circulation, easing muscle and joint tension when applied externally. Its clean, penetrating aroma supports nervous-system calm during respiratory stress. Antimicrobial volatiles reduce microbial load in air and tissues without requiring internal essential-oil use. Overall, Balsam Fir functions as a clarifying, aromatic respiratory herb best suited for inhalation, diffusion, and topical application.

---

## Primary Uses

- Chest congestion and mucus
- Muscle aches, back pain, arthritis
- Gentle expectorant and decongestant
- Local inflammation of skin or joints
- Mental fatigue and low mood related to illness

---

## Scientific Backing

Contains borneol, limonene, α-pinene, β-pinene, and camphene, compounds associated with antimicrobial, expectorant, and mild analgesic effects. Purified "Canada balsam" was historically used in optical science, reflecting its stability and purity.

---

## 🪵 Forms Available

- Essential oil (diffusion, diluted topical)
- Resin (salves, balms)
- Dried needles (steam, bath, light tea)
- Liniments and chest rubs

---

## 🧴 How to Use / Dosage

**Steam:** 3–5 drops essential oil in hot water; inhale 5–10 minutes
**Topical:** Dilute EO to 1–3% in carrier oil; apply to muscles or joints
**Tea:** 1 tsp chopped needles; steep 10 minutes (light, aromatic)
**Bath:** Handful of needles in hot bath for respiratory and muscle ease

---

## ⌛ Expected Results

- Breathing ease: immediate to 1–2 days
- Muscle relaxation: minutes to hours
- Mood uplift: same day
- Inflammation support: several days to 1–2 weeks

---

## ⚠ Caution Level: ◍ Caution

- Essential oil must always be diluted
- Avoid internal use of essential oil
- Strong aromatics may irritate sensitive airways
- Not suitable for infants or young children
- Avoid during pregnancy and breastfeeding
- Asthma-prone individuals should use steam gently

---

## Gender-Specific Safety (GS)

**Men — ● Safe**
Appropriate for topical and aromatic use for muscle soreness and congestion.
**Women — ● Safe**
Well tolerated in diluted forms; avoid heavy exposure if scent-sensitive.
**Pregnancy / Nursing — ● Avoid**

Essential oils are too stimulating; safety data insufficient.

---

## Same / Similar Results

- White Pine Needles
- Spruce
- Eucalyptus
- Peppermint
- Camphor (stronger; use cautiously)

---

## Shelf Life / Potency After Preparation

- Dried needles: 1 year airtight (aroma fades first)
- Essential oil: 3–4 years, cool and dark
- Resin salves: 1–2 years depending on base oils
- Prepared tea: Use within 24 hours refrigerated

---

## Herbal Reflections of Balsam Fir

Balsam Fir brings the forest directly into the breath — crisp, grounding, and steady. It softens the places where tension gathers, whether in weary lungs, tight joints, or an overworked mind. More than a remedy, it reminds the body how to breathe deeply and recover gently, teaching renewal through simplicity and clarity.

---

**Herbal Confidence Index** 🌿 🌿 🌿 🌿 (4/5 green stars — a dependable aromatic ally for respiratory clarity and muscular comfort; gentle, uplifting, and best suited for seasonal and topical support.)

# BLACK CARDOON

★★★

*Cynara cardunculus var. ferocis*

**Black Cardoon** is a robust Mediterranean bitter that awakens the liver, moves bile, and steadies digestion after heavy meals. Rich in cynarin and related phenolics, it supports hepatic clearance, bile flow, and lipid metabolism, easing fullness and metabolic stagnation.

A wild cousin of globe artichoke, Cardoon has been cultivated since Roman times for both food and medicine. Its thistle flowers still provide vegetable rennet for traditional cheeses, reflecting its long role at the intersection of kitchen and clinic.

---

## Core Herbal Category — Black Cardoon

**Primary Core: Liver & Detoxification Support herb** with (bitter, choleretic action that stimulates bile flow and supports liver and gallbladder function)

**Secondary Cores:** Digestive Support herb · Metabolic & Blood Sugar Support herb · Circulatory & Cardiovascular herb

---

## How It Works

Black Cardoon activates bitter receptors, triggering increased bile production and improved fat digestion. This choleretic effect helps decongest the liver and gallbladder while enhancing metabolic efficiency. Antioxidant compounds support vascular and hepatic protection. The result is improved digestive flow, lipid balance, and metabolic clarity rather than stimulation or purging.

---

## Primary Uses

- Liver support and detoxification
- Cholesterol and lipid balance
- Bile flow stimulation
- Digestive sluggishness and fullness

---

## Scientific Backing

Research on Cardoon and related artichoke species shows hepatoprotective, antioxidant, and LDL-lowering effects. Cynarin is associated with bile production and lipid metabolism support.

---

## 🌿 Forms Available

- Dried leaf
- Tincture
- Capsules
- Digestive bitters blends

---

## How to Use / Dosage

- **Tea:** 1–2 tsp dried leaf, 10–15 minutes before meals
- **Tincture:** 1–2 mL, 2–3× daily before meals
- **Capsules:** Follow label instructions

---

## ⏳ Expected Results

- Digestive improvement: 3–7 days
- Liver and cholesterol support: 2–4 weeks

---

## ⚠ Caution Level: Caution

- Strong bitter action may overstimulate bile
- Avoid with gallstones or bile-duct obstruction unless supervised
- Large doses may cause cramping or loose stools
- Avoid during pregnancy and breastfeeding
- Discontinue if abdominal pain occurs

---

## Gender-Specific Safety (GS)

**Men — Safe**
Supports liver, cholesterol, and digestion when used short-term.
**Women — Safe**
Well tolerated at moderate doses; avoid prolonged daily use.
**Pregnancy / Nursing — Avoid**
Strong bitter and bile-stimulating action is not appropriate.

---

## Same / Similar Results

- Artichoke Leaf
- Dandelion Root
- Milk Thistle

● Gentian

---

## 📦 Shelf Life / Potency After Preparation

- Dried leaf: 1 year airtight (bitterness declines after 9–12 months)
- Tincture: 3–5 years, stable potency
- Capsules: 1–2 years unopened; 6 months after opening
- Prepared tea: Use within 24 hours refrigerated

---

## 💬 Herbal Reflections of Cardoon

Black Cardoon carries the wild bitterness of open hillsides, restoring movement where heaviness settles. It reminds the body that bitterness, when balanced, clears stagnation and invites lightness. Less refined than artichoke yet deeply effective, it teaches that cleansing often begins with awakening.

## ★ Herbal Confidence Index

🌿 🌿 🌿 🌿 (4/5 green stars — a potent wild liver bitter offering deep digestive and metabolic support; best used mindfully and in defined courses.)

# TEASEL ROOT

★★★★

*Dipsacus fullonum*

**Teasel Root** is a mover and mender for deep musculoskeletal patterns. Traditionally used for chronic joint stiffness, old injuries, and long recoveries, it supports circulation into connective tissues and restores strength gradually rather than suppressing pain.

Known in East Asian medicine as "Xu Duan" — "restore what is broken" — Teasel has long been associated with bones, tendons, and low-back weakness. Its rugged reputation reflects its slow, thorough, and restorative nature.

---

## Core Herbal Category — Teasel Root

**Primary Core: Anti-Inflammatory & Pain Support herb** with (deep connective-tissue-stimulating action that supports tendon, ligament, and joint recovery)

**Secondary Cores:** Circulatory & Cardiovascular herb · Nervines (Nervous System Support) herb

---

## How It Works

Teasel Root stimulates circulation into deep connective tissues, supporting nourishment and repair of tendons, ligaments, and joints. Improved blood flow clears stagnation and metabolic waste, easing chronic stiffness. Its tonic effect supports nerve-muscle coordination and gradual structural strengthening. Rather than rapid suppression, Teasel promotes steady remodeling and functional recovery.

---

## Primary Uses

- Chronic joint pain and stiffness
- Long-term injury recovery
- Hip, knee, and spinal weakness
- Persistent muscle tension
- Nervous-system fatigue during healing

---

## Scientific Backing

Contains iridoid glycosides (including loganin) with anti-inflammatory and antioxidant activity. Animal and laboratory studies suggest connective-tissue and bone-supportive effects. Human clinical data remain limited.

## 📦 Forms Available

- Tincture
- Dried root (decoction)
- Capsules
- Powder
- Topical infused oil

---

## ⏱ How to Use / Dosage

- **Tincture:** 10–30 drops up to 3× daily
- **Capsules:** 500 mg, 1–2× daily with meals
- **Topical:** Massage infused oil into affected areas
- **Poultice:** Warm root with oil for stubborn joints

---

## ⌛ Expected Results

- Joint and tissue support: 1–3 weeks
- Topical relief: 2–7 days
- Mobility improvement: gradual and cumulative

---

## ⚠ Caution Level: ● Caution

- May cause dizziness, nausea, or overstimulation at high doses
- Can intensify detox reactions in sensitive individuals
- Use cautiously with autoimmune conditions
- Avoid during pregnancy and breastfeeding
- Start low and increase gradually

---

## 🧬 Gender-Specific Safety (GS)

**Men — ● Safe**
Appropriate for joint and recovery support at moderate doses.
**Women — ● Safe**
Well tolerated short-term; start low if sensitive.
**Pregnancy / Nursing — ● Avoid**
Stimulating and detoxifying actions are not appropriate.

---

## 🔄 Same / Similar Results

● Devil's Claw

- Turmeric
- Ashwagandha
- Burdock Root
- Boswellia

---

## Shelf Life / Potency After Preparation

- Dried root: 2–3 years sealed
- Tincture: 4–6 years
- Powder: 1 year airtight
- Infused oil: 12–18 months

---

## Herbal Reflections of Teasel Root

Teasel Root awakens what has gone dormant, stirring circulation where injury and time have settled in. It teaches that true repair comes through movement and patience, guiding the body back toward strength rather than quick relief.

---

## Herbal Confidence Index

🌿 🌿 🌿 🌿 (4/5 green stars — a respected structural tonic for chronic stiffness and long recovery; powerful yet best used deliberately.)

# TURKEY RHUBARB

★★★★

*Rheum palmatum*

**Turkey Rhubarb** is a strong, directive purgative used sparingly to relieve stubborn constipation and clear digestive stagnation. Its anthraquinone-rich root stimulates bowel movement and is sometimes used in short cleansing protocols. Historically traded along Silk Road routes and used for centuries in Asian and Western pharmacopeias, it remains an herb of purposeful use — effective when needed, but inappropriate for routine use.

---

## 🌿 Core Herbal Category — Turkey Rhubarb

**Primary Core: Digestive System Support** herb with (anthraquinone-rich, stimulant-laxative principles that promote short-term bowel movement and colon clearance)
**Secondary Cores:** Liver & Detoxification herb · Metabolic & Blood Sugar Support herb

---

## 🌿 How It Works

Turkey Rhubarb stimulates the large intestine to increase peristalsis, leading to evacuation within hours. Bitter constituents also promote digestive secretions and may increase bile flow, which can reduce heaviness from sluggish digestion. Because its action is forceful, repeated use can weaken bowel tone and contribute to dependency, dehydration, and electrolyte loss. It is a short-term tool for acute stagnation — not a daily digestive herb.

---

## 🌱 Primary Uses

- Occasional stubborn constipation (short-term)
- Digestive heaviness with sluggish elimination
- Short cleanse protocols under structured use

---

## 🧪 Scientific Backing

Contains anthraquinones (including rhein and emodin) responsible for laxative effects, with tannins that provide some astringent balance. Research includes preclinical antimicrobial and anti-inflammatory signals, but its most established use remains bowel stimulation.

## 📦 Forms Available

- Capsules / tablets
- Powder
- Dried root (decoction)
- Tincture
- Combination cleanse formulas

---

## ⏱ How to Use / Dosage

**Internal use must be brief and low-dose only.**

- **Capsules:** 200–500 mg only when needed
- **Tincture:** 5–10 drops before bed (not nightly)
- **Decoction:** Small amount simmered 10–15 minutes (occasional only)

Hydrate well. Stop if cramping is significant.

---

## ⌛ Expected Results

- Bowel movement: 6–24 hours
- Relief of heaviness: 1–3 days (spaced use only)

Not intended for ongoing use.

---

## ⚠ Caution Level: ● Avoid (routine use) / ● Caution (rare, supervised use)

Turkey Rhubarb is a stimulant laxative and carries meaningful risk with misuse.

**Avoid** if you have: pregnancy/nursing, children/teens, IBD (Crohn's/UC), colitis, IBS-D, intestinal obstruction, unexplained abdominal pain, kidney disease, dehydration, electrolyte imbalance, or active bleeding hemorrhoids/fissures.

**Do not use long-term** due to dependency and electrolyte loss risk.

---

## 🧬 Gender-Specific Safety (GS)

**Men — ● Caution**

Rare, short-term use only; not for ongoing "cleansing."

**Women — ● Avoid**

Routine use should be limited due to cramping sensitivity and fluid/electrolyte risks; avoid around menstruation.

**Pregnancy / Nursing — ● Avoid**

Not appropriate due to strong stimulant-laxative action and safety concerns.

---

## 🔄 Same / Similar Results

- Yellow Dock (gentler bowel/liver support)
- Cascara (stimulant laxative; still not for long-term use)
- Slippery Elm (soothing, non-stimulant)
- Marshmallow Root (soothing, non-stimulant)
- Triphala (gentler regulation)

---

## Shelf Life / Potency After Preparation

- Dried root: 3–4 years airtight, dark
- Powder: 1–1.5 years (loses potency faster)
- Capsules: 2–3 years sealed
- Tincture: 5–7 years
- Prepared decoction: 24 hours refrigerated

## DIY Recipe — Occasional Rhubarb-Ginger Decoction (Rare Use Only)

¼ tsp Turkey Rhubarb + ½ tsp ginger
Simmer 10 minutes, strain, take before bed **no more than once every several days**.

## Herbal Reflections of Turkey Rhubarb

Turkey Rhubarb is not a daily helper — it is an emergency key. It clears stuckness, then steps back so gentler herbs can rebuild rhythm. Its wisdom is restraint: clear what must be cleared, then return to nourishment, hydration, and steady digestive tone.

**Herbal Confidence Index** (4/5 green stars — highly effective for short-term constipation relief, but limited by dependency and electrolyte risks; best reserved for rare, purposeful use.)

# USNEA

★★★★

*Usnea barbata*

**Usnea** is a slow-growing forest lichen valued for steady antimicrobial and tissue-supportive use, especially for respiratory catarrh and external wound care. As a lichen (a fungal–algal partnership), it grows deliberately and should be harvested ethically — primarily from windfall. Traditionally used as a wound dressing and for stubborn infections, modern interest centers on usnic acid and related compounds.

---

## Core Herbal Category — Usnea

**Primary Core: Immune System Support** herb with (broad antimicrobial action that supports the body in resisting bacterial overgrowth)
**Secondary Cores:** Respiratory Support herb · Skin & Tissue Repair herb · Digestive Support herb

---

## How It Works

Usnea supports immune defense through usnic acid and related constituents that can inhibit certain bacteria and help reduce microbial load. This is most relevant for upper respiratory congestion and surface-level infections where steady antimicrobial pressure is helpful. Topically, it supports clean tissue repair. Internal use should be short-course only due to rare liver sensitivity concerns associated with concentrated preparations.

---

## Primary Uses

- Respiratory/sinus congestion with suspected bacterial load
- External wound cleansing and tissue support
- Fungal skin patches (topical)
- Short-term immune reinforcement

---

## Scientific Backing

Preclinical studies show antibacterial activity (including against certain resistant organisms) with antifungal and antiviral signals. Human clinical evidence is limited, so it is best used as an adjunct rather than a standalone solution for serious infection.

---

## 📦 Forms Available

- Alcohol tincture (best extraction for key constituents)
- Salves and infused oils (topical)
- Dried lichen (primarily for external washes)

---

## How to Use / Dosage

- **Tincture:** 10–30 drops, 1–2× daily for short courses
- **Topical:** Salve/infused oil 1–3× daily
- **External wash:** Simmer gently 15–20 minutes; use as a rinse

---

## ⌛ Expected Results

- Topical support: 1–3 days
- Respiratory support: 3–7 days depending on severity

Use in short courses, then stop.

---

## ⚠ Caution Level: Caution

Usnea contains usnic acid and may cause stomach upset. Rare liver irritation has been reported, especially with concentrated or prolonged internal use.

Avoid internal use if you have liver disease or take hepatotoxic medications. Stop immediately if unusual fatigue, nausea, dark urine, or right-upper abdominal discomfort appears. Use only ethically sourced material.

---

## Gender-Specific Safety (GS)

**Men — Caution**

Short-course use only; avoid if liver-compromised.

**Women — Caution**

Short-course use only; avoid if liver-compromised.

**Pregnancy / Nursing — Avoid**

Not appropriate due to limited safety data.

---

## Same / Similar Results

- Calendula (topical tissue support)
- Yarrow (topical cleansing support)
- Goldenseal (strong antimicrobial; short-term)

- Thyme (respiratory antimicrobial support)
- Oregano Oil (strong; not for sensitive users)

---

## 📦 Shelf Life / Potency After Preparation

- Dried lichen: 2–3 years airtight, dark
- Powder: 1 year
- Salve/infused oil: ~1 year
- Tincture: 5–7 years
- Prepared wash/decoction: 48 hours refrigerated

---

## 🛠 DIY Recipe — Usnea Antiseptic Wash (External)

1 tbsp Usnea simmered in 1 cup water for 20 minutes.
Cool, strain, refrigerate. Use within 48 hours.

---

## 💬 Herbal Reflections of Usnea

Usnea works like quiet armor — steady, protective, and patient. It holds the line while tissues recover and immunity regains coordination. Its ecology teaches restraint and respect: use only what is needed, harvest ethically, and let slow-growing medicine remain available for the future.

---

## ★ Herbal Confidence Index

🌿 🌿 🌿 🌿 (4/5 green stars — strong topical and short-course antimicrobial ally; limited by sustainability concerns and rare internal liver sensitivity.)

# VIDANGA

★★★★

(*Embelia ribes*)

**Vidanga** is a classic Ayurvedic gut cleanser used in short cycles to address intestinal imbalance, including parasite concerns and sluggish digestion. The peppery berries sharpen digestive fire (agni), reduce bloating, and appear in traditional "Krimighna" formulas. Its strength is best expressed in focused protocols with clear start/stop timing rather than continuous use.

---

## 🌿 Core Herbal Category — Vidanga

**Primary Core: Digestive System Support** herb with (antiparasitic cleansing action that supports intestinal balance and elimination)
**Secondary Cores:** Immune Support herb · Skin & Tissue Repair herb · Metabolic & Blood Sugar Support herb

---

## 🌿 How It Works

Vidanga supports gut cleansing by creating an unfavorable environment for certain parasites and dysbiotic microbes while encouraging elimination. This can reduce internal irritation and may support clearer skin when digestive imbalance is contributing. Its warming nature increases digestive activity. Because it is strong and drying, it works best in short cycles followed by restoration.

---

## 🌱 Primary Uses

- Parasite-cleansing protocols (short cycles)
- Bloating, indigestion, sluggish digestion
- Skin issues linked to digestive imbalance
- Metabolic sluggishness

---

## 🧪 Scientific Backing

Contains embelin, associated with anti-helminthic activity, plus antimicrobial and antioxidant signals. Evidence is still developing; its strongest support remains traditional use aligned with known pharmacology.

---

## 📦 Forms Available

- Powder
- Capsules
- Tincture
- Ayurvedic blends (Krimighna formulas)

---

## How to Use / Dosage

- **Powder:** 1–3 g daily with warm water
- **Capsules:** 250–500 mg, 1–2× daily
- **Tincture:** 15–30 drops, 1–2× daily

Use **7–10 day cycles**, then stop. Rebuild afterward.

---

## ⌛ Expected Results

- Digestive lightness: within days
- Protocol effect: 7–10 days
- Skin clarity from gut correction: 2–4 weeks with diet support

---

## ⚠ Caution Level: ▨ Caution

Avoid during pregnancy and breastfeeding. May irritate sensitive stomachs or increase acidity and can cause cramping or loose stools at higher doses. Not for continuous use — cycles only. Stop if burning, nausea, or persistent cramping develops.

---

## 🧬 Gender-Specific Safety (GS)

**Men — ● Caution**
Short-cycle use; reduce dose if cramping or loose stools occur.
**Women — ● Caution**
Short-cycle use; avoid if prone to diarrhea or significant acidity.
**Pregnancy / Nursing — ● Avoid**
Not appropriate due to stimulating cleansing action and limited safety data.

---

## 🔄 Same / Similar Results

● Neem ● Black Walnut Hull ● Clove (irritating for some) ● Wormwood (strong; short-cycle use) ● Myrrh (drying; short-term)

---

## 📦 Shelf Life / Potency After Preparation

- Whole berries: 3–4 years airtight, dark
- Powder: 1–1.5 years
- Capsules: ~1 year
- Tincture: 5–7 years
- Prepared tea: 24 hours refrigerated

---

## 🛠 DIY Recipe — Vidanga-Triphala Cycle Blend (Short Course)

1 tsp Vidanga powder + 1 tsp Triphala in warm water at bedtime
Use **7–10 days**, then stop and restore.

---

## 💬 Herbal Reflections of Vidanga

Vidanga clarifies rather than comforts. It corrects microbial imbalance and creates room for digestion to regain order. Its strength demands timing: a focused cycle, then replenishment. Used this way, Vidanga becomes a disciplined reset that makes healthier rhythms possible.

---

## ★ Herbal Confidence Index 🌿 🌿 🌿 🌿 (**4/5 green stars** — a time-tested Ayurvedic cleanser best used in short, intentional cycles due to its stimulating nature.)

# OATSTRAW

★★★★

*Avena sativa*

**Oatstraw** is one of the most nourishing and restorative nervines in Western herbal medicine. Rather than sedating or stimulating the nervous system, it rebuilds and strengthens nerve tissue itself, making it uniquely valuable for exhaustion, burnout, nerve weakness, and long-term stress depletion.

Traditionally prepared as a mineral-rich infusion, Oatstraw has been relied upon to restore vitality after illness, emotional strain, overwork, or aging. Its gentle yet profound action supports the myelin sheath, nerve endurance, and overall nervous system resilience, helping the body recover stability rather than merely masking symptoms.

---

### Core Herbal Category — Oatstraw

**Primary Core:** Nervous System Support (Nervines) herb (trophic nervine that rebuilds and strengthens nerve tissue and myelin integrity)

**Secondary Cores:** Fatigue Recovery · Mineral Replenishment · Stress Resilience · Musculoskeletal Support

---

### How It Works

Oatstraw works by supplying bioavailable minerals—particularly silica, magnesium, calcium, and trace elements—alongside calming phytochemicals that nourish nerve tissue and support myelin sheath integrity. This combination strengthens nerve signaling, improves stress tolerance, and restores depleted nervous reserves without sedation. Its rebuilding action supports long-term recovery rather than short-term symptom relief.

---

### Primary Uses

- Rebuilds and nourishes depleted nerves
- Supports recovery from chronic stress, burnout, or illness
- Improves nerve endurance and stress tolerance
- Supports peripheral nerve health and mild neuropathy
- Reduces nervous exhaustion and irritability
- Strengthens hair, skin, nails, and connective tissue through mineral support

---

### Scientific Backing

Oatstraw contains flavonoids, saponins, alkaloids, and a dense mineral profile shown to support nervous system stability and stress resilience. Research supports its role in calming nervous excitability, reducing fatigue, and improving cognitive endurance under stress. Its mineral content contributes to nerve conduction, connective tissue integrity, and long-term nervous system health.

---

### How to Use (Dosage)

**Infusion (Preferred):**
Steep 1–2 Tbsp dried Oatstraw in 1 quart hot water for 4–8 hours; drink throughout the day.
**Tea:**
1–2 tsp per cup, 2–3× daily for gentle support.
**Tincture:**
2–4 mL, up to 3× daily for fatigue or nervous depletion.
**Capsules:**
500–1,500 mg daily (less effective than infusion).

---

### Caution Level — Safe

Extremely gentle and well tolerated. Suitable for long-term use. Gluten-sensitive individuals should ensure gluten-free sourcing, as the green tops are naturally low in gluten but may be cross-contaminated.

---

### Gender-Specific Safety

**Men:** Safe — supports stress resilience, nerve endurance, and recovery from exhaustion.
**Women:** Safe — excellent for burnout, emotional depletion, and long-term nervous balance.
**Pregnancy/Nursing:** Safe — traditionally used as a nourishing tonic when properly sourced.

---

### Expected Results

• Nervous calming: several days
• Improved stress tolerance: 1–2 weeks
• Nerve strength and endurance: 3–6 weeks
• Mineral repletion benefits: cumulative over time

---

### Long-Term Rebuilding Protocol (Clinical Use)

Oatstraw is best understood as a **rebuilding tonic**, not a quick-fix remedy. For deep nervous depletion, it is traditionally used daily for **4–12 weeks** or longer.
**Best results occur when:**
• Taken as a long-steeped infusion rather than capsules
• Used consistently rather than intermittently
• Combined with adequate rest, hydration, and nutrition
This makes Oatstraw especially valuable for individuals recovering from prolonged stress, caregiving fatigue, emotional trauma, chronic illness, or age-related nervous decline.

---

### Mineral Profile & Synergy Notes

Oatstraw is particularly rich in **silica, magnesium, calcium, and trace minerals**, which support nerve conduction, muscle relaxation, and connective tissue strength.
It pairs especially well with:• **Nettle Seed** — mineral depth and adrenal support• **Milky Oats** —

acute nervous soothing• **Skullcap** — calming without depletion• **Bamboo Silica** — structural reinforcement

---

🔄 **Same / Similar Results**

⚪ Lemon Balm · ⚪ Skullcap · ⚪ Milky Oats · ⚪ Nettle Seed

---

**Shelf Life / Potency After Preparation**

Dried herb: 1–2 years · Infusion: 24–36 hours refrigerated · Tincture: 4–5 years

**Herbal Reflections of Oatstraw**

Oatstraw restores what stress quietly erodes, rebuilding steadiness where nerves have frayed and endurance where vitality has thinned. Its medicine is patience and nourishment — a reminder that true strength returns through restoration, not force.

---

**Herbal Confidence Index** 🌿 🌿 🌿 🌿 *(4/5 — A foundational trophic nervine for rebuilding nerve strength, resilience, and l vitality.)*

# PURPLE DEAD NETTLE

★★★

*Lamium purpureum*

Often dismissed as a weed, **Purple Dead Nettle** is a mild, nourishing herb that supports seasonal reactivity, lymphatic flow, and surface tissue comfort. Traditionally used as a fresh-leaf poultice for minor cuts and rashes and as tea for sinus puffiness and throat irritation, it offers gentle antioxidant and calming support without heaviness. Despite the name, it is not a stinging nettle; its soft mint-family leaves signal a friendly, food-like spring ally.

---

## Core Herbal Category — Purple Dead Nettle

**Primary Core: Immune System Support** herb with (mild lymphatic-moving, anti-inflammatory action that helps reduce seasonal reactivity and congestion)
**Secondary Cores:** Skin & Tissue Repair herb · Liver & Detoxification herb · Nutritive & Restorative herb

---

## How It Works

Purple Dead Nettle supports immune balance by providing plant antioxidants that calm inflammatory irritation and gently assist lymphatic movement. This may reduce seasonal stuffiness and "puffiness" patterns by supporting fluid flow and tissue calm. Topically, its mild astringent and soothing properties support minor skin recovery. As a nutrient-dense spring green, it offers supportive minerals and plant compounds that strengthen resilience over time.

---

## Primary Uses

- Seasonal congestion and mild allergy reactivity
- Minor cuts, scrapes, and irritated skin (topical)
- Lymphatic sluggishness/puffiness patterns
- Mild throat irritation
- Gentle nutritive support as a spring tonic

---

## Scientific Backing

Contains phenolics and flavonoids associated with antioxidant, anti-inflammatory, and mild antimicrobial activity. Evidence is preliminary but aligns with traditional use for gentle tissue support and seasonal comfort.

---

## 🌿 Forms Available

- Dried herb
- Fresh leaf (poultice)
- Tincture
- Infused oil (topical)

---

## ☕ How to Use / Dosage

- **Tea:** 1 tsp dried herb per cup, 1–2× daily
- **Tincture:** 10–20 drops, 2–3× daily
- **Poultice:** crush fresh leaves and apply to minor irritation
- **Infused oil:** apply topically 1–2× daily

---

## ⏳ Expected Results

- Less nasal/throat irritation: 1–3 days
- Lighter puffiness/flow: ~1 week
- Skin steadiness: 2+ weeks with consistency

---

## ⚠ Caution Level: ● Safe

Food-like and generally gentle.

- Very large amounts may cause mild digestive upset
- Those sensitive to mint-family plants should trial cautiously
- Use only clean, correctly identified plants (avoid roadside/treated areas)

---

## Gender-Specific Safety (GS)

**Men — ● Safe**
Supportive for seasonal reactivity and mild skin issues.
**Women — ● Safe**
Generally gentle; appropriate for most adults as tea or topical.
**Pregnancy / Nursing — ● Caution**
Limited research; occasional tea is usually mild, but avoid heavy daily use unless guided.

---

## 🔄 Same / Similar Results

● Nettle Leaf
● Cleavers

- Plantain Leaf
- Mullein
- Yarrow

---

## 📦 Shelf Life / Potency After Preparation

- Dried herb: 1 year (best potency within 9–12 months)
- Tincture: 3–5 years
- Infused oil: 6–12 months (discard if cloudy/rancid)
- Prepared tea: 24 hours refrigerated

---

## 🛠 DIY Recipe — Allergy-Relief Tea Blend

1 part Purple Dead Nettle
1 part Mullein
½ part Nettle Leaf
½ part Chamomile
Steep 1 Tbsp in 2 cups hot water 10–15 minutes. Sip during flare-ups.

---

## 💬 Herbal Reflections of Purple Dead Nettle

Purple Dead Nettle is quiet medicine—steady, nourishing, and reliable. It doesn't force change; it supports the body's own cleanup and calm, especially during seasonal transitions. Its lesson is humility: small plants can offer consistent help when used regularly and with patience.

---

## ★ Herbal Confidence Index

🌿🌿🌿 (3/5 green stars — gentle, food-like spring support for seasonal reactivity, lymph flow, and minor skin comfort; mild but dependable through consistency.)

# CISTANCHE TUBULOSA

★★★★★

*Cistanche tubulosa*

**Cistanche** is a deep restorative tonic traditionally used to rebuild endurance, libido, and resilience during depletion. Revered across East Asian traditions for supporting healthy aging, stamina, and foundational vitality, it is best suited to those who feel chronically tired, cold, and overextended. Rather than a quick stimulant, it supports steadier recovery over time. Modern interest focuses on its phenylethanoid glycosides and their roles in fatigue resistance and neuroprotective support.

---

## Core Herbal Category — Cistanche

**Primary Core: Nutritional & Tonic Support** with (deep yang-tonifying, essence-nourishing action that rebuilds foundational energy, endurance, and long-term resilience)
Secondary Cores: Endocrine & Hormonal Regulation · Nervous System Regulation (Nervines) · Immune Support & Modulation · Foundational Regulation & Terrain Support.

---

## How It Works

Cistanche supports vitality by nourishing endurance systems rather than stimulating them. Its tonic constituents support recovery from fatigue, steadier stress tolerance, and healthy hormonal signaling. This can translate into improved stamina, libido, and cognitive steadiness in depleted states. It also supports immune resilience during long-term stress by strengthening baseline recovery capacity. The overall pattern is **rebuilding**: gradual, cumulative improvements with consistent, moderate use.

---

## Primary Uses

- Low stamina and endurance in depleted states
- Libido and reproductive vitality support
- Fatigue-related low focus/mental steadiness
- Recovery support after chronic overexertion
- Resilience support during long-term stress

---

## Scientific Backing

Contains echinacoside and acteoside (phenylethanoid glycosides) studied for antioxidant, neuroprotective, and anti-fatigue effects. Research includes signals for energy-metabolism support and cellular resilience; human evidence is still emerging but aligns with long-standing traditional tonic use.

---

## 🍵 Forms Available

- Capsules/tablets (often standardized extract)
- Powder
- Tincture
- Tea/decoction (traditional; less common)

---

## ⏱ How to Use / Dosage

- **Capsules/Powder:** 500–1500 mg daily (morning is best)
- **Tincture:** typically 1–3 mL/day (follow label)

Use consistently for several weeks; avoid stacking multiple strong tonics at high doses.

---

## ⌛ Expected Results

- Energy and steadier focus: 1–2 weeks
- Endurance and recovery tone: 3–4 weeks
- Deeper restoration: gradual with sustained use

---

## ⚠ Caution Level: ● Caution

Use mindfully if you have:

- Hormone-sensitive conditions
- Autoimmune conditions or immunosuppressant therapy
- Significant insomnia, heat agitation, or overstimulation patterns

Avoid during pregnancy and breastfeeding due to limited safety data.
Stop if persistent agitation, headache, or digestive upset occurs.

---

## 🧬 Gender-Specific Safety (GS)

**Men — ● Safe**
Well suited for stamina and vitality support when used moderately.
**Women — ● Caution**
Often tolerated, but warming tonics may aggravate heat/insomnia in sensitive individuals.
**Pregnancy / Nursing — ● Avoid**

Not appropriate due to limited safety data and tonic intensity.

---

## 🔄 Same / Similar Results

- Tongkat Ali
- Panax Ginseng
- Epimedium
- Ashwagandha
- Maca

---

## 📦 Shelf Life / Potency After Preparation

- Powder: 1–1.5 years airtight, cool, dry
- Capsules/tablets: 2–3 years unopened
- Tincture: 4–6 years
- Brewed tea: 24 hours refrigerated

---

## 🛠 DIY Recipe — Cistanche Vitality Blend

1 tsp Cistanche powder + ½ tsp Maca in warm nut milk.
Use in the morning for steady support (avoid late-day use if sleep is sensitive).

---

## 💬 Herbal Reflections of Cistanche

Cistanche is patient strength—restoration that arrives by rebuilding the foundation. It supports the kind of energy that doesn't spike and crash, but grows steadier with time. For the depleted and overextended, it teaches that true vitality is cultivated, not forced, and that resilience can be restored through consistent, measured nourishment.

---

## ★ Herbal Confidence Index

🌿 🌿 🌿 🌿 🌿 (5/5 green stars — a premier restorative tonic with strong traditional reputation and promising modern support; exceptionally useful for depletion, stamina, and healthy aging when used responsibly and consistently.)

# CLEOME

★★★

*Cleome gynandra*

**Cleome** (African spider plant) is a nutrient-dense leafy green used as food-as-medicine in African and Asian traditions. Cooked as a daily vegetable, it offers carotenoids, minerals, and plant antioxidants that support steady nourishment, mild digestive "clearing," and resilience during recovery. Its strength is not in dramatic effects, but in consistent rebuilding—warm meals that restore tissue tone and support the body's natural rhythms.

---

## Core Herbal Category — Cleome

**Primary Core: Nutritional & Tonic Support** herb with (mineral-rich, food-based action that rebuilds strength while supporting gentle elimination)
**Secondary Cores:** Digestive Support herb · Skin & Tissue Repair herb · Women's Health herb · Immune Support herb

---

## How It Works

Cleome supports the body primarily through **nutrient delivery**—vitamins, minerals, fiber, and protective plant compounds that strengthen tissues over time. Its mild bitter and fibrous qualities can support digestion and regular elimination, easing "heaviness" patterns without stimulant action. Antioxidant constituents help calm low-grade inflammatory irritation, which can support skin and overall recovery when used as a consistent dietary green.

---

## Primary Uses

- Nutritive rebuilding (general weakness or depletion)
- Daily digestive support and regularity (food-based)
- Skin and eye nutrition support (dietary)
- Mild "spring tonic" style support through cooked greens

## Scientific Backing

Cleome is studied for nutrient density and antioxidant activity, with early research signals for anti-inflammatory and liver-supportive patterns. Most reliable benefit remains its role as a **high-value medicinal food** rather than a strong medicinal extract.

---

## Forms Available

- Fresh leaves (cooked in stews/soups)

• Dried leaf (tea or powdered food additive)
• Powder (mixed into meals)

---

## ⏱ How to Use / Dosage

• **Food use:** ½–1 cup cooked leaves, several times per week or daily
• **Powder:** 1–3 g/day mixed into meals
Cooking improves digestibility and reduces bitterness; avoid relying on large raw servings.

---

## ⌛ Expected Results

• Digestive comfort and steadier elimination: 1–2 weeks
• Skin/eye nutrition support: 3–6 weeks with consistent use
• Rebuilding strength: gradual with regular food use

---

## ⚠ Caution Level: ● Safe

Generally safe as a cooked food.
• Large amounts (especially raw) may cause digestive upset
• If prone to kidney stones or oxalate sensitivity, favor **cooked** use and moderate portions
• Use clean, properly identified plants (avoid roadside/treated areas)

---

## Gender-Specific Safety (GS)

**Men — ● Safe**
Nutritive cooked green appropriate for regular use.
**Women — ● Safe**
Food-based support; traditional postpartum use exists, but keep claims modest and food-level.
**Pregnancy / Nursing — ● Caution**
Food portions when cooked are generally reasonable; avoid concentrated "medicinal dosing" (strong powders/extract-like use) due to limited safety data.

---

## Same / Similar Results

● Moringa Leaf
● Amaranth Leaf
● Purslane
● Spinach (food-level)

- Dandelion Leaf (food/tea)

---

## 📦 Shelf Life / Potency After Preparation

- Fresh leaves: refrigerate 2–4 days
- Dried leaf/powder: ~1 year airtight
- Prepared tea: 24 hours refrigerated
- Frozen cooked leaves: 2–3 months

---

## 🛠 DIY Recipe — Cleome Green Soup

1 cup Cleome leaves + onion + garlic + pinch of turmeric.
Simmer 15–20 minutes; blend if desired. Use as a nourishing weekly or daily meal.

---

## 💬 Herbal Reflections of Cleome

Cleome's medicine is the medicine of a bowl—warm, mineral-rich, and steady. It nourishes without pushing, supports without overstating, and rewards consistency. In traditions where food and medicine live together, Cleome stands as proof that healing can be practical, shared, and built one meal at a time.

**★ Herbal Confidence Index** 🌿 🌿 🌿 (3/5 green stars — reliable medicinal food with gentle nutritive and digestive value; best through consistent cooked use rather than concentrated dosing.)

# CHINESE SKULLCAP

★★★★★

*Scutellaria baicalensis • Huang Qin*

**Chinese Skullcap** (Huang Qin) is a classic bitter-cool root used to clear inflammatory "heat" patterns, especially in the lungs and upper respiratory tract. It is valued for supporting immune balance, calming irritated tissues, and assisting liver stress patterns linked to inflammation. Unlike *Scutellaria lateriflora* (a nervine), Huang Qin is primarily an anti-inflammatory and heat-clearing herb used in structured formulas and appropriate dosing windows.

---

## Core Herbal Category — Chinese Skullcap

**Primary Core:** Respiratory System Support herb with (cooling, flavonoid-rich root action that calms inflamed airways and clears heat irritation)
**Secondary Cores:** Immune Support herb · Liver & Detoxification herb · Nervines (Nervous System Support) herb

---

## How It Works

Chinese Skullcap works through flavonoids (notably baicalin/baicalein) that support **inflammation regulation** and help calm irritated respiratory tissues. It can reduce inflammatory "heat" signals while still supporting appropriate immune defense. It also supports liver stress patterns associated with inflammation. Its "nervine" role here is indirect—by lowering inflammatory tension, it may reduce the restless, wired feeling that can accompany inflammatory stress.

---

## Primary Uses

- Hot, irritated cough/throat heat patterns
- Inflammation-calming immune support
- Liver stress patterns linked to heat/inflammation
- Damp-heat style patterns in traditional frameworks (used appropriately)

---

## Scientific Backing

Contains baicalin and baicalein with studied anti-inflammatory, antioxidant, antimicrobial signals and hepatoprotective activity. Evidence is strongest for inflammation modulation and respiratory irritation support; clinical outcomes vary by condition and formulation.

---

## 🍵 Forms Available

- Capsules/tablets
- Tincture
- Decoction (root simmered 20–30 minutes)

---

## ⏱ How to Use / Dosage

- **Capsules:** follow label; typical ranges vary widely by extract strength
- **Tincture:** 30–60 drops, 2–3× daily (short courses)
- **Decoction:** commonly 3–9 g root simmered 20–30 minutes (traditional use)

Use in defined phases, not indefinite high dosing.

---

## ⌛ Expected Results

- Respiratory heat/irritation easing: 3–10 days (pattern-dependent)
- Calmer inflammatory tone: 2–4 weeks with structured use

---

## ⚠ Caution Level: ▨ Caution

- Avoid prolonged high-dose use without guidance
- Use cautiously with immunosuppressants or autoimmune therapies
- Use cautiously with liver-metabolized medications
- May cause digestive upset in sensitive individuals

Stop if unusual fatigue, persistent nausea, or worsening symptoms occur.

---

## 🧬 Gender-Specific Safety (GS)

**Men — ● Caution**

Generally tolerated; use structured dosing and avoid long high-dose use with complex meds.

**Women — ● Caution**

Generally tolerated; caution with heavy cooling if constitution is very cold/weak.

**Pregnancy / Nursing — ● Avoid**

Not appropriate due to limited safety data and potency as a bitter-cool medicinal root.

## 🔄 Same / Similar Results

● Andrographis (acute immune support)
● Oregon Grape Root (damp-heat/microbial patterns)
● Licorice Root (harmonizing support)
● Goldenseal (strong; short-term)

- Thyme (respiratory antimicrobial support)

---

## 📦 Shelf Life / Potency After Preparation

- Dried root: ~2 years airtight
- Capsules/powder: 1–2 years
- Tincture: 3–5 years
- Decoction: 48 hours refrigerated (best same day)

---

## 🛠 DIY Recipe — Cooling Respiratory Decoction

5 g Chinese Skullcap + 3 g Licorice Root.
Simmer 25 minutes; sip warm up to 2× daily during heat-type irritation.

---

## 💬 Herbal Reflections of Chinese Skullcap

Huang Qin is disciplined medicine—cooling, clarifying, and precise. It does not numb; it restores proportion. When inflammation runs hot and tissues feel raw, it offers a calmer immune rhythm and steadier breathing. Used responsibly, it is a quiet instructor in balance: cool what is overactive, support what is strained, and return the system to order.

**★ Herbal Confidence Index** 🌿 🌿 🌿 🌿 🌿 (5/5 green stars — cornerstone bitter-cool root with deep traditional credibility and strong research interest; powerful inflammation and respiratory "heat" support when used correctly.)

# CISSUS QUADRANGULARIS

★★★★

*Cissus quadrangularis*

**Cissus (Hadjod)** is a traditional structural-support herb long used in Ayurvedic practice for assisting the recovery of bones and connective tissues after strain or injury. Historically valued as a "bone-joiner," it has been used for generations to support comfort, tissue repair processes, and the gradual return of function—particularly in cases where recovery feels prolonged. In modern use, Cissus is commonly taken in standardized capsule form to ensure consistency and ease of use.

---

## Core Herbal Category — Cissus

**Primary Core: Anti-Inflammatory & Pain Support herb** with (bone- and connective-tissue–restorative action that supports structural repair and reduces inflammatory discomfort)
**Secondary Cores:** Digestive Support herb · Metabolic & Blood Sugar Support herb · Immune Support herb

---

## How It Works

Cissus supports structural repair by assisting collagen-related rebuilding and helping the body maintain a healthier inflammatory response during recovery. This can support comfort and mobility while tissues remodel. It may also support digestion and nutrient utilization, which indirectly supports repair by improving access to building materials. The overall effect is steady, functional restoration when paired with appropriate movement and rehabilitation.

---

## Primary Uses

- Recovery support after sprain/strain and joint irritation
- Structural rebuilding support during fracture recovery (adjunct)
- Inflammatory discomfort support (wear-and-tear patterns)
- Digestive and metabolic support as a secondary benefit

---

## Scientific Backing

Research includes preclinical and some human studies exploring bone metabolism markers, inflammation modulation, and joint comfort outcomes. Evidence varies by extract type and dosing;

strongest use remains as an adjunct to proper rehab and nutrition.

---

## 🍵 Forms Available

- Capsules/standardized extract
- Dried stem (decoction)
- Topical paste/poultice (traditional use)

---

## ⏱ How to Use / Dosage

- **Capsules/extract:** commonly 500–1000 mg, 1–2× daily (follow label)
- **Decoction:** 1 Tbsp dried stem simmered 20 minutes; 1–2× daily (short courses)
- **Topical:** short-course poultice to tender areas (avoid broken skin)

---

## ⌛ Expected Results

- Comfort/mobility support: 2–4 weeks
- Structural tone with continued rehab: 4–8 weeks

---

## ⚠ Caution Level: ◍ Caution

- May cause digestive upset in some users
- Some report restlessness/insomnia—avoid late-day dosing if sensitive
- Use cautiously with diabetes medications (may influence glucose)
- Avoid during pregnancy and breastfeeding due to limited safety data

Take breaks during long-term use (cycle use).

---

## 🧬 Gender-Specific Safety (GS)

**Men — ● Safe**

Generally tolerated; monitor sleep and digestion.

**Women — ● Safe**

Generally tolerated; monitor sleep and digestion.

**Pregnancy / Nursing — ● Avoid**

Not appropriate due to limited safety data and metabolic activity.

---

## 🔄 Same / Similar Results

● Horsetail (silica support)

● Turmeric (inflammation support)

● Boswellia (joint comfort)

● Comfrey (external only; safety limits)

🔘 Moringa (nutritive support)

---

## 📦 Shelf Life / Potency After Preparation

- Dried stem: ~2 years
- Capsules/extract: ~2 years sealed
- Decoction: 36–48 hours refrigerated (best fresh)

---

## 🛠 DIY Recipe — Cissus Recovery Tea (Short Course)

1 Tbsp dried Cissus stem + 2 cups water.
Simmer 20 minutes, strain. Use 1× daily during early recovery phases.

---

## 💬 Herbal Reflections of Cissus

Cissus is repair-minded medicine—quiet, structural, and consistent. It supports the body's patient work of rebuilding what was strained or weakened. Its lesson is steady effort: tissue restores through time, nutrition, movement, and measured support. Cissus helps hold that process together.

---

## ★ Herbal Confidence Index

🌿 🌿 🌿 🌿 (4/5 green stars — dependable structural-repair ally with strong traditional reputation; best as a supportive tool alongside rehab and nutrition.)

# MUIRA PUAMA

★★★★

*Ptychopetalum olacoides*

**Muira Puama** is a traditional Amazonian herb long used to support nervous system resilience, vitality, and reproductive health. Often referred to as "Potency Wood," it has been valued for generations as a restorative tonic for fatigue, low libido, and diminished physical or mental drive. Indigenous use focused on strengthening the body's response to stress while promoting circulation, nerve tone, and overall vitality.

Rather than acting as a stimulant, Muira Puama works gradually—supporting the nervous system, improving circulation, and helping restore functional balance in cases of depletion or prolonged stress. In modern use, it is commonly taken as capsules, tinctures, or powdered extracts for consistent, cumulative support.

---

### Core Herbal Category — Muira Puama

**Primary Core: Nervous System Support (Nervines)** herb with (tonic and mildly stimulating actions that support nerve resilience, mental clarity, and stress recovery)
**Secondary Cores:** Endocrine & Hormonal Regulation herb · Circulatory & Cardiovascular Support herb · Nutritional, Tonic & Longevity Support herb

---

### How It Works

Muira Puama supports the nervous system by promoting circulation to nerve tissues and helping modulate the body's response to stress. Its active compounds are believed to influence neurotransmitter activity and vascular tone, contributing to improved mental clarity, mood balance, and physical responsiveness.

By supporting both circulation and nerve signaling, it may enhance energy levels, improve libido, and assist in restoring functional balance in cases of fatigue or stress-related depletion. Its effects are typically gradual and build with consistent use over time.

---

### Primary Uses

- Nervous system fatigue and stress recovery
- Low libido and reduced vitality
- Mild cognitive fatigue and mental fog
- Circulatory support (especially peripheral circulation)

• General tonic support for physical and mental endurance

---

### Scientific Backing

Preliminary research and traditional use suggest Muira Puama may support nervous system function, libido, and cognitive performance through its effects on circulation and neurotransmitter activity. Evidence is still emerging, and most benefits are supported by traditional use and observational data rather than large-scale clinical trials.

---

### Forms Available

• Capsules / standardized extracts
• Tinctures (liquid extract)
• Powdered bark

---

### How to Use / Dosage

• Capsules: typically 500–1000 mg daily (follow product label)
• Tincture: 20–40 drops, 1–2 times daily
• Powder: small measured amounts in beverages

Best taken consistently for cumulative effects. Avoid taking late in the evening if sensitive to mild stimulation.

---

### Expected Results

• Mild energy and clarity: 3–7 days
• Nervous system support: 2–4 weeks
• Libido and vitality support: 3–6 weeks
• Full tonic effects: 6–8 weeks

---

### Caution Level: Caution

• May cause mild stimulation—avoid if highly sensitive to stimulants
• Use caution with blood pressure or cardiovascular medications
• Not recommended for severe anxiety or agitation states
• Avoid use late in the evening if it affects sleep
• Limited data in pregnancy—avoid use

---

### Gender-Specific Safety (GS)

Men — Safe
Commonly used for vitality and libido support; monitor if sensitive to stimulation

Women — Safe

May support energy, mood, and circulation; use moderate dosing

Pregnancy / Nursing — ● Avoid
Insufficient safety data—avoid use

---

### 🔄 Same / Similar Results

- Tongkat Ali
- Maca
- Ashwagandha
- Rhodiola
- Ginseng

---

### Shelf Life / Potency After Preparation

- Capsules: 1.5–2 years sealed
- Tincture: 2–3 years
- Powder: ~1 year airtight

---

### 🛠 DIY Recipe — Vitality Support Tonic Blend

½ tsp Muira Puama powder + ½ tsp Maca + warm almond milk.
Blend well and consume in the morning.

---

### 💬 Herbal Reflections of Muira Puama

Muira Puama restores through awakening—reviving what has been dulled by fatigue, stress, or prolonged strain. It works not by force, but by rekindling responsiveness—supporting the body's natural rhythm of energy, clarity, and vitality. It reminds us that strength is not always about intensity, but about restoring connection between the body and its capacity to respond.

---

### ⭐ Herbal Confidence Index

🌿 🌿 🌿 🌿 (4/5 green stars — a strong traditional nervine and vitality tonic with reliable supportive effects; best suited for gradual restoration of energy, circulation, and functional resilience)

# MORINGA LEAF

★★★★★

*Moringa oleifera*

**Moringa Leaf** is a highly nutrient-dense medicinal food used across Ayurvedic and African traditions to support nourishment and recovery. Its leaves provide vitamins, minerals, amino acids, and antioxidants that help rebuild depleted tissues and support steady energy over time. Moringa's best strength is consistency—regular use as food or powder for foundational wellness rather than dramatic, fast effects.

---

## Core Herbal Category — Moringa Leaf

**Primary Core: Nutritional & Tonic Support** herb with (exceptionally nutrient-dense, food-based action that supports cellular repair and whole-body nourishment)
**Secondary Cores:** Immune Support herb · Metabolic & Blood Sugar Support herb · Liver & Detoxification herb · Circulatory & Cardiovascular herb

---

## How It Works

Moringa works mainly by delivering concentrated nutrition—minerals, vitamins, amino acids, and antioxidant compounds that support cellular function and tissue repair. This steady nourishment can improve energy availability, immune resilience, and metabolic balance over time. Antioxidants help reduce oxidative stress, easing inflammatory burden and supporting normal liver processing. When used consistently, Moringa functions as a foundational restorative herb that supports the body's rebuilding processes rather than stimulating the system.

---

## Primary Uses

- Whole-body nourishment during depletion or low dietary quality
- Steady energy and resilience support (food-based)
- Metabolic support (blood sugar and lipids) as part of diet and routine
- Antioxidant support for immune and cardiovascular resilience

---

## Scientific Backing

Studies on *Moringa oleifera* support antioxidant and anti-inflammatory activity, with research interest in metabolic support (glucose and lipids) and liver-protective signals. Strength of effects varies by preparation and dose; the most reliable benefit remains its role as a consistent nutritive food herb.

---

## Forms Available

- Dried leaf powder
- Capsules
- Tea (dried leaf infusion)
- Whole dried leaf

---

## How to Use / Dosage

- **Powder:** ½–1 tsp daily in food, smoothies, or warm water
- **Tea:** 1–2 tsp dried leaf steeped 5–10 minutes
- **Capsules:** follow label (extract strength varies)

Start low if digestion is sensitive.

---

## Expected Results

- Digestive comfort and steadier energy: 3–10 days
- Improved nutritional "tone" and resilience: 2–4 weeks
- Deeper restorative benefits: 4–8 weeks with consistent use

---

## ⚠ Caution Level: Caution

Generally well tolerated, but:

- High doses may cause digestive upset
- May lower blood sugar—use caution if on diabetes medications
- Use caution with blood-pressure medications if prone to low BP
- Choose clean sourcing (avoid contaminants)

---

## Gender-Specific Safety (GS)

**Men — Safe**

Excellent daily nutritive herb; monitor if on glucose-lowering meds.

**Women — Safe**

Supports nutrition and iron intake as part of diet; monitor if on glucose meds.

**Pregnancy / Nursing — Caution**

Cooked/food-level leaf use is generally reasonable; avoid concentrated extracts or high-dose powders without professional guidance.

---

## 🔄 Same / Similar Results

- Nettle Leaf
- Spirulina
- Chlorella
- Alfalfa Leaf
- Burdock Leaf (nutritive adjunct)

---

## 📦 Shelf Life / Potency After Preparation

- Powder: ~1 year airtight, cool, dry
- Capsules: 1.5–2 years sealed
- Whole dried leaf: ~1 year
- Prepared tea: 24 hours refrigerated

---

## 🛠 DIY Recipe — Moringa Superfood Smoothie

½ tsp Moringa powder + banana + nut milk + handful of greens.
Use daily or several times weekly for steady nourishment.

---

## 💬 Herbal Reflections of Moringa Leaf

Moringa is restoration through nourishment—quiet, steady, and complete. It doesn't push the body; it supplies what the body needs to rebuild. Its lesson is simple: when the foundations are strong—minerals, vitamins, and consistent daily care—resilience returns naturally.

---

## ★ Herbal Confidence Index

🌿 🌿 🌿 🌿 🌿 (5/5 green stars — cornerstone nutritive herb with excellent consistency and broad usefulness; best as a daily food-based restorative.)

# GOJI BERRY

★★★★★

***Lycium barbarum***

**Goji Berry (Wolfberry)** is a classic longevity fruit used in Traditional Chinese Medicine as a gentle daily tonic for vitality, immune resilience, and eye nourishment. Rich in carotenoids (including zeaxanthin), polysaccharides, and antioxidants, it supports long-term tissue protection and steady energy when used consistently as food.

---

## Core Herbal Category — Goji Berry

**Primary Core:** Nutritional & Tonic Support
*with (blood-nourishing, antioxidant action that supports long-term vitality and eye resilience)***Secondary Cores:** Liver & Detoxification herb · Immune Support herb · Adaptogen Support herb

---

## How It Works

Goji supports the body through carotenoids and antioxidants that help protect eye and vascular tissues from oxidative stress. Its polysaccharides support balanced immune signaling and recovery. Goji's traditional "blood and yin" nourishment translates practically into steady tissue support and resilience when used as a consistent food. Liver-supportive effects are gentle and indirect, helping the body manage metabolic stress rather than acting as a purge.

---

## Primary Uses

- Eye nourishment and protective support (food-based, long-term)
- Immune resilience and antioxidant support
- Gentle vitality and stamina support
- Daily tonic use during stress and aging patterns

---

## Scientific Backing

Research supports antioxidant effects, immune modulation signals, and the role of zeaxanthin in eye support. Clinical results vary by dose and preparation; the strongest and safest use remains regular dietary inclusion.

---

## Forms Available

- Dried berries
- Juice/concentrate
- Powder
- Extract products (vary widely)

---

## How to Use / Dosage

- **Dried berries:** 1–2 Tbsp daily (snacks, soups, teas)
- **Tea:** steep berries 5–10 minutes; eat berries afterward
- **Powder/extract:** follow label; avoid excessive dosing

---

## Expected Results

- Energy and steadier mood: 3–10 days
- Eye/skin/immune support: 2–4 weeks
- Longevity-tonic benefits: gradual with consistent use

---

## Caution Level: Caution

- May interact with warfarin and other blood thinners
- May lower blood sugar—monitor if on diabetes meds
- Choose unsulfured, clean sourcing
- Avoid high-dose extracts unless guided

---

## Gender-Specific Safety (GS)

**Men — Safe**
Appropriate as a daily food tonic; caution if on blood thinners or diabetes meds.
**Women — Safe**
Food-level use is typically well tolerated; caution with blood thinners/diabetes meds.
**Pregnancy / Nursing — Caution**
Food-level amounts are generally reasonable; avoid concentrated extracts or high therapeutic dosing without professional guidance.

---

## Same / Similar Results

- Bilberry
- Amla

- Schisandra Berry
- Rosehip
- Sea Buckthorn

---

## 📦 Shelf Life / Potency After Preparation

- Dried berries: 1–2 years airtight
- Powder: ~1 year
- Tincture/extract: 3–5 years
- Prepared tea: 24 hours refrigerated

---

## 🛠 DIY Recipe — Goji Vision Tea

1 Tbsp Goji + optional chrysanthemum.
Steep 10 minutes; drink and eat berries.

---

## 💬 Herbal Reflections of Goji Berry

Goji is gentle longevity—sweet, steady, and best used like a daily habit. It supports the eyes and immune system without strain, reminding us that the strongest tonics often work quietly, building protection and resilience over time.

## ⭐ Herbal Confidence Index

🌿 🌿 🌿 🌿 🌿 (5/5 green stars — cornerstone longevity food herb with excellent safety and consistency; especially strong for eye nourishment and antioxidant resilience.)

# WHITE SPRUCE

★★★★

*Picea glauca*

**White Spruce** is an evergreen ally traditionally used for respiratory support, topical wound care, and seasonal resilience. Its needles and resin provide aromatic compounds that can loosen congestion and support clearer breathing through steam or light tea. Resin-based preparations have long been used externally for minor skin issues when prepared correctly.

---

## 🌿 Core Herbal Category — White Spruce

**Primary Core: Respiratory System Support** herb with (aromatic, resinous principles that help ease cough and support mild chest congestion relief)
**Secondary Cores:** Immune Support herb · Skin & Tissue Repair herb · Musculoskeletal & Pain-Relief herb

---

## 🌿 How It Works

White Spruce works primarily through aromatic volatile compounds that support airway comfort and help loosen mucus when used as steam or a light needle infusion. Externally, properly prepared resin salves create a protective barrier and provide mild antimicrobial support for minor skin irritation. Its warming aromatics also support localized comfort when used topically on muscles, but essential oils must always be diluted.

---

## 🌱 Primary Uses

- Mild chest congestion and cough support (steam/light tea)
- Seasonal immune resilience (adjunct)
- Minor skin support via resin salve (external)
- Muscle comfort via diluted topical preparations

---

## 🧪 Scientific Backing

Conifer needles contain terpenes and antioxidants; resin and essential-oil components show antimicrobial activity in preclinical research. Traditional use is strong; internal essential-oil use is not appropriate.

---

## Forms Available

- Fresh/dried needles (tea, steam)
- Resin (salves)
- Essential oil (aromatherapy, diluted topical)
- Infused oils

---

## How to Use / Dosage

- **Tea:** 1–2 tsp chopped needles; steep in hot (not boiling) water 10 minutes
- **Steam:** needles in hot water; inhale 5–10 minutes
- **Salve:** resin in oil/beeswax base; apply externally
- **Essential oil:** external only; 1–2% dilution for topical use

---

## Expected Results

- Breathing comfort: same day to 48 hours
- Topical skin support: 1–3 days
- Seasonal resilience: 1–2 weeks with consistent supportive care

---

## ⚠ Caution Level: Caution

- Essential oil must be diluted; external only
- Resin may irritate sensitive skin—patch test
- Avoid internal resin use unless professionally guided
- Avoid prolonged heavy internal use if kidney-irritation prone

---

## Gender-Specific Safety (GS)

**Men — Safe**
Aromatic/topical use is generally safe; keep internal tea light and short-term.
**Women — Safe**
Aromatic/topical use generally safe; keep internal tea light and short-term.
**Pregnancy / Nursing — Avoid**
Not recommended due to strong volatile oils/resins; do not use essential oils topically during pregnancy/nursing.

---

## Same / Similar Results

Pine Needles

- Spruce (other species)
- Mullein Leaf (lung soothing)
- Eucalyptus (stronger; use correctly)
- Frankincense (topical resin support)

---

## 📦 Shelf Life / Potency After Preparation

- Dried needles: best 9–12 months airtight
- Resin salves: 1–2 years (oil base dependent)
- Essential oil: ~2 years; oxidized oils should not be used on skin
- Prepared tea: 24 hours refrigerated

---

## 🛠 DIY Recipe — White Spruce Lung Tea

1 tsp needles (optional mullein). Steep 10–12 minutes in hot water. Sip warm.

---

## 💬 Herbal Reflections of White Spruce

White Spruce is forest clarity—steady, bracing, and protective. It supports the breath through clean aromatics and supports the skin through well-made resin preparations. It teaches endurance: simple medicine, used carefully, can carry people through cold seasons with quiet strength.

---

## ★ Herbal Confidence Index 🌿 🌿 🌿 🌿 (4/5 green stars — dependable evergreen for respiratory steam/tea and topical resin care; excellent tradition and practical usefulness when used safely.)

# DANSHEN

★★★★

*Salvia miltiorrhiza*

**Danshen (Red Sage)** is a respected Traditional Chinese Medicine root used to support healthy circulation and microcirculation. It is commonly used for vascular "stagnation" patterns, stress-related tightness, and cardiovascular resilience. Modern research focuses on tanshinones and salvianolic acids and their antioxidant and vascular-support activity. Because it can influence clotting and blood pressure, safety and medication awareness are essential.

---

## Core Herbal Category — Danshen

**Primary Core: Cardiovascular System Support** herb with (microcirculation-supporting action that assists healthy blood flow and vascular resilience)
**Secondary Cores:** Liver & Detoxification herb · Nervines (Nervous System Support) herb · Anti-Inflammatory Support herb

---

## How It Works

Danshen supports microcirculation by helping maintain healthy vascular tone and endothelial function. Its antioxidant compounds help protect tissues from oxidative stress linked to vascular strain. By reducing inflammatory burden and easing stress-driven tension patterns, it can support steadier circulation and calmer cardiovascular load. This is not a "quick fix" herb—benefits tend to build with consistent use, movement, and hydration.

---

## Primary Uses

- Microcirculation and vascular resilience support
- Stress-related chest tightness patterns (non-emergency support)
- Recovery support for circulation tone (adjunct to lifestyle)
- Calm support where vascular tension and stress overlap

## Scientific Backing

Tanshinones and salvianolic acids are studied for antioxidant activity, endothelial support, and circulation-related effects. Clinical outcomes vary by extract type and condition; medication interactions are the primary safety concern.

---

## Forms Available

- Standardized extract capsules/tablets
- Root slices (decoction)
- Tincture
- Combination formulas (often with Hawthorn)

---

## How to Use / Dosage

- **Decoction:** 1–2 tsp dried slices simmered 20–30 minutes; up to 2× daily
- **Tincture:** 1–2 mL up to 3× daily (verify strength)
- **Capsules/extract:** follow label (standardization varies)

Use in courses (often 4–8 weeks) unless professionally directed otherwise.

---

## Expected Results

- Warmer extremities/microcirculation tone: 1–2 weeks
- Reduced "stagnation" sensations and tension: 2–4 weeks
- Cardiovascular resilience support: 4–12 weeks with routine care

---

## Caution Level: Caution

- **Do not combine with anticoagulants/antiplatelets** (warfarin, aspirin, clopidogrel) without medical supervision
- Discontinue at least **2 weeks before surgery**
- Use caution with low blood pressure or BP medications
- Avoid in pregnancy and breastfeeding

Stop if unusual bruising, bleeding, dizziness, or weakness occurs.

---

## Gender-Specific Safety (GS)

**Men — Caution**

Generally safe in moderate doses, but medication interactions are significant.

**Women — Caution**

May increase menstrual flow in some; avoid if prone to heavy bleeding.

**Pregnancy / Nursing — Avoid**

Blood-invigorating activity is not appropriate.

---

## Same / Similar Results

Hawthorn

- Grape Seed (OPCs)
- Pine Bark (OPCs)
- Gotu Kola
- Bilberry

---

## 📦 Shelf Life / Potency After Preparation

- Dried root slices: 2–3 years airtight
- Capsules/extract: 1–2 years (follow expiry)
- Tincture: 4–5 years
- Decoction: 24–48 hours refrigerated (best fresh)

---

## 🛠 DIY Recipe — Danshen-Hawthorn Tea (If Med-Safe)

Simmer Danshen slices + Hawthorn berries 20 minutes. Sip 1 cup daily.
**If on blood thinners or before surgery: do not use.**

---

## 💬 Herbal Reflections of Danshen

Danshen is the smoother of flow—supporting the vessels' ability to relax and the tissues' ability to receive nourishment. It pairs well with daily walking, hydration, and stress reduction, teaching that circulation improves when rhythm and routine return.

---

## ★ Herbal Confidence Index 🌿 🌿 🌿 🌿 (4/5 green stars — reliable circulation and endothelial support with strong tradition and research interest; excellent when used consistently with careful medication awareness.)

# EUCALYPTUS

★★★★

*Eucalyptus globulus*

**Eucalyptus** is a sharp, aromatic respiratory herb best known for steam inhalation, rubs, and properly diluted topical use. Its volatile oils—especially 1,8-cineole (eucalyptol)—support easier breathing by loosening thick mucus and reducing upper-airway irritation. Because the essential oil is potent and can be toxic if misused, Eucalyptus belongs to the "strong but useful" category: effective when used correctly, risky when used carelessly.

---

## Core Herbal Category — Eucalyptus

**Primary Core: Respiratory System Support** herb with (aromatic, volatile-oil action that helps loosen mucus and ease congested breathing)
**Secondary Cores:** Immune Support herb · Skin & Tissue Repair herb (topical) · Musculoskeletal & Pain-Relief herb (topical)

---

## How It Works

Eucalyptus works through volatile oils that help thin and mobilize mucus, supporting clearer airflow and easier expectoration. Inhaled aromatics can reduce the sensation of congestion and support more comfortable breathing. Topically, properly diluted preparations provide warming, counterirritant comfort and mild antimicrobial support on intact skin. Because the essential oil is highly concentrated, safe outcomes depend on correct dilution and correct route of use.

---

## Primary Uses

- Chest congestion and thick mucus support (steam, rubs)
- Sinus heaviness and "stuffy head" support (steam)
- Seasonal respiratory comfort (short-term)
- Muscle/joint comfort (properly diluted topical)
- External antimicrobial support for minor skin issues (intact skin only)

## Scientific Backing

Eucalyptus oils and 1,8-cineole are widely studied for mucolytic effects, respiratory comfort, and antimicrobial activity. Evidence supports short-term symptom relief for congestion and respiratory irritation. Essential oil safety is the main limiting factor.

---

## 🌿 Forms Available

- Essential oil (steam, diffuser, diluted topical)
- Dried leaf (tea or steam)
- Chest rubs and balms
- Inhalers/diffusers
- Standardized products (label-dependent)

---

## ⏱ How to Use / Dosage

**Steam inhalation (common):**
- 1–2 drops essential oil in a bowl of hot water (not boiling). Inhale 5–10 minutes.

**Topical (intact skin only):**
- Dilute to **1–2%** for most adults (about 1–2 drops per teaspoon carrier oil).
- Chest rubs/balms: follow label directions.

**Leaf tea (short-term only):**
- ½–1 tsp dried leaf steeped 10 minutes. Use briefly and moderately.

---

## ⌛ Expected Results

- Steam relief: within minutes
- Congestion and cough comfort: hours to 1–2 days
- Topical muscle comfort: 10–30 minutes

(Best results with rest, hydration, and warm fluids.)

---

## ⚠ Caution Level: ▨ Caution

- **Essential oil is NOT for internal use** (do not swallow)
- Keep away from eyes and mucous membranes
- Use extra caution with asthma/COPD sensitivity (can irritate)
- Not appropriate for young children without professional guidance
- Never apply undiluted oil to skin
- Avoid use near infants and small children (diffusion and topical)

---

## Gender-Specific Safety (GS)

**Men — Caution**

Safe when used correctly (steam/diluted topical). Avoid heavy leaf tea or concentrated products if prone to reflux or stomach irritation.

**Women — Caution**
Safe when used correctly (steam/diluted topical). Avoid strong internal dosing; discontinue if irritation or tightness occurs.
**Pregnancy / Nursing — Avoid**
Essential oil use (steam/topical) and medicinal dosing should be avoided during pregnancy/nursing due to volatility and limited safety margins. Do not use near infants.

---

## Same / Similar Results

- Peppermint (steam/topical)
- Pine Needle (steam/tea)
- Thyme (respiratory support)
- Mullein Leaf (lung soothing)
- Camphor (external only; strong)

---

## Shelf Life / Potency After Preparation

- Dried leaf: best within 1 year airtight
- Essential oil: ~2–3 years (oxidized oil can irritate—discard if "off")
- Balms/salves: 1–2 years (oil base dependent)
- Prepared tea: 24 hours refrigerated

---

## DIY Recipe — Eucalyptus Steam Bowl

1–2 drops eucalyptus oil in hot water. Inhale 5–10 minutes.
**Do not use for children** and do not exceed drops.

---

## Herbal Reflections of Eucalyptus

Eucalyptus is clarity by aroma—quick, sharp, and effective when the breath feels blocked. It is not a "gentle herb," but it can be a reliable ally when used correctly and briefly. Its lesson is precision: the right dose, the right route, and the right respect.

---

## Herbal Confidence Index

(4/5 green stars — fast, effective aromatic decongestant and topical support herb; high usefulness with correct handling, but safety demands careful use.)

# CASCARA SAGRADA

★★★

*Rhamnus purshiana*

**Cascara Sagrada** is a stimulant laxative bark used for short-term constipation relief. It works reliably, but it is not a daily regulator and not a "colon tonic." Its value is **occasional rescue** for sluggish bowels—especially when paired afterward with gentler, restorative bowel supports to prevent dependency.

---

## Core Herbal Category — Cascara Sagrada

**Primary Core: Digestive System Support** herb with (stimulant-laxative action that promotes bowel movement through short-term colon stimulation)
**Secondary Cores:** Liver & Detoxification herb · Gallbladder Support herb

---

## How It Works

Cascara works through anthraquinone glycosides (cascarosides) that stimulate the colon to increase motility and reduce water reabsorption, producing a softer stool and more complete evacuation. It can also increase bile-driven elimination indirectly by moving the intestinal tract. Because it stimulates rather than strengthens bowel tone, it should be used briefly and followed by hydration, fiber, and demulcent support.

---

## Primary Uses

- Occasional constipation
- Short-term "stuck" elimination patterns
- Temporary bowel clearing during sluggish digestion
- Short course use in constipation-focused protocols

---

## Scientific Backing

Cascara's cascarosides are well documented as stimulant laxatives. Research supports effectiveness for short-term constipation, while long-term use is associated with electrolyte imbalance and reduced bowel tone. Safe use depends on **properly aged bark** and short duration.

---

## 🌿 Forms Available

- Capsules (aged bark)
- Tincture (aged bark extract)
- Loose bark tea (aged bark only)

---

## ⏱ How to Use / Dosage

- **Capsules:** 300–500 mg aged bark at bedtime as needed
- **Tea:** ½–1 tsp aged bark steeped 10–15 minutes (use sparingly)
- **Tincture:** per label (strength varies)

**Never use fresh bark.** Use only short-term.

---

## ⏳ Expected Results

- Bowel movement: typically 6–12 hours after dose
- Best for occasional use, not daily "regularity"

---

## ⚠ Caution Level: ● Caution

- Use short-term only (generally ≤ 7 days)
- Can cause cramping, diarrhea, dehydration
- Risk of electrolyte imbalance (low potassium) with overuse
- Avoid with intestinal obstruction, IBD flares, severe hemorrhoids, unexplained abdominal pain
- Medication caution: diuretics, corticosteroids, digoxin/heart meds, anticoagulants (via electrolyte shifts)

---

## 🧬 Gender-Specific Safety (GS)

**Men — ● Caution**
Short-term only; avoid if dehydrated, electrolyte-sensitive, or on heart/diuretic medications.
**Women — ● Caution**
Short-term only; discontinue if cramping is strong or if bowel urgency becomes excessive.
**Pregnancy / Nursing — ● Avoid**
Not recommended due to stimulant-laxative action and risk to infant via breast milk.

---

## 🔄 Same / Similar Results

● Senna Leaf
● Turkey Rhubarb (stronger purgative)

- Slippery Elm (restorative stool-softening support)
- Marshmallow Root (demulcent support)
- Triphala (gentler regulation)

---

## 📦 Shelf Life / Potency After Preparation

- Properly aged bark: 2–3 years airtight
- Capsules: follow expiry (often ~2 years)
- Tincture: 4–5 years
- Prepared tea: 24 hours refrigerated (best made fresh)

---

## 🛠 DIY Recipe — "Gentler" Cascara Night Tea (Short Course)

½ tsp aged cascara bark + chamomile. Steep 10 minutes.
Use only as needed; do not use nightly or long-term.

---

## 💭 Herbal Reflections of Cascara Sagrada

Cascara is a tool, not a lifestyle. It helps the body move when it has become stuck, but it does not build long-term strength in the colon. Its wisdom is restraint: use it briefly, then restore the bowel's natural rhythm with hydration, fiber, and gentler allies.

---

## ★ Herbal Confidence Index

🌿 🌿 🌿 (3/5 green stars — reliable short-term laxative bark; effective but dependency/electrolyte risk keeps it in the "rescue" category.)

# SENNA LEAF

★★★

*Senna alexandrina*

**Senna Leaf** is a dependable, fast-acting stimulant laxative used for occasional constipation and short-term bowel clearing. It is effective, but it works by stimulating the colon—so it should not be used habitually. Like Cascara, Senna belongs on the "emergency shelf," followed by gentler, restorative bowel supports.

---

## Core Herbal Category — Senna Leaf

**Primary Core: Digestive System Support** herb with (short-term colon-stimulating action that promotes bowel movement and evacuation)
**Secondary Cores:** Liver & Detoxification herb · Gallbladder Support herb

---

## How It Works

Senna works through sennosides that stimulate the large intestine and reduce water reabsorption, creating a softer stool and stronger peristalsis. This can reliably produce a bowel movement within hours. Because the mechanism is stimulatory, repeated use can weaken bowel tone and increase dependency risk. Best practice is short, intentional use with hydration and post-use bowel restoration (fiber and demulcents).

---

## Primary Uses

- Occasional constipation (short-term)
- Short-course bowel clearing (when appropriate)
- Temporary elimination support during acute sluggishness

---

## Scientific Backing

Senna's sennosides are widely recognized for laxative efficacy. Evidence supports short-term use, while long-term use is linked to electrolyte imbalance, cramping, and reduced natural motility.

---

## Forms Available

- Dried leaf (tea)
- Capsules/tablets
- Liquid extracts
- Included in "detox/slimming" teas (often overused)

---

## How to Use / Dosage

- **Tea:** ½ tsp dried leaf steeped 10–15 minutes; take at night
- **Capsules:** per label (start low)
- **Tincture/extract:** per label

Use only as needed and avoid frequent dosing.

---

## Expected Results

- Relief: usually within 6–12 hours
- Best for occasional use, not ongoing regulation

---

## Caution Level: Caution

- Short-term use only (generally ≤ 7 days)
- Can cause cramping, urgency, diarrhea, dehydration
- Risk of low potassium and electrolyte imbalance
- Avoid with IBD, obstruction, severe hemorrhoids, unexplained abdominal pain
- Medication caution: diuretics, digoxin/heart meds, corticosteroids, medications affected by potassium shifts

---

## Gender-Specific Safety (GS)

**Men — Caution**
Short-term only; avoid if electrolyte-sensitive or on heart/diuretic medications.
**Women — Caution**
Short-term only; may worsen cramping in sensitive individuals—stop if severe.
**Pregnancy / Nursing — Avoid**
Not recommended due to stimulant-laxative action and potential infant exposure via breast milk.

---

## Same / Similar Results

Cascara Sagrada

- Turkey Rhubarb (stronger purgative)
- Slippery Elm
- Marshmallow Root
- Triphala

---

## Shelf Life / Potency After Preparation

- Dried leaf/powder: 1–2 years airtight
- Capsules/tablets: ~2 years (follow expiry)
- Tincture: 4–5 years
- Prepared tea: 12–24 hours refrigerated (best fresh)

---

## DIY Recipe — Senna "Softened" Night Tea (Occasional)

½ tsp Senna + peppermint. Steep 10 minutes.
Use rarely; hydrate well; follow with demulcent support.

---

## Herbal Reflections of Senna Leaf

Senna is decisive—and that is both its gift and its warning. It can relieve painful stagnation quickly, but it should never replace daily habits that build bowel health. Its place is occasional and intentional, followed by gentler herbs that restore comfort and tone.

---

## Herbal Confidence Index

(3/5 green stars — highly effective short-term stimulant laxative; reliable for rescue use but not suitable for routine long-term support.)

# AJWAIN

★★★★

*Trachyspermum ammi*

**Ajwain** also called **(Carom Seed)** is a pungent, warming aromatic seed used as both spice and medicine for fast relief of gas, bloating, and intestinal cramping. Its thymol-rich volatile oils give it strong carminative and antimicrobial activity, making it a classic "after-meal" helper—especially for heavy foods, legumes, and sluggish digestion. Used correctly and in small amounts, Ajwain is dependable, quick, and culturally time-tested.

---

## Core Herbal Category — Ajwain

**Primary Core: Digestive System Support herb** with (warming, carminative action that reduces gas, bloating, and digestive spasm)
**Secondary Cores:** Antimicrobial Support herb · Respiratory Support herb · Metabolic & Blood Sugar Support herb

---

## How It Works

Ajwain stimulates digestive secretions and helps relax intestinal smooth muscle, easing spasms and trapped gas. Its thymol-rich aromatics help discourage unwanted microbes in the gut and can support clearer breathing when used as gentle steam or aroma. When taken in modest culinary-to-medicinal amounts, Ajwain improves digestive "flow" without heavy sedation or harsh purging.

---

## Primary Uses

- Gas, bloating, indigestion after meals
- Intestinal cramping and digestive spasm
- Appetite support when digestion feels "cold/sluggish"
- Mild respiratory congestion support (steam/aroma)
- Microbial-balancing support (short course)

---

## Scientific Backing

Ajwain's thymol and related volatile oils are associated with antimicrobial activity and antispasmodic, carminative effects. Evidence aligns strongly with traditional use for post-meal discomfort, gas, and cramping.

---

## 🌿 Forms Available

- Whole seeds
- Ground powder
- Capsules / digestive blends
- Essential oil (external only; very concentrated)

---

## ⏱ How to Use / Dosage

**Culinary use:** add to legumes/heavy meals as a spice.
**Chewed seeds (fast relief):** ¼–½ tsp after meals, then sip warm water.
**Tea:** ½ tsp seeds simmered 5–7 minutes in 1 cup water; sip warm.
**Steam/aroma:** lightly crush seeds, add to hot water, inhale gently 3–5 minutes.

---

## ⏳ Expected Results

- Gas/cramping relief: 15–30 minutes
- "Settled stomach" after meals: same day
- Microbial-balancing support: 3–7 days (short course)

---

## ⚠ Caution Level: Caution

(Adjusted for realistic safety: food-safe, but strong and irritating at higher doses.)

- Can worsen heartburn/GERD in sensitive people
- Avoid high-dose medicinal use with active ulcers
- Use caution with blood thinners/antiplatelet drugs

## Gender-Specific Safety (GS)

**Men — Safe**
Generally safe in culinary and standard tea/seed doses.
**Women — Safe**
Generally safe in culinary and standard tea/seed doses; reduce dose if reflux occurs.
**Pregnancy / Nursing — Caution**
Food amounts are acceptable; avoid medicinal/high-dose use and avoid essential oil use.

---

## Same / Similar Results

- Fennel Seed
- Ginger

● Peppermint
● Caraway
● Oregano Oil (strong; not a daily digestive)

---

## 📦 Shelf Life / Potency After Preparation

● Whole seeds: 2–3 years airtight
● Powder: 9–12 months (aroma fades first)
● Tea: best same day; up to 12–24 hours refrigerated
● Essential oil: ~2 years (discard if harsh/oxidized)

---

## 🛠 DIY Recipe — Ajwain Gas-Relief Tea

½ tsp ajwain + pinch of fennel. Simmer 6 minutes. Strain and sip warm after meals.

---

## 💬 Herbal Reflections of Ajwain

Ajwain is the "quick correction" spice—small, strong, and direct. It restores comfort when meals sit heavy, when gas becomes pressure, and when the gut needs warmth and movement. Its strength is speed and simplicity: a pinch, a cup, a breath—then relief.

★ **Herbal Confidence Index** 🌿 🌿 🌿 🌿 (4/5 green stars — fast, reliable carminative and antimicrobial seed; excellent in small doses, but intensity keeps it out of the "unlimited" category.)

# ALLSPICE

★★★★

*Pimenta dioica*

**Allspice** is a warming aromatic berry used as both culinary spice and gentle medicine. Rich in eugenol-like aromatic compounds, it supports digestion, eases mild cramping, and offers topical comfort for sore muscles when infused into oil. It is not a stimulant laxative; its digestive value comes from relaxing spasm, improving comfort after meals, and warming circulation.

---

## Core Herbal Category — Allspice

**Primary Core: Digestive System Support** herb with (warming aromatic action that eases gas, mild cramping, and post-meal heaviness)
**Secondary Cores:** Musculoskeletal & Pain-Relief herb (topical) · Circulatory & Cardiovascular herb · Nervines (Nervous System Support) herb

---

## How It Works

Allspice supports digestion through aromatic compounds that stimulate gentle digestive activity and relax intestinal spasm, easing gas and cramping. As a warming circulatory spice, it promotes comfortable movement in cold, tight tissues. Used topically (infused oil/compress), it provides warming comfort for sore muscles and minor aches by increasing local circulation and calming discomfort.

---

## Primary Uses

- Post-meal gas, bloating, mild cramping
- Cold, sluggish digestion patterns
- Mild menstrual cramp comfort (tea as spice)
- Muscle soreness (topical compress/infused oil)
- "Cold weather" tension and stiffness support

---

## Scientific Backing

Allspice contains aromatic phenolics (including eugenol-related compounds) associated with antimicrobial and analgesic activity. Evidence supports digestive spasm relief and topical comfort effects consistent with traditional use.

---

## 🌿 Forms Available

- Whole berries
- Ground spice
- Tea blend ingredient
- Infused oil (topical)
- Essential oil (external only; very concentrated)

---

## How to Use / Dosage

**Tea:** ½–1 tsp crushed berries steeped 10–15 minutes; drink after meals.
**Culinary:** use as warming spice in food.
**Topical:** warm compress or infused oil on sore muscles (intact skin).
**Essential oil:** external only, diluted.

---

## ⌛ Expected Results

- Digestive comfort: 20–45 minutes
- Warming/circulatory feel: within an hour
- Topical muscle comfort: 10–30 minutes

---

## ⚠ Caution Level: Caution

(Adjusted for essential oil potency and eugenol sensitivity.)
- Large internal doses may cause nausea/irritation
- Use caution with blood thinners/antiplatelet therapy
- Essential oil is **external only** and must be diluted
- Avoid applying concentrated preparations to sensitive skin

---

## Gender-Specific Safety (GS)

**Men — Safe**
Normal culinary and tea use is well tolerated.
**Women — Safe**
Normal culinary and tea use is well tolerated.
**Pregnancy / Nursing — Caution**

Food amounts are acceptable; avoid medicinal/high-dose use and avoid essential oil use.

---

## 🔄 Same / Similar Results

- Ginger
- Cinnamon
- Clove (stronger)
- Nutmeg (low doses only)
- Cardamom

---

## 📦 Shelf Life / Potency After Preparation

- Whole berries: 3–4 years airtight
- Ground spice: 6–12 months (aroma fades)
- Tea: best same day
- Infused oil: ~1 year (oil-base dependent)

---

## 🛠 DIY Recipe — Allspice Settle Tea

1 tsp crushed berries + optional ginger slice. Steep 15 minutes. Sip after meals.

---

## 💬 Herbal Reflections of Allspice

Allspice is comfort with quiet strength—warming the belly, easing tension, and smoothing the edges of cold, heavy meals. It's a household ally: more subtle than clove, gentler than pepper, and dependable when digestion needs warmth and calm.

---

## ★ Herbal Confidence Index 🌿🌿🌿🌿

(4/5 green stars — versatile warming digestive and topical comfort spice; strong usefulness with good safety in normal doses.)

# AMERICAN GINSENG

★★★★★

*Panax quinquefolius*

American Ginseng is a cooling, restorative adaptogen prized for calm energy, steady focus, and recovery from stress or illness. Unlike more stimulating ginseng types, it supports resilience without pushing the nervous system. It is best suited for people who feel depleted, overworked, or "run down," especially when heat, irritability, or overstimulation are not desired.

---

## Core Herbal Category — American Ginseng

**Primary Core: Nutritional & Tonic Support** herb with (cooling adaptogenic action that rebuilds depleted energy and supports calm resilience)
**Secondary Cores:** Nervines (Nervous System Support) herb · Immune Support herb · Metabolic & Blood Sugar Support herb · Cognitive Support herb

---

## How It Works

American Ginseng works by modulating stress response and supporting energy metabolism without overstimulation. Its ginsenosides help the body adapt to physical and mental stress, supporting steadier endurance and clearer thinking. It also supports immune balance and can improve metabolic efficiency, including healthier glucose handling in some individuals. Over time, it restores "reserve energy"—helping stamina, recovery, and mental clarity build gradually.

---

## Primary Uses

- Stress resilience and fatigue recovery
- Calm energy and endurance support
- Cognitive clarity, focus, and mental stamina
- Immune support during depletion
- Metabolic balance support (including blood sugar steadiness)

---

## Scientific Backing

American Ginseng is studied for adaptogenic effects, cognitive support, immune modulation, and metabolic balance. Key compounds include ginsenosides (notably Rb1) associated with neuroprotective and calming adaptogenic activity.

---

## 🌿 Forms Available

- Sliced dried root (decoction)
- Powder
- Capsules
- Tincture
- Standardized extracts (varied strengths)

---

## ⏱ How to Use / Dosage

**Decoction:** 1–2 tsp chopped root simmered 15–20 minutes (morning/midday).
**Tincture:** 30–60 drops up to 2× daily (avoid late day if sleep-sensitive).
**Capsules/extract:** follow label; start low.
**Cycle use:** 3–6 weeks on, then 1 week off (helps keep effects balanced).

---

## ⌛ Expected Results

- Calm energy and stress steadiness: 7–14 days
- Focus and mental stamina: 1–2 weeks
- Immune/metabolic support: 2–4 weeks
- Deep restoration: 4–8 weeks consistent use

---

## ⚠ Caution Level: ● Caution

- May lower blood sugar—monitor if on diabetes medication
- Avoid combining with heavy stimulants/high caffeine
- Can disturb sleep if taken late
- Use breaks for long-term continuous use
- Source responsibly (wild populations are vulnerable)

---

## Gender-Specific Safety (GS)

**Men — ● Safe**
Generally well tolerated; monitor blood sugar if medicated.
**Women — ● Safe**
Generally well tolerated; monitor blood sugar if medicated.
**Pregnancy / Nursing — ● Caution**
Use only with professional guidance due to metabolic effects and limited safety data in

concentrated forms.

---

## 🔄 Same / Similar Results

- Ashwagandha (more grounding; not cooling)
- Eleuthero (gentle endurance)
- Rhodiola (more stimulating; use cautiously)
- Schisandra (adaptogenic; liver support)
- Asian Ginseng (more stimulating)

---

## 📦 Shelf Life / Potency After Preparation

- Dried root: 3–5 years airtight
- Powder: 1–2 years
- Tincture: 5+ years
- Decoction: 24 hours refrigerated (best fresh)

---

## 🛠 DIY Recipe — American Ginseng Calm-Focus Tonic

Simmer 1 tsp sliced root in 2 cups water for 20 minutes. Sip morning or midday.
(Use 2–3× per week for steady resilience.)

---

## 💬 Herbal Reflections of American Ginseng

American Ginseng is quiet strength—cooling, steady, and restorative. It does not push the body; it rebuilds it. Over time, it teaches the system how to hold pressure without breaking, restoring a calm endurance that feels like true recovery.

---

## ★ Herbal Confidence Index

🌿 🌿 🌿 🌿 🌿 (5/5 green stars — cornerstone adaptogen for calm resilience, cognitive steadiness, and deep restoration; powerful yet gentle when used wisely.)

# ARJUNA

★★★★

*Terminalia arjuna*

**Arjuna** is a classic cardiac tonic that helps the heart work smarter, not harder. Its bark concentrates triterpenoid saponins (including arjunolic and arjunic acids), flavonoids, and tannins that support myocardial tone, healthy blood pressure, lipid balance, and microcirculation. Herbalists reach for Arjuna when the chest feels "overworked and under-recovered," using it to steady pulse quality, ease exertional fatigue, and support calm cardiovascular endurance.

Beyond the heart, Arjuna offers gentle antioxidant and adaptogenic support that helps the body meet stress without excess strain. Traditionally paired with Hawthorn for vascular resilience, Ashwagandha for stress load, or CoQ10 (nutraceutical) for cellular energy support, Arjuna works best alongside breath work, walking, hydration, and lighter evening meals.

Rooted in Ayurveda for over 2,500 years, Arjuna appears in classical texts as a "guardian of the heart," traditionally prepared as bark decoctions (*kashaya*) or milk decoctions (*ksheerapāka*). Riverside trees symbolized protection and endurance—mirroring the herb's steady, structural action on the heart itself.

---

## Core Herbal Category — Arjuna

*(Terminalia arjuna)*

**Primary Core: Cardiovascular System Support** herb with *(heart-tonifying principles that strengthen cardiac muscle and support healthy blood pressure)*

**Secondary Cores:** Nervous System Support herb · Circulatory Support herb · Metabolic Balance Support herb

---

## How It Works

Arjuna works by delivering tannins, flavonoids, and triterpenoid glycosides that help tone and strengthen cardiac muscle fibers. These compounds support vessel elasticity and endothelial function, promoting smoother circulation and steadier blood pressure. Antioxidant activity reduces oxidative stress in cardiovascular tissues, while metabolic effects assist lipid balance. Through gentle tonic action, Arjuna builds endurance and long-term heart resilience rather than rapid stimulation.

---

## 🌱 Primary Uses

- Cardiac tone & myocardial support
- Healthy blood pressure & pulse quality
- Circulatory comfort, angina patterns, exercise endurance
- Lipid balance (adjunct to diet & movement)
- Calm resilience under cardiovascular stress

---

## Scientific Backing

Arjuna bark contains arjunolic and arjunic acids, arjungenin, polyphenols, and flavonoids with cardiotonic, antioxidant, and endothelial-supportive actions. Small clinical studies suggest improved exercise tolerance and reduced angina frequency. Evidence is supportive but evolving; outcomes are strongest when paired with lifestyle foundations such as movement, nutrition, and sleep.

---

## Forms Available

- Bark chips (decoction)
- Powder (*churna*)
- Capsules / standardized extract
- Tincture / liquid extract
- Traditional milk decoction (*ksheerapāka*)

---

## How to Use

**Milk Decoction (*Ksheera Pāka*):**
1 tsp bark powder + ½ cup water + ½ cup milk
Simmer 8–10 minutes until reduced to ~½ cup. Strain and sip warm once daily.
**Basic Decoction:**
Simmer 1–2 tsp bark chips in 10–12 oz water for 15–20 minutes; strain.
**Capsules / Tincture:**
Use standardized products as directed.

---

## ⚠ Caution Level: Caution

- Not a substitute for prescribed cardiac care
- Coordinate use if taking BP medications, antiarrhythmics, anticoagulants, or antiplatelets
- May modestly lower blood pressure and influence platelet activity
- Avoid during pregnancy unless professionally supervised
- Discontinue 1–2 weeks before surgery
- Seek immediate care for worsening chest pain, dizziness, or palpitations

---

## 👫 Gender-Specific Safety (GS)

**Men:** Generally safe — supports cardiovascular tone and calm stamina.

**Women:** Generally safe — helpful for stress-influenced cardiovascular fluctuations.

**Pregnancy/Nursing:** Use with caution — avoid unless professionally supervised; limited safety data for higher doses.

---

## ⏳ Expected Results

- Reduced "cardiac awareness," calmer stamina: 1–2 weeks
- Improved exercise comfort & steadier pulse: 2–4 weeks
- Lipid/endothelial support: 6–8+ weeks (best with diet & movement)

---

## 🛠 DIY Recipe — Arjuna Ksheera Pāka

- 1 tsp Arjuna bark powder
- ½ cup water
- ½ cup milk (or plant milk)

Simmer uncovered 8–10 minutes until reduced to ~½ cup.
Strain and sip warm once daily (evening preferred).

---

## 🔄 Same / Similar Results

- Hawthorn
- Danshen
- Grape Seed / Pine Bark (OPCs)
- Motherwort
- Ashwagandha

---

## 📦 Shelf Life & Potency After Preparation

- Bark chips: 2–3 years (airtight, cool, dry)
- Powder (*churna*): 9–12 months
- Decoction/tea: Best within 12–24 hours
- Tincture: 4–6 years
- Milk decoction: Consume same day

---

## 🗨 Herbal Reflections of Arjuna

Arjuna offers a quiet, steady form of strength—supporting the physical heart while calming the emotional load that often accompanies cardiovascular strain. Its medicine is structural rather than stimulating, building resilience layer by layer.

Distinct among cardiac herbs, Arjuna unites myocardial toning with vessel protection, a dual action confirmed by centuries of Ayurvedic use and growing modern research. For those seeking long-term cardiovascular stability and emotional grounding, Arjuna stands as a reliable and enduring ally.

---

## ★ Herbal Confidence Index

🌿 🌿 🌿 🌿

**4 / 5** — A long-revered Ayurvedic heart tonic that strengthens cardiac muscle, supports healthy circulation and blood pressure, and promotes emotional steadiness. Arjuna earns its ancient title as the "protector of the heart" through calm endurance rather than force.

# CHUCHUHUASI

★★★★

*Maytenus krukovii*

**Chuchuhuasi** is a powerful Amazonian tonic bark traditionally used to restore strength, ease deep musculoskeletal pain, and support recovery from physical depletion. Native to Peru and Brazil, its Quechua name—often translated as "trembling back"—reflects its long-standing role in relieving joint stiffness, back pain, and rheumatic discomfort. The bark is most commonly prepared as a decoction or alcohol infusion to extract its warming, resinous compounds. Within Amazonian medicine, Chuchuhuasi is regarded as a fortifying tonic rather than a quick analgesic. It is used after illness, injury, or prolonged fatigue to rebuild strength, improve mobility, and support immune resilience. Its reputation extends to libido and hormonal vitality, particularly when depletion follows stress or physical strain.

---

## Core Herbal Category — Chuchuhuasi

*(Maytenus krukovii)*
**Primary Core: Anti-Inflammatory & Pain Support** herb with (joint-tonifying, warming principles that reduce stiffness and inflammation)
**Secondary Cores:** Immune Support herb · Nervous System Support herb · Hormonal & Endocrine Support herb

---

## How It Works

Chuchuhuasi works by calming inflammatory processes within joints and connective tissues through resinous compounds, tannins, and triterpenoids. These constituents support improved circulation to muscles and joints, helping ease stiffness and soreness. Mild nervous-system toning contributes to improved stress tolerance and physical recovery. Through steady tonic use, the herb promotes durability, flexibility, and predictable musculoskeletal relief.

---

## Primary Uses

- Joint, muscle, and back pain relief
- Rheumatic stiffness and inflammation
- Post-illness or post-injury recovery
- Immune vitality and tonic support
- Libido and stamina support during depletion

## 🧪 Scientific Backing

Chuchuhuasi contains mayteine, triterpenoids, and tannins associated with anti-inflammatory, analgesic, and immune-modulating activity. Traditional evidence is strong, though modern human clinical studies remain limited.

📚 *Journal of Natural Products · Phytomedicine · Brazilian Journal of Pharmacognosy*

---

## 🌿 Forms Available

- Dried bark (decoctions, powders)
- Alcohol tinctures (traditional preparations)

---

## 🧴 How to Use

- **Decoction:** Simmer 1–2 tsp dried bark in 2 cups water for 20–30 minutes; drink up to 1 cup twice daily
- **Traditional tincture:** Taken in small measured doses; follow professional guidance
- **Use in cycles:** 2–4 weeks on, 1 week off

---

## ⚠ Caution Level: ● Caution

- Avoid during pregnancy (traditional uterine-stimulating use)
- May cause digestive upset in sensitive individuals
- Monitor carefully if using immune-modulating or anti-inflammatory medications
- Discontinue if unusual reactions occur

---

## 🧬 Gender-Specific Safety (GS)

**Men:** ● Generally Safe — Supports joint comfort, stamina, and vitality

**Women:** ● Generally Safe — Helpful for pain and fatigue recovery

**Pregnancy/Nursing:** ● Avoid — Insufficient safety data; traditional cautions apply

---

## ⌛ Expected Results

- Joint and muscle comfort: 3–7 days
- Improved mobility and recovery: 1–2 weeks
- Stamina and vitality support: 1–3 weeks

---

## 🛠 DIY Recipe — Chuchuhuasi Decoction

- 1½ tsp dried bark

Simmer 25–30 minutes → Strain → Drink 1–2 cups daily

---

## 🔄 Same / Similar Results

Cat's Claw · Turmeric · Devil's Claw · Muira Puama

---

## Shelf Life & Potency After Preparation

- Dried bark: 3–5 years
- Powder: 1–2 years
- Tincture: 5–7+ years
- Decoction: Use within 24 hours

---

## Herbal Reflections of Chuchuhuasi

Chuchuhuasi is a medicine of endurance—warming, grounding, and restorative. It does not rush relief but rebuilds strength where pain and fatigue have taken hold. Among musculoskeletal tonics, it stands apart for its deep structural support and long-term resilience. Used respectfully, it restores movement, confidence, and physical steadiness.

---

**Herbal Confidence Index:** (4 / 5)

*A potent Amazonian tonic bark supporting joints, stamina, and immune resilience through steady, restorative action.*

# DULSE

★★★★

*Palmaria palmata*

**Dulse** is a mineral-rich red sea vegetable traditionally consumed along the cold Atlantic coasts of Ireland, Iceland, Canada, and Northern Europe. Valued as both food and medicine, it provides concentrated iodine, iron, potassium, and trace minerals that modern diets often lack. Its mild, savory flavor allows for regular use as nourishment rather than short-term therapy.
In herbal nutrition, Dulse supports thyroid signaling, mineral replenishment, and gentle detoxification. Unlike stimulant herbs, it works slowly and steadily, rebuilding reserves at the cellular level and supporting blood, skin, hair, and metabolic balance.

---

## Core Herbal Category — Dulse

*(Palmaria palmata)*
**Primary Core: Nutritional & Tonic Support** herb with (mineral-replenishing principles that restore cellular nutrient balance)
**Secondary Cores:** Hormonal & Endocrine Support herb · Kidney & Urinary Support herb · Digestive Support herb

---

## How It Works

Dulse works by supplying highly bioavailable minerals that support thyroid signaling, red blood cell formation, and cellular energy production. Its iodine content assists endocrine communication, while polysaccharides support gentle detoxification through renal pathways. Digestive toning improves nutrient absorption, allowing long-term rebuilding rather than quick stimulation.

---

## Primary Uses

- Thyroid and endocrine nourishment
- Mineral and trace-element replenishment
- Blood and iron support
- Gentle detoxification
- Skin, hair, and nail strengthening

---

## 🧪 Scientific Backing

Dulse contains iodine, iron, potassium, antioxidants, and polysaccharides associated with endocrine support and cellular protection.

📚 *Marine Drugs · Journal of Applied Phycology*

---

## 🌿 Forms Available

• Dried whole leaves or flakes
• Powder (food or capsules)
• Culinary seaweed blends

---

## 🧂 How to Use

• Flakes: 1–2 tsp daily on food
• Powder: 500–1,000 mg daily
• Culinary use in soups, grains, vegetables

---

## ⚠ Caution Level: 🟠 Caution

• High iodine content — avoid excess
• Use moderately in thyroid disorders
• Source from clean waters only

---

## 🧬 Gender-Specific Safety (GS)

**Men:** 🟢 Generally Safe
**Women:** 🟢 Generally Safe — Especially helpful for low iron
**Pregnancy/Nursing:** 🟡 Use With Caution — Food-level use only

---

## ⏳ Expected Results

• Energy and thyroid support: 7–10 days
• Mineral replenishment: 4–8 weeks

---

## 🌿 Herbal Reflections of Dulse

Dulse reminds us that nourishment itself can be medicine. Quiet, steady, and deeply rebuilding, it restores what modern life depletes. As a daily tonic food, it bridges nutrition and herbalism with uncommon elegance.

⭐ **Herbal Confidence Index:** 🌿 🌿 🌿 🌿 (4 / 5) Reliable, mineral-rich nutritive sea vegetable that supports long-term nourishment and metabolic balance, with excellent safety when used in moderate amounts.

# ELEUTHERO

★★★★★

*Eleutherococcus senticosus*

**Eleuthero** is a foundational adaptogenic root long valued for building long-term stamina, immune strength, and resistance to physical and mental stress. Native to Northeast Asia and widely studied in Russian herbal and sports medicine, it earned the nickname "Siberian Ginseng" for its endurance-building qualities—though it is gentler and less stimulating than true ginsengs. Rather than producing a quick surge of energy, Eleuthero strengthens baseline capacity, making it especially useful during chronic fatigue, recovery from illness, and sustained mental or physical demand.

Traditionally used by laborers, soldiers, and athletes, Eleuthero supports consistent performance under pressure while protecting against burnout. Its value lies in normalization—helping the body meet stress efficiently without pushing it beyond sustainable limits.

---

## 🌿 Core Herbal Category — Eleuthero

*(Eleutherococcus senticosus)*
**Primary Core: Adaptogens** herb with (tonic principles that increase stress resistance and sustainable endurance)
**Secondary Cores:** Immune Support herb · Nervous System Support herb · Metabolic Balance Support herb

---

## 🌿 How It Works

Eleuthero works by supporting coordination between the adrenal glands, immune system, and nervous system. Its eleutherosides improve cellular energy efficiency and oxygen utilization, particularly during exertion. Rather than stimulating, the herb strengthens adaptive response, allowing the body to remain balanced under ongoing physical or emotional stress. Over time, this results in steadier energy, improved focus, and enhanced resilience.

---

## 🌱 Primary Uses

- Long-term stress resilience
- Physical stamina and endurance
- Mental clarity under pressure

• Immune recovery after illness or exhaustion
• Support during demanding routines

---

## 🧪 Scientific Backing

Research demonstrates Eleuthero's ability to improve work capacity, immune response (notably natural killer cell activity), cognitive performance under stress, and fatigue resistance. It has been extensively studied in Soviet and post-Soviet sports and occupational medicine.

📚 *Journal of Ethnopharmacology · Planta Medica · International Journal of Sports Nutrition*

---

## 🌿 Forms Available

• Dried root (tea or decoction)
• Tincture
• Capsules
• Standardized extracts (eleutherosides)

---

## 🧴 How to Use

• **Decoction:** Simmer 1–2 tsp dried root in 2 cups water for 20 minutes; drink up to 2 cups daily
• **Tincture:** 30–60 drops once or twice daily (morning/early afternoon)
• **Capsules/Extracts:** Follow standardized dosing
• **Cycle:** Use 3–6 weeks, then take a 1-week break

---

## ⚠ Caution Level: ● Caution

• May mildly raise blood pressure in some individuals
• Avoid late-day use (may disrupt sleep)
• Avoid during acute infections or fever
• Use caution with stimulant, sedative, or cardiac medications
• Avoid during pregnancy unless professionally supervised

---

## 🧬 Gender-Specific Safety (GS)

**Men:** ● Generally Safe — Supports stamina, focus, and endurance
**Women:** ● Generally Safe — Helpful for fatigue, immune recovery, and stress balance
**Pregnancy/Nursing:** ● Use With Caution — Limited safety data; avoid unless supervised

---

## ⏳ Expected Results

• Improved stress tolerance: 7–10 days

• Increased stamina and endurance: 2–4 weeks
• Immune and cognitive support: 2–3 weeks

---

## 🛠 DIY Recipe — Eleuthero Endurance Decoction

• 1½ tsp dried Eleuthero root
• Optional: 1 tsp Licorice root
Simmer 20 minutes → Strain → Drink in the morning

---

## 🔄 Same / Similar Results

● Ashwagandha · ● Rhodiola Rosea · ● Gynostemma · ● Panax Ginseng

---

## 📦 Shelf Life & Potency After Preparation

• Dried root: 3–5 years
• Powdered extract: ~2 years
• Capsules: 1–2 years
• Tincture: 5+ years
• Decoction: Best within 24 hours

---

## 🌿 Herbal Reflections of Eleuthero

Eleuthero is the working person's adaptogen—quiet, steady, and deeply protective. It does not force energy but builds it patiently, reinforcing the body's ability to endure stress without collapse. Among adaptogens, it stands as one of the most reliable allies for sustainable performance and long-term resilience.

⭐ **Herbal Confidence Index:** 🌿 🌿 🌿 🌿 🌿 (5 / 5)

*A cornerstone adaptogen for stamina, immune defense, and stress resilience—effective without overstimulation.*

# GYNOSTEMMA

★★★★★

*Gynostemma pentaphyllum*

**Gynostemma,** also known as **Jiaogulan**, is a revered adaptogenic vine native to southern China and Southeast Asia. Often called the **"Herb of Immortality,"** it is traditionally consumed as a daily tea in longevity regions where vitality and cardiovascular health are notably strong. Though sometimes compared to ginseng, Gynostemma is gentler, cooling, and more self-regulating in nature.

Rich in gypenosides—structurally similar to ginsenosides—Gynostemma supports endurance, metabolic balance, immune strength, and emotional steadiness. Its appeal lies in its ability to energize when depleted and calm when overstimulated, making it exceptionally well suited to modern stress patterns.

---

## Core Herbal Category — Gynostemma

*(Gynostemma pentaphyllum)*

**Primary Core: Adaptogens herb** with (longevity-tonifying principles that strengthen whole-body resilience)

**Secondary Cores:** Cardiovascular Support herb · Metabolic Balance Support herb · Immune Support herb

---

## How It Works

Gynostemma works by modulating stress hormone signaling while protecting vascular and mitochondrial tissues from oxidative strain. Its gypenosides support lipid metabolism, insulin sensitivity, and immune regulation. Rather than stimulating or sedating, the herb restores balance, helping multiple systems function efficiently over time.

---

## Primary Uses

- Longevity and vitality support
- Cardiovascular and cholesterol balance
- Stress regulation and emotional steadiness
- Blood-sugar and metabolic support
- Immune system strengthening

## 🧪 Scientific Backing

Research shows Gynostemma supports cortisol regulation, lipid metabolism, mitochondrial energy production, insulin sensitivity, and immune modulation. Its gypenosides share functional similarities with ginseng compounds while remaining gentler and more adaptable.

📚 *Journal of Medicinal Food · Phytomedicine · Chinese Journal of Integrative Medicine*

---

## 🌿 Forms Available

- Dried leaf tea
- Powdered standardized extract
- Capsules
- Longevity and adaptogen blends

---

## 🧴 How to Use

- **Tea:** Steep 1–2 tsp dried leaf in hot water for 5–10 minutes; drink 1–3 cups daily
- **Extracts/Capsules:** Use standardized gypenoside formulas as directed
- **Cycle:** 6–8 weeks on, 1 week off for long-term use

---

## ⚠ Caution Level: 🟠 Caution

- May lower blood pressure or blood sugar
- Monitor if using antihypertensive or antidiabetic medications
- Avoid during pregnancy (insufficient safety data)
- Periodic breaks recommended with prolonged use

---

## 🧬 Gender-Specific Safety (GS)

**Men:** 🟢 Generally Safe — Supports stamina, cardiovascular balance, and clarity

**Women:** 🟢 Generally Safe — Helpful for stress regulation and metabolic support

**Pregnancy/Nursing:** 🟡 Use With Caution — Avoid concentrated extracts; tea only under guidance

---

## ⏳ Expected Results

- Emotional balance and energy: 3–7 days
- Stress resilience and focus: 1–2 weeks
- Metabolic and cardiovascular benefits: 2–4+ weeks

---

## 🛠 DIY Recipe — Gynostemma Longevity Tea

• 1 tsp Gynostemma leaf
• Optional: ½ tsp Licorice root or Lemon peel
Steep 7–10 minutes → Drink 1–2 times daily

---

## Same / Similar Results

Eleuthero · Ashwagandha · Rhodiola Rosea · Schisandra

---

## Shelf Life & Potency After Preparation

• Dried leaves: ~2 years
• Powdered extract: 2+ years
• Capsules: 1–2 years
• Prepared tea: 12–24 hours

## Herbal Reflections of Gynostemma

Gynostemma's medicine is balance itself—energizing without agitation and calming without dullness. It harmonizes the heart, metabolism, immune system, and emotional body, making it one of the most complete longevity tonics known. Its quiet power explains why it has been cherished for generations as a daily ally for sustained health. **Herbal Confidence Index:** (5 / 5)

*A premier longevity adaptogen supporting cardiovascular health, metabolic balance, immune strength, and calm vitality.*

# MARSHMALLOW

★★★★★

*Althaea officinalis*

**Marshmallow** is a soft, soothing herb traditionally used to calm inflammation, ease dry coughs, and protect irritated mucous membranes. Native to Europe, Western Asia, and North Africa, its primary medicinal value lies in the root, which is rich in mucilage—a thick, gel-like polysaccharide that coats, cools, and shields inflamed tissues when taken internally or applied externally.

Used for centuries in Western herbalism as well as Greek and Arabic medicine, Marshmallow is deeply hydrating and cooling in nature. It is especially valuable for conditions marked by dryness, heat, and irritation—whether in the throat, lungs, stomach, bladder, or skin—making it one of the most gentle and universally supportive herbs in traditional practice.

---

## Core Herbal Category — Marshmallow

*(Althaea officinalis)*
**Primary Core: Digestive System Support** herb with (demulcent mucilage that soothes and protects irritated mucosal tissues)
**Secondary Cores:** Respiratory Support herb · Kidney & Urinary System Support herb · Skin Support herb

---

## How It Works

Marshmallow works by releasing soothing mucilage that forms a protective coating over irritated tissues. This demulcent action reduces friction, inflammation, and exposure to digestive acids or environmental irritants, allowing damaged mucosa to heal more efficiently. In the respiratory tract, it moistens dry tissues and calms cough reflexes. In the urinary system, it eases irritation by cooling inflamed linings and reducing heat and discomfort. Through gentle protection rather than stimulation, Marshmallow restores comfort and tissue integrity.

---

## Primary Uses

- Soothes sore throat and dry, irritated cough
- Coats and calms inflamed stomach lining (gastritis, ulcers)

- Eases urinary tract irritation and burning
- Calms skin irritation, rashes, and minor burns
- Gently relieves dry constipation

---

## 🧪 Scientific Backing

Marshmallow Root contains high levels of mucilaginous polysaccharides that form a protective film over mucous membranes, reducing irritation and supporting tissue repair. Research supports its traditional use for dry coughs, gastritis, ulcers, urinary tract irritation, and mild skin inflammation.

📚 *Journal of Ethnopharmacology · Avicenna Journal of Phytomedicine*

---

## 🌿 Forms Available

- Dried root (best for cold infusion)
- Powder (capsules, smoothies)
- Tincture
- Poultices, salves, and topical preparations

---

## 🧴 How to Use

**Cold Infusion (preferred method):**
1–2 Tbsp dried Marshmallow root
8–10 oz cold water
Soak 4–8 hours (or overnight), strain, drink 1–3× daily
**Hot Tea:**
Steep in hot water (less mucilage, still soothing)
**Topical:**
Apply poultice or salve to burns, rashes, or irritated skin

---

## ⚠ Caution Level: ● Safe (Mild Advisory)

- Extremely gentle and well tolerated
- High mucilage content may slow medication absorption — separate doses by ~2 hours
- May mildly lower blood sugar — monitor if on diabetes medication
- Avoid very heavy doses with intestinal blockage
- Safe for children; pregnancy generally safe (leaf is often gentler)

---

## 🧬 Gender-Specific Safety (GS)

**Men:** ● Generally Safe — Excellent for throat, gut, urinary, and skin support
**Women:** ● Generally Safe — Helpful for gastritis, urinary irritation, and dry cough

**Pregnancy/Nursing:** Generally Safe — Food-level use and cold infusions well tolerated

---

## ⌛ Expected Results

- Throat, urinary, and digestive soothing: within hours
- Mucosal healing and comfort: 3–7 days with consistent use

---

## DIY Recipe — Marshmallow Cold Infusion

1 Tbsp Marshmallow root
8 oz cold water
Soak overnight → Strain in the morning
Drink 1–2 cups daily for throat, gut, or bladder support

---

## Same / Similar Results

Slippery Elm · Licorice Root · Plantain Leaf · Comfrey (topical; internal caution)

---

## Shelf Life / Potency After Preparation

- Dried root: 2–3 years
- Powder: 1–2 years
- Tincture: 4–6 years
- Cold infusion: Best within 24 hours
- Topical salve: ~1 year

---

## Herbal Reflections of Marshmallow

Marshmallow embodies gentle healing. Wherever heat, dryness, or irritation take hold, it brings cooling moisture and protection. Rather than suppressing symptoms, it shields tissues so the body can repair itself naturally.

This nurturing quality is why Marshmallow is trusted for children, elders, and those recovering from illness. Foundational in digestive, respiratory, and urinary formulas, it offers calm restoration—quietly reminding the body how to heal.

**Herbal Confidence Index:** (5 / 5)

*A cornerstone demulcent for the throat, lungs, stomach, and urinary tract. Exceptionally safe, deeply soothing, and essential for foundational herbal education.*

# PAU D'ARCO

★★★★

*Tabebuia impetiginosa*

**Pau d'Arco** is the inner bark of a towering rainforest tree native to Central and South America. Known traditionally as *taheebo* or *lapacho*, it has been used for centuries by Indigenous healers as a cleansing and protective remedy during times of infection, inflammation, and chronic weakness. Its reputation as a strengthening "protector herb" reflects its long-standing role in supporting resilience under harsh environmental and physiological conditions.

The bark's primary bioactive compounds—lapachol and beta-lapachone—exhibit antifungal, antibacterial, antiviral, and anti-inflammatory activity in laboratory studies. Traditionally prepared as a decoction, Pau d'Arco has been used for fungal overgrowth, respiratory congestion, inflammatory discomfort, and immune depletion. In modern herbal practice, it remains respected as a cleansing, immune-supportive herb when used in measured cycles.

---

## Core Herbal Category — Pau d'Arco

*(botanical synonym: Handroanthus impetiginosus)*
**Primary Core: Antimicrobial Support** herb with (antifungal and antimicrobial principles that assist the body in resisting pathogenic overgrowth)
**Secondary Cores:** Liver Support herb · Anti-Inflammatory Support herb · Respiratory Support herb

---

## How It Works

Pau d'Arco works by supplying naturally occurring quinones that inhibit the growth of certain fungi, bacteria, and viruses. These compounds support immune defense while helping reduce inflammatory signaling in tissues. The herb also assists hepatic detoxification pathways involved in blood filtration and metabolic waste processing. Through measured, time-limited use, Pau d'Arco promotes immune balance, reduced microbial burden, and clearer respiratory and circulatory function.

---

## Primary Uses

- Supports resistance to fungal overgrowth (including Candida)
- Strengthens immune response during chronic or recurrent infections

• Reduces inflammation and inflammatory discomfort
• Assists liver-supported detoxification
• Supports respiratory and systemic resilience

---

## 🧪 Scientific Backing

Laboratory and preclinical studies document Pau d'Arco's activity against *Candida albicans*, select bacteria, parasites, and inflammatory pathways via lapachol and beta-lapachone. Evidence supports antimicrobial and anti-inflammatory potential, though large-scale human trials remain limited.

📚 *Journal of Ethnopharmacology · Planta Medica · Antimicrobial Agents and Chemotherapy*

---

## 🌿 Forms Available

• Dried inner bark (decoctions)
• Capsules
• Tinctures / liquid extracts
• Traditional Amazonian preparations

---

## How to Use

**Decoction (preferred method):**
1–2 Tbsp dried inner bark
Simmer in 4 cups water for 15–20 minutes
Strain → Drink 1–2 cups daily
**Capsules / Tincture:**
Use standardized products as directed
**Cycling:**
Use 1–2 weeks on, followed by 1 week off to avoid excess accumulation of active compounds.

---

## ⚠ Caution Level: Caution

• May cause nausea or digestive irritation at higher doses
• Long-term continuous use is not recommended
• Use caution with anticoagulants, antiplatelet drugs, or chemotherapy agents
• Discontinue if gastrointestinal discomfort develops
• Avoid during pregnancy and nursing

---

## Gender-Specific Safety (GS)

**Men:** Generally Safe — Supports immune cleansing and microbial balance
**Women:** Generally Safe — Useful for fungal and inflammatory support
**Pregnancy/Nursing:** Avoid — Insufficient safety data; traditional avoidance advised

## ⌛ Expected Results

- Symptom relief during infections: 3–5 days
- Fungal load reduction & immune balance: 2–4 weeks (with cycling)
- Reduced inflammatory burden: gradual and cumulative

---

## 🛠 DIY Recipe — Pau d'Arco Antifungal Decoction

2 Tbsp Pau d'Arco bark
4 cups water
Optional: cinnamon stick or 2–3 cloves
Simmer 20 minutes → Strain → Drink 1–2 cups daily

---

## 🔄 Same / Similar Results

● Olive Leaf · ● Oregon Grape Root · ● Black Walnut Hull · ● Goldenseal (short-term use only)

---

## 📦 Shelf Life / Potency After Preparation

- Dried bark: 3–5 years
- Capsules: 1–2 years
- Tincture: 5–7+ years
- Decoction: Best within 24–36 hours

---

## 🌿 Herbal Reflections of Pau d'Arco

Pau d'Arco carries the cleansing strength of the rainforest—firm but disciplined. It addresses microbial excess and inflammatory stagnation without forcing the body, making it valuable in longer-term cleansing and immune-rebuilding strategies.

While modern herbalism offers many "detox" trends, Pau d'Arco remains a sober, time-tested ally when resilience, patience, and balance are required. Used respectfully and in cycles, it supports internal clarity and steady recovery rather than quick suppression.

⭐ **Herbal Confidence Index:** 🌿 🌿 🌿 🌿 (4 / 5)

*A respected antimicrobial and immune-supportive bark with strong traditional use and supportive research. Effective when used cyclically and with attention to safety considerations.*

# SHILAJIT

★★★★★

*Asphaltum punjabianum*

Ancient Mineral Resin of Strength and Vitality

**Shilajit** is not a plant but a rare herbo-mineral resin that seeps from high-altitude rocks in the Himalayas and other mountain ranges, formed over centuries by the slow decomposition of plants and microbes. Sticky, dark, and tar-like in texture, it has long been revered in Ayurveda as a rasayana — **a rejuvenating substance that restores strength, endurance, and resilience. Traditionally called the "Destroyer of Weakness," Shilajit is seen as a potent ally for stamina, mental clarity, and deep tissue repair, especially in those depleted by stress, age, or illness. What sets Shilajit apart is its rich composition of more than 80 trace minerals, fulvic acid, and humic substances, which work together to enhance energy metabolism, detoxification, and cellular regeneration. Modern herbalists and researchers alike regard it as a broad-spectrum adaptogen, supporting sexual vitality, immunity, cognitive function, and recovery from fatigue.** In both ancient texts and modern practice, **Shilajit is celebrated as a bridge between earth and body** — a dense, restorative essence that feeds resilience from the deepest levels upward.

---

## Core Herbal Category — Shilajit

*(Asphaltum / Mineral Pitch)*

**Primary Core: Adaptogens herb** with (energy-restorative principles that support longevity, stamina, and stress resilience)

**Secondary Cores:** Hormonal & Endocrine Support **herb** · Nervous System Support **herb** · Nutritive Support **herb**

---

## How It Works

Shilajit works by supplying bioavailable minerals and fulvic compounds that enhance cellular energy production.

These compounds improve mitochondrial efficiency and physical stamina over time.

The herb supports hormonal signaling by nourishing endocrine tissues and adaptive stress response.

Its mineral-rich profile assists nervous-system nourishment and cognitive clarity.

Through steady use, Shilajit restores vitality, resilience, and long-term metabolic strength.

---

## 🌱 Primary Uses

- Boosts stamina, energy, and physical performance
- Enhances memory and brain function
- Supports testosterone and libido in men
- Strengthens immunity and detox pathways
- Aids nutrient absorption and anti-aging

---

## 🧪 Scientific Backing

Research shows Shilajit:

- Enhances **mitochondrial energy output**
- Raises **testosterone** in men (clinical evidence)
- Improves **cognitive protection** against oxidative stress
- Reduces **inflammation** via fulvic acid
- Supports **nutrient transport** and absorption

📚 *Journal of Ethnopharmacology* • *Andrologia* • *Phytotherapy Research*

---

## 🍃 Forms Available

- Purified resin (strongest and most traditional)
- Capsules / powders
- Tinctures and adaptogenic blends

---

## 🧂 How to Use

- **Resin (best method):**

Dissolve pea-sized amount (300–500 mg) in warm water or milk
1–2× daily

- **Powder/Capsules:**

250–500 mg per dose

- **Timing:**

Morning or early afternoon
May be taken with meals for better absorption

- **Cycle:**

6–8 weeks on → 1–2 weeks off

---

## ⚠️ Caution Level: Caution

- Only use **purified, lab-tested** Shilajit
- Avoid raw/unprocessed forms (risk of heavy metals)
- Not recommended for individuals with **gout**
- Avoid in **pregnancy** and **hemochromatosis**
- May interact with blood pressure or diabetes medications

---

## Gender-Specific Safety (GS)

**Men:** Generally Safe — Beneficial for vitality, testosterone, endurance, and immunity.

**Women:** Generally Safe — Supports energy, cognition, and nutrient absorption; avoid high doses if prone to excess heat.

**Pregnancy/Nursing:** Avoid — Not recommended due to hormonal, detox, and mineral-concentration effects.

---

## Expected Results

- Increased energy & mental clarity: **3–7 days**
- Hormonal & testosterone support: **2–4 weeks**
- Enhanced stamina & recovery: **2–3 weeks**

---

## DIY Recipe — Shilajit Vitality Tonic

- Pea-sized amount of Shilajit resin
- Warm milk or nut milk
- Optional: ½ tsp Ashwagandha
- Optional: honey + cinnamon

Stir until dissolved → Drink in the morning or midday for energy and focus.

---

## Same/Similar Results

**Ashwagandha** – Stress resilience + deep vitality

**Tongkat Ali** – Testosterone & energy enhancer

**Panax Ginseng** – Stamina & cognitive clarity

**Maca Root** – Libido & hormonal balance

---

## Shelf Life / Potency After Preparation

- **Purified resin:** 3–5+ years
- **Powder/Capsules:** 1–2 years
- **Tinctures:** 3–5 years
- **Prepared tonic:** Best consumed immediately (within 2–4 hours)

---

## Herbal Reflections of Shilajit

Shilajit stands at the crossroads between earth and vitality—a resin formed by time, pressure, and the transformation of ancient herbal material. Its strength lies not in superficial stimulation but in supporting the body's deepest systems.

By enhancing mitochondrial function, Shilajit reawakens the bioenergy that stress, age, and depletion diminish. Its fulvic-acid-rich matrix enhances nutrient absorption, detoxifies cells, supports hormones, and sharpens the mind.

While timeless in tradition, its true value today lies in purity and proper preparation—only clean, well-tested resin delivers its profound rejuvenating effect.

---

## Herbal Confidence Index

**(5 / 5)**

A revered Himalayan substance that restores strength, stamina, and clarity by nourishing cells at the deepest level. Shilajit enhances testosterone, detoxification, energy metabolism, and nutrient absorption, earning its place among the greatest longevity tonics in natural medicine.

# SKULLCAP

★★★★★

*Scutellaria lateriflora*

**Skullcap is a soothing nervine herb long valued in Western and Traditional Chinese Medicine for its calming effects on the nervous system.** The two most common types used medicinally are American Skullcap (Scutellaria lateriflora) and Chinese Skullcap (Scutellaria baicalensis). While Chinese Skullcap is often used for its anti-inflammatory and immune-boosting properties, **American Skullcap is best known for its ability to quiet the mind, relax the body, and relieve anxiety and stress-induced tension.**
**Traditionally used for treating insomnia, nervous exhaustion, tremors, and muscle spasms, Skullcap supports emotional balance, eases nervous irritability, and restores depleted nerves. It's a go-to herb for those struggling with mental restlessness, especially at night.**

---

### Core Herbal Category — Skullcap
*(Scutellaria lateriflora)*

**Primary Core: Nervous System Support (Nervines) (Nervous System Support) herb** with (calming, restorative flavonoid action that settles nervous tension and supports emotional balance)
**Secondary Cores:** Sleep Support **herb** · Musculoskeletal Support **herb**

---

## How It Works

Skullcap works by calming overactive nervous-system signaling and easing mental agitation.
Its flavonoid compounds help reduce stress-related tension in both mind and body.
The herb supports emotional balance by gently stabilizing mood and nervous response.
Muscle-relaxing action helps release physical tightness linked to chronic stress.
Through restorative nervous-system support, Skullcap promotes relaxation, clarity, and recovery.

---

## Primary Uses

• Eases anxiety and emotional stress
• Supports restful sleep and insomnia relief
• Calms nervous tension and irritability
• Relieves muscle spasms and mild tremors
• Restores and nourishes the nervous system

---

## Forms Available — Skullcap

• Dried aerial parts (for tea, infusion, or blends)
• Tincture / liquid extract (most reliable and commonly used form)
• Capsules (powdered herb or standardized extract)
• Glycerite (excellent option for children or alcohol-sensitive individuals)
• Fresh plant tincture (preferred by many herbalists for strong nervine action)
• Tea blends (paired with Passionflower, Lemon Balm, Chamomile, or Hops for calming synergy)

---

## How to Use

**Tea:**
• 1–2 tsp dried Skullcap
• Steep in hot water for **10 minutes**
• Use 2–3× daily for anxiety, or once in the evening for sleep
**Tincture:**
• 20–40 drops, up to 3× daily
**Forms:**
• Liquid extracts
• Combination formulas with other nervines

## Scientific Backing

Research confirms that Skullcap:
• Exhibits **anxiolytic** (anti-anxiety) effects
• Enhances **GABA activity** in the brain
• Offers mild **sedative and neuroprotective** benefits
• Helps restore healthy sleep without dependency
*Journal of Ethnopharmacology* • *Alternative Medicine Review*

---

## Caution Level: Caution

• Best used in moderate doses; long-term use should be cycled
• Avoid combining with alcohol or sedative drugs
• Ensure the correct species (**American Skullcap**)—avoid toxic substitutes

• Avoid during pregnancy unless advised by a professional

---

## 👥 Gender-Specific Safety (GS)

**Men:** 🟢 Generally Safe — Excellent for tension, anxiety, and sleep imbalance.
**Women:** 🟢 Generally Safe — Helpful for emotional overwhelm, nervous exhaustion, and stress-related tension.
**Pregnancy/Nursing:** 🟡 Mild Caution — Not preferred unless supervised; gentler nervines may be better.

---

## ⏳ Expected Results

- Noticeable calming: **30–60 minutes**
- Improved sleep: **same night** or within 1–3 days
- Nervous system rebuilding: **5–7 days** of consistent use

---

## 🛠 DIY Recipe — Skullcap Sleepy-Time Tea

- 1 tsp dried Skullcap
- 1 tsp Lemon Balm
- Steep in 10 oz hot water for 10 minutes

Drink 30 minutes before bed for restful sleep.

---

## 🌿 Same/Similar Results

🟢 **Lavender** – Relaxes the nervous system & promotes sleep onset (aromatic calming herb)
🟢 **Passionflower** – Eases anxiety & insomnia (GABA enhancer)
🟢 **Lemon Balm** – Uplifts mood & calms nervous tension
🟢 **Valerian Root** – Strong sedative & muscle relaxant
🟡 **Hops** – Deep sedative; stronger sleep herb

---

## 📦 Shelf Life / Potency After Preparation

- **Dried herb:** 2–3 years
- **Tincture:** 4–6 years
- **Capsules:** 1–2 years
- **Tea (prepared):** Best within **24 hours** refrigerated

---

## Herbal Reflections of Skullcap

Skullcap is one of the most reliable herbs for easing the weight of stress, emotional strain, and overactivity of the mind. Its magic lies in its ability to calm without clouding—creating mental spaciousness and quieting the chatter of anxious thoughts.

Traditionally used for nervous tics, tremors, trauma recovery, and chronic tension, Skullcap doesn't merely sedate. It **nourishes** the nervous system, giving the body what it needs to rebuild balance and inner steadiness.

For those carrying grief, exhaustion, or the tightness of long-term stress, Skullcap offers peace, rest, and gentle repair.

## Herbal Confidence Index

**(5 / 5)**

A premier nervine tonic that quiets the mind, eases anxiety, restores the nervous system, and supports deep restorative sleep without fog or dependence. Skullcap offers calm, steadiness, and emotional ease—making it a cornerstone herb for stress relief and mental resilience.

# YERBA MATÉ

★★★★

*Ilex paraguariensis*

**Yerba Mate** is a South American evergreen whose leaves brew a steady, clear lift—alert but grounded. Rich in naturally occurring xanthines (caffeine, theobromine, theophylline), chlorogenic acids, and saponins, it supports mental focus, sustained energy, mood, digestion, and metabolic tone without the abrupt crash often associated with coffee. Herbalists traditionally use it as a daytime tonic for cognitive endurance, physical stamina, and antioxidant defense.

Rooted in Guaraní tradition and later adopted by Jesuit missions ("Jesuit tea"), Yerba Mate is as much ritual as remedy. Shared from a gourd (*mate*) through a metal straw (*bombilla*), it represents fellowship and continuity. Traditional preparations include hot infusions and *tereré* (cold-brewed mate, especially in Paraguay). Modern air-dried ("sin humo") varieties are now preferred for their cleaner flavor and reduced smoke exposure. Beyond physiology, Yerba Mate remains a cultural anchor—uniting clarity, nourishment, and social connection.

---

## Core Herbal Category — Yerba Maté

*(Ilex paraguariensis)*
**Primary Core: Nervous System Support (Nervines)** herb with (stimulating principles that enhance alertness and cognitive endurance)
**Secondary Cores:** Metabolic Balance Support herb · Digestive Support herb · Cardiovascular Support herb

---

## How It Works

Yerba Mate works by stimulating the central nervous system through naturally occurring xanthines, increasing alertness, focus, and sustained mental performance. Its chlorogenic acids and polyphenols provide antioxidant protection that helps moderate inflammatory and oxidative stress. Bitter compounds and saponins support digestive activity and lipid metabolism. Through balanced stimulation rather than sharp excitation, Yerba Mate promotes mental clarity, physical stamina, and steady circulatory tone.

---

## Primary Uses

- Enhances alertness, focus, and mental stamina

• Supports physical endurance and daytime energy
• Aids digestion through bitter stimulation
• Provides antioxidant protection
• Supports healthy metabolic and circulatory tone

---

## 🧪 Scientific Backing

Yerba Mate contains polyphenols, chlorogenic acids, saponins, and xanthines that contribute to antioxidant, metabolic, and cognitive effects. Research supports benefits for alertness, lipid metabolism, digestive stimulation, and antioxidant defense.
📚 *Journal of Agricultural and Food Chemistry · Phytotherapy Research · Nutrition & Metabolism*

---

## 🌿 Forms Available

• Loose-leaf tea
• Tea bags
• Powdered extracts
• Capsules
• Bottled / ready-to-drink preparations
• Traditional gourd & bombilla use

---

## 🧉 How to Use

**Traditional Method:**
Fill gourd ~⅓ with dried leaves, moisten with cool water, then add hot (not boiling) water. Sip through a bombilla; refill multiple times.
**Modern Infusion:**
Steep 1–2 tsp dried leaves in hot water for 5–10 minutes; strain before drinking.
**Cold Brew (*Tereré*):**
Steep leaves in cool water; drink chilled, often with citrus or herbs.
Best used earlier in the day.

---

## ⚠ Caution Level: 🟠 Caution

• Contains caffeine — may cause insomnia, anxiety, or palpitations
• Use cautiously with arrhythmias or uncontrolled hypertension
• Avoid excessive daily intake
• Traditional smoke-dried mate consumed very hot has been associated with increased cancer risk; modern air-dried ("sin humo") products reduce this concern
• Limit use during pregnancy and nursing

---

## Gender-Specific Safety (GS)

**Men:** Generally Safe — Supports energy, stamina, digestion, and circulation
**Women:** Generally Safe — Beneficial for focus and daytime energy; monitor caffeine sensitivity
**Pregnancy/Nursing:** Use With Caution — Small, occasional amounts may be acceptable; avoid high intake

---

## Expected Results

- Increased alertness and digestive stimulation: hours to days
- Improved stamina and metabolic tone: 2–4 weeks with regular use

---

## DIY Recipe — Yerba Mate Citrus Refresher

Brew strong Yerba Mate → Chill
Add fresh lemon and orange juice
Serve over ice with mint for a cooling, energizing tonic

---

## Same / Similar Results

Green Tea · Guarana · Matcha · Black Tea · Kola Nut

---

## Shelf Life / Potency After Preparation

- Dried leaf: 1–2 years
- Powder/extract: 1–2 years
- Bottled mate: follow manufacturer guidance
- Brewed tea: best within 24 hours refrigerated

---

## Herbal Reflections of Yerba Mate

Yerba Mate occupies a rare position in herbal medicine—stimulating yet grounding, energizing yet socially centering. Its balanced chemistry delivers clarity without chaos and stamina without collapse.

Whether shared in a circle or brewed alone, Yerba Mate reminds us that energy is not merely fuel, but rhythm. When used thoughtfully, it sharpens attention, supports vitality, and connects individuals to both tradition and community.

---

**Herbal Confidence Index:** (4 / 5)

*A respected nervine stimulant that enhances focus, endurance, and metabolic tone while offering strong antioxidant support. Best used with moderation and awareness of caffeine sensitivity.*

# LEMONGRASS

★★★★

*Cymbopogon citratus*

**Lemon Grass** is a fragrant tropical grass widely used in both culinary and medicinal traditions across Asia, Africa, and South America. Known for its crisp citrus aroma and refreshing taste, **Lemon Grass is much more than a kitchen herb—it's a proven remedy for calming the nerves, reducing fevers, aiding digestion, and combating infections. Traditionally steeped as a tea or used in poultices, its active compounds (notably citral) exhibit anti-inflammatory, antifungal, antibacterial, and mild sedative effects.**

In folk medicine, **Lemon Grass has long been valued for relieving colds, indigestion, and insomnia. Modern research has confirmed its potential as a gentle yet effective herb to soothe the stomach, support immunity, and reduce oxidative stress. It's also used in essential oil form to uplift the mood, freshen the air, or repel insects.**

---

## Core Herbal Category — Lemongrass

*(Cymbopogon citratus)*

**Primary Core: Digestive System Support herb** with (aromatic carminative principles that ease bloating, gas, and digestive tension)

**Secondary Cores:** Antimicrobial Support **herb** · Anti-Inflammatory Support **herb** · Nervous System Support **herb**

---

## How It Works

Lemongrass works by stimulating digestive secretions and relaxing intestinal muscle tension.
Its aromatic oils help reduce gas, cramping, and sluggish digestion.
Natural antimicrobial compounds assist the body in resisting unwanted microbial growth.
The herb calms low-grade inflammation that contributes to digestive and muscular discomfort.
Through gentle nervous-system support, Lemongrass promotes relaxed digestion and emotional ease.

---

## Primary Uses

- Digestive relief
- Mild anxiety and nervous tension

• Fever and cold remedy
• Anti-inflammatory and antimicrobial support

---

## How to Use

**Tea:**
• 1–2 tsp dried or fresh chopped Lemongrass
• Steep 10–15 minutes in hot water
• Use 1–3× daily for digestion, tension, or immune support
**Fresh stalk:**
Simmer in broths, soups, or decoctions for digestion & immune strength
**Essential oil:**
Aromatic or topical use only
• Always dilute before applying to skin

---

## DIY Recipe — Soothing Lemongrass Herbal Tea

• 1 tsp Lemongrass
• ½ tsp Chamomile
• ¼ tsp Ginger
Steep 10 minutes → Strain → Drink for calm nerves and bloating relief.

---

## Scientific Backing

Lemongrass contains **citral, geraniol, and limonene**, compounds known for:
• Antibacterial action (E. coli & Staph aureus)
• Anti-inflammatory effects
• Mild sedative properties (GABA modulation)
• Relaxation and sleep support
*NCBI • Journal of Advanced Pharmaceutical Technology & Research*

---

## Forms Available

• Fresh stalk
• Dried herb
• Tea bags
• Essential oil
• Tincture
• Capsules

## ⚠ Caution Level: Safe (Mild Use Advisory)

- Essential oil can irritate skin if undiluted
- Avoid strong medicinal doses in pregnancy
- May slightly lower blood pressure
- Monitor if allergic to grasses
- Large amounts may irritate stomach in sensitive individuals

## Gender-Specific Safety (GS)

**Men:** Generally Safe — Helpful for digestion, tension, and inflammation.
**Women:** Generally Safe — Particularly supportive for stress, digestion, and cleansing.
**Pregnancy/Nursing:** Mild Caution — Avoid concentrated doses and essential oil; small culinary amounts are typically fine.

## Expected Results

- Digestive and mood benefits: **30–60 minutes**
- Immune & anti-inflammatory support: **1–2 weeks**

## Same/Similar Results

- Chamomile
- Lemon Balm
- Peppermint
- Ginger

## Shelf Life / Potency After Preparation

- **Dried Lemongrass:** 1–2 years
- **Fresh stalk:** Refrigerated 1–2 weeks
- **Essential oil:** 2–4 years (kept cool and dark)
- **Tea (brewed):** Best within **24 hours** refrigerated

## 🌿 Herbal Reflections of Lemongrass

Lemongrass is a quietly powerful healer—aromatic, uplifting, and deeply supportive. Its citrus brightness lifts the spirit, while its antimicrobial and anti-inflammatory chemistry works behind the scenes to cleanse and restore.

It eases stress, settles digestion, reduces internal heat, and refreshes the mind, making it ideal for evening unwinding or daytime clarity. Under its light, refreshing aroma lies a steady, dependable ally for emotional calm, digestive ease, and whole-body renewal.

## ⭐ Herbal Confidence Index

🌿🌿🌿🌿 **(4 / 5)**

A fragrant digestive and circulatory tonic that refreshes the body and mind. Lemongrass calms bloating, eases tension, supports detoxification, and lifts the spirit with its bright citrus aroma—a soothing antimicrobial ally offering clarity, balance, and clean renewal from within.

# ALKANET

★★★

*Alkanna tinctoria*

**Alkanet Root** is best recognized for its deep crimson pigment, long prized as a natural dye, yet its role in traditional medicine runs deeper than color alone. For centuries, it has been infused into oils and salves to soothe irritation, cool inflammation, and support the healing of minor wounds and burns. With its grounding, cooling energy, Alkanet has served as both a cosmetic enhancer and a protective skin ally, helping calm redness while imparting a subtle vibrancy when used in topical preparations.

Beyond its practical applications, Alkanet carries a thread of folk and ceremonial significance. Herbalists and healers once added it to ointments and charms, believing it could shield the body and spirit from negative influences while restoring balance to the skin. Though its internal use is limited due to safety considerations, Alkanet continues to hold a respected place in external herbal practice, blending beauty with protection in the timeless tradition of root-based remedies.

---

## Core Herbal Category — Alkanet Root

*(Alkanna tinctoria)*

**Primary Core: Lymphatic & Skin Support herb** with (soothing, protective principles that calm irritation and support surface tissue integrity)
**Secondary Cores:** Anti-Inflammatory Support **herb** · Antimicrobial Support **herb**
**Important Note:** Traditionally used **externally** in oils, salves, and cosmetic preparations.

---

## How It Works

Alkanet Root works by releasing soothing compounds that calm irritated and inflamed skin.
Its protective action helps support surface tissue repair and barrier integrity.
Natural anti-inflammatory constituents reduce redness and localized swelling.
Mild antimicrobial activity assists in keeping minor skin disruptions clean.

---

## Primary Uses

- Natural dye for oils, salves, and balms
- Soothes skin irritations and inflammation
- Used in ceremonial, protective, and cosmetic blends

## Scientific Backing

Alkanet Root contains **naphthoquinone derivatives** (especially **alkannin**) which show:
- Mild **anti-inflammatory** activity
- Mild **antimicrobial** effects
- Strong **pigmenting** action for external preparations

Validated primarily for:
- Skin-soothing topical formulas
- Natural coloring agent in cosmetic/herbal preparations

*Journal of Ethnopharmacology* • Cosmetic & phytochemical analyses

## Forms Available

- Infused oils
- Ointments & salves
- Powdered root

## How to Use

Used externally only.
- Infuse dried root in oil for 1–2 weeks
- Strain and use as a base for salves, balms, or ceremonial blends
- Add small amounts of powder to cosmetics for color

**Essential Note:** Alkanet is not used internally in modern herbal practice.

## Caution Level: Caution

- **External use only** — internal use discouraged due to pyrrolizidine alkaloids (PAs)
- Avoid during pregnancy and breastfeeding
- Do not apply to **open wounds** or broken skin
- Individuals with **liver disease** should avoid any contact use without guidance
- Always use **cosmetic-grade** or purified forms
- Essential to avoid ingestion of oils or preparations

## Gender-Specific Safety (GS)

**Men:** Generally Safe — For external, cosmetic, or ritual use only.

**Women:** Generally Safe — Avoid high concentrations on sensitive skin.

**Pregnancy/Nursing:** 🔴 Avoid — Due to PA alkaloids and limited safety data.

---

## ⏳ Expected Results

• Skin soothing: **1–3 days** of regular topical application
• Coloring effects: **Immediate** in oils, balms, and salves

---

## 🛠 DIY Recipe — Alkanet-Infused Oil

• 1 tbsp dried Alkanet Root
• 1 cup olive or almond oil
Place in a sealed jar → let sit **1–2 weeks**, shaking occasionally.
Strain → Use as a base for protective balms, salves, and natural dye blends.

---

## 🌿 Same/Similar Results

🟢 Calendula — Skin healing & anti-inflammatory
🟢 Plantain Leaf — Wound soothing & drawing action
🟡 Comfrey Root — Strong topical repair (caution internally)
🟢 Chamomile — Calming and anti-inflammatory
🟡 Yarrow — Astringent wound care

---

## 📦 Shelf Life / Potency After Preparation

• **Dried root:** 2–3 years
• **Infused oil:** 1 year (cool, dark storage)
• **Ointments/salves:** 6–12 months
• **Powder:** Up to 2 years

---

## 🌿 Herbal Reflections of Alkanet Root

Alkanet Root bridges the worlds of healing, beauty, and ritual. Its deep crimson pigment has symbolized vitality, protection, and sacredness for centuries. In salves and oils, it adds both color and gentle soothing action for dry, irritated, or inflamed skin.

Though limited to external use, its value is far from minor—Alkanet reminds us that herbal medicine is not only biochemical, but symbolic, artistic, and ceremonial. Its presence in an oil or balm transforms the blend both visually and energetically, carrying a quiet protective quality honored in folk traditions.

**Herbal Confidence Index** 🌿 🌿 🌿 **(3 / 5)** A traditional external-use herb valued for its natural red pigment and mild skin-healing qualities. Best used topically in salves, oils, and ceremonial blends. Gentle, useful, but niche—Alkanet Root remains a respected cosmetic and protective ally in herbal practice.

# SEA BUCKTHORN

★★★★★

*Hippophae rhamnoides*

---

Sea Buckthorn is a resilient shrub native to cold coastal and alpine regions of Europe and Asia, long valued in traditional systems for its ability to support tissue repair, vitality, and recovery. Its vivid orange berries are rich in vitamin C, carotenoids, flavonoids, and a unique fatty acid profile—including omega-7—making it one of the most nutritionally and structurally supportive herbs for skin and mucosal health.

Often referred to as a "restorative superfruit," Sea Buckthorn has been used for generations to nourish epithelial tissues, support circulation, and promote recovery following strain, dryness, or depletion. Both the berry and its oils (from pulp and seed) contribute to its effects—supporting barrier integrity, tissue moisture, and gradual regeneration from within and without. In modern use, it is commonly taken as oils, capsules, powders, or topical preparations for consistent and cumulative benefit.

---

**Core Herbal Category — Sea Buckthorn**

Primary Core: Lymphatic & Skin Support herb with (omega-rich, antioxidant, and mucosal-repair actions that support barrier integrity and cellular renewal)

Secondary Cores: Immune Support herb · Digestive Support herb · Circulatory & Cardiovascular herb · Liver & Metabolic Balance herb · Women's Health herb · Foundational / Systemic Support

---

**How It Works**

Sea Buckthorn works by delivering a rare combination of fatty acids—especially omega-7—along with carotenoids and flavonoids that nourish epithelial tissues and support both skin and mucosal repair. These compounds help strengthen cellular membranes, improve moisture retention, and protect tissues from oxidative stress.

Its antioxidant profile supports immune signaling and vascular resilience, while gentle metabolic and hepatic support assists lipid balance and detoxification pathways. Through consistent use, Sea Buckthorn promotes tissue integrity, circulation, and gradual cellular renewal.

---

**Primary Uses**

- Supports skin repair, hydration, and barrier function
- Nourishes mucosal tissues (digestive, respiratory, urogenital)
- Supports digestive lining and dryness-related imbalance
- Promotes cardiovascular and circulatory health

• Strengthens immune resilience
• Supports liver and metabolic balance
• Provides antioxidant protection against oxidative stress

---

### Scientific Backing

Sea Buckthorn contains omega-7 fatty acids, carotenoids, flavonoids, and vitamin C that contribute to antioxidant, lipid-modulating, and tissue-repair effects. Research supports benefits for skin hydration, mucosal integrity, immune balance, and cardiovascular health. Outcomes are typically cumulative and depend on preparation (oil vs. berry extract) and consistency of use.

---

### Forms Available

• Cold-pressed berry or seed oil (internal & topical)
• Capsules / softgels
• Juice or concentrate
• Powdered berry
• Topical creams, serums, and salves

---

### How to Use / Dosage

Internal:
• ½–1 tsp oil daily or 500–1000 mg in capsules
• Powders or juices may be added to food or beverages

Topical:
• Apply oil directly or diluted in a carrier oil
• Blend into creams or skin-repair formulas

Introduce gradually if digestion is sensitive. Best used consistently for cumulative benefit.

---

### Expected Results

• Topical comfort: 3–7 days
• Skin and tissue nourishment: 2–4 weeks
• Mucosal and systemic support: 4–8 weeks
• Cardiovascular and metabolic support: 6–8 weeks

---

### Caution Level: Caution

• May influence bleeding tendency—use caution with anticoagulants/antiplatelet medications
• Excess internal oil may cause loose stools
• May mildly affect blood pressure or blood sugar—monitor if on related medications
• Introduce slowly if sensitive to acidic fruits or rich oils

• Strong pigment may temporarily stain skin or fabric
• During pregnancy, food-level use is reasonable; avoid high-dose oils without guidance

🧬 **Gender-Specific Safety (GS)**

Men — 🟢 Safe
Supports cardiovascular health and tissue repair; monitor if on blood thinners

Women — 🟢 Safe
Often helpful for skin and mucosal dryness patterns; monitor if on blood thinners

Pregnancy / Nursing — 🟡 Caution
Food-level use is generally acceptable; avoid concentrated supplementation without guidance

🔄 **Same / Similar Results**

🟢 Rosehip
🟢 Amla
🟢 Goji Berry
🟢 Evening Primrose Oil
🟢 Calendula (topical tissue support)

---

📦 **Shelf Life / Potency After Preparation**

⚫ Cold-pressed oil: 9–12 months (refrigerated preferred)
⚫ Capsules: 1–2 years sealed
⚫ Powder: ~1–2 years airtight
⚫ Juice/concentrate: 1–2 weeks refrigerated
⚫ Topical blends: 6–12 months

---

🛠 **DIY Recipe — Gentle Repair & Radiance Oil**

1 tsp Sea Buckthorn oil + 2 Tbsp jojoba oil
Blend and apply a few drops nightly (avoid light fabrics)

---

💬 **Herbal Reflections of Sea Buckthorn**

Sea Buckthorn restores through nourishment—supplying what is dry, strained, or depleted with the materials needed for repair. Its strength lies not in force, but in consistency—supporting tissues, protecting cells, and building resilience over time. It reflects a simple principle of healing: when the body is properly nourished, restoration follows.

⭐ **Herbal Confidence Index**

🌿 🌿 🌿 🌿 🌿 (5/5 green stars — a cornerstone regenerative herb rich in omega-7, carotenoids, and antioxidants; exceptional for skin, mucosal, and cellular support when used consistently)

# LICORICE ROOT

★★★★★

*Glycyrrhiza glabra*

**Licorice Root** has long been regarded as one of the most effective soothing herbs for the throat, stomach, and digestive lining. For centuries, it has been used when tissues feel inflamed, irritated, or overworked—whether from acid reflux, gastritis, lingering cough, or voice strain. Its naturally sweet, demulcent constituents coat mucous membranes in a protective layer, offering immediate comfort while creating favorable conditions for tissue repair and hydration. This dual action—relief paired with restoration—has secured Licorice's place in traditional medical systems across Europe, Asia, and the Middle East.

Beyond its direct soothing effects, Licorice Root is widely valued for its harmonizing role in herbal formulas. It softens the intensity of stronger herbs while contributing its own anti-inflammatory and protective influence. Herbalists frequently include Licorice as part of short-term recovery protocols involving rest, warm fluids, and gentle nourishment. When used appropriately, it remains one of the most versatile protectors of irritated tissues in the herbal tradition.

---

## Core Herbal Category — Licorice Root

*(Glycyrrhiza glabra)*
**Primary Core: Digestive System Support** herb with (demulcent and anti-inflammatory principles that protect irritated tissues and support digestive lining integrity)
**Secondary Cores:** Throat & Respiratory Comfort Support herb · Formula Harmonization Support herb · Anti-Inflammatory Support herb

---

## How It Works

Licorice Root works by coating mucosal tissues with soothing polysaccharides that reduce friction and irritation. Its key constituent, glycyrrhizin, along with supportive flavonoids, helps calm inflammation and supports repair of the digestive and respiratory linings. Licorice also assists in regulating gastric secretions and protecting tissues from irritation related to stress or dietary imbalance. In formulas, it enhances tolerance and synergy, helping herbs work together more smoothly.

---

## Primary Uses

- Reflux, gastritis, and ulcer-related irritation
- Hoarseness, voice strain, and dry or irritated cough
- Hydration and protection of mucous membranes
- Formula harmonization and irritation buffering

## 🧪 Scientific Backing

Licorice Root contains glycyrrhizin, glycyrrhetinic acid, flavonoids, and mucilaginous compounds associated with anti-inflammatory, anti-ulcer, and mucosal-protective effects.
Deglycyrrhizinated Licorice (DGL) removes most glycyrrhizin while preserving mucosal benefits, making it better suited for longer-term gastrointestinal use.
Clinical and traditional evidence supports its use for:

- Gastric and esophageal irritation
- Ulcer support and lining protection
- Throat and respiratory membrane comfort

📚 *Journal of Ethnopharmacology* · *Phytomedicine* · DGL clinical research

---

## 🌿 Forms Available

- DGL chewable tablets (preferred for reflux and ulcer support)
- Standardized extracts (glycyrrhizin content labeled)
- Dried root slices (tea or decoction)
- Syrups and lozenges for throat comfort

---

## 🧴 How to Use

**DGL for digestive support:**

- Chew 1–2 tablets
- 15–20 minutes before meals and before bed
- Use for 2–4 weeks

**Tea (short-term soothing):**

- Simmer 1–2 tsp dried root in 10–12 oz water for 10–15 minutes
- Often combined with Marshmallow or Slippery Elm

**Lozenges/Syrups:**

- Useful for hoarseness, dry cough, and throat irritation

---

## ⚠ Caution Level: 🟠 Caution

- Glycyrrhizin may raise blood pressure, promote fluid retention, and lower potassium when used in excess
- Avoid whole-root Licorice with:
  - Hypertension
  - Heart or kidney disease
  - Diuretics, digoxin, or corticosteroids
- Prefer DGL for chronic digestive conditions
- Avoid during pregnancy unless professionally supervised
- Discontinue 1–2 weeks before surgery

## 👥 Gender-Specific Safety (GS)

**Men:** ⚪ Caution — Moderate use advised; monitor blood pressure with whole-root forms
**Women:** ⚪ Caution — Appropriate for short-term mucosal support; avoid prolonged high-dose use
**Pregnancy/Nursing:** ⚫ Avoid — Hormonal and circulatory effects warrant avoidance unless directed by a clinician

---

## ⏳ Expected Results

- Throat and voice comfort: same day–3 days
- Reflux or meal-related irritation: 3–7 days (DGL)
- Ulcer or lining repair: 2–4+ weeks
- Voice strain recovery: 1–5 days

---

## 🛠 DIY Routine — Gentle Mucosal Support

**Before meals:**
- Chew 1–2 DGL tablets 20 minutes before eating

**Evening tea:**
- 1 tsp Licorice root + Marshmallow or Slippery Elm
- Simmer 10–15 minutes → sip warm

---

## 🔄 Same / Similar Results

⚪ Marshmallow Root · ⚪ Slippery Elm · ⚪ Plantain Leaf · ⚪ Chamomile · ⚪ Aloe Vera (inner gel)

---

## 📦 Shelf Life / Potency After Preparation

- DGL tablets: ~2 years
- Dried root: 2–3 years
- Extracts/powders: 1–2 years
- Syrups/lozenges: ~1 year
- Prepared tea: best within 24 hours (refrigerated)

---

## 🌿 Herbal Reflections of Licorice Root

Licorice Root offers protection where tissues have been worn thin—by stress, acidity, or overuse. Its sweetness reflects its role: buffering, unifying, and restoring balance rather than forcing change.

While Marshmallow and Slippery Elm cool and moisten, Licorice adds structure, helping tissues seal, stabilize, and recover.
As both a remedy and a harmonizer, it stands among the most indispensable herbs in classical practice—gentle in action when used correctly, yet deeply effective in restoring comfort and cohesion.

---

**Herbal Confidence Index:** (5 / 5)
*A foundational harmonizing herb that protects mucous membranes, calms inflammation, and supports digestive and respiratory comfort. Licorice Root remains an essential cornerstone of classical herbal medicine when used with discernment and respect.*

# REISHI

★★★★★

*Ganoderma lucidum*

**Reishi** is the quiet architect of balance in traditional medicine—**an adaptogenic mushroom prized for steadying the immune system, easing stress, and supporting healthy sleep and recovery. Its glossy "varnished" cap earned it names like "Lingzhi" and the "Mushroom of Immortality," reflecting centuries of use for longevity, resilience, and calm.**
Beyond folklore, Reishi offers a grounded, day-by-day lift: **less jittery than stimulants, gentler than sedatives, and deeply restorative. Its polysaccharides and triterpenes are studied for immune modulation, normalized inflammatory response, and support for the heart, liver, and lungs**—making it a reliable base note in wellness formulas rather than a flashy soloist.

### Core Herbal Category — Reishi

*(Ganoderma lucidum)*

**Primary Core: Immune System Support** herb with (adaptogenic polysaccharide and triterpene principles that balance immune response and support long-term stress tolerance)

**Secondary Cores:** Nervous System Restoration Support herb · Cardiometabolic Support herb · Liver Support herb

---

## How It Works

Reishi works by supplying beta-glucans and triterpenes that help regulate immune activity rather than overstimulating it.

These compounds support nervous system calm and improve the body's ability to adapt to chronic stress.

The herb assists liver function by supporting detoxification and antioxidant defense pathways.

Its cardiometabolic actions help maintain healthy circulation and lipid balance under stress.

Through steady adaptogenic action, Reishi promotes resilience, recovery, and long-term vitality.

---

## 🌱 Primary Uses

- Stress resilience, calm mood & improved sleep
- Balanced immune support (not overstimulating)
- Supports healthy inflammatory response (joints, airways)
- Circulation & cholesterol balance
- Gentle liver support and detox tone

---

## 🧪 Scientific Backing

Reishi contains:

- Beta-glucans (polysaccharides): immune modulation, balanced defense
- Ganoderic acids (triterpenes): anti-inflammatory, antioxidant, hepatoprotective
- Adaptogenic compounds: normalize stress signals & fatigue

Clinical notes:

- Improved sleep quality & reduced nighttime wakefulness
- Better energy stability & mood regulation
- Enhanced respiratory & cardiovascular tone
- Liver-protective and antioxidant actions

📚 *Journal of Ethnopharmacology* • *Mycological Research* • *Phytomedicine*

---

## ☕ Forms Available

- Sliced or powdered fruiting body (tea/decoction)
- Standardized extracts (polysaccharide/triterpene)
- Tinctures (dual-extraction preferred)
- Capsules or powders for drinks

---

## 🧂 How to Use

Decoction:

- 3–5 g sliced Reishi
- Simmer 30–45 minutes, covered
- Sip 1 cup in evening; refrigerate remainder up to 48 hours

Extracts & Capsules:

- Follow standardized dosage labels for triterpene or polysaccharide content

Powder:

- Add to evening tea, coffee substitutes, or warm oat milk blends

---

## ⚠️ Caution Level: 🟢 Safe (Mild Use Advisory)

• Generally very safe—even with long-term use
• Mild caution with anticoagulants
• May gently lower blood pressure
• Avoid during pregnancy/nursing unless supervised
• Stop 1–2 weeks before surgery

---

## 👥 Gender-Specific Safety (GS)

Men: 🟢 Safe — Excellent for stress, sleep, circulation & immune tone.
Women: 🟢 Safe — Supports hormonal resilience, mood balance & restorative sleep.
Pregnancy/Nursing: 🟡 Mild Caution — Insufficient human research; use only with professional guidance.

---

## ⏱️ Expected Results

• Stress/calm support: 3–7 days
• Improved sleep depth: 1–2 weeks
• Immune & respiratory modulation: 2–4 weeks
• Joint/airway inflammatory support: 3–6 weeks

---

## 🛠️ DIY Recipe — Reishi Night Tea

Add 3–5 g sliced Reishi to 3 cups water.
Simmer 30–45 minutes (lid on), strain.
Sip 1 cup in evening; store remainder for up to 48 hours.
*Optional: Add oat milk + cinnamon for a calming night tonic.*

---

## 🔄 Same/Similar Results

🟢 Turkey Tail
🟢 Maitake
🟢 Cordyceps
🟢 Astragalus
🟡 Chaga (use caution: oxalates / anticoagulant concerns)

---

## 📦 Shelf Life / Potency After Preparation

- Dried slices: 2–3 years
- Powder: 1–2 years
- Capsules/extracts: 2 years (unopened)
- Tincture (dual-extract): 4–5 years
- Prepared decoction: 48 hours refrigerated

## 💬 Herbal Reflections of Reishi

Reishi is the quiet lantern of herbal medicine—never flashy, always profound. Its power lies in consistency: fewer restless nights, fewer internal "fires," fewer immune missteps, and better emotional steadiness. Where stimulating adaptogens push, Reishi guides. Where the nervous system frays, Reishi smooths. Its value is often seen in what never becomes a problem. This is the true magic of a long-term tonic—steadiness, protection, and a deeply rooted calm that strengthens both body and spirit.

## ⭐ Herbal Confidence Index

🌿 🌿 🌿 🌿 🌿 (5 / 5)

A sacred immune and longevity mushroom revered for millennia. Reishi calms the nervous system, supports deep sleep, modulates immunity, nurtures cardiovascular and liver health, and restores inner equilibrium. A cornerstone herb for long-term vitality, peace, and resilience.

# LION'S MANE

★★★★★

*Hericium erinaceus*

**Lion's Mane** (*Hericium erinaceus*) is a distinctive medicinal mushroom named for its cascading white spines that resemble a lion's mane. Long revered in Traditional Chinese Medicine and modern herbal practice, it is valued as a nootropic and nerve-supportive tonic rather than a stimulant. Lion's Mane works gradually, supporting cognitive clarity, memory recall, and emotional balance by nourishing the nervous system itself.

Modern research has identified unique compounds in Lion's Mane—**hericenones** (from the fruiting body) and **erinacines** (from the mycelium)—that stimulate nerve growth factor (NGF). This activity may encourage the repair and regeneration of neurons, making Lion's Mane useful not only for memory support, but also for long-term brain resilience, focus, and neurological integrity.

---

## Core Herbal Category — Lion's Mane

*(Hericium erinaceus)*

**Primary Core: Nervous System Support (Nervines)** herb with (neurotrophic and nerve-supportive principles that promote neuronal repair and cognitive resilience)

**Secondary Cores:** Cognitive Support herb · Emotional Balance & Stress Resilience Support herb

---

## How It Works

Lion's Mane works by stimulating nerve growth factor (NGF) activity through its unique hericenones and erinacines. These compounds support the repair and regeneration of neurons and strengthen neural communication pathways. By nourishing brain tissue and synaptic function, the herb enhances memory, focus, and cognitive clarity. Its calming influence also supports emotional balance by stabilizing stress-related nervous system activity. Through sustained neuro-supportive action, Lion's Mane promotes long-term brain health and mental resilience.

---

## Primary Uses

- Supports memory and cognitive performance
- Encourages nerve repair and regeneration
- Promotes focus and sustained mental clarity
- Calms mild anxiety and emotional imbalance
- Strengthens overall neurological resilience

---

## 🧪 Scientific Backing

Lion's Mane contains **hericenones** (fruiting body) and **erinacines** (mycelium), both shown to stimulate nerve growth factor (NGF) production.
Research indicates potential benefits for:

- Cognitive support in mild cognitive impairment
- Reduced symptoms of anxiety and depression
- Neuroprotection against age-related degeneration
- Support for peripheral nerve injury and neuropathy
- Gut–brain axis modulation via microbiome support

📚 *Phytotherapy Research · Journal of Agricultural and Food Chemistry · International Journal of Medicinal Mushrooms*

---

## 🍵 Forms Available

- Powder (whole mushroom or extracts)
- Capsules
- Dual-extract tinctures
- Dried pieces for tea or decoction

---

## 🧴 How to Use

**Tea / Decoction:**

- 1 tbsp dried Lion's Mane
- Simmer 30 minutes in 3 cups water
- Strain and drink 1 cup daily

**Powder / Capsules:**

- 500–1500 mg daily (depending on extract strength)
- Best taken in the morning or early afternoon

**Tincture:**

- Dual-extract tinctures offer broad-spectrum neuro-support

---

## ⚠ Caution Level: ● Safe (Mild Use Advisory)

- Generally well tolerated, including long-term use
- Mild digestive upset may occur initially or at higher doses
- May mildly influence platelet activity — use caution with anticoagulants or before surgery
- Avoid if allergic to mushrooms
- Limited pregnancy and lactation data — use with professional guidance

---

## 👥 Gender-Specific Safety (GS)

**Men:** ● Generally Safe — Supports memory, nerve repair, and cognitive endurance

**Women:** ● Generally Safe — Helpful for focus, mood balance, and stress-related cognitive fatigue
**Pregnancy/Nursing:** ● Mild Caution — Insufficient data; avoid concentrated extracts without supervision

---

## ⌛ Expected Results

- Cognitive clarity and focus: 7–14 days
- Mood balance and stress resilience: 2–3 weeks
- Nerve repair and neuropathy support: 4–8 weeks
- Gut–brain support: 1–2 months
- Full cognitive and neurological benefits: 8–12 weeks of consistent use

---

## 🛠 DIY Recipe — Lion's Mane Brain Tea

- 1 tbsp dried Lion's Mane
- 3 cups water

Simmer 30 minutes → strain → drink 1 cup daily
Optional: add cinnamon or lemon for flavor and synergy

---

## 🔄 Same / Similar Results

● Bacopa · ● Gotu Kola · ● Ashwagandha · ● Rhodiola · ● Ginkgo

---

## 📦 Shelf Life / Potency After Preparation

- Dried mushroom: 2–3 years
- Powder: 1–2 years
- Capsules: ~2 years unopened
- Alcohol tincture: 4–5 years
- Prepared decoction: up to 48 hours refrigerated

---

## 💬 Herbal Reflections of Lion's Mane

Lion's Mane is both guardian and gardener of the mind. Rather than forcing stimulation, it restores neurological pathways through nourishment and repair. Its effects are subtle at first, but deeply structural over time—clearing cognitive fog, strengthening memory, and stabilizing emotional response.
Unlike fast-acting nootropics, Lion's Mane works quietly and persistently, rebuilding resilience from within. For students, elders, creatives, or anyone recovering from stress, injury, or cognitive fatigue, it becomes a steady companion in clarity, grounding, and long-term neurological health.

🌟 **Herbal Confidence Index**

🌿 🌿 🌿 🌿 🌿 **(5 / 5)**

*A premier neurotrophic mushroom that supports nerve regeneration, cognitive clarity, emotional balance, and long-term brain resilience. Lion's Mane stands among the most important modern allies for neurological restoration and sustained mental health.*

# MAITAKE

★★★★★

*Grifola frondosa*

**Maitake**, often called the "hen of the woods," is a prized mushroom of both kitchen and apothecary. Traditionally gathered from the bases of oak trees, its layered, feathery fronds have been valued for centuries as food and medicine. Rich in beta-glucans and other polysaccharides, Maitake supports the body's ability to respond to modern stressors such as blood-sugar fluctuation, immune imbalance, and metabolic strain. Its dual role as a nourishing food and therapeutic tonic makes it one of the most approachable medicinal mushrooms for daily use.

What distinguishes Maitake from many other medicinal mushrooms is its gentle, regulatory intelligence. Rather than forcing sharp physiological shifts, it works with existing systems—supporting insulin sensitivity, balancing appetite signals, and strengthening immune readiness without overstimulation. For those seeking resilience without risk, Maitake offers a steady, food-like ally that integrates easily into meals or supplement routines, reflecting the essence of functional nutrition: nourishment that is both sustaining and protective.

---

## Core Herbal Category — Maitake

*(Grifola frondosa)*

**Primary Core: Immune System Support** herb with (beta-glucan and polysaccharide principles that support immune balance and healthy glucose metabolism)

**Secondary Cores:** Blood Sugar Balance Support herb · Cardiovascular Support herb

---

## How It Works

Maitake works by supplying beta-glucans that help regulate immune signaling without overstimulation. These compounds also support insulin sensitivity and healthy glucose handling. Maitake assists metabolic efficiency by improving cellular communication involved in nutrient use and energy balance. Its cardiovascular support helps maintain healthy lipid profiles and circulation. Through steady immune and metabolic modulation, Maitake promotes long-term systemic balance.

---

## Primary Uses

- Supports healthy blood-sugar and lipid balance
- Promotes immune modulation and seasonal resilience
- Encourages healthy blood-pressure tone and circulation
- Aids natural weight balance through satiety and steady energy

## 🧪 Scientific Backing

Maitake contains highly active beta-glucans, including **D-fraction** and **X-fraction**, studied for immune-modulating and metabolic effects.
Research highlights include:

- Improved insulin sensitivity and glucose regulation
- Support for healthy lipid profiles
- Balanced immune response (neither overstimulating nor suppressive)
- Enhanced natural killer (NK) cell and macrophage activity
- Promising early human data for cardiometabolic support

📚 *International Journal of Medicinal Mushrooms · Journal of Clinical Biochemistry & Nutrition · Nutrition Research*

---

## 🍵 Forms Available

- Fresh or dried fronds (culinary use)
- Powdered fruiting body
- Standardized extracts (D-fraction / X-fraction)
- Dual-extract tinctures

---

## 🧂 How to Use

**Culinary:**

- Add fresh or dried Maitake to soups, stir-fries, or broths

**Broth / Decoction:**

- 20–30 g dried Maitake
- 8 cups water
- Simmer 45–60 minutes; strain
- Refrigerate up to 3 days or freeze

**Extracts:**

- Capsules or tinctures: follow standardized D-fraction/X-fraction dosing
- Best taken consistently with meals

---

## ⚠ Caution Level: 🟠 Caution

- Generally safe and well tolerated
- May potentiate hypoglycemic or antihypertensive medications
- Discontinue 1–2 weeks before surgery (mild platelet activity possible)
- Limited safety data during pregnancy and lactation
- Rare mushroom allergies may occur

---

## 👥 Gender-Specific Safety (GS)

**Men:** 🟢 Generally Safe — Supports metabolic steadiness, immune tone, and cardiovascular balance

**Women:** 🟢 Generally Safe — Helpful for blood-sugar regulation, immune modulation, and weight balance

**Pregnancy/Nursing:** 🟡 Mild Caution — Insufficient data; use only with practitioner guidance

---

## ⏳ Expected Results

• Meal-to-meal metabolic steadiness: 1–2 weeks
• Glycemic and lipid improvements: 4–8 weeks
• Immune tone and seasonal support: 2–4 weeks
• Appetite balance and weight support: gradual, ongoing

---

## 🛠 DIY Recipe — Savory Maitake Metabolic Broth

• 20–30 g dried Maitake
• 8 cups water
• Onion and garlic (optional)

Simmer 45–60 minutes, covered.
Sip 1–2 cups with meals daily.

---

## 🔄 Same / Similar Results

🟢 Reishi
🟢 Turkey Tail
🟢 Shiitake
🟡 Gymnema (caution with blood-sugar medication)
🟢 Ceylon Cinnamon

---

## 📦 Shelf Life / Potency After Preparation

• Dried Maitake: 2–3 years
• Powder: 1–2 years
• Capsules: ~2 years unopened
• Alcohol tincture: 4–5 years
• Prepared broth/decoction: up to 3 days refrigerated

---

## 💬 Herbal Reflections of Maitake

Maitake feels like discipline disguised as nourishment—steady, grounding, and quietly corrective. It does not spike energy or force metabolic change. Instead, it smooths the daily extremes: sugar surges, immune dips, and the fatigue that follows instability. Over time, its benefits reveal themselves through subtle but meaningful shifts—steadier meals, calmer cravings, and more consistent energy.

Reishi softens the spirit; Lion's Mane clears the mind. Maitake strengthens the centerline—the metabolic and immune core that quietly shapes resilience and daily vitality.

---

### 🌟 Herbal Confidence Index

🌿 🌿 🌿 🌿 🌿 **(5 / 5)**

*A deeply nourishing immune and metabolic tonic prized for blood-sugar balance, cardiovascular support, and fortified resilience. Maitake exemplifies functional nourishment—steady, protective, and sustaining long-term equilibrium.*

# CATUABA BARK

★★★★

Erythroxylum catuaba

**Catuaba Bark** is a treasured tonic from the Brazilian rainforest, long celebrated for its energizing, mood-lifting, and aphrodisiac qualities. **Indigenous Tupi tribes have used it for generations to enhance stamina, improve mental clarity, and restore vitality during fatigue.** Today, **herbalists recognize Catuaba not only for its reputed effects on libido but also for its ability to gently support the nervous system, reduce anxiety, and promote restful sleep.**

**This herb's unique compounds—catuabine alkaloids—are believed to stimulate circulation to the brain and pelvic region, helping balance mood, strengthen memory, and increase physical endurance.** Gentle yet restorative, Catuaba stands out as a natural herb of renewal, confidence, and mental resilience.

---

## Core Herbal Category — Catuaba Bark

*(Erythroxylum catuaba)*

**Primary Core: Nervous System Support (Nervines)** herb with (alkaloid-rich, nervine tonic principles that restore neural vitality, ease fatigue, and support cognitive resilience)
**Secondary Cores:** Libido & Vitality Support herb · Adaptogenic Stress Support herb

---

## How It Works

Catuaba Bark works by supplying alkaloid compounds that support healthy neural signaling and nervous-system tone.

These compounds are traditionally associated with easing fatigue and restoring mental and physical vitality.

The herb assists circulatory flow to peripheral tissues, supporting its traditional use for libido and reproductive vigor.

Its adaptogenic-leaning action helps the body cope with stress-related fatigue and depletion.

Through steady nervine and circulatory support, Catuaba Bark promotes long-term vitality and resilience.

---

## Primary Uses

• Supports healthy libido and sexual vitality
• Enhances energy, endurance, and resilience
• Reduces mild anxiety, tension, and mental fatigue
• Promotes restorative sleep (especially stress-related insomnia)
• Supports memory, concentration, and mental clarity

---

## Scientific Backing

Catuaba contains unique alkaloids—catuabine A, B, and C—linked to its nerve-tonic and vitality-supporting effects.

**Research shows:**
• Mild central nervous system stimulation
• Neuroprotective & antioxidant activity
• Improved circulation to cerebral & pelvic vessels
• Adaptogenic support for low mood & fatigue

Human clinical research is limited, but Catuaba's long historical use forms a strong evidence base.

*Journal of Natural Medicines • Phytotherapy Research • Brazilian Journal of Pharmacognosy*

---

## Forms Available

• Tincture (fast-acting nerve & libido tonic)
• Capsules / powder (steady daily support)
• Tea / decoction (traditional Amazonian method)

---

## How to Use / Dosage

Tincture: 1–2 dropperfuls (1–2 mL), 1–2× daily
Tea: 1 tsp bark simmered 10–15 minutes in 1½ cups water
Capsules: 400–600 mg (follow product label)
Best: Morning or early afternoon to avoid sleep disruption.

---

## Caution Level: Caution

• May cause mild insomnia if taken late
• Avoid with stimulants or high-caffeine beverages
• Use caution with hypertension or heart conditions
• Avoid during pregnancy and nursing

• Very mild overstimulation possible in sensitive users

## 👥 Gender-Specific Safety (GS)

Men: 🟢 Safe — Supports libido, circulation, stamina, and mood without hormonal interference.
Women: 🟢 Safe — Enhances libido, reduces stress fatigue, clears mental fog, and supports calmer sleep.
Pregnancy / Nursing: 🔴 Avoid — Stimulating properties and insufficient data.

## ⏱ Expected Results

- Energy & mental clarity: 1–3 days
- Libido & stamina: 1–2 weeks
- Mood elevation & calm focus: 3–10 days
- Sleep improvement (stress-related): 5–7 days

## 🛠 DIY Recipe — Catuaba Vitality Tea

- 1 tsp dried Catuaba bark
- Simmer 10–15 minutes in 1½ cups water
- Strain and drink warm (morning or early afternoon)

Optional: Cinnamon or honey for warmth & smoothness.

## 🔄 Same / Similar Results

🟢 Muira Puama — libido + nerve tonic
🟢 Damiana — uplifting relaxant
🟢 Maca Root — hormone balance + stamina
🟢 Ginseng — energizing adaptogen

## 📦 Shelf Life / Potency After Preparation

- Dried bark: 2–3 years
- Powder/capsules: 2 years unopened
- Alcohol tincture: 4–6 years
- Prepared tea/decoction: 2–3 days refrigerated

## 💭 *Herbal Reflections of Catuaba Bark*

Catuaba is the bark of renewal—a tonic that lifts the spirit as gently as it strengthens the body. It energizes without forcing, clarifies without strain, and rekindles confidence without agitation. Its medicine is courage through calmness, endurance through balance, circulation through harmony.

Indigenous healers long described it as "the bark that gives strength to the old and youth to the weary." In an age of stress overload, emotional fatigue, and low vitality, Catuaba reminds us that strength can return through warmth, circulation, and quiet nerve nourishment.

## 🌟 Herbal Confidence Index

🌿 🌿 🌿 🌿 (4 / 5)

A balanced Amazonian aphrodisiac and nerve tonic. Catuaba supports libido, clarity, mood, and resilience with clean, sustainable energy. Its effects are reliable yet gentle, falling just short of cornerstone status due to limited modern clinical trials and variability between individuals. Still, it remains one of the most trusted rainforest botanicals for restoring vitality and emotional steadiness.

# TURKEY TAIL

★★★★★

Trametes versicolor

**Turkey Tail is a classic gut–immune ally**, named for its fan-shaped, multicolored bands that mirror a wild turkey's tail. **Long simmered as a daily tea, it's rich in beta-glucans and distinctive polysaccharopeptides that help the immune system stay responsive without tipping into overdrive**. Gentle and food-like, Turkey Tail fits easily into steady routines rather than crisis moments.

Where it really shines is at the intersection of gut health and immune tone. **Its prebiotic fibers support a friendlier microbiome environment, which in turn influences resilience, regularity, and overall comfort.** Think of it as a quiet trainer: consistent, non-stimulating, and reliable over weeks—ideal for people who want year-round support they can sip without noticing any buzzy edges.

---

## Core Herbal Category — Turkey Tail

(Trametes versicolor)

**Primary Core: Immune System Support** herb with (polysaccharide-rich principles that support balanced immune signaling and host defense resilience)

**Secondary Cores:** Gut Restoration Support herb · Longevity & Vitality Support herb · Antioxidant Defense Support herb

---

## How It Works

Turkey Tail works by supplying polysaccharopeptides and beta-glucans that help regulate immune response rather than overstimulating it.

These compounds support communication between immune cells and enhance adaptive immune readiness.

The herb promotes gut health by supporting beneficial microbiota and intestinal immune function.

Its antioxidant activity helps protect cells from oxidative stress associated with aging and immune burden.

---

### Primary Uses

- Immune modulation and seasonal wellness
- Gut support (prebiotic polysaccharides; post-antibiotic routines)
- Recovery & resilience when run down
- General antioxidant tone

---

### Scientific Backing

Turkey Tail provides beta-glucans and PSP/PSK studied for immune modulation, microbial balance, and antioxidant effects. Early human data and extensive traditional use point to benefits for gut-immune crosstalk and recovery; quality and extract standardization matter.

---

### Forms Available

- Decoction (dried fronds simmered as tea)
- Powder/capsules (standardized extracts)
- Dual-extract tinctures (water + alcohol)

---

## How to Use (Dosage & Methods)

Turkey Tail is most effective when taken consistently over time.

• **Capsules / Powder:**

Take **1–3 grams daily** with food. Can be divided into two doses for easier digestion.

• **Tea / Decoction:**

Simmer **1–2 teaspoons** of dried Turkey Tail in **2 cups of water** for **20–30 minutes**.
Drink **1 cup, 1–2× daily**.

• **Tincture:**

Use **2–4 mL** up to **2× daily**.

**Note:** Best taken for **4–8 weeks** to support immune balance and long-term wellness.

---

### ⚠ Caution Level : Caution

Generally well tolerated. Use caution with autoimmune conditions or immunotherapies (consult a professional). Possible interactions with immunomodulating or anticoagulant medications. Insufficient data in pregnancy/lactation. Discontinue 1–2 weeks before surgery.

---

## 🚹 🚺 Gender-Specific Safety (GS)

**Men:** 🟢 Safe — supports immune defense, stamina, liver function, and post-illness recovery with no hormonal concerns.
**Women:** 🟢 Safe — beneficial for stress-related fatigue, immune balance, and detoxification without disrupting hormonal cycles.
**Pregnancy/Nursing:** 🟡 Caution — limited research; occasional tea under professional guidance may be acceptable, but avoid long-term or high-dose use.

---

## ⏳ Expected Results

- Gut comfort/regularity: **1–2 weeks**
- Seasonal immune tone: **2–4 weeks**
- Recovery/stamina: **3–6 weeks**, gradual

---

## 🛠 DIY — Turkey Tail Daily Decoction

- Add **6–8 g dried Turkey Tail** to **5 cups water**
- Simmer **30–45 minutes**, covered
- Strain; drink **1 cup daily**
- Refrigerate up to **3 days**

---

## 🔄 Same/Similar Results

🟢 Maitake
🟢 Reishi
🟢 Shiitake
🟢 Astragalus
🟡 Chaga (caution: high oxalates)

---

## 🗨 Herbal Reflections of Turkey Tail

Turkey Tail is one of nature's quiet defenders — a mushroom that works beneath the surface, fortifying resilience rather than offering quick, flashy effects. Long revered in Chinese medicine and validated by modern research, it builds immune stability from the inside out.

Unlike energizing or calming herbs, Turkey Tail moves silently, strengthening the body's foundation so recovery, endurance, and balance return naturally. It is a bridge between ancient wisdom and modern immunology — proof that slow, steady reinforcement remains one of the wisest paths to lifelong vitality.

---

## ★ Herbal Confidence Index: 🌿🌿🌿🌿🌿

(5/5 green stars — a foundational immune-supporting mushroom with exceptional polysaccharide richness; strengthens microbiome integrity, long-term immunity, and recovery. Gentle yet potent, a cornerstone herb for daily vitality and defense.)

# RHODIOLA

★★★★★

*Rhodiola rosea*

**Rhodiola** is an alpine adaptogen traditionally used in northern and high-altitude regions to help people meet cold climates, long workdays, and sustained mental strain. Its root concentrates **rosavins** and **salidroside**—compounds studied for supporting stress tolerance, perceived energy, and emotional steadiness. Unlike sedating herbs, Rhodiola carries a bright, lifting profile that many experience as clean motivation rather than nervous stimulation.
Best used earlier in the day, Rhodiola pairs well with focused work, training blocks, and periods of heavy cognitive load. It helps smooth task initiation, supports endurance under pressure, and complements calming evening tonics such as Reishi or magnesium. With consistent use over days to weeks, many notice fewer energy dips and a steadier internal "gear" throughout the day.

---

## 🌿 Core Herbal Category — Rhodiola

*(Rhodiola rosea)*
**Primary Core: Adaptogens** herb with (neuroendocrine-balancing principles that enhance stress tolerance and support mental and physical performance)
**Secondary Cores:** Cognitive Support herb · Mood Balance Support herb · Physical Endurance Support herb

---

## 🌿 How It Works

Rhodiola works by modulating stress-response pathways within the nervous and endocrine systems. Its active compounds help balance cortisol signaling and improve cellular energy efficiency. The herb enhances mental clarity and focus during periods of fatigue or cognitive strain. Its mood-supportive action stabilizes emotional response under prolonged stress. Through adaptogenic regulation, Rhodiola supports stamina, resilience, and recovery.

---

## 🌱 Primary Uses

- Anti-fatigue support; mental and physical stamina
- Stress resilience and mood steadiness
- Focus, task initiation, and productivity
- Exercise capacity and recovery support

---

## 🧪 Scientific Backing

Modern research confirms Rhodiola's reputation as a premier **endurance adaptogen**.
Clinically supported findings include:

- Standardized extracts (3% rosavins / 1% salidroside) improving fatigue, cognitive performance, and mood under stress
- Reduced perceived exertion and enhanced work efficiency in randomized trials
- Cortisol modulation without overstimulation
- Improved mitochondrial energy output for physical endurance
- Neuroprotective effects under stress and hypoxic conditions

Rhodiola performs best with **daily morning use**, allowing gradual adaptogenic buildup.

---

## 🧴 Forms Available

- Standardized extract capsules or tablets
- Tincture
- Powder (bitter; best lightly blended into warm water or tea)

---

## 📏 How to Use / Dosage

**Standardized Extract:** 200–400 mg once daily (morning)
**Tincture:** 1–2 mL once or twice daily; avoid evenings
**Powder:** 200–300 mg mixed into warm water or tea
⛔ **Avoid after 2 PM** — may disturb sleep.

---

## ⏱ Expected Results

- Energy and focus: 3–7 days
- Stress buffering and mood steadiness: 2–3 weeks
- Exercise capacity and endurance: 1–2 weeks

---

## ⚠ Caution Level: ▨ Use With Caution

Rhodiola is potent and mildly stimulating.

Use cautiously if you:
- Are sensitive to stimulants, anxiety, or insomnia
- Experience palpitations or labile blood pressure
- Take antidepressants, anxiolytics, or thyroid medication
- Have bipolar disorder or uncontrolled hypertension
- Use strong stimulants (coffee, guarana, pre-workouts)

Avoid during pregnancy and nursing.

---

## 👥 Gender-Specific Safety (GS)

**Men:** ▨ Generally Safe — Supports stamina, focus, clarity, and stress tolerance. Start low if stimulant-sensitive.

**Women:** ▨ Use With Caution — Highly effective but stimulating. Some experience mild agitation, headaches, or cycle sensitivity at higher doses. Begin low and monitor response.

**Pregnancy/Nursing:** ▨ Avoid — Cortisol modulation and insufficient safety data.

---

## Same / Similar Results

▨ Panax Ginseng (stronger stimulation; BP/glucose effects)
▨ Eleuthero
▨ Schisandra
▨ Ashwagandha (calming; evening-friendly)
▨ Cordyceps

---

## 🧪 Shelf Life / Potency After Preparation

- Dried root: ~2 years (airtight, cool, dark)
- Powder: ~1 year
- Capsules / standardized extracts: 2–3 years
- Tincture: 5+ years
- Prepared tea: Best within 24 hours (refrigerated)

Alcohol-based extracts retain potency best.

---

## 🛠 DIY Recipe — Rhodiola Morning Tonic

- 200–300 mg standardized Rhodiola powder
- Stir into warm water or mild tea
- Add honey or lemon if desired
- Take **once in the morning only**

Provides clean mental uplift and stress buffering for the day.

---

## 🗨 Herbal Reflections of Rhodiola

Rhodiola is the herb of endurance—born from wind-scoured cliffs and frozen terrain where only the hardiest plants survive. It carries mountain resilience within its root, offering strength that rises slowly, steadily, and cleanly.

Traditionally known as the "golden root," Rhodiola supported hunters, travelers, scholars, and healers who required clarity under pressure. Today, it serves those navigating modern exhaustion—long workdays, emotional strain, and cognitive overload.

Energetically, Rhodiola refines the stress response. It does not hype the system; it harmonizes it. At the right dose, it restores natural rhythm: awake, steady, and capable.

---

## ⭐ Herbal Confidence Index

**🌿🌿🌿🌿🌿 (5 / 5)**

A premier adaptogen for physical endurance, mental clarity, and emotional resilience. Exceptional reliability, deep historical use, and strong scientific support—requiring respect for its potency. A true **Cornerstone Adaptogen** when used wisely.

# HOLY BASIL

★★★★★

*Ocimum tenuiflorum*

**Holy Basil** (Ocimum sanctum)—known in Ayurveda as **Tulsi**, meaning "the incomparable one"—is a sacred herb revered for centuries as a protector of health and spirit. In India, it is planted near homes and temples not only for its fragrance but for its role in purifying the air, strengthening the body, and calming the mind.

Modern research confirms Holy Basil as a true adaptogen—helping the body resist stress, balance blood sugar, and support immune and adrenal function. Its aromatic leaves contain **eugenol**, **rosmarinic acid**, and **ursolic acid**, compounds that soothe inflammation while gently supporting clarity and emotional balance.

Unlike caffeine-based tonics, Tulsi restores energy without overstimulation, nurturing a steady sense of peaceful vitality. It is both a healer and a spiritual ally—an herb that uplifts the heart, steadies the breath, and encourages balance in both body and mind.

---

## Core Herbal Category — Holy Basil

*(Ocimum sanctum / Ocimum tenuiflorum)*

**Primary Core: Adaptogens** herb with (neuroendocrine-balancing and antioxidant principles that enhance stress tolerance and emotional stability)

**Secondary Cores:** Immune Strengthening Support herb · Respiratory Comfort Support herb · Metabolic Balance Support herb

---

## How It Works

Holy Basil works by modulating stress-response pathways that influence cortisol balance and nervous-system tone. Its phytochemicals support emotional steadiness and mental clarity during prolonged stress. The herb enhances immune readiness through antioxidant and immunomodulating actions. Its aromatic and warming qualities support respiratory comfort and airway clarity. Through metabolic support, Holy Basil helps stabilize energy levels and glucose regulation.

---

## Primary Uses

- Stress resilience, calm focus, balanced mood
- Respiratory comfort (throat and chest)
- Glycemic and inflammatory balance support

- Gentle digestive and liver support
- Aromatic uplift for emotional clarity

---

## 🧪 Scientific Backing

Holy Basil is one of Ayurveda's most documented tonics.
**Supported actions include:**

- Presence of eugenol, rosmarinic acid, ursolic acid, and polyphenols
- Demonstrated adaptogenic effects in human and animal studies
- Cortisol regulation and stress buffering
- Improved glycemic control and lipid balance in early trials
- Antioxidant, anti-inflammatory, and antimicrobial activity
- Support for normal respiratory function and mucosal comfort
- Traditional and clinical use for mood steadiness and mental clarity

Holy Basil is generally considered safe for daily, long-term use when taken in moderate amounts.

---

## 🧴 Forms Available

- Tea or infusion (fresh or dried leaf)
- Tincture or dual-extract
- Capsules or powder (standardized extracts)
- Fresh leaves for culinary or traditional use

---

## 📏 How to Use

**Tea:** 1–2 tsp dried Tulsi, steep 10–12 minutes; 1–3× daily
**Tincture:** 2–4 mL up to twice daily
**Capsules:** 300–600 mg standardized extract
**Evening use:** Encourages calm sleep without sedation

---

## ⏱ Expected Results

- Calm focus and respiratory ease: 3–7 days
- Stress resilience and mood steadiness: 2–3 weeks
- Blood-sugar and lipid tone: 4–8 weeks
- Emotional and spiritual uplift: often immediate

---

## ⚠ Caution Level: ▨ Use With Mild Caution

Holy Basil is among the safest adaptogens.
Use caution if:

- Taking hypoglycemic medications (may enhance effect)
- Using anticoagulants or antiplatelet drugs

• Preparing for surgery (discontinue 1–2 weeks prior)
Avoid high-dose supplementation during pregnancy due to limited modern clinical data.

---

## 👥 Gender-Specific Safety (GS)

**Men:** ● Safe — Excellent for stress, mood, immune, and respiratory support.
**Women:** ● Safe — Supports emotional balance, cycle-related stress, and endocrine harmony.
**Pregnancy/Nursing:** ● Caution — Traditional use supports small culinary or tea-level intake; modern data limited. Avoid concentrated extracts unless advised by a professional.

---

## Same / Similar Results

● Ashwagandha — calming adaptogen
● Rhodiola — energizing adaptogen (morning use)
● Lemon Balm — mood and nervous-system support
● Schisandra — stress resilience and liver support
● Green Tea — clarifying antioxidant tonic

---

## Shelf Life & Potency After Preparation

• Dried leaf: 1–1.5 years (airtight, dark)
• Powder: 6–9 months
• Tincture: 4–5 years
• Prepared tea: Best within 24 hours (refrigerated)
• Fresh leaves: 3–5 days refrigerated
Tulsi loses aromatic potency quickly—store tightly sealed.

---

## DIY Recipe — Tulsi-Ginger Breath Tea

• 1–2 tsp dried Tulsi
• 3–4 fresh ginger slices
• Steep 10–12 minutes
• Add lemon or honey if desired
Use 1–2× daily for respiratory ease and emotional grounding.

---

## 💬 Herbal Reflections of Holy Basil

Holy Basil is more than a plant—it is a living sanctuary. Across centuries it has stood at the threshold of homes and temples, believed to protect not only the body but the spirit. Its fragrance calms the restless mind; its tea softens the weight of stress; its presence invites clarity, devotion, and centered breath.

Tulsi does not stimulate—it harmonizes.
It teaches balance through gentleness.
It reminds the weary that peace is a form of strength, and serenity its own medicine.
In a world full of noise, Holy Basil is the herb of stillness—a fragrant guardian of resilience and inner quiet.

---

## ⭐ Herbal Confidence Index

🌿🌿🌿🌿🌿 **(5 / 5)**
Holy Basil earns a perfect score for its exceptional safety, broad utility, and deep restorative power. A cornerstone adaptogen for stress, mood, immunity, and spiritual grounding—gentle, protective, and enduring.

# BOSWELLIA

★★★★★

*Boswellia serrata*

**Boswellia,** also known as Indian frankincense, is the aromatic resin of hardy desert trees long valued for easing heat, swelling, and stiffness in the body. Traditional systems of medicine in India and the Middle East prized it for calming inflamed joints, irritated airways, and digestive flare-ups—making it a steady ally wherever pain and restriction interfered with daily life. Rather than dulling the senses, Boswellia works with the body's natural processes, gently cooling areas of excess inflammation so movement feels freer and breathing comes easier. Its resin has been burned in temples, blended in tonics, and infused into oils for centuries as both a spiritual and physical medicine.

In modern practice, standardized extracts rich in **boswellic acids** bring this ancient remedy into clearer focus. Clinical studies confirm its usefulness for arthritis, asthma, and inflammatory bowel conditions—offering steady relief without the sedation common to pharmaceuticals. Because it supports mobility, comfort, and clarity of breath without fogging the mind, Boswellia has become a trusted daytime herb for people seeking to stay active while managing chronic inflammation. In this way, it continues to serve as both ancient healer and modern anchor for resilience.

---

## Core Herbal Category — Boswellia

**Primary Core: Anti-Inflammatory & Pain Support** herb with (resin-based, leukotriene-modulating action that supports joint comfort and tissue mobility)

**Secondary Cores:** Respiratory Tonic herb · Digestive Comfort herb · Sacred Aromatic Resin herb

---

## How It Works

Boswellia works by modulating inflammatory signaling pathways that contribute to joint stiffness and tissue discomfort. Its resin compounds calm excessive inflammatory activity without suppressing healthy tissue repair. By easing inflammatory congestion, it supports respiratory comfort and freer breathing. Its grounding aromatic qualities also promote digestive ease and systemic balance. Together, these actions support flexible movement, clearer respiration, and sustained musculoskeletal comfort.

---

## 🌱 Primary Uses

• Healthy joint comfort and mobility
• Airway ease and exercise breathing
• Digestive comfort (non-sedating)
• General inflammatory tone support

---

## 🧪 Scientific Backing

Standardized Boswellia extracts—especially those rich in **AKBA (acetyl-11-keto-β-boswellic acid)**—are studied for supporting normalized inflammatory responses via **5-LOX and related pathways**. Clinical trials report improvements in joint function, walking distance, airway comfort, and recovery from exertion, often with excellent tolerability when quality-controlled extracts are used.

---

## 🍵 Forms Available

• Standardized capsules or tablets (boswellic acids / AKBA %)
• Tincture (less common; resin-based)
• Topical creams and balms (localized comfort)
• Traditional raw resin (rarely chewed internally today)

---

## How to Use (Dosage & Methods)

Boswellia is best taken **consistently** to reduce inflammation and support joint comfort.
**• Capsules / Tablets:**
300–500 mg, 2–3× daily, standardized to 30–40% boswellic acids
**• Resin / Powder:**
¼–½ tsp daily, mixed into warm water, honey, or herbal blends
**• Tincture:**
2–4 mL, 1–2× daily
**Note:** Benefits typically build over **2–4 weeks** of steady use.

---

## ⚠ Caution Level: Caution

• May cause mild digestive upset, nausea, or reflux in sensitive individuals
• Use caution with anticoagulants, NSAIDs, or inflammation-modulating medications
• Those with ulcers or chronic reflux should begin with food-level doses
• Avoid during pregnancy and breastfeeding (possible uterine stimulation)

- Consult a practitioner if managing autoimmune conditions or preparing for surgery

---

## 🚹 🚺 Gender-Specific Safety (GS)

**Men:** 🟢 Safe
Well tolerated for joint pain, inflammation, and respiratory support.
Use mild caution if on blood thinners or with ulcer history.
**Women:** 🟡 Caution
Helpful for joint discomfort, autoimmune flares, and menstrual inflammation.
Use cautiously if taking anticoagulants or experiencing heavy menstrual flow.
Take with food if prone to reflux.
**Pregnancy / Nursing:** 🔴 Avoid
Not recommended due to possible uterine stimulation and limited safety data.

---

## ⏱ Expected Results

- Joint and airway comfort: **7–14 days**
- Mobility and endurance confidence: **3–6 weeks**
- Digestive comfort: **1–2 weeks** with regular use

---

## 🛠 DIY Recipe — Boswellia Mobility Balm

- Warm 2 tbsp shea butter + 1 tbsp jojoba oil in a double boiler
- Stir in 1 tsp Boswellia extract powder until evenly suspended
- Cool fully and apply a pea-sized amount to sore joints 2–3× daily

---

## 🔄 Same / Similar Results

🟢 Turmeric (Curcuma)
🟢 Ginger
🟢 Corydalis
🟢 White Willow
🟡 Devil's Claw (GI and medication cautions)

---

## 💬 Herbal Reflections of Boswellia

Boswellia is the ancient resin of renewal, once carried by caravans through desert winds and burned as sacred incense in temples of healing. Long before modern science understood inflammation, healers recognized its smoke and resin as medicine—easing pain, cleansing the spirit, and opening the breath of life.
In the body, Boswellia moves like calm fire—reducing inflammation, soothing joints, and restoring

mobility where stiffness and heat have settled. Unlike chemical anti-inflammatories, its wisdom is measured: it quiets pain without silencing the body's healing voice. Boswellia teaches that true relief comes through balance, not suppression.

Even today, its fragrance carries echoes of sacred places, bridging old-world tradition with modern science. Each golden tear of resin represents renewal—steadfast, grounding, and profoundly restorative.

## Herbal Confidence Index

**(5 / 5)**

A powerful anti-inflammatory resin revered for soothing joint pain, arthritis, and chronic inflammation without harsh side effects. Boswellia supports flexibility, respiratory comfort, and cellular protection while grounding the body in calm strength—one of nature's most reliable allies for pain relief, balance, and renewal.

# HORSE CHESTNUT

★★★★

*Aesculus hippocastanum*

**Horse Chestnut** is a powerful circulatory restorative renowned for strengthening the veins and improving blood flow throughout the body. Its active compound, **aescin**, helps tone and protect fragile blood vessels, reduce swelling, and relieve symptoms of varicose veins, hemorrhoids, and chronic leg fatigue. Herbalists rely on it to restore elasticity to vascular tissue, ease inflammation, and support lymphatic drainage. Whether taken internally as a standardized extract or applied externally as a cream or gel, Horse Chestnut renews vitality in the body's lower circulation—restoring rhythm, movement, and relief where stagnation once lived.

Historically, Horse Chestnut was revered in traditional European medicine as **"the architect of the body's rivers,"** symbolizing harmony within the blood's pathways. Originating in the Balkan regions, it spread across Europe as a trusted remedy for tired legs and venous weakness. Early healers observed that it did not force blood to move—it guided it, refining the body's natural flow back into balance. Its message endures: movement is medicine. When life's currents begin to flow again, heaviness fades, energy awakens, and the body remembers what harmony feels like.

---

## Core Herbal Category — Horse Chestnut

*(Aesculus hippocastanum)*

**Primary Core:** Cardiovascular System Support herb with (venotonic and capillary-strengthening principles that support healthy blood flow and vascular integrity)

**Secondary Cores:** Anti-Inflammatory Support herb · Edema & Fluid Balance Support herb

---

## How It Works

Horse Chestnut works by supplying **aescin and related saponins** that strengthen vein walls and improve venous tone. These compounds stabilize capillaries, reducing fluid leakage into surrounding tissues. The herb supports healthy upward blood flow—especially in the lower extremities—helping counter stagnation. Its anti-inflammatory effects calm vascular irritation and tissue swelling. Through improved venous efficiency and fluid balance, Horse Chestnut restores circulation comfort and resilience.

---

## 🌱 Primary Uses

- Strengthens vein walls and supports circulation
- Relieves swelling, heaviness, and varicose vein discomfort
- Supports hemorrhoids and chronic venous insufficiency
- Reduces inflammation and fluid retention
- Enhances capillary tone and lymphatic drainage

---

## 🧪 Scientific Backing

Horse Chestnut seeds contain **aescin**, a well-studied saponin clinically shown to:

- Improve venous return
- Reduce edema and leg swelling
- Restore capillary integrity
- Reduce inflammation within vessel walls

Clinical trials consistently support its effectiveness for **varicose veins, hemorrhoids, and chronic venous insufficiency**, with outcomes often comparable to prescription therapies when **standardized extracts** are used. Safety remains strong under proper formulation and dosing.

---

## 🍵 Forms Available

- Standardized seed extract (capsules or tablets)
- Topical gels and creams for varicose veins and swelling
- Professionally prepared tincture (internal use only)

---

## 📏 How to Use / Dosage

**Internal (standardized extract):**

- 100–150 mg aescin-standardized extract daily (divided doses), or as labeled

**Topical:**

- Apply Horse Chestnut gel or cream 2× daily to swollen or heavy legs

**Important:**

⚠️ **Never use raw seeds, leaves, or bark internally** — they contain toxic **esculin** unless properly processed.

---

## ⚠ Caution Level: 🟠 Use with Caution

- Use **only standardized extracts** — raw plant parts are toxic
- May cause mild nausea, itching, or dizziness
- Use caution with blood thinners, antiplatelet drugs, or diabetes medications

- Avoid during pregnancy and breastfeeding
- Discontinue 1–2 weeks before surgery
- Kidney or liver disorders require professional supervision

---

## 🚹 🚺 Gender-Specific Safety (GS)

**Men:** ⚪ Caution
Generally safe when standardized extracts are used.
Avoid with anticoagulants or circulation-sensitive conditions.

**Women:** ⚪ Caution
Helpful for varicosities, swelling, and heaviness.
Avoid with heavy bleeding or clotting disorders unless supervised.

**Pregnancy / Nursing:** ● Avoid
Internal use not recommended.
Topical gels may be acceptable **only** with professional guidance.

---

## ⌛ Expected Results

- Reduced swelling and heaviness: **2–3 weeks**
- Improved vein tone: **4–6 weeks**
- Varicose vein or hemorrhoid improvement: **8–12 weeks**
- Topical soothing: **minutes to hours**

---

## 🛠 DIY Recipe — Circulation Revival Balm

- 2 tbsp Horse Chestnut extract gel
- 1 tbsp witch hazel
- 5 drops lavender essential oil

Mix well and apply to legs, ankles, or varicose areas twice daily to encourage circulation and reduce inflammation.

---

## 🔄 Same / Similar Results

● Gotu Kola
● Hawthorn
⚪ Butcher's Broom
● Ginkgo Biloba

## Shelf Life / Potency After Preparation

- Standardized capsules: **2–3 years** (cool, dry storage)
- Topical gels/creams: **12–18 months** after opening
- Tincture: **3–5 years**
- Homemade balms: **3–4 months refrigerated**

## Herbal Reflections of Horse Chestnut

Horse Chestnut is the architect of the body's rivers, restoring flow where stagnation has taken hold. Long honored as the healer of the tired leg, it strengthens the hidden channels through which vitality moves.
It does not push the blood—it guides it, allowing rhythm and movement to return naturally. As circulation renews itself, heaviness fades, energy rises, and harmony quietly re-enters the body.
Horse Chestnut reminds us that when flow is restored, life follows.

## Herbal Confidence Index

**(4 / 5)**
A time-honored vascular tonic renowned for strengthening veins, reducing varicose discomfort, and restoring healthy circulation. Reliable, effective, and safe when standardized—an essential ally for chronic venous stagnation and lower-body heaviness.

# PYGEUM

★★★★

*Prunus africana*

**Pygeum** is a time-tested bark traditionally used to support prostate comfort and urinary flow, especially in men over 40. Originating in African herbal medicine, its use later evolved into standardized extracts now studied for easing nocturia (night urination), weak urinary stream, urgency, and incomplete emptying—issues that can quietly erode restful sleep and daytime confidence. The bark's phytosterols and triterpenes help soothe inflammation and improve bladder tone, restoring a healthier rhythm within the lower urinary tract and easing age-related strain. Beyond the "plumbing," Pygeum's appeal lies in its gentle, functional relief without sedation. Many users report fewer nighttime awakenings, steadier urinary flow during the day, and renewed comfort and control in daily life. Unlike stronger pharmaceutical options, Pygeum offers gradual, natural support that aligns with long-term wellness goals. Its ability to ease strain without harsh side effects has made Pygeum a trusted ally for men's health—bridging traditional wisdom with modern clinical validation.

---

## Core Herbal Category — Pygeum

*(Prunus africana)*
**Primary Core: Kidney & Urinary Support** herb with (phytosterol-rich principles that support prostate tissue balance and healthy urinary flow)
**Secondary Cores:** Anti-Inflammatory Support herb · Mild Hormone Modulation Support herb

---

## How It Works

Pygeum works by delivering phytosterols and triterpenes that help reduce inflammatory activity within prostate tissue. These compounds ease pressure on the bladder and urethra, supporting healthier urinary flow and reducing urgency. Pygeum assists in regulating excess prostate tissue signaling associated with age-related changes while gently modulating androgen activity without hormonal suppression. Through combined anti-inflammatory and tissue-supportive effects, it promotes long-term prostate comfort and urinary function.

---

## Primary Uses

- Lower urinary tract symptoms (LUTS) associated with BPH
- Nocturia (nighttime urination) and weak urinary stream
- Pelvic and prostate comfort with improved post-void ease

## 🧪 Scientific Backing

Standardized Pygeum extracts (commonly standardized to ~14% sterols/sterolins) demonstrate human clinical evidence for improving:

• Nocturia frequency
• Urinary flow rate
• Residual urine volume
• Pelvic and prostate comfort

Proposed mechanisms include:

• Reduction of prostate inflammation
• Improved local circulation
• Mild modulation of 5-alpha-reductase pathways
• Support of bladder tone and detrusor relaxation

Best outcomes are consistently observed with **daily use over several weeks**.

---

## Forms Available

• Standardized extract capsules (dosage based on sterol content)
• Tincture (less common; quality varies by source)
• Encapsulated powder blends (often combined with Saw Palmetto or Nettle Root)

---

## How to Use / Dosage

**Standardized Extract:**

• 50–100 mg Pygeum extract daily (or per label), taken with food

**Tincture:**

• 1–2 mL, 1–2× daily (verify quality and standardization)

**Timing Notes:**

• Evening use may support nocturia reduction
• Consistent daily use improves long-term outcomes

---

## ⚠ Caution Level: Caution

• Generally well tolerated
• Possible mild gastrointestinal upset—take with food
• Use caution with anticoagulants or antiplatelet medications
• Intended primarily for adult men with LUTS
• Avoid during pregnancy or lactation
• Discontinue 1–2 weeks before surgery

---

## 🚹 🚺 Gender-Specific Safety (GS)

**Men:** Generally Safe
Well-tolerated support for prostate health, nocturia, urinary flow, and pelvic comfort.
Mild digestive effects may occur but typically resolve quickly.
Commonly paired with **Saw Palmetto** or **Stinging Nettle Root** for synergistic benefit.
**Women:** Caution
Not traditionally a women's herb. May support bladder tone, but mild hormone receptor activity warrants caution.
Avoid with hormone-sensitive conditions unless supervised.
**Pregnancy / Nursing:** Avoid
Due to hormonal modulation and insufficient safety data, internal use is not recommended.
Gentler urinary herbs such as **Corn Silk** or **Marshmallow Root** are preferred alternatives.

---

## ⌛ Expected Results

- Reduced nighttime frequency: **2–3 weeks**
- Improved flow and urgency comfort: **3–6 weeks**
- Sleep quality and urinary rhythm stabilization: **4–8 weeks**

---

## DIY Recipe — Evening Pygeum Support Tonic

- Take a standardized Pygeum capsule with dinner
- Or open capsule into 8–10 oz warm chamomile tea or plain water
- Pair with:
- Reduced evening fluid intake after 7 PM
- Gentle pelvic-floor relaxation or breathing exercises

---

## Same / Similar Results

Saw Palmetto
Stinging Nettle Root
Pumpkin Seed
Beta-Sitosterol (use cautiously with lipid-lowering medications)
Maritime Pine Bark

---

## Shelf Life / Potency After Preparation

- Standardized capsules: **2–3 years** (cool, dry storage)
- Tincture: **3–5 years** (alcohol preserves sterols well)
- Powder blends: **1–2 years**
- Opened capsules added to warm drinks: consume immediately

## 💬 Herbal Reflections of Pygeum

Pygeum carries the quiet confidence of an old forest tree—grounded, patient, and steady. Its bark medicine offers relief not through force, but through balance: easing urgency, smoothing flow, and lifting strain from a system often burdened by time and stress.

Rather than aggressively altering hormones, Pygeum tends the terrain—cooling inflammation, opening pathways, and restoring rhythm. Its greatest teaching is patience. Like the tree itself, Pygeum works slowly and dependably, returning peace to the night, comfort to the day, and confidence to the body's natural balance.

## ★ Herbal Confidence Index

🌿 🌿 🌿 🌿 **(4 / 5)**

A respected male tonic bark supporting prostate health, hormonal steadiness, and healthy urinary flow. Rooted in African healing traditions and reinforced by modern research, Pygeum remains a dependable long-term ally for men's wellness and restorative balance.

# GUDUCHI (GILOY)

★★★★★

*Tinospora cordifolia*

**Guduchi**, one of the most celebrated herbs in Ayurveda, often referred to as **Amrita**, meaning "nectar of immortality." With its heart-shaped leaves and climbing vine structure, Guduchi has long been treasured for promoting vitality, resilience, and whole-body rejuvenation. Traditional healers have used it to strengthen immunity, combat fever, and restore balance during recovery from illness or exhaustion.

Revered as a **Rasayana** (rejuvenator), Guduchi is said to sharpen the mind, calm the nerves, and support longevity. It has been traditionally employed to detoxify the blood, regulate blood sugar, and improve digestion. In Indian households, Guduchi is frequently combined with other herbs to enhance energy and resistance to seasonal illness, earning its place as a foundational herb of holistic wellness.

---

## 🌿 Core Herbal Category — Guduchi

*(Tinospora cordifolia)*

**Primary Core: Immune System Support** herb with (rasayana and immunomodulating principles that strengthen systemic resilience and support long-term vitality)

**Secondary Cores:** Liver & Detox Support herb · Metabolic Balance Support herb · Digestive Harmony Support herb

---

## 🌿 How It Works

Guduchi works by supplying alkaloids, diterpenes, and polysaccharides that help regulate immune response and enhance adaptive resilience. These compounds support liver detoxification pathways while protecting tissues from oxidative stress. Guduchi assists metabolic balance by improving glucose handling and cellular energy regulation. Its bitter-tonic qualities stimulate digestion, improve nutrient assimilation, and reduce metabolic stagnation.

---

## 🌱 Primary Uses

- Boosts immunity and resistance to infections
- Reduces chronic fever and inflammatory burden
- Supports liver function and detoxification
- Helps regulate blood sugar levels
- Promotes digestive balance and reduces acid buildup

- Enhances energy, focus, and longevity

---

## 🧪 Scientific Backing

Guduchi contains alkaloids (including berberine and magnoflorine), diterpenoid lactones, and polysaccharides.
Studies demonstrate **immunomodulatory, antioxidant, anti-inflammatory, antidiabetic, and hepatoprotective** effects.
Clinical findings support its role in reducing recurrent infections, improving white blood cell activity, regulating blood glucose, and restoring vitality after illness.

---

## 🍵 Forms Available

- Fresh or dried stem (for decoctions/teas)
- Powder (churna)
- Capsules and tablets
- Guduchi Satva (starch extract)
- Tincture or liquid extract

---

## 🍵 How to Use

**Tea / Decoction:**
- Add 1 tsp dried Guduchi stem powder to 2 cups water
- Simmer until reduced to 1 cup
- Strain and drink once daily

**Powder (Churna):**
- ½–1 tsp daily with warm water or honey

**Capsules/Tablets:**
- Follow standardized product dosing

**Tincture / Liquid Extract:**
- 20–40 drops, 1–2× daily

**Guduchi Satva (Starch Extract):**
- ½–1 tsp in warm water as a post-illness restorative

---

## ⚠ Caution Level: 🟠 Caution

- Generally safe but avoid during pregnancy or lactation unless supervised
- May lower blood sugar—use caution with diabetes medications

• Overuse may cause constipation in sensitive individuals

## 🚹 🚺 Gender-Specific Safety (GS)

**Men:** ● Safe
Widely regarded as a safe long-term rejuvenating tonic supporting immunity, metabolism, liver health, and endurance.
Men with autoimmune conditions should consult a practitioner.
**Women:** ● Safe
Traditionally used for inflammation, immune support, fatigue, and stress.
Use caution with autoimmune disorders.
**Pregnancy / Nursing:** ● Caution
Insufficient safety data—avoid unless supervised by a qualified practitioner.
Avoid high-dose extracts.

## ⌛ Expected Results

• **1–2 weeks:** Increased energy, reduced fatigue
• **3–4 weeks:** Improved digestion, clearer skin, stronger immunity
• **6–8 weeks:** Noticeable blood sugar and liver improvements

## 🛠 DIY Recipe — Guduchi Immunity Decoction

• 1 tsp dried Guduchi stem powder
• Boil in 2 cups water until reduced to 1 cup
• Strain and drink warm once daily
👉 Optional: add Tulsi + ginger for enhanced immune support

## 🔄 Same / Similar Results

● Ashwagandha · ● Amla · ● Licorice Root · ● Ginseng · ● Tulsi (Holy Basil)

## 🧴 Shelf Life / Potency After Preparation

• Dried stem: 2 years
• Powder (churna): 12–18 months
• Guduchi Satva: 1–2 years (airtight container)
• Capsules/Tablets: Follow product expiration

• Prepared decoction: Refrigerate up to 48 hours

---

## 🗨 Herbal Reflections of Guduchi

Guduchi stands apart as a true rejuvenator—often called the **Ayurvedic lifesaver** for its unusually broad healing spectrum. Unlike single-system herbs, it works across immunity, metabolism, digestion, and vitality, making it one of the rare herbs suitable for long-term use. Its unique starch extract (Guduchi Satva) restores strength after illness in a way few other herbs can match. Less widely known is its traditional use for sharpening memory and calming anxiety, confirming Guduchi's role as a bridge between physical restoration and mental clarity.

---

## ★ Herbal Confidence Index

🌿 🌿 🌿 🌿 🌿 **(5 / 5)**

A revered Ayurvedic rejuvenator known as **Amrita** ("the nectar of immortality"). Guduchi fortifies vitality, purifies the blood, balances metabolism, and strengthens immune and liver function—an enduring symbol of resilience, clarity, and longevity.

# PLEURISY ROOT

★★★★

*Asclepias tuberosa*

**Pleurisy Root** is a warming, lung-strengthening herb traditionally used to ease chest congestion, break up thick mucus, and relieve the painful breathing associated with pleurisy, bronchitis, and deep respiratory infections. It supports healthy lung expansion, reduces tightness, and gently stimulates expectoration without overstimulating the system.

Long valued by Indigenous healers and American Eclectic physicians, Pleurisy Root was considered one of the most dependable **pulmonary expectorants**—an herb that helps the lungs open, release lodged mucus, and breathe more freely. Its warming, sweat-inducing nature made it a central remedy for respiratory distress throughout the 18th and 19th centuries.

---

## Core Herbal Category — Pleurisy Root

*(Asclepias tuberosa)*

**Primary Core:** Respiratory System Support herb with (warming, antispasmodic principles that support bronchial relaxation and the release of lodged mucus)

**Secondary Cores:** Warming Diaphoretic Support herb · Anti-Inflammatory Lung Support herb

---

## How It Works

Pleurisy Root works by gently relaxing bronchial tissues, allowing constricted airways to open more freely. Its warming compounds encourage productive expectoration, helping clear thick or stagnant mucus from the lungs. The herb promotes mild perspiration, supporting the body's natural fever response during respiratory illness. Its anti-inflammatory action calms irritated pleural tissues, easing dry or painful breathing.

---

## Primary Uses

- Eases pleurisy and painful breathing
- Breaks up thick, sticky mucus
- Relieves chest congestion and tightness
- Supports bronchitis and deep coughs
- Encourages gentle sweating during fever

• Helps lungs expand more comfortably

---

## 🧪 Scientific Backing

Pleurisy Root contains asclepiadin, resins, flavonoids, and cardiac-like glycosides associated with:
• Expectorant and bronchodilating effects
• Mild diaphoretic (sweat-inducing) action
• Reduced pleural inflammation
• Improved lung circulation and oxygenation
Eclectic medical literature strongly documents its use for pleurisy, bronchitis, influenza-related chest pain, and painful productive coughs. Modern research is limited but supports its expectorant and inflammatory-modulating effects.

---

## 🍵 Forms Available

• Dried root (tea/decoction)
• Tincture (most common form)
• Capsules or powders
• Respiratory herbal blends

---

## ▧ How to Use

**Tincture:**
• 1–2 mL up to 3× daily during acute chest congestion
**Tea / Decoction:**
• 1 tsp root in 1½ cups water
• Simmer 15–20 minutes
• Drink 1–2× daily
**Capsules:**
• Follow standardized dosing
⚠ **Use short-term only** for active respiratory conditions; not a daily tonic.

---

## ⚠ Caution Level: ▨ Caution

• Avoid during pregnancy (possible uterine stimulation)
• Do not combine with digitalis/heart medications or strong sedatives
• Use caution with arrhythmias or low blood pressure
• High doses may cause nausea or vomiting

- Not for long-term daily use

**Safer daily lung tonics:** Mullein, Elecampane, Lungwort

---

## 🚹 🚺 Gender-Specific Safety (GS)

**Men:** ⚪ Caution

Safe short-term for pleurisy, bronchial tightness, or congestion.
Avoid with heart medications or arrhythmias.

**Women:** ⚪ Caution

Helpful for chest tightness and stuck mucus.
Avoid during heavy menstrual bleeding or when combining strong diaphoretics.

**Pregnancy / Nursing:** ⚫ Avoid

Not recommended due to cardiac-like glycosides and uterine stimulation.
Avoid while nursing (may irritate infant digestion).

---

## ⌛ Expected Results

- Chest tightness relief: **1–3 days**
- Improved mucus movement: **3–5 days**
- Deeper respiratory comfort: **5–10 days**
- Pleuritic pain relief: noticeable within several doses

---

## 🛠 DIY Recipe — Pleurisy Root Lung-Opening Tea

- 1 tsp Pleurisy Root
- 1 tsp Mullein Leaf
- ½ tsp Thyme

Simmer 15 minutes in 2 cups water.
Sip warm 2–3× daily during congestion or pleuritic pain.

---

## 🔄 Same / Similar Results

⚪ Mullein Leaf · ⚪ Elecampane · ⚪ Lobelia (low-dose) · ⚪ Thyme · ⚪ Wild Cherry Bark

---

## 🍬 Shelf Life / Potency After Preparation

- Dried root: 2–3 years (cool, dark storage)
- Tincture: 4–5 years
- Powder: 1 year (airtight container)

• Prepared tea/decoction: 36–48 hours refrigerated

---

## 🗨 Herbal Reflections of Pleurisy Root

Pleurisy Root is the herb of the deep breath—softening pain, easing tightness, and restoring movement to a chest locked by inflammation or fear. It invites warmth, release, and expansion where breathing has become guarded. Its medicine reminds the body how to open again, restoring comfort with every inhale.

---

## ★ Herbal Confidence Index

🌿 🌿 🌿 🌿 **(4 / 5)**

A dependable respiratory opener for pleurisy, deep coughs, and chest tightness—potent, time-tested, and highly effective when used respectfully and short-term.

# GRAPE SEED

★★★★

*Vitis vinifera*

**Grape Seed** extract is prized for its concentration of oligomeric proanthocyanidins (OPCs)—**powerful antioxidants that strengthen capillaries, improve circulation, and protect collagen. Traditionally linked with cardiovascular and skin health, this extract is often chosen to ease heavy legs, support eye comfort after long hours, and enhance overall tissue resilience. It provides subtle yet visible benefits, showing up in smoother skin, less swelling, and improved vascular tone over time.**

Because OPCs help stabilize collagen and capillary walls, Grape Seed sits at the intersection of beauty, circulation, and vision health. Taken daily, it functions like a supportive baseline—backing up lifestyle habits such as hydration, walking, and balanced nutrition. With consistent use, it offers long-term protective benefits for both appearance and inner vascular strength.

---

## Core Herbal Category — Grape Seed

*(Vitis vinifera)*

**Primary Core:** Cardiovascular System Support herb with (oligomeric proanthocyanidin–rich principles that strengthen capillaries, support endothelial integrity, and promote healthy blood flow)

**Secondary Cores:** Antioxidant Defense Support herb · Skin & Collagen Restoration Support herb

---

## How It Works

Grape Seed works by supplying proanthocyanidins that help protect and reinforce blood vessel walls.

These compounds support endothelial function and improve microcirculatory efficiency.

Its strong antioxidant activity helps neutralize free radicals that contribute to vascular and tissue aging.

The herb supports collagen stability, benefiting skin elasticity and connective tissue strength.

Through combined vascular and antioxidant action, Grape Seed promotes circulation resilience and tissue protection.

---

## Primary Uses

- Strengthens capillaries and blood vessels
- Supports healthy circulation and reduces swelling
- Enhances skin elasticity and collagen integrity
- Protects cells from oxidative damage
- Promotes eye and retinal health
- Supports recovery from venous insufficiency (tired, heavy legs)

---

## Scientific Backing

Grape Seed extract contains high levels of OPCs—antioxidants shown to support collagen repair, stabilize blood vessels, and reduce oxidative stress.

Clinical studies demonstrate benefits for:

- Improving circulation and capillary strength
- Supporting venous insufficiency
- Enhancing skin elasticity and reducing inflammation
- Providing retinal protection from oxidative stress

---

## Forms Available

- Capsules and tablets (standardized OPC extract)
- Liquid extract / tincture
- Powder for smoothies
- Topical creams for skin elasticity
- Combined formulas for cardiovascular or skin support

---

## How to Use (Dosage & Methods)

Typical dose: **100–300 mg daily** of standardized Grape Seed extract (containing OPCs).

- Take with food to support absorption
- Consistency is important—benefits increase over time

---

## Caution Level

● Generally safe and well tolerated.

● May mildly thin the blood—use caution if taking anticoagulants or preparing for surgery.

Avoid exceeding recommended doses without professional guidance.

---

## Gender-Specific Safety (GS)

**Men:**

● Safe and commonly used for circulation, vascular health, and antioxidant protection.

**Women:**
Safe for daily use; beneficial for swelling, vein support, and skin clarity.
**Pregnancy / Nursing:**
Use only with professional supervision due to limited safety research, though mild dietary exposure is generally considered low-risk.

---

## Expected Results (Timeline)

- **1–2 weeks:** Reduced leg fatigue, lighter circulation
- **3–6 weeks:** Improved skin tone, less puffiness, stronger vascular support
- **8–12 weeks:** Maximum antioxidant and collagen-protective effects

---

## Same/Similar Results

**Bilberry** — Eye & capillary support
**Hawthorn** — Circulatory strengthening
**Gotu Kola** — Collagen + vein health
**Horse Chestnut** — Varicose vein and swelling relief
**Schisandra** — Antioxidant and tissue protection

---

## DIY Recipe

**Circulation & Skin-Tone Support Blend**

- 1 tsp honey
- 1 tsp lemon juice
- ¼–½ tsp Grape Seed powder

Mix into warm water and drink once daily to support vascular tone and skin clarity.

---

## Shelf Life / Potency After Preparation

- Capsules & powder: **2 years** if kept cool and dry
- Liquid extract: **3–4 years** when stored properly
- Once mixed into beverages: consume immediately

---

## Herbal Reflections of Grape Seed

Grape Seed stands apart as one of nature's most concentrated antioxidant sources, offering protection that goes far beyond simple circulation support. Unlike herbs that work quickly and fade, Grape Seed builds a steady, long-term foundation for vascular strength, collagen resilience, and oxidative defense. It pairs well with lifestyle improvements and is especially valuable in modern times when environmental stressors are high.

Few herbs can match its combined benefits for skin, circulation, and vision, making it a quiet but powerful cornerstone in daily wellness.

### Herbal Confidence Index — Grape Seed: ★★★★

Potent antioxidant and vascular-support herb that strengthens circulation and tissue integrity, with strong reliability and excellent long-term safety when used appropriately.

# PINE BARK

★★★★

*Pinus pinaster*

**Pine Bark extract**, often marketed under the name **Pycnogenol®**, is a powerful antioxidant derived from the bark of the French maritime pine. For centuries, it has been used in European folk medicine to ease circulation, reduce swelling, and support wound healing. Modern science identifies it as a rich source of procyanidins—compounds that stabilize capillaries, strengthen veins, and protect collagen from oxidative stress. This makes Pine Bark especially valued for cardiovascular wellness, microcirculation support, and skin vitality.

Beyond its vascular benefits, Pine Bark has gained recognition for improving cognitive function, eye health, and athletic recovery. Its ability to increase nitric oxide production supports healthy blood flow, enhancing stamina, reducing leg heaviness, and improving oxygen delivery to tissues throughout the body.

---

**Core Herbal Category — Pine Bark**

**Primary Core: Cardiovascular System Support** herb with (capillary-protective, flow-enhancing polyphenols that support vascular integrity and tissue perfusion)

**Secondary Cores:** Antioxidant Defense herb · Skin & Collagen Health herb · Cognitive Support herb

## How It Works

Pine Bark works by strengthening capillary walls and supporting healthy vascular tone, allowing blood to move efficiently through the smallest vessels. Its polyphenols protect the endothelial lining and reduce oxidative stress that weakens microcirculation. Improved microvascular flow enhances oxygen and nutrient delivery to tissues, reinforcing skin structure, collagen maintenance, and cognitive clarity over time.

---

## Primary Uses

- Enhances circulation and vein strength
- Supports skin elasticity and collagen protection
- Reduces leg heaviness, swelling, and microvascular stress
- Promotes eye comfort and retinal health
- Aids cognitive function and endurance recovery

---

## 🧪 Scientific Backing

Clinical research on **Pycnogenol®** demonstrates benefits in chronic venous insufficiency, diabetic retinopathy, and cardiovascular health. Studies confirm its strong antioxidant capacity, nitric-oxide-enhancing effects, and connective-tissue protection. Human trials report reduced leg edema, improved skin hydration and elasticity, enhanced circulation, and better athletic recovery.

---

## Forms Available

- Standardized capsules or tablets (50–100 mg)
- Powdered extract (for mixing)
- Combination formulas (with Vitamin C, Grape Seed, or Bilberry)

---

## How to Use (Dosage & Methods)

Pine Bark is most effective when taken consistently.

- **Capsules / Tablets:** 50–100 mg, 1–2× daily (standardized to Pycnogenol® or procyanidins)
- **Powder:** ¼ tsp daily in water, juice, or smoothies
- **Tincture:** 1–2 mL, 1–2× daily

*Note:* Best results appear after 3–6 weeks of steady use.

---

⚠ **Caution Level:** **Caution**
Generally well tolerated. Rare GI upset or dizziness may occur.
Use caution with anticoagulants or antiplatelet medications.
Discontinue 1–2 weeks before surgery.
Limited safety data in pregnancy or breastfeeding.

---

## Gender-Specific Safety — Pine Bark (Pycnogenol®)

**Men — Safe**
Supports circulation, endothelial health, joint comfort, and antioxidant defense. Mild blood-thinning effects possible at higher doses; use moderation if on anticoagulants or aspirin therapy.
**Women — Safe**

Supports circulation, skin radiance, and vascular tone. May help with menstrual discomfort related to vascular fragility. No known estrogenic effects. Monitor dosing if prone to heavy bleeding.

**Pregnancy / Nursing — Caution**

Limited clinical data. Avoid concentrated extracts unless guided by a qualified practitioner. Gentler antioxidants such as Rooibos, Rosehip, or Nettle are preferred.

---

## DIY Recipe — Pine Bark Circulation Elixir

- 50–100 mg Pine Bark extract powder
- 8 oz water
- Add citrus juice for absorption
  Drink once daily with food.

---

## Same / Similar Results

Grape Seed · Bilberry · Horse Chestnut · Gotu Kola · Witch Hazel (external only)

---

## Shelf Life / Potency — Pine Bark

- **Dried Bark:** 2–3 years (airtight, cool, dark)
- **Tincture / Liquid Extract:** 4–6 years
- **Capsules / Powder:** 1–2 years
- **Prepared Tea:** 24–48 hours refrigerated

---

## Herbal Reflections of Pine Bark

Pine Bark works as a quiet shield—reinforcing vessels and connective tissues from within. Its strength is cumulative, not forceful, rewarding patience with steadier circulation, lighter legs, clearer skin tone, and enduring resilience. It is a companion herb to movement, hydration, and consistency, amplifying the body's natural repair rhythms.

**Herbal Confidence Index:** **(4 / 5)**

A modern antioxidant powerhouse rooted in ancient forest medicine. Pine Bark Extract protects blood vessels, enhances circulation, supports skin and cognition, and reinforces graceful aging through steady, reliable action.

# ECHINACEA

★★★★★

*Echinacea purpurea*

**Echinacea** is one of the most widely recognized immune-supporting herbs, **traditionally used by Native American tribes for infections, snakebites, and wound healing. Today it is best known as a first-line defense during colds, flu, and seasonal immune challenges**. Its purple coneflower blossoms and roots contain polysaccharides, alkamides, and caffeic acid derivatives that stimulate immune response, helping the body to respond quickly to pathogens and strengthen overall resistance.

**Beyond its role in acute illness, Echinacea is also valued for its anti-inflammatory and antioxidant actions. Herbalists often recommend it to shorten the duration of colds, ease sore throats, and provide relief for respiratory discomfort.** While not intended for indefinite daily use, **Echinacea excels as a short-term "booster herb", giving the immune system the quick push it needs during times of stress, exposure, or infection.** Its reputation as a fast-acting immune ally makes it one of the most trusted and dependable herbs in both traditional and modern herbal practice.

## Core Herbal Category — Echinacea

**Primary Core: Immune System Support** herb with (immune-activating, response-modulating action that supports the body's early defense mechanisms)

**Secondary Cores:** Respiratory Support herb · Lymphatic Support herb · Skin & Wound Support herb

## How It Works

Echinacea works by stimulating immune cell activity and supporting a rapid, organized response to external challenges. It helps activate macrophages and other frontline defenders while modulating excessive immune strain. The herb supports lymphatic movement, aiding the clearance of metabolic debris and immune byproducts. Its immune-directing action benefits respiratory tissues during periods of stress. Topically and internally, it supports tissue defense and repair in the skin.

---

## *Primary Uses*

- Stimulates immune response during cold and flu
- Helps shorten duration/severity of infections

- *Provides respiratory and throat comfort*
- Supports wound healing and skin protection

---

## 🔬 Scientific Backing

Echinacea activates white blood cells, enhances phagocytosis, and modulates cytokine response. Research shows generally favorable results when taken at the first sign of symptoms, often shortening cold duration and improving immune alertness.

---

## 🍵 Forms Available

- Dried root/aerial parts (tea or decoction)
- *Standardized capsules/tablets*
- *Liquid extract/tincture*
- *Lozenges and throat sprays*

---

## 📘 How to Use (Dosage)

**Tincture:** 1–2 mL every 2–3 hours during acute symptoms (first 24–48 hours), then 2–3× daily
**Tea (root):** Simmer 1–2 tsp dried root in 8 oz water for 10–15 min; drink 2–3× daily
**Capsules:** Follow product-standardized instructions (commonly 300–500 mg, 2–3× daily during onset)
**Topical:** Use infused oils/salves for minor skin irritation or wound support
👉 **Best Strategy:** Begin immediately at the first sign of illness.
Not intended for daily use longer than 6–8 weeks.

---

## ⏱ Expected Results

- **1–3 days:** Relief of throat irritation, boosted immune alertness
- **1–2 weeks:** Shortened duration of colds/infections

- **3–6 weeks:** Improved resilience with cyclical use

---

## ⚠ Caution Level: Caution

- Avoid if allergic to Asteraceae (ragweed, chamomile, yarrow)
- May interact with immunosuppressant medication
- *Rare rash or digestive upset possible*
- *Not for continuous long-term daily use*
- Use cautiously with autoimmune conditions

---

## Gender-Specific Safety — Echinacea

### Men — Safe

Well tolerated during colds, infections, or seasonal exposure. Mild GI upset or tingling may occur (especially with E. angustifolia).
Use caution with autoimmune disease.

### Women — Safe

Well tolerated for short-term immune activation. Non-hormonal and gentle.
Women with autoimmune disorders should use periodically, not daily.

### Pregnancy / Nursing — Caution

Generally regarded as one of the safer herbs during pregnancy, but use should be:

- *Occasional*
- *Moderate*
- *Not continuous*

Breastfeeding: start with small amounts; watch infant for mild digestive sensitivity.
Safer everyday immune herbs: **Nettle, Rooibos, Ginger.**

---

## Shelf Life / Potency After Preparation

**Tincture:** 4–6 years (stored cool, dark)

- **Dried Root:** 1–2 years (airtight jar, low humidity)
- **Prepared Tea:** Best within 24 hours (refrigerated)
- **Homemade Syrups/Blends:** 2–4 weeks (refrigerated)
- **Capsules/Tablets:** 2–3 years (check manufacturer date)

Potency declines sharply with heat, moisture, and light exposure.

---

## *DIY Recipe — Immune-Boosting Echinacea Tea*

- Simmer **1–2 tsp dried root** in **8 oz water for 10–15 minutes**
- Strain and drink warm **2–3× daily** at symptom onset
  Add **lemon + honey** for throat relief

---

## *Same/Similar Results*

*Elderberry Astragalus Andrographis Goldenseal (sustainability caution) Garlic (raw may irritate stomach)*

---

## *Herbal Reflections of Echinacea*

Echinacea feels like a sentry standing guard—it doesn't work in the background like nutritive tonics but steps forward when the body sounds the alarm. Its strength is in its immediacy, especially when taken at the very first tingle of a sore throat or heaviness behind the eyes.

Unlike herbs that build over months, Echinacea shines during acute need. For those who face frequent colds or winter exposures, it offers not just relief, but a sense of readiness and resilience. It teaches timing, precision, and the art of supporting the body's defenses right when they are needed most.

**Herbal Confidence Index**

(4 / 5 — A fast-acting immune "sentry" that shines when taken at the very first sign of illness. Echinacea is a trusted short-term ally for colds, flu, and acute infections, offering strong support when used promptly and wisely rather than as a daily long-term tonic.)

# SOLOMON'S SEAL

★★★★★

*Polygonatum biflorum*

**Solomon's Seal** is a favorite for joints, tendons, and ligaments that feel dry, creaky, or overused. Herbalists reach for it when tissues need glide and lubrication—supporting synovial fluid, fascia, and the soft-tissue matrix so movement feels more like it should. It shines after sprains, repetitive strain, or weekend overuse: not a painkiller, but a restorer that helps tissues track properly again when paired with gentle movement, hydration, and smart rest.

Beyond easing wear-and-tear, many use the moistening rhizome for tendon sheaths, bursae, and "clicky" joints that need coaxing back to smooth mechanics. Known across northern woodlands, Solomon's Seal has a long record in Indigenous North American and European folk medicine for musculoskeletal comfort and convalescence. Its name nods to folklore: the rhizome's round leaf-scar "seals" were likened to King Solomon's signet, a symbol of wisdom and repair. In apothecaries and cottage lore alike, it stood for setting things right—quiet, steady restoration over quick fixes.

---

**Core Herbal Category — Solomon's Seal**

**Primary Core: Anti-Inflammatory & Pain Support** herb with (steroidal saponin principles that lubricate joints, restore connective tissue tone, and ease musculoskeletal tension)

**Secondary Cores:** Connective Tissue Support herb · Anti-Inflammatory Support herb · Joint Lubrication Support herb

---

### *How It Works*

Solomon's Seal works by nourishing and restoring connective tissues that support joints, tendons, and ligaments. Its tissue-rebuilding properties help improve elasticity and resilience within the musculoskeletal system. The herb supports natural joint lubrication, allowing smoother movement and reduced friction. By calming inflammatory stress, it aids recovery from wear and strain. This restorative action promotes long-term structural balance and mobility.

---

### *Primary Uses*

- Tendon and ligament comfort; promotes healthy glide
- Supports joint lubrication for dry or creaky joints
- Helps recovery after sprains or repetitive strain
- Soothes irritated connective-tissue sheaths

- Useful for bursae inflammation and soft-tissue wear

---

## 🧪 Scientific Backing

Traditional use highlights Solomon's Seal's affinity for soft-tissue restoration and synovial support. While modern laboratory literature is limited, clinical herbalists consistently report improved range of motion, reduced creakiness, and stronger tendon resilience with steady use. It remains a cornerstone herb in connective-tissue, sports-injury, and rehabilitation-support formulas.

---

## *Forms Available*

- *Tincture (most common)*
- *Decoction (low simmer of dried rhizome)*
- Topical preparations: infused oil or liniment for localized support

---

## How to Use (Dosage)

***Tincture:***

- *10–30 drops (0.5–1 mL), 2–3× daily*
- For sprains or tendon irritation, smaller doses taken more frequently work best

***Decoction:***

- 1 tsp chopped rhizome simmered in 1 cup water for 15 minutes
- *Drink 1–2× daily*

***Topical:***

- Massage infused oil or liniment 2–3× daily over affected areas
- Best paired with gentle, consistent range-of-motion work

---

## *Expected Results*

- Smoother movement / less creak: 1–3 weeks
- Tendon and ligament comfort: 3–6+ weeks with rehabilitation

- Post-sprain stability and confidence: gradual, ongoing improvement

---

⚠️ **Caution Level:** 🟢 **Safe (Mild Use Advisory)**

- Generally well tolerated when properly prepared
- Large doses may cause mild digestive upset
- Avoid in pregnancy unless guided by a professional
- Ensure reputable species sourcing to avoid adulterants

---

## 🚹 🚺 Gender-Specific Safety — Solomon's Seal

🟢 **Men — Safe**
Well tolerated in tincture, decoction, or topical form. Offers steady soft-tissue support without hormonal effects. Those with sensitive digestion should begin with smaller doses.

🟢 **Women — Safe**
Supportive for overuse injuries, postpartum tendon strain, and joint dryness. Mild digestive upset may occur at higher doses.

🟡 **Pregnancy / Nursing — Caution**
Limited research—avoid systemic use unless professionally guided.
Topical external preparations are generally acceptable.

---

## 🛠️ DIY Recipe — Tendon-Glide Liniment

- *1 tsp Solomon's Seal tincture*
- *1 tsp Arnica oil*

Massage gently along tender or inflamed areas 2–3× daily.
Pair with light physical therapy or mobility work.

---

## 🔄 *Same / Similar Results*

🟢 Comfrey (external only) · 🟢 Boswellia · 🟢 Turmeric · 🟢 Devil's Claw · 🟢 Ginger

---

## ⏳ Shelf Life / Potency After Preparation

- **Dried Rhizome:** 2 years (cool, dry storage)

- **Tincture:** 4–5 years (excellent potency retention)
- **Infused Oil:** 1 year refrigerated; ~6 months at room temperature
- **Decoction:** Refrigerate 48 hours; freeze portions for 1–2 months

---

## 🗨 Herbal Reflections of Solomon's Seal

Solomon's Seal is the whisperer of joints and soft tissue—more oil can than hammer. Its mellow, mucilaginous rhizome restores glide where tissues should slide: tendons in tight sheaths, ligaments tugged by overuse, joints dried by inflammation or strain. Rather than forcing a fix, it coaxes hydration back into connective tissue and calms irritated insertions.
Think of it as a background harmonizer: small, frequent doses over weeks, paired with respectful movement. It layers beautifully with arnica or comfrey for sprains, turmeric or ginger for systemic inflammation, and marshmallow for dryness. Used patiently, Solomon's Seal trades bravado for longevity—returning ease, lubrication, and quiet strength to the body's working hinges.

---

**Herbal Confidence Index:**
🌿 🌿 🌿 🌿 🌿 **(5 / 5)** — A master-level restorative herb for tendons, ligaments, and joints. Solomon's Seal hydrates, aligns, and rehabilitates connective tissues with quiet intelligence. Its safety, consistency, and deep nourishment make it one of the finest long-term allies for structural healing.

# *BILBERRY*

★★★★★

*Vaccinium myrtillus*

**Bilberry** is a small, intensely colored European cousin of the blueberry, renowned for its rich anthocyanins that nourish the eyes, blood vessels, and delicate capillaries. Long used in European folk and clinical herbalism**, Bilberry supports night vision, visual comfort under strain, and healthy microcirculation to the retina and other fine vascular beds.** It has become a favorite herb for readers, drivers, screen workers, and elders who want to preserve clarity and ease of sight. **Beyond the eyes, Bilberry's deep pigments act as powerful antioxidants that protect collagen-rich tissues throughout the body. Herbalists turn to it for strengthening fragile capillaries, easing leg heaviness or varicose tendencies, and supporting healthy circulation in people managing blood sugar or metabolic stress.** Gentle, food-like, and versatile, Bilberry is both a protective daily berry and a targeted ally for eye and vascular resilience.

---

## 🌿 Core Herbal Category — Bilberry

**Primary Core: Cardiovascular System Support** herb with (capillary-strengthening, vision-supportive anthocyanins that protect retinal and vascular tissue)
**Secondary Cores:** Antioxidant Defense herb · Vein & Capillary Strength herb · Metabolic & Blood Sugar Support herb

---

## How It Works

Bilberry works by strengthening small blood vessels and improving circulation to delicate tissues, particularly within the eyes. Its anthocyanins help protect the retina from oxidative stress and support visual clarity. By reinforcing capillary walls, the herb promotes stable blood flow and vascular resilience. Improved microcirculation supports metabolic efficiency at the cellular level. This balanced vascular support contributes to both eye function and blood sugar stability.

## 🌱 Primary Uses

- Supports night vision and visual comfort under strain (reading, screens, night driving)
- Strengthens fragile capillaries (eyes, skin, veins)
- Helps ease leg heaviness and vein discomfort (varicose-prone legs)
- Provides broad-spectrum antioxidant protection for collagen and connective tissue
- Supports healthy blood sugar and microvascular health in metabolic stress

---

## 🧪 Scientific Backing

Bilberry berries are rich in anthocyanins and other flavonoids that:

- Improve capillary integrity and reduce fragility

• Support retinal circulation and protect photoreceptor cells
• Exhibit strong antioxidant and anti-inflammatory actions
• Help maintain healthy blood flow in microvascular beds
Studies and traditional use both support Bilberry's role in night-vision support, vascular tone, and antioxidant protection—especially when used consistently over time.

---

## Forms Available

• Fresh or frozen berries (food and smoothies)
• Dried berries (tea or decoction)
• Standardized capsules/tablets (anthocyanin-rich extract)
• Tincture or liquid extract
• Combined eye-support formulas (with Eyebright, Ginkgo, etc.)

---

## How to Use (Dosage)

**Food (Everyday Support):**
• ½–1 cup fresh or frozen Bilberries (or mixed dark berries) daily as food
**Tea / Decoction:**
• 1–2 tsp dried berries in 1 cup water
• Simmer gently 10–15 minutes, then steep covered 10 minutes
• Drink 1–2× daily for eye and vessel support
**Capsules (Standardized Extract):**
• 80–160 mg standardized extract (often 25% anthocyanosides)
• 1–2× daily with meals
**Tincture:**
• 1–2 mL, 1–2× daily
• Best taken with food for long-term vascular support

---

## Expected Results

• Eye comfort under strain: 1–2 weeks
• Night-vision support: 4–8 weeks of consistent use
• Vein/capillary tone and leg comfort: 4–12 weeks
• Antioxidant and metabolic support: gradual, cumulative over months

---

## Caution Level: Safe (Mild Use Advisory)

• Generally very safe as a food-like herb
• High-dose extracts may mildly thin the blood — use caution with anticoagulants or antiplatelet meds
• May enhance blood sugar–lowering efforts; monitor levels if on diabetes medications
• Excessive intake may cause mild digestive looseness in sensitive individuals

---

### Gender-Specific Safety — Bilberry

**Men — Safe**

Well tolerated and beneficial for eye strain, circulation, capillary strength, and metabolic support.
• Use extra awareness if taking blood thinners or multiple cardiovascular medications.

**Women — Safe**

Supports visual comfort, vein tone (including varicose-prone legs), and collagen integrity.
• Generally safe across life stages, with the same mild cautions regarding blood thinners and diabetes meds.

**Pregnancy / Nursing — Mild Caution**

• Food-level use (berries in meals) is considered safe and nourishing.
• High-dose extracts or tinctures should be used cautiously and ideally with professional guidance.

---

## Shelf Life / Potency After Preparation

• Dried Berries: 1–2 years (airtight, dark, cool)
• Standardized Capsules: 2–3 years (follow manufacturer's date)
• Tincture: 4–5 years (cool, dark storage)
• Prepared Tea/Decoction: Best within 24 hours refrigerated

Anthocyanin potency drops with heat, light, and long storage; protect from those for best results.

---

## DIY Recipe — Eye & Vein Support Berry Tea

• 1 tsp dried Bilberries
• 1 tsp dried Blueberries or Hawthorn berries (optional)
• 1 cup hot water

Simmer gently for 10–15 minutes, then cover and steep another 10 minutes.
Drink 1–2× daily, especially during periods of eye strain or heavy standing/walking days.

---

## Same/Similar Results

Goji Berry • Blueberry • Grape Seed Extract • Hawthorn • Eyebright

## Herbal Reflections of Bilberry

Bilberry feels like twilight medicine for the eyes and vessels—protecting the places where light, blood, and perception meet. It doesn't rush; instead, it quietly reinforces the tiny capillaries that keep vision clear, legs light, and tissues resilient. Used regularly, it teaches the value of slow, consistent care.

## Herbal Confidence Index

(4 / 5 — A gentle yet powerful microcirculation and eye-health ally. Bilberry's anthocyanin-rich profile protects capillaries, supports night vision, and strengthens vascular tissues throughout the body. Best as a long-term, food-like protector rather than a quick-fix remedy.)

# KANNA

★★★★

*Sceletium tortuosum*

**Kanna** offers clear-headed calm rather than knock-you-out sedation—**a steadying lift that takes the edge off without dulling focus**. People reach for it when stress feels loud but thinking, speaking, and working still matter, making it a favorite for social ease, "Sunday scaries," public speaking, and desk-time jitters. In practice it can soften anxious rumination, brighten low mood, and release jaw or shoulder tension, with a day-friendly composure that pairs well with breath work or a short walk. Chewed, sublingual, or taken as tea or tincture, effects are typically felt within minutes to an hour.

Alongside this immediate composure, Kanna can support resilience over time—**helping some users ride out cravings, ease irritability, and rebuild baseline good mood during stressful seasons**. It is best used at modest doses to keep clarity intact; modern practitioners commonly caution against combining it with serotonergic medications.

Known in southern Africa as *kougoed* ("chew-good"), Kanna has been prepared and chewed by Khoi and San peoples for centuries, traditionally fermented to mellow bitterness and enhance effect before communal use for mood, stamina, and social connection. Early Cape accounts describe its trade and ritual value; modern research highlights mesembrine-type alkaloids (SERT modulation and PDE-4 pathways) consistent with its calming-yet-clear profile. Today it appears as standardized extracts, teas, and chews—an herb that bridges ancient convivial use and contemporary stress care without the fog.

---

## Core Herbal Category — Kanna

Primary Core: **Nervous System Support (Nervines)** herb with (calming, mood-modulating alkaloids that support emotional resilience and mental balance)

Secondary Cores: Mood & Emotional Balance herb · Cognitive Support herb

---

## How It Works

Kanna supports neurotransmitter balance within the nervous system, calming stress responses while preserving clarity. Its alkaloids promote emotional steadiness, reduce nervous tension, and help maintain focus during periods of pressure. The result is composed, day-friendly calm without sedation or cognitive dulling.

---

## Primary Uses

- Daytime anxious stress and social ease
- Mood steadiness without drowsiness

• Focus under pressure; gentle lift in outlook

---

## 🧪 Scientific Backing

Kanna contains mesembrine-type alkaloids that influence serotonin reuptake and PDE-4 pathways. Standardized extracts show benefits for stress reduction, emotional steadiness, and calmer cognitive performance. Effects may appear within 30–120 minutes and can build gradually with consistent, modest use.

---

## Forms Available

• Standardized extract capsules or tablets
• Sublingual powder or chew (traditional kougoed)
• Tincture (standardized strength preferred)

---

## ⚠ Caution Level: Caution

**• Do not combine with SSRIs, SNRIs, MAOIs, or antidepressant/anti-anxiety medications**
• High doses may cause headache, nausea, emotional flattening, or overstimulation
• Avoid with bipolar disorder, schizophrenia, or severe mood instability
• Avoid alcohol or sedatives
• Avoid during pregnancy or breastfeeding
• Always begin with very low doses

---

## Gender-Specific Safety (GS)

**Men:** Caution — Preserves clarity while easing tension; avoid if using psychiatric medications.
**Women:** Caution — Helpful for emotional strain; start very low to prevent nausea or oversedation.
**Pregnancy/Nursing:** Avoid — Psychoactive alkaloids are not considered safe.

---

## Expected Results

• Calm, clear focus: 30–120 minutes
• Mood steadiness: several days to 2 weeks
• Social ease: often same day

---

## How to Use (Dosage)

• Sublingual powder: **25–75 mg**, effects in 20–45 minutes
• Capsules/extract: **50–150 mg**, once or twice daily
• Chewable kougoed: pea-sized pinch, chewed slowly

• Tincture: **0.5–1 mL**, up to 2× daily
👉 Always start at the lowest effective dose

---

## ♻ Shelf Life / Potency

• Dried herb/powder: ~2 years
• Capsules: 2–3 years
• Tincture: 3–5 years
• Homemade lozenges: 2–3 months refrigerated

---

## 🛠 DIY Recipe — "Calm Focus" Kanna Lozenge

Mix **100–200 mg** Kanna powder with **1 tsp raw honey**.
Dry thinly, cut into pea-sized pieces.
Dissolve **one lozenge** under the tongue as needed (max 2× daily).

---

## 💬 Herbal Reflections of Kanna

Kanna is a mood-softener rooted in South African desert wisdom, traditionally chewed as *kougoed* to smooth worry, brighten spirit, and ease conversation. Its touch is clear rather than heavy — mental noise quiets, tension releases, and the day feels more workable.

Where Kava slows and St. John's Wort asks for weeks, Kanna often works in the moment, offering composure without fog. Used respectfully, it supports ease rather than escape.

---

## ✿ Herbal Confidence Index

🌿 🌿 🌿 🌿 (4 / 5) — A refined mood-balancing succulent that eases anxiety, softens tension, and supports calm focus when used with proper dosing and medication awareness.

# MULUNGU

★★★★

*Erythrina mulungu*

**Mulungu** is a traditional South American healing tree, native to Brazil and other parts of the Amazon, where its bark and flowers have been used for centuries by Indigenous healers as a calming remedy. **Known as a natural sedative, Mulungu has long been turned to for anxiety, insomnia, stress relief, and even support during emotional upheaval.** Its gentle yet profound influence on the nervous system makes it one of the most respected herbal allies for restoring peace of mind and restful sleep in tropical folk medicine.

**Beyond its sedative effects, Mulungu is also valued for its ability to lower blood pressure, ease palpitations, and calm the overworked heart.** Traditional use often placed it in contexts of community healing, where stress, conflict, or grief needed soothing. **Modern research continues to explore its alkaloids, such as erythravine, which interact with brain receptors to produce relaxation without heavy side effects.** In an anxious and overstimulated world, Mulungu remains a botanical symbol of tranquility—an herb that helps the mind slow down, the body unclench, and the spirit find stillness again.

---

## Core Herbal Category — Mulungu

Primary Core: **Nervous System Support (Nervines)** herb with (deeply relaxing, nervous-system-quieting compounds that reduce excitatory signaling and promote restorative calm)
Secondary Cores: Sleep Support herb · Cardiovascular (Stress-Induced) Support herb · Emotional Restoration herb

---

### How It Works

Mulungu calms overactive nervous system signaling, helping the body shift out of heightened stress states. Its alkaloids promote mental quiet, physical relaxation, and smoother sleep onset without stimulant effects. By reducing stress-driven tension, it indirectly supports cardiovascular balance and emotional recovery from prolonged strain.

---

### Primary Uses

- Calms anxiety, agitation, and emotional overload
- Supports relaxation and restorative sleep

- Helps reduce stress-related hypertension and palpitations
- Relieves muscle tension and restlessness
- Supports emotional settling after prolonged stress or trauma

---

## 🧪 Scientific Backing

Mulungu contains erythrinian alkaloids (including erythravine) associated with nervous-system calming, muscle relaxation, reduced anxiety-related tension, mild blood-pressure lowering, and improved sleep quality. Traditional Amazonian use is extensive for insomnia, agitation, emotional overload, and stress-induced cardiovascular discomfort. Modern research continues to explore its sedative and anxiolytic mechanisms.

---

## Forms Available

- Tincture (preferred for absorption)
- Standardized capsules (bark extract)
- Decoction (traditional; very bitter)

---

## How to Use (Dosage)

**Tincture:** 1–2 mL in water, evening use only (start with 0.5–1 mL)
**Capsules:** Follow standardized dosing (often 200–400 mg), 30–60 minutes before bed
**Decoction:** ½–1 tsp dried bark simmered 10–15 minutes (use cautiously)
**Timing:** Nighttime only

---

## ⚠ Caution Level: Use with Caution

- Strong sedative — may cause drowsiness, dizziness, or slowed reaction time
- Avoid alcohol, benzodiazepines, opioids, sleep meds, or other sedatives
- May lower blood pressure; use caution with hypotension or BP medications
- Avoid driving or machinery use after dosing
- Avoid during pregnancy or breastfeeding
- Long-term use: cycle (2–3 weeks on, 1 week off)

---

## Gender-Specific Safety (GS)

**Men:** Caution — Effective for anxiety and sleep; monitor BP, drowsiness, and morning heaviness.
**Women:** Caution — Helpful for tension-based insomnia; monitor for grogginess or hypotension.
**Pregnancy/Nursing:** Avoid — Sedative alkaloids + insufficient safety data.

---

## Expected Results

- Wind-down ease: first night–1 week
- Improved sleep quality: 1–2 weeks
- Tension relief: several days–2 weeks

---

## DIY Recipe — Evening Unwind Drops

- Mulungu tincture: 1–2 mL
- Passionflower tincture: 1 mL

Mix in water 30–60 minutes before bed. Reduce dose if overly sedating.

---

## Same / Similar Results

Passionflower · Lemon Balm · Chamomile
Valerian (dose carefully) · Kava (short-term only)

---

## Shelf Life / Potency

- Dried bark: 2–3 years
- Tincture: 4–5 years
- Capsules: 2 years unopened; 1 year opened
- Decoction: Use within 48 hours refrigerated

---

## Herbal Reflections of Mulungu

Mulungu feels like dusk settling over a restless nervous system — steady, grounding, and quieting. It slows the inner tempo without force, offering relief rather than collapse. Compared to lighter nervines it moves deeper; compared to heavy sedatives it remains humane. Used with respect, Mulungu teaches the body how to exhale again.

---

## Herbal Confidence Index

(4 / 5 — A deeply calming Amazonian sedative for anxiety, emotional overload, and insomnia. When used wisely, it softens nervous tension and promotes restorative sleep without harshness.)

# COLEUS FORSKOHLII

★★★★

*Plectranthus barbatus*

**Coleus forskohlii is a member of the mint family native to India, long used in Ayurvedic medicine for supporting heart health, respiratory function, and metabolic balance.** Its root contains the compound forskolin, which stimulates the enzyme adenylate cyclase, increasing levels of cyclic AMP (cAMP) in cells. **This action improves cellular signaling, influencing cardiovascular, respiratory, and metabolic processes.**
**What makes Coleus forskohlii unique is its ability to support healthy blood pressure, enhance circulation, and improve breathing capacity, while also showing promise for aiding weight management and thyroid function.** In **Ayurveda, it was traditionally used for heart conditions, asthma, and digestive complaints, but modern research has expanded its recognition as a versatile herb that works at a cellular level.**

---

## 🌿 Core Herbal Category — Coleus forskohlii

**Primary Core:** **Cardiovascular System Support** herb with *(vasodilatory, signal-activating compounds that support healthy blood flow and cellular communication)*
**Secondary Cores:** Metabolic Activation herb · Respiratory Opening herb · Thyroid & Energy Regulation herb

---

## How It Works

Coleus forskohlii works by supporting cellular signaling pathways that encourage blood vessel relaxation and efficient circulation. This vasodilatory action helps improve oxygen and nutrient delivery throughout the body. By supporting metabolic activation, the herb assists energy utilization at the cellular level. Its respiratory-opening influence supports freer airflow and oxygen exchange. These combined actions contribute to balanced cardiovascular performance and energy regulation.

---

## 🌱 Primary Uses

- Supports healthy blood pressure regulation
- Improves circulation and heart function
- Enhances respiratory function (asthma, bronchial tightness)
- Aids metabolism, thyroid health, and weight management

● Supports energy balance through improved cAMP signaling

---

## Scientific Backing

Forskolin has been studied for:
- Vasodilation and healthy blood pressure regulation
- Increased fat metabolism via elevated cAMP
- Bronchodilatory effects useful for asthma
- Thyroid-stimulating properties (T3/T4 support)
- Potential intraocular pressure reduction in glaucoma

Clinical evidence varies by extract quality but shows promise for metabolic and cardiovascular activation.

---

## Forms Available

● Standardized extract capsules (root)
● Tincture (less common)
● Powdered root for encapsulation or teas

---

## How to Use (Dosage)

**Capsules (standardized extract):**
- 100–250 mg extract daily (typically standardized to 10–20% forskolin)
- Take with food to reduce stomach irritation

**Tincture:**
- 1–2 mL, up to 2× daily
- Best taken with meals

**Tea / Hot infusion:**
- 1 tsp dried root in 1 cup hot water
- Steep covered 10–12 minutes
- Drink 1× daily for metabolic and circulatory support

**Cycles:**
- 8–12 weeks on, followed by 2–4 weeks off

---

## Caution Level: ● Caution

- May lower blood pressure or increase heart rate
- Use caution with antihypertensive meds or low BP
- May enhance effects of blood thinners or thyroid meds
- Large doses may cause dizziness, rapid heartbeat, or stomach burning
- Avoid during pregnancy/breastfeeding

• Discontinue 1–2 weeks before surgery
• Avoid if you have ulcers, active bleeding disorders, or serious heart disease

---

## 🚹 🚺 Gender-Specific Safety — Coleus forskohlii

### 🟠 Men — Caution

Supports metabolism, circulation, bronchial opening, and energy.
Avoid or use medically supervised if taking:
• BP meds
• Blood thinners
• Thyroid meds
• Acid-reflux meds
Begin low-dose with food; monitor dizziness or heart-pounding.

### 🟠 Women — Caution

Helpful for metabolism, thyroid, and circulation.
Avoid or use carefully if you have:
• Heavy menstrual flow
• Fibroids
• Anemia
• Low BP or acid sensitivity
Do not combine with stimulants or weight-loss stacks.

### 🔴 Pregnancy / Nursing — Avoid

Not safe due to:
• Blood pressure–lowering effects
• Uterine-stimulating potential
• Circulatory changes

---

## ⏱ Expected Results

1–2 weeks: Early metabolic and energy improvements
2–4 weeks: Circulation & BP support
6–8 weeks: Weight-management support
Days–1 week: Respiratory ease
8–12 weeks: Full systemic benefits

---

## 🛠 DIY Recipe — Metabolic & Circulatory Support Tonic

• 1 tsp dried Coleus forskohlii root
• OR ½ tsp powdered extract

• 1 cup hot water
Steep 10–12 minutes. Add lemon + ½ tsp raw honey.
Optional: add cinnamon or ginger for thermogenic lift.
Drink in the morning for gentle metabolic activation.

---

## 🔄 Same/Similar Results

- Hawthorn
- Motherwort
- Ginkgo
- Garlic

---

## ⏳ Shelf Life / Potency After Preparation

• **Dried root:** 1–2 years in airtight container
• **Powdered root:** 1 year (store cool/dark)
• **Capsules:** Follow expiration — typically 1–2 years
• **Tincture:** 3–5 years (alcohol preserves potency)
• **Tea (prepared):** Best within 24 hours (refrigerated)
Potency fades faster with heat, light, and air exposure.

---

## 💬 Herbal Reflections of Coleus forskohlii

Coleus is not a forceful stimulant — it's a **signal clarifier**, awakening circulation, breath, and metabolism through improved cellular communication. It reminds vessels to open instead of forcing them, helps lungs widen without strain, and lifts energy without jitter.
It is a bridge between ancient Ayurvedic intuition and modern metabolic science — supporting clean flow, brighter vitality, and better responsiveness throughout the body.
Used with grounding habits (hydration, minerals, rest), Coleus becomes a steady catalyst for better rhythm and renewed momentum.

---

## ⭐ Herbal Confidence Index: 🌿 🌿 🌿 🌿 (4 / 5)

*A metabolic and cardiovascular activator prized for supporting thyroid function, fat metabolism, circulation, and respiratory ease. A focused herb that restores clarity, movement, and vitality when the system feels slow or congested.*

# GOLDENSEAL

★★★★

*Hydrastis canadensis*

**Goldenseal** is a perennial woodland herb native to North America, prized for centuries by Indigenous peoples and later adopted by European settlers. Its golden-yellow root, rich in berberine, earned it a reputation as one of the most potent natural antimicrobials, digestive tonics, and mucous membrane healers. Traditionally, it was used to support skin, eyes, ulcers, and respiratory complaints.

What makes Goldenseal distinct is its broad-spectrum action. It clears infection, tones inflamed mucosa, and strengthens digestive resilience. Though once overharvested and endangered in the wild, cultivated Goldenseal remains a powerful ally, often paired with Echinacea for immune defense.

---

## Core Herbal Category — Goldenseal

**Primary Core: Antimicrobial Support** herb with *(berberine-rich, antimicrobial principles that support mucous membrane tone and microbial balance)*

**Secondary Cores:** Digestive Restoration · Immune Activation · Topical Infection Care

### How It Works

Goldenseal supports microbial balance along mucous membranes while toning and strengthening the tissues they protect. Its berberine content creates an inhospitable environment for pathogens without destroying tissue integrity. It restores digestive lining function, reinforces immune readiness at mucosal entry points, and supports localized defense when used topically.

---

## Primary Uses

- Fights bacterial, fungal, and protozoal infections
- Soothes inflamed mucous membranes (sinus, throat, stomach, intestines)
- Supports immune defense during acute colds and flu
- Aids healing of ulcers and gastritis

- Useful topically for wounds, rashes, and gum infections

---

## 🔬 Scientific Backing

Goldenseal contains berberine, hydrastine, and canadine—compounds shown to exert antimicrobial, anti-inflammatory, and immune-modulating effects. Research confirms effectiveness against several pathogens and reduction of mucosal inflammation. Because it may disrupt gut flora and stress liver enzymes, Goldenseal is intended **for short-term use only**.

---

## Forms Available

- Root powder or capsules
- Tincture or liquid extract
- Topical salves, washes, irrigations
- Combination formulas (especially with Echinacea)

---

## How to Use

**Tincture:** 10–15 drops, 2–3× daily for **7–10 days only**
**Capsules/Powder:** 250–500 mg, 2× daily, short-term use
**Topical:** Wash, mouth rinse, or poultice on infected tissue
**Important:** Goldenseal is not a daily immune tonic. Use only for acute, short-duration infections.

---

## ⚠ Caution Level: Caution

Goldenseal is powerful and must be used sparingly. Avoid if pregnant, nursing, or using blood-pressure, diabetes, antibiotic, or liver-metabolized medications. May cause dryness, constipation, or elevated liver enzymes with misuse.

---

## Gender-Specific Safety — Goldenseal

**Men — Caution**
May alter liver enzymes, lower blood sugar, dry mucous membranes, worsen GERD, or aggravate gallbladder conditions. Use short-term only; avoid stacking with other strong antimicrobials.
**Women — Caution**

May worsen heavy menstrual flow or tissue dryness and mildly stimulate uterine circulation. Avoid with hormonal medications, blood thinners, diabetes meds, or gallbladder sensitivity. Not ideal for vaginal yeast unless paired with demulcent herbs.

● **Pregnancy / Nursing — Avoid**

Berberine crosses the placenta and enters breast milk, potentially affecting infant liver and digestion. Avoid entirely.

*Safer alternatives:* Marshmallow Root, Chamomile, Cranberry, Echinacea, Garlic (condition-dependent).

---

## Expected Results

- Topical infection relief: within days
- Sinus discomfort reduction: 3–5 days
- Digestive mucosa support: 1–2 weeks (short-term, monitored)

---

## DIY Recipe — Goldenseal Mouth Rinse

Steep ½ tsp Goldenseal root powder in hot water for 15 minutes, strain, cool, and use as a gargle or rinse 2–3× daily for throat, gum, or oral infection. Do not swallow large amounts.

---

## Same / Similar Results

Oregon Grape Root · Barberry · Echinacea · Myrrh

---

## Shelf Life / Potency After Preparation

- Dried root: 2–3 years (airtight, cool, dark)
- Tincture: 4–5 years
- Powder: 1–2 years
- Prepared rinse/wash: Use within 24 hours (refrigerated)

---

## Herbal Reflections — Goldenseal

Goldenseal is one of nature's great defenders—its golden root symbolizing purification and resolve. It acts swiftly, tightening and restoring tissues overwhelmed by infection or stagnation. Yet its strength demands respect. This is not a daily tonic but a rescue herb, best reserved for moments of true need. Used wisely and briefly, it clears, resets, and reinforces the body's defenses with decisive precision.

---

## Herbal Confidence Index (4 / 5 — Cornerstone Antimicrobial)

A potent antimicrobial and mucous-membrane tonic valued for infection clearing, digestive repair, and immune reinforcement. Strong, effective, and deeply respected — best used **short-term and intentionally**.

# FENNEL SEED

★★★★★

*Foeniculum vulgare*

**Fennel Seed** has been treasured since ancient Egyptian, Roman, and Greek times for soothing digestion, freshening breath, and easing cramping. Its sweet, licorice-like flavor makes it both a culinary spice and a medicinal staple. Known as a classic carminative, fennel reduces bloating, gas, and indigestion while gently supporting stomach and intestinal comfort.

Beyond digestion, fennel has long been valued for lactation support, cough relief, and hormonal balance. Its seeds contain aromatic oils, flavonoids, and mild phytoestrogens that provide a calming, balancing influence throughout the body.

---

## Core Herbal Category — Fennel Seed

**Primary Core: Digestive System Support** herb with *(aromatic, smooth-muscle–relaxing action that eases gas, cramping, and digestive tension)*

**Secondary Cores:** Women's Hormonal Support · Respiratory Comfort · Lactation Support

---

## How It Works

Fennel Seed relaxes digestive smooth muscle and disperses trapped gas, easing bloating and cramping. Its aromatic compounds support efficient digestive movement after meals and extend gently into respiratory tissues, supporting freer breathing. Mild phytoestrogenic activity helps ease cyclical abdominal discomfort, while its nutritive influence supports healthy milk flow during lactation.

---

## Primary Uses

- Relieves bloating, gas, and indigestion
- Eases menstrual cramping and abdominal tension
- Freshens breath and soothes oral tissues
- Supports lactation in nursing mothers
- Eases mild coughs, throat tension, and chest tightness

## Scientific Backing

Fennel Seed contains anethole, fenchone, estragole, and other volatile oils with antispasmodic, anti-inflammatory, and digestive-soothing effects. Research supports its use for infant colic, IBS-related gas and tension, mild hormone-balancing effects, and bronchial relaxation.

---

## Forms Available

- Whole or ground seeds (culinary or medicinal)
- Herbal tea (infusion)
- Capsules or tinctures
- Essential oil *(aromatherapy or diluted topical use only — never internal)*

---

## How to Use

**Tea:** Crush 1 tsp seeds; steep 10 minutes; drink after meals
**Chewed seeds:** ¼–½ tsp after meals for digestion and breath
**Tincture:** 1–2 mL, up to 3× daily
**Lactation:** 1 cup light tea once or twice daily; avoid concentrated forms
*Essential oil must never be taken internally.*

---

## Caution Level: Safe (with mild cautions)

Generally safe when used appropriately. Excessive or prolonged high-dose use may cause hormonal effects or photosensitivity. Avoid concentrated use during pregnancy. Women with estrogen-sensitive conditions should use moderate amounts only. May interact with seizure medications or certain antibiotics. Essential oil must always be diluted; internal use is unsafe.

---

## Gender-Specific Safety — Fennel Seed

**Men — Safe**
Supports digestion, gas relief, and mild respiratory comfort. Avoid very high or concentrated doses.
**Women — Caution**
Contains mild phytoestrogens (primarily anethole). Use caution with estrogen-sensitive conditions

(fibroids, endometriosis), hormone-driven cancer history, or very heavy menstrual flow. Culinary use and moderate tea are generally safe.

**Pregnancy / Nursing — Mild Caution**

**Pregnancy:** Light tea acceptable for gas or nausea; avoid strong teas, tinctures, and essential oils.

**Nursing:** Traditionally used as a galactagogue; excessive intake may cause infant digestive upset, sleepiness, or milk-flavor changes. Use lightly and discontinue if sensitivity appears.

---

## Expected Results

- Gas and bloating relief: within hours
- Menstrual cramp relief: 1–3 days
- Lactation support: 1–2 weeks

---

## DIY Recipe — Fennel Seed Digestive Tea

Crush 1 tsp fennel seeds and steep in 1 cup hot water for 10 minutes. Drink after meals to reduce gas, bloating, and intestinal cramping.

---

## Same / Similar Results

Caraway · Anise · Dill Seed · Chamomile

---

## Shelf Life / Potency After Preparation

- Whole seeds: 2–3 years
- Ground seeds: 6–12 months
- Tincture: 3–5 years
- Prepared tea: Best within 12 hours

Store airtight, away from heat and sunlight.

---

## Herbal Reflections — Fennel Seed

Fennel Seed carries the warmth of ancient kitchens and early apothecaries. Its sweet aroma has comforted digestion for millennia, easing gas, cramping, and stagnation without force. This is a herb of harmony rather than confrontation—nurturing, reliable, and gentle enough for the young, the old, and those with sensitive digestion. Used wisely, fennel restores digestive rhythm, lightness, and quiet resilience.

---

## Herbal Confidence Index (5 / 5 — Cornerstone Digestive Herb)

A warm, aromatic classic for gas, bloating, cramping, lactation support, and respiratory ease. Gentle enough for regular use, yet powerful enough to meaningfully transform digestive comfort.

# CLEAVERS

★★★★

*Galium aparine*

**Cleavers** is a gentle yet effective herb long prized in European folk medicine for cleansing and stimulating the lymphatic system. Recognizable by its clinging stems, it has been used for swollen lymph nodes, skin eruptions, and sluggish elimination. Traditionally taken fresh as a spring tonic, Cleavers helps clear accumulated wastes after winter.
Modern herbalists value Cleavers as a mild diuretic and urinary tract ally, helping flush toxins and reduce inflammation in cystitis and kidney irritation. Its gentle nature allows longer-term use and makes it useful for eczema, psoriasis, and acne when lymphatic stagnation contributes to flares.

---

## 🌿 Core Herbal Category — Cleavers

**Primary Core: Lymphatic & Skin Support herb** with *(cooling, fluid-moving action that supports lymph flow and gentle waste removal)*
**Secondary Cores:** Skin Clarity · Urinary Tract Support · Inflammation Cooling · Spring Cleansing

---

## How It Works

Cleavers gently stimulates lymphatic movement, helping clear stagnant fluids and metabolic byproducts. Its cooling nature soothes inflammatory heat while supporting detox pathways. By improving lymph flow, it indirectly supports clearer skin and reduced congestion. The herb also promotes urinary elimination, supporting fluid balance and gentle cleansing during seasonal transitions.

---

## 🌱 Primary Uses

- Supports lymphatic drainage; reduces swollen glands
- Helps clear chronic skin eruptions (eczema, psoriasis, acne)
- Aids mild urinary tract irritation and kidney congestion
- Acts as a gentle spring detoxifying tonic

- Reduces puffiness and fluid retention

---

## Scientific Backing

Early research on Cleavers demonstrates diuretic, anti-inflammatory, and antioxidant activity. Traditional use is supported by evidence of mild lymphatic circulation enhancement, reduction of inflammatory markers, gentle immune modulation, and increased urinary flow—validating its historical role as a cooling eliminative herb.

---

## Forms Available

- Fresh juice (traditional spring tonic)
- Cold-water infusion
- Dried herb infusion (tea)
- Tincture or liquid extract
- Capsules *(less effective than fresh or infusion forms)*

---

## How to Use

**Cold infusion (preferred):** Steep 1–2 tsp fresh or dried Cleavers in cold water overnight; strain and sip throughout the day.
**Warm infusion:** Steep 1–2 tsp dried herb in warm water for 10–15 minutes.
**Tincture:** 2–4 mL, up to 2× daily.
**Fresh juice:** 1–2 tsp freshly pressed juice diluted in water.
Adequate hydration is essential, as Cleavers increases urination.

---

## Caution Level: Caution

Cleavers is gentle but mildly diuretic. Use caution if dehydrated, prone to low blood pressure, using prescription diuretics, managing chronic kidney disease, or during pregnancy or breastfeeding (insufficient safety data). Increase water intake during use.

---

## Gender-Specific Safety — Cleavers

**Men — Safe**
Supports lymphatic drainage, urinary clarity, and skin detoxification. Use caution only with dehydration, very low blood pressure, or concurrent diuretic use.

**Women — Caution**
Helpful for PMS swelling, sluggish lymphatics, acne, and puffiness. Use caution with very low blood pressure, heavy menstrual bleeding, or urinary sensitivity. Moderate tea or tincture use is appropriate; avoid excessive long-term dosing.

**Pregnancy / Nursing — Avoid**
Due to its lymph-moving and diuretic action, Cleavers may be overly stimulating. Safer alternatives include Nettle Leaf or Marshmallow Root.

---

## Expected Results

- Increased urination / gentle detoxification: several days
- Reduction in swollen lymph nodes: 1–3 weeks
- Skin clarity and improved tone: 3–6 weeks

---

## DIY Recipe — Cleavers Spring Tea

Add 1–2 tsp fresh or dried Cleavers to cool water, steep overnight, strain, and sip the following day as a cooling lymphatic tonic.

---

## Same / Similar Results

Red Clover · Nettle · Burdock Root · Dandelion

---

## Shelf Life / Potency After Preparation

- Dried herb: ~1 year (potency declines quickly)
- Tincture: 3–4 years
- Cold infusion / tea: Use within 24 hours (refrigerated)
- Fresh herb: Best used immediately or frozen short-term

Cleavers is most potent when fresh; active compounds diminish significantly once dried.

---

## Herbal Reflections — Cleavers

Cleavers moves quietly through the body like water through reeds—cooling, cleansing, and restoring flow where stagnation has taken hold. Gathered in early spring, it symbolizes renewal and gentle release. Rather than forcing elimination, Cleavers encourages the body to let go with patience and softness. Used wisely, it teaches cleansing without conflict and renewal without strain.

---

## Herbal Confidence Index (4 / 5)

A cooling lymphatic and urinary tonic that reduces swelling, clarifies skin, and supports gentle detoxification. Mild yet effective, Cleavers excels when cleansing is needed with grace rather than force.

# MUGWORT

★★★★

*Artemisia vulgaris*

**Mugwort** is among the most ancient and storied herbs in natural medicine, revered for stimulating circulation, balancing digestion, and supporting women's reproductive health. As a warming nervine and bitter tonic, it calms nervous tension while awakening digestive and hepatic function. Herbalists have long used Mugwort for menstrual irregularity, mild anxiety, insomnia, and digestive sluggishness. Its aromatic oils and bitter compounds encourage gentle detoxification, ease cramping, and release lingering tension in both body and mind.

Beyond medicine, Mugwort carries deep ritual and cultural significance. Known historically as the "Witch's Herb," it was burned for protection, placed beneath pillows for dream work, and carried by travelers against fatigue. In Chinese and Japanese medicine, dried Mugwort is used in **moxibustion**, where it is burned near acupuncture points to stimulate circulation and healing response. Mugwort remains a plant of medicine and mystery—bridging physiology, intuition, and tradition.

---

## Core Herbal Category — Mugwort

**Primary Core:** Nervous System Support (Nervines) herb with *(warming, aromatic bitterness that stimulates digestion while gently regulating nervous system tone)*
**Secondary Cores:** Women's Reproductive Support · Circulatory Activation · Dreamwork & Energetic Support

---

### How It Works

Mugwort stimulates digestive secretions through bitter compounds that enhance appetite and assimilation. Its warming aromatic oils gently tone the nervous system—easing tension while maintaining alertness. By activating circulation, it supports pelvic and peripheral blood flow, contributing to menstrual regulation and reproductive rhythm. Its nervine action also enhances inner awareness and vivid dream states.

---

## Primary Uses

- Stimulates digestion and appetite
- Helps regulate menstruation and ease cramping

- Calms nervous tension; supports vivid or lucid dreams
- Enhances circulation and mild detoxification
- Supports emotional grounding and intuitive clarity

---

## Scientific Backing

Mugwort contains flavonoids, sesquiterpene lactones, essential oils, and bitters responsible for its digestive, circulatory, and nervine effects. Research on moxibustion in traditional East Asian medicine demonstrates improved circulation, pain reduction, and enhanced healing response. While controlled studies on dream enhancement are limited, centuries of consistent traditional use support these effects.

---

## Forms Available

- Dried herb tea (infusion)
- Tincture or liquid extract
- Smudging bundles (traditional use)
- Pillow stuffing for dream support
- Dried herb for moxibustion (TCM / Kampo)

---

## How to Use

**Tea:** Steep 1 tsp dried Mugwort in hot water for 5–10 minutes; use at bedtime for dream support or daytime for digestion.
**Tincture:** 1–2 mL once or twice daily; avoid long-term daily use.
**Topical / moxibustion:** Use only under professional guidance.
*Start low—individual sensitivity varies.*

---

## Caution Level: Caution

Avoid during pregnancy due to strong uterine-stimulating effects. May worsen insomnia, agitation, or nervous overstimulation in sensitive individuals. Can provoke allergic reactions in those sensitive to ragweed or other Asteraceae plants. Excess intake may overstimulate digestion or the nervous system. Avoid high-dose tinctures, long-term use, and use in epilepsy or seizure disorders.

---

## 🚹 🚺 Gender-Specific Safety — Mugwort

**Men — Caution**
Generally safe in moderate amounts for digestion, circulation, and dreamwork. Use caution with ragweed allergy, seizure disorders, or very sensitive digestion. Avoid long-term or high-dose use.

**Women — Caution**
Traditionally used to regulate cycles and ease PMS stagnation. Use caution with heavy bleeding, fibroids, uterine sensitivity, or hormone-triggered migraines. Moderate tea is usually tolerated; avoid overuse.

**Pregnancy / Nursing — Avoid**
A strong emmenagogue and uterine stimulant. Avoid entirely during pregnancy and nursing due to volatile oil transfer into milk, possible infant digestive upset, and allergy sensitization.
*Prefer:* Chamomile, Lemon Balm, or Ginger.

---

## ⏳ Expected Results

- Improved digestion: within days
- Nervine / dream activity: same night to several nights
- Menstrual balance: 1–2 cycles
- Circulatory warming: minutes to days

## 🛠 DIY Recipe — Mugwort Dream Tea

Steep 1 tsp dried Mugwort in hot water for 10 minutes. Drink before bed to support dream recall and clarity. Optional: blend with Chamomile or Lavender for gentler effects.

---

## 🔄 Same / Similar Results

Chamomile · Lemon Balm · Wormwood

---

## 🧪 Shelf Life / Potency After Preparation

- Dried herb: 1–2 years
- Tincture: 4–5 years

- Smudge bundles: 3–5 years
- Prepared tea: Best within 12 hours

Store dried herb away from heat and sunlight to preserve volatile oils.

---

## Herbal Reflections — Mugwort

Mugwort is a herb of thresholds—stirring digestion, circulation, and inner perception simultaneously. Its bitterness awakens the body while its aromatics soften the mind. Mugwort does not work casually; it shifts internal rhythms and clears stagnation. Used with respect, it realigns cycles, rekindles intuition, and restores creative flow.

---

## Herbal Confidence Index 🌿 🌿 🌿 🌿 (4 / 5 — Cornerstone Nervine-Bitter)

A classic nervine and digestive bitter valued for dream enhancement, circulatory warming, tension relief, and women's reproductive balance. Deep-working and effective when used thoughtfully.

# MULLEIN FLOWER

★★★

*Verbascum thapsus*

**Mullein flowers** are the soft, golden blossoms of the Mullein plant, long valued for their gentle yet precise soothing properties. Unlike the leaf, which focuses primarily on respiratory support, the flowers possess distinct anti-inflammatory and analgesic compounds that make them especially useful for ear comfort, nerve irritation, and localized pain. Traditionally infused into warm oil, Mullein flowers have been trusted for generations as one of the safest and most effective herbal allies for ear discomfort, irritation, or congestion.
Across Europe and North America, herbalists have relied on Mullein flower oil to calm inflamed tissues, soften congestion, and bring warmth to sensitive areas without overstimulation. Their action is subtle but targeted, offering relief where irritation lingers. Mullein flowers remind us that gentle remedies can restore comfort, ease, and balance when applied with care.

---

## Core Herbal Category — Mullein Flower

**Primary Core: Anti-Inflammatory & Pain Support** herb with (soothing, nerve-calming compounds that ease localized irritation and tissue sensitivity)
**Secondary Cores:** Pain Modulation · Ear & Eustachian Tube Support · Lymphatic Comfort

### How It Works

Mullein Flower calms irritated nerves and soothes inflamed tissues at a localized level. Its gentle anti-inflammatory action reduces discomfort associated with sensitivity and congestion, while its nerve-calming influence helps balance pain perception without systemic stimulation. When applied to the ear and surrounding tissues, it supports comfort by encouraging gentle drainage and tissue relaxation, also easing lymphatic congestion in nearby structures.

---

## Primary Uses

- *Supports comfort during ear irritation*
- Helps ease congestion in the ear canal and Eustachian tube
- Provides localized anti-inflammatory support
- Offers mild analgesic relief for nerve irritation

- Commonly used in combination ear oils (e.g., with garlic oil)
- Soothes tenderness from mild injury, swelling, or inflammation

---

## *Scientific Backing*

Mullein flowers contain iridoid glycosides, saponins, flavonoids, and volatile oils that contribute to their calming, anti-inflammatory, and analgesic properties. Research and clinical herbal practice note antimicrobial activity when flowers are infused in oil, reduction of localized inflammation, and nerve-soothing effects. Traditional use for ear discomfort (including otitis-related irritation) is well established in Western herbalism, with growing modern validation.

---

## *Forms Available*

- Fresh or dried flower-infused oil (classic preparation)
- *Tincture (less common)*
- *Salves or ointments*
- Ear-oil blends (often combined with garlic or St. John's Wort)

---

## *How to Use*

**Ear oil (classic use):** Warm oil gently (never hot). Apply 1–3 drops into the ear canal, lie on the opposite side for 5–10 minutes. Use 1–2× daily as needed.
**Topical use:** Apply a small amount to tense or inflamed areas for soothing warmth.
**Tincture:** Rarely used alone; typically combined with nervines or topical formulas.

---

## *Caution Level: Generally Safe*

Do not use in the ear if the eardrum is perforated. Seek professional evaluation if a severe ear infection is suspected. Intended primarily for external or aural use; internal use should be professionally formulated. Always warm oil gently before application to avoid discomfort.

---

## *Gender-Specific Safety (GS)*

- **Men:** Safe for topical and aural use
- **Women:** Safe; commonly used for nerve and ear comfort
- **Pregnancy:** Safe for external use
- **Nursing:** Safe for external use on adults
- **Children:** Use with caution — diluted, gently warmed oil preferred

---

## *Expected Results*

- *Ear comfort: 10–30 minutes*
- *Nerve soothing: within hours*
- *Inflammation reduction: 1–3 days*
- *Swelling ease (topical): 1–2 days*
- Eustachian tube comfort: gradual, 2–5 days

---

## *DIY Recipe — Mullein Flower Ear-Comfort Oil*

Combine ½ cup dried Mullein flowers with 1 cup olive or jojoba oil. Warm gently in a double boiler for 2–3 hours, then strain through cheesecloth.
**Use:** Apply 1–3 drops into the ear for soothing inflammation or discomfort.

## *Same / Similar Results*

- Garlic Oil — antimicrobial ear support
- St. John's Wort Oil — nerve-soothing topical support
- Calendula Oil — anti-inflammatory tissue support
- Lavender Oil — calming nerve support
- Chamomile Oil — gentle anti-inflammatory action

---

## *Shelf Life / Potency After Preparation*

- *Flower-infused oil: ~1 year*
- *Dried flowers: 1–2 years*
- *Tincture: 4–5 years*

Store oils in a cool, dark place. Potency declines rapidly with heat or light exposure.

---

## Herbal Reflections — Mullein Flower

Mullein flowers embody softness—golden, delicate, and quietly powerful. Their medicine arrives not with force, but with warmth and reassurance, easing irritation and calming restless nerves. For generations, healers recognized the flower's gift for bringing peace to inflamed tissues and sensitive spaces. Mullein Flower teaches that some of the most effective healing comes through gentleness, patience, and steady comfort.

---

## Herbal Confidence Index (4 / 5)

*A gentle yet highly effective local anti-inflammatory and nerve-soothing remedy, prized for ear comfort, tissue sensitivity, and calming support. Safe, precise, and deeply trusted when used correctly.*

# BLACK COHOSH

★★★★

*Actaea racemosa*

**Black Cohosh**—known to early American healers as *"Woman's Root"*—has been a cornerstone of female medicine for centuries. Native American tribes, including the Cherokee and Iroquois, used its dark, knotted root to ease menstrual cramping, childbirth pain, and the transitions of womanhood. By the 19th century, it entered the U.S. Pharmacopeia as a primary remedy for female complaints and rheumatic pain.

Medicinally, Black Cohosh acts as a neuroendocrine-modulating and anti-inflammatory herb that supports hormonal rhythm without supplying hormones directly. It relaxes uterine tension, reduces hot flashes, and steadies emotional fluctuation during menopause. Its nervine qualities support sleep, mood balance, and calm during endocrine change. Grounded in tradition and supported by modern research, Black Cohosh remains a botanical bridge between ancient wisdom and contemporary women's health.

---

## Core Herbal Category — Black Cohosh

**Primary Core: Reproductive & Women's Health Support herb** with *(neuroendocrine-modulating action that supports hormonal signaling and reproductive rhythm balance)*

**Secondary Cores:** Nervine Stabilization · Anti-Inflammatory Support · Menopause & PMS Balancing

### How It Works

Black Cohosh supports communication between the nervous system and hormonal centers, helping regulate reproductive signaling during cyclical and transitional phases. Its neuroendocrine influence stabilizes mood and nerve responsiveness, while its anti-inflammatory action eases pelvic and musculoskeletal tension. Together, these effects support adaptation during PMS, perimenopause, and menopause, promoting steadier hormonal balance and physical comfort.

---

## Primary Uses

- Eases menopausal hot flashes and night sweats
- Relieves menstrual cramping, PMS, and uterine tension

- Supports emotional balance during hormonal transitions
- Helps with sleep disturbances linked to endocrine fluctuation

---

## Scientific Backing

Black Cohosh contains triterpene glycosides, aromatic acids, and phytoestrogen-like compounds that influence serotonin signaling, thermoregulation, and neuroendocrine balance. Clinical research suggests it may reduce the frequency and intensity of hot flashes, improve mood and sleep quality, and ease menstrual tension. Its action is **modulating rather than hormone-replacing**, supporting balance without acting as estrogen.

---

## Forms Available

- Dried root (decoctions, tinctures, capsules)
- Standardized extracts (commonly used in menopause formulations)

---

## How to Use

**Tea (decoction):** Simmer 1 tsp dried root in 1 cup water for 10–15 minutes; drink once daily.
**Tincture:** 1–2 mL up to 2× daily for hormonal or mood support.
**Capsules:** 40–80 mg standardized extract or 250–500 mg whole root daily.
Black Cohosh works best when used consistently for several weeks.

---

## Caution Level: Caution

Avoid during pregnancy or breastfeeding due to uterine-stimulating potential. Avoid with known liver disease or liver sensitivity. Do not use with hormone-sensitive cancers (breast, ovarian, uterine) unless medically supervised. Use caution when taking HRT, birth control, or SERMs. Excessive intake may cause headache, dizziness, nausea, or abdominal discomfort. Use only reputable products—adulteration has occurred in commercial preparations.

---

## Gender-Specific Safety — Black Cohosh

**Men — Mild Caution**
Generally safe for short-term, moderate use for nervous tension, muscle tightness, stress-related

insomnia, or mild joint discomfort. Avoid with hormone-sensitive conditions, low testosterone, or hormone-related cancer history.

**Women — Caution**

Highly valued for hot flashes, night sweats, PMS cramping, mood fluctuation, and perimenopausal symptoms. Use caution with liver disorders, hormone-sensitive cancers, fibroids, endometriosis, very heavy bleeding, or active hormonal medication use. Typical use is 3–6 months with standardized extracts.

**Pregnancy / Nursing — Avoid**

Traditionally contraindicated due to uterine effects. Avoid strong tinctures or extracts during nursing.

---

## Expected Results

- Hot flash reduction: 2–4 weeks
- PMS relief: 1–2 cycles
- Mood balance and sleep support: several weeks

---

## DIY Recipe — Black Cohosh Decoction

Simmer 1 tsp dried root in 1 cup water for 20 minutes. Drink ½ cup twice daily for hormonal and nervine support.

---

## Same / Similar Results

Dong Quai · Red Clover · Chaste Tree (Vitex)

---

## Shelf Life / Potency After Preparation

- Dried root: 2–3 years
- Tincture: 5+ years
- Capsules: 1–2 years
- Prepared decoction: 24–48 hours (refrigerated)

## Herbal Reflections — Black Cohosh

Black Cohosh moves in harmony with the cycles of womanhood—grounding, steadying, and deeply attuned to transition. It softens the waves of menopause, calms cramping, and restores rhythm where balance has faltered. Known to Indigenous healers as a root of renewal, it reflects resilience during profound change, reminding us that clarity and stability are often revealed—not lost—during transformation.

---

## Herbal Confidence Index (4 / 5)

A deeply grounding women's tonic valued for easing menopausal transition, menstrual discomfort, hormonal turbulence, and nervine tension. Black Cohosh supports emotional balance and physiological renewal with quiet strength.

# ASHITABA

★★★★★

*Angelica keiskei*

**Ashitaba,** known as the "Tomorrow Leaf," is a vibrant green herb native to Japan and celebrated for its remarkable regenerative capacity. Its name reflects its ability to regrow new leaves rapidly after harvest—a living symbol of renewal and vitality. Medicinally, Ashitaba is valued as a longevity tonic that supports cellular regeneration, circulation, immune resilience, and metabolic balance. Its unique chalcones—xanthoangelol and 4-hydroxyderricin—contribute antioxidant, anti-inflammatory, and tissue-repair–supportive effects.

Historically used by Buddhist monks and Japanese islanders to sustain stamina and clarity during fasting or meditation, Ashitaba earned a reputation as a daily herb of endurance and longevity. In modern herbalism, it is recognized as a youth-preserving superfood rich in chlorophyll, potassium, vitamin B12–like activity, and antioxidants that help counter oxidative stress. Its long cultural history bridges ancient wisdom with contemporary science of cellular renewal.

---

## 🌿 Core Herbal Category — Ashitaba

**Primary Core: Nutritional & Tonic Support** herb with *(chalcone-rich, cellular-renewal-supportive action that promotes tissue regeneration and systemic resilience)*

**Secondary Cores:** Immune Strengthening · Metabolic Support · Digestive Nourishment

---

### How It Works

Ashitaba supports cellular renewal processes that contribute to tissue repair and long-term vitality. Its bioactive chalcones enhance metabolic efficiency and antioxidant defense, while nourishing digestive function to improve nutrient assimilation. Through sustained nutritional and regenerative support, it strengthens immune resilience and promotes systemic balance associated with healthy aging.

---

## 🌱 Primary Uses

- Promotes cellular regeneration and tissue repair
- Supports immune strength and resilience
- Aids digestion and liver detoxification

- Helps balance blood sugar and lipid levels
- Boosts energy, stamina, and mental clarity

---

## 🧪 Scientific Backing

Ashitaba chalcones (xanthoangelol and 4-hydroxyderricin) demonstrate potent antioxidant and anti-inflammatory activity, improved glucose tolerance and insulin sensitivity, liver-protective effects, DNA protection from oxidative stress, cholesterol-lowering activity, and enhanced cellular regeneration. Emerging research supports benefits for metabolic syndrome, liver health, and longevity, aligning with its traditional role as a daily vitality tonic.

---

## 🍵 Forms Available

- Powder (smoothies, capsules, teas)
- Fresh or dried leaves (infusions, salads)
- Extracts and tinctures
- Tablets and functional beverages

## 🧭 How to Use — Ashitaba

**Tea:** Steep 1–2 tsp dried leaf in 1 cup hot water for 10 minutes; drink 1–2× daily.
**Capsules/Powder:** 500–1,000 mg daily with food for long-term vitality.
**Tincture:** 1–2 mL, 1–2× daily for circulation and immune tone.
Most effective when used consistently for several weeks.

---

## ⚠️ Caution Level: 🟢 Safe

Generally well tolerated. Mild digestive activation (looser stools) may occur initially. May mildly enhance circulation and lower blood sugar; monitor if using blood thinners or diabetes medications. Daily use is typically safe for most adults.

---

## Gender-Specific Safety — Ashitaba

**Men — Safe**
Supports energy, liver function, blood sugar regulation, immune resilience, and healthy aging. Monitor blood sugar or clotting if on related medications.

**Women — Safe (Mild Caution)**
Used for hormonal balance, menstrual regularity, skin clarity, and immune support. Use moderation with very heavy cycles, fibroids, estrogen-dominant patterns, or significant blood sugar instability.

**Pregnancy — Avoid**
Medicinal use should be avoided due to possible uterine stimulation (Angelica family), detoxifying chalcones, and insufficient safety data.

**Nursing — Mild Caution**
Light dietary amounts likely safe; avoid medicinal doses. Monitor for infant digestive sensitivity.

---

## Expected Results

- Digestive and energy improvement: 3–7 days
- Skin and vitality benefits: 2–4 weeks
- Deep cellular and immune support: 1–3 months

---

## DIY Recipe — "Tomorrow Tonic Smoothie"

Blend 1 tsp Ashitaba powder with banana, pineapple, and coconut water; optional fresh ginger. Drink in the morning for energy, clarity, and digestive support.

---

## Same / Similar Results

Moringa · Spirulina · Matcha Green Tea · Gotu Kola

---

## Shelf Life / Potency After Preparation

- Dried leaf: ~2 years

- Powder: 1–2 years (airtight)
- Tincture: 4–6 years
- Fresh juice: 24–48 hours (refrigerated)
- Capsules: 1–2 years

---

## 💭 Herbal Reflections — Ashitaba

Ashitaba embodies renewal—a plant that teaches persistence through regeneration. Rather than forcing stimulation or sedation, it harmonizes nourishment and repair, strengthening from within. Its wisdom reminds us that true longevity is built through steady renewal, not haste.

## 🌟 Herbal Confidence Index

🌿 🌿 🌿 🌿 🌿 **(5 / 5)**

A rare longevity herb prized for regenerative power and nutritional richness. Supports cellular renewal, liver health, circulation, and energy through unique chalcones and antioxidants—truly living up to its name, "Tomorrow's Leaf."

# SHATAVARI

★★★★★

*Asparagus racemosus*

**Shatavari**—"she who possesses a hundred husbands"—is Ayurveda's premier female tonic, revered for nourishing and balancing the reproductive system across all stages of life. Traditionally used to support fertility, ease PMS and menopausal transitions, and restore vitality postpartum, Shatavari is especially suited to dry, depleted patterns. Rather than stimulating, it provides moistening, rebuilding nourishment that steadies hormones, digestion, and immunity during stress. Classical Ayurvedic texts describe Shatavari as a daily **rasayana** (rejuvenative), sustaining reproductive strength from menarche through menopause and recovery after birth. Historically prepared as powders in warm milk or ghee, it remains a cornerstone of women's care today, with modern formats preserving its lineage while fitting contemporary routines. Modern herbalists also value Shatavari as a gentle adaptogen that supports the gut–nervous system axis and pairs well with allies like Ashwagandha or Raspberry Leaf during hormonal transitions.

---

## 🌿 Core Herbal Category — Shatavari

**Primary Core: Reproductive & Women's Health Support** herb with *(deeply nourishing, endocrine-modulating action that supports reproductive tissues and hormonal resilience)*
**Secondary Cores:** Hormonal Balance · Adaptogenic Nourishment · Digestive Soothing · Immune Support

---

### How It Works

Shatavari nourishes and tones reproductive tissues while supporting balanced hormonal signaling. Its adaptogenic qualities help buffer stress that can disrupt reproductive function. The herb's soothing nature supports digestive comfort and nutrient assimilation, indirectly strengthening immune resilience. This integrated nourishment promotes long-term reproductive vitality and systemic balance.

---

## 🌱 Primary Uses

- Balances female hormones and fertility
- Eases PMS, menstrual irregularities, and menopausal shifts

- Supports digestion, immunity, and stress resilience
- Acts as a gentle, rebuilding adaptogen

---

## 🧪 Scientific Backing

Shatavari contains shatavarins, steroidal saponins, and mild phytoestrogenic compounds studied for menopausal comfort, lactation support, immune modulation, gastrointestinal soothing, and hormonal stabilization. Its traditional rasayana use aligns with modern findings that emphasize restorative, nourishing effects rather than direct hormonal replacement.

---

## ☕ Forms Available

- Dried root powder (traditional; often taken in warm milk or ghee)
- Capsules or tablets
- Tincture or extract

---

## 🧭 How to Use — Shatavari

**Tea/Milk:** Simmer 1 tsp powdered root in warm water or milk for 5–10 minutes; drink 1× daily.
**Capsules/Powder:** 500–1,000 mg daily for women's vitality and moisture balance.
**Tincture:** 1–2 mL, 1–2× daily for adrenal steadiness and reproductive nourishment.
Best results occur with steady use over several weeks.

---

## ⚠️ Caution Level: 🟢 Safe (Mild Awareness)

Generally well tolerated. Use mild caution with estrogen-sensitive conditions (certain cancers, fibroids, endometriosis), very heavy menstrual bleeding, or asparagus allergy (Asparagaceae family). High doses may cause mild bloating or loose stools. Pregnancy and nursing use should follow professional guidance.

---

## 👨 👩 Gender-Specific Safety — Shatavari

🟢 **Men — Safe**

Supports stress resilience, digestion, immune balance, and nervous-system nourishment. Does not feminize men or significantly alter testosterone at typical doses. Mild caution for sluggish digestion or loose stools at higher doses.

**Women — Safe**

Highly valued for hormonal balance, fertility nourishment, PMS relief, perimenopause and menopause support, vaginal dryness, and emotional steadiness. Use mild caution with strong estrogen dominance, active fibroids/endometriosis, PCOS with high estrogen, or very heavy bleeding.

**Pregnancy — Mild Caution / Professional Guidance**

Traditionally used in Ayurveda, but modern practice advises supervision due to hormonal modulation and limited Western clinical data. Avoid medicinal dosing without guidance.

**Nursing — Generally Safe (Mild Caution)**

A traditional galactagogue. Moderate daily use is often beneficial; avoid high-alcohol tinctures. Monitor infants for gas or loose stools with higher doses.

---

## Expected Results

- Menstrual support: 1–2 cycles
- Fertility and hormonal balance: weeks to months
- Stress and immune support: with consistent use

---

## DIY Recipe — Shatavari Tonic Milk

Stir 1 tsp powdered Shatavari into warm milk with honey or cardamom. Drink nightly for nourishment, hormonal balance, and restorative calm.

---

## Same / Similar Results

Maca Root · Ashwagandha · Dong Quai

---

## Shelf Life / Potency After Preparation

- Root powder: 1–2 years (airtight)
- Capsules/tablets: 1–2 years
- Tincture: 4–6 years
- Prepared milk tonic: consume immediately; refrigerate up to 24 hours

- Ghee preparations: 6–12 months refrigerated

---

## 💭 Herbal Reflections — Shatavari

Shatavari is replenishment in root form—moistening, steady, and protective. Where stress and dryness thin the body's reserves, it restores the capacity to receive nourishment again. Its medicine is continuity rather than drama: small, consistent support that accumulates into stability. As a classical rasayana, Shatavari embodies feminine resilience across life stages, teaching that when nourishment comes first, balance follows naturally.

---

## ⭐ Herbal Confidence Index 🌿 🌿 🌿 🌿 🌿 (5 / 5)

Ayurveda's supreme rejuvenator for women. Restores hormonal balance, supports fertility, eases menopausal discomfort, and nourishes dryness and depletion with steady, rebuilding care.

# BAOBAB

★★★★★

*Adansonia digitata*

**Baobab fruit pulp** is a nutrient-dense superfood rich in vitamin C, prebiotic fiber, and polyphenols that supports digestion and regularity, feeds a healthy gut microbiome, and fortifies immune defenses while providing steady, non-stimulating energy. Its gentle acidity and mineral profile—especially potassium and magnesium—support hydration and electrolyte balance, while antioxidants temper oxidative stress and nourish skin and connective tissue. The naturally tangy powder dissolves easily in water, smoothies, or yogurt, and its vitamin C enhances iron absorption when paired with iron-rich foods.

Native to sub-Saharan Africa, the baobab is known as the "tree of life," revered for drought resilience, water-storing trunks, and extraordinary longevity. For centuries, communities have used the fruit ("monkey bread") in cooling drinks and porridges, simmered the leaves as nourishing greens, and pressed the seeds for oil. Naturally dried on the tree, the pulp offers exceptional flavor and shelf stability—carrying a heritage of resilience into modern kitchens and apothecaries.

---

## *Core Herbal Category — Baobab*

**Primary Core: Nutritional & Tonic Support** herb with (vitamin- and mineral-dense nourishment that supports immune resilience and foundational vitality)

**Secondary Cores:** Digestive Strength · Antioxidant Protection · Electrolyte Replenishment

---

### *How It Works*

Baobab delivers concentrated vitamins, minerals, and soluble fiber that nourish cells and support immune readiness. Its antioxidants protect tissues from oxidative stress, while prebiotic fiber improves gut comfort and nutrient absorption. A natural electrolyte profile supports hydration and metabolic balance, promoting steady energy and foundational nourishment.

---

## *Primary Uses*

- Boosts immunity (high natural vitamin C)
- Supports digestion and gut microbiome health
- *Provides daily antioxidant protection*

- *Hydrates and replenishes electrolytes*

---

## Scientific Backing

Baobab pulp demonstrates extremely high antioxidant capacity, prebiotic soluble fiber that improves microbiome diversity and regularity, anti-inflammatory effects that reduce oxidative stress markers, and natural electrolyte balance from potassium, calcium, and magnesium. Modern research validates its gut-restoring, immune-supportive, and metabolic benefits, aligning with its traditional role as a foundational food-medicine.

---

## Forms Available

- *Powder (most common; dissolves easily)*
- *Fresh fruit pulp (where available)*
- *Capsules or standardized extracts*

---

## How to Use — Baobab

**Powder:** 1–2 tsp daily mixed into water, juice, or smoothies.
**Capsules:** 500–1,000 mg daily for antioxidant and immune support.
**Food Use:** Stir into yogurt, oatmeal, or herbal blends for added fiber and minerals.
*Gentle enough for daily, long-term use.*

---

## Caution Level: Safe

One of the safest nutritive herbal foods. Mild cautions: very high doses may cause temporary bloating from soluble fiber; may gently improve insulin sensitivity—monitor with diabetes medications.

---

## Gender-Specific Safety — Baobab

**Men — Safe**
Supports digestion, vitality, immune strength, and electrolyte balance. Excessive intake may cause mild bloating.
**Women — Safe**

Supportive for fatigue, immune weakness, digestive sluggishness, and nutrient depletion. Fiber may require gradual introduction.

**Pregnancy & Nursing — Mild Caution**

Food-level use is generally safe; begin with small amounts. High vitamin C or fiber may cause stomach sensitivity or alter milk flavor in sensitive infants.

---

## *Expected Results*

- *Energy and vitality: several days*
- Digestive comfort and regularity: 1–3 weeks
- Immune resilience: with consistent daily use

---

## *DIY Recipe — Baobab Vitamin Smoothie*

Blend 1 tbsp baobab powder with orange juice and ½ banana; optional ginger or pineapple for digestive lift.

---

## *Same / Similar Results*

Camu Camu · Acerola Cherry · Rosehip

---

## *Shelf Life / Potency After Preparation*

- *Powder: 2–3 years (airtight, cool, dry)*
- *Capsules/extracts: 1–2 years*
- *Fresh pulp: several weeks refrigerated*
- Mixed beverages: consume within 24 hours

---

## *Herbal Reflections — Baobab*

Baobab is endurance made edible—cooling, hydrating, and quietly fortifying. Its fiber feeds the microbiome, minerals replenish deeply, and antioxidants support daily renewal without stimulation. As a true "tree of life," it teaches balance and sufficiency: steady replenishment as the foundation of wellness.

---

## ⭐ Herbal Confidence Index 🌿 🌿 🌿 🌿 🌿 (5 / 5)

*A cornerstone nutritive superfruit celebrated for safety, digestibility, and universal benefit—strengthening digestion, immunity, energy, and hydration with gentle, daily restorative power.*

# MACA ROOT

★★★★★

*Lepidium meyenii*

**Maca** is a non-stimulating adaptogen traditionally used to support baseline energy, stress resilience, libido, and hormonal harmony. Rather than forcing stimulation, it rebuilds endurance gradually—supporting mood under pressure, smoother stamina, and reproductive tone in both men and women. When used consistently, Maca provides a steady lift without the jitter or crash associated with stimulants.

Cultivated for millennia on the Andean plateau—often above 12,000 feet—Maca served as both food and medicine, sustaining communities through harsh climates and long winters. In Incan tradition, it fortified warriors and stored well as a staple crop. Roasted roots were eaten daily, giving rise to the modern nickname "Peruvian ginseng," though Maca is botanically distinct. Traditional color strains (yellow, red, black) are valued for subtle differences, and modern preparations may be raw or gelatinized for digestibility—each reflecting the same lineage of resilience.

---

## 🌿 Core Herbal Category — Maca

**Primary Core: Endocrine & Hormonal Support** herb with *(endocrine-balancing, vitality-building nourishment that supports stress resilience and hormonal communication)*
**Secondary Cores:** Hormonal Balance · Reproductive Vitality · Mood & Stress Resilience · Foundational Energy

---

## How It Works

Maca supports adaptive communication between the endocrine system and the stress response, stabilizing hormonal signaling without overstimulation. Its nourishing compounds enhance resilience to physical and emotional stress, promoting consistent energy, balanced mood, and reproductive vitality. This adaptogenic action builds endurance gradually and sustainably.

---

## 🌱 Primary Uses

- Boosts energy and stamina
- Enhances libido and fertility
- Supports hormonal balance (men and women)

- Improves mood, stress tolerance, and emotional steadiness

---

## Scientific Backing

Maca contains macaenes, macamides, amino acids, and sterols associated with improved sexual function, fertility support in both genders, enhanced energy metabolism, and improved mood and stress tolerance. Modern research aligns with its long-standing use as a daily nutritive adaptogen that works cumulatively over time.

---

## Forms Available

- Powder (smoothies, warm drinks, food)
- Capsules or tablets
- Roasted root (traditional food form)

---

## How to Use — Maca Root

**Powder:** 1–3 tsp daily mixed into smoothies, oatmeal, yogurt, or warm drinks. Start with ½–1 tsp and increase gradually.
**Capsules/Tablets:** Follow label directions (often equivalent to 1–3 tsp powder daily).
**Timing:** Best taken earlier in the day with food. Works cumulatively—consistent daily use over weeks produces the best results.

---

## Caution Level: Safe (Mild Awareness)

Generally well tolerated. Use mild awareness with thyroid disorders (trace goitrogens), hormone-sensitive conditions (fibroids, PCOS, estrogen dominance), or adrenal sensitivity—start low and titrate slowly. High doses may cause mild digestive upset, restlessness, or sleep disruption. Avoid large concentrated extracts with uncontrolled hypertension.

---

## Gender-Specific Safety — Maca Root

**Men — Safe**
Supports energy, stamina, libido, fertility, mood balance, and endocrine resilience. Mild caution for

restlessness or anxiety at high doses.

**Women — Caution**

Supports PMS comfort, fertility, perimenopause/menopause transitions, libido, and emotional resilience. Use caution with PCOS, fibroids, endometriosis, estrogen dominance, or very heavy cycles. High doses may cause breast tenderness, acne, or cycle shifts.

**Pregnancy — Avoid**

Not recommended due to endocrine-modulating effects.

**Nursing — Avoid**

May affect milk production or infant sensitivity.

---

## Expected Results

- Energy lift: days
- Libido support: weeks
- Hormonal balance: months with steady use

---

## DIY Recipe — Maca Energy Shake

Blend 1 tbsp Maca powder with milk or plant milk, cocoa powder, and honey for a warming, grounding daily tonic.

---

## Same / Similar Results

Ashwagandha · Shatavari · Rhodiola · Panax Ginseng
Tongkat Ali · Tribulus

---

## Shelf Life / Potency After Preparation

- Powder: 1–2 years (airtight)
- Capsules/tablets: 1–2 years
- Roasted root: up to 2 years (cool, dry)
- Prepared drinks: consume within 24 hours refrigerated

---

## 💬 Herbal Reflections — Maca Root

Maca teaches durable vitality—steady endurance rather than quick bursts. Grown where wind is thin and soil is spare, it reminds us that stamina is cultivated slowly. With routine use, rest, and nourishment, Maca becomes not a spark but a stable flame—supporting resilience that lasts.

---

## ⭐ Herbal Confidence Index 🌿 🌿 🌿 🌿 🌿 (5 / 5)

A revered Andean adaptogen that rebuilds stamina, hormonal harmony, libido, fertility, and emotional resilience through gentle, cumulative nourishment.

# SUMA ROOT

★★★★★

*Pfaffia paniculata*

**Suma** is a broad-spectrum adaptogen traditionally used to support endurance, recovery, and stress balance without stimulation. Rather than pushing energy, it helps restore baseline capacity—supporting calm stamina, steadier drive, and improved resilience during long rebuilds from fatigue, illness, or overtraining. Many describe its effect as feeling "filled back in" rather than revved. Native to the Amazon basin and known locally as *para tudo* ("for everything"), Suma has been used as a daily fortifier in food-like tonics and convalescent broths. Though sometimes called "Brazilian ginseng," it is not a true ginseng; its value lies in converging qualities—nourishment, endocrine support, circulatory ease, and sustainable strength. This heritage still shapes modern use: slow, steady, and paired with rest, protein, and movement.

---

## 🌿 Core Herbal Category — Suma

**Primary Core: Adaptogens** herb with *(broad-spectrum, vitality-restoring action that supports endocrine balance and physical resilience under stress)*
**Secondary Cores:** Hormonal Balance · Circulatory Activation · Immune Fortification · Endurance & Physical Recovery

---

## How It Works

Suma supports adaptive balance within the endocrine system, helping the body respond more efficiently to physical and environmental stressors. Its restorative compounds encourage steady energy output and improved recovery after exertion. By supporting circulation, it enhances nutrient and oxygen delivery to tissues, contributing to immune fortification during periods of demand. The overall effect is improved endurance, resilience, and recovery capacity.

---

## 🌱 Primary Uses

- Boosts stamina, endurance, and recovery
- Supports hormonal balance (men and women)
- Enhances circulation and daily vitality

- Strengthens immune resilience under stress

---

## Scientific Backing

Suma contains ecdysteroids, saponins, and organic germanium associated with improved athletic performance and muscle recovery, immune modulation, enhanced oxygen utilization and circulation, and mild endocrine support. Research supports its traditional role as a broad-spectrum strengthening tonic rather than a stimulant.

---

## Forms Available

- Dried powdered root (capsules, smoothies)
- Decoction or tea
- Tincture or extract

---

## How to Use — Suma Root

**Tea/Decoction:** Simmer 1 tsp powdered or sliced root in 1 cup water for 10–15 minutes; drink 1× daily.
**Capsules/Powder:** 500–1,000 mg daily to support vitality and hormone tone.
**Tincture:** 1–2 mL, 1–2× daily as an adaptogenic tonic.
Works gradually; best results come with consistent daily use. Often cycled 3–4 weeks on, 1 week off.

---

## Caution Level: Caution (Moderate Awareness)

Generally well tolerated, but awareness is advised due to plant sterols and ecdysteroids. Use caution or seek guidance with hormone-sensitive conditions, hypertension, liver disorders, or concurrent hormone therapy, steroids, or stimulant supplements. Rare effects at high doses include digestive warmth, restlessness, or mild acne.
**Pregnancy & nursing: Avoid.**

---

## Gender-Specific Safety — Suma Root

**Men — Safe**

Supports stamina, athletic recovery, libido, hormone tone, stress resilience, and immune strength. Mild androgen-like activity may enhance vitality without destabilizing hormones. Avoid very high doses if hypertensive or using stimulants.

**Women — Caution**

Helpful for energy, libido, thyroid/adrenal support, and mood stability. Use caution with PCOS, fibroids, endometriosis, or estrogen-dominant cycles. High doses may cause mild acne, cycle shifts, or overstimulation; reduce or discontinue if headaches or irritability occur.

**Pregnancy & Nursing — Avoid**

Hormone-modulating effects and lack of safety data.

---

## Expected Results

- Energy lift: days
- Hormonal and balance effects: weeks
- Fatigue recovery and endurance: with long-term consistency

---

## DIY Recipe — Suma Root Energy Tonic

Simmer 1 tsp powdered Suma in hot water or warm milk for 10 minutes. Sweeten with honey for a grounding, strengthening daily tonic.

---

## Same / Similar Results

Ginseng · Maca Root · Ashwagandha

---

## Shelf Life / Potency After Preparation

- Powder: 1–2 years (airtight, cool, dry)
- Capsules: 1–2 years
- Tincture: 3–5 years
- Prepared decoction: refrigerate; use within 48 hours

---

## 💬 Herbal Reflections — Suma Root

Suma restores the quiet strength behind endurance—the place stress depletes first. Its medicine is structural rather than forceful, helping effort translate into lasting capacity. With rhythm and consistency, Suma makes strength sustainable, reminding us that resilience grows from rooted stability, not adrenaline surges.

---

## ⭐ Herbal Confidence Index 🌿 🌿 🌿 🌿 (4 / 5)

A reliable adaptogen for stamina, recovery, immune strength, and hormonal resilience. Suma supports sustainable energy for those worn down by chronic stress or physical demand—steady, cumulative, and tonifying.

# MARAL ROOT

★★★★★

*Rhaponticum carthamoides*

**Maral Root** is a performance-leaning adaptogen traditionally used to support stamina, recovery, and focus under physical load. It helps the body convert stress into adaptation—improving recovery, sustaining drive, and reducing post-effort crash without stimulant overstimulation. Its ecdysteroid-rich chemistry aligns with natural protein synthesis support and physical resilience. Native to Siberian alpine regions, Maral Root earned its name from observations of maral deer seeking the roots during demanding seasons. Folk use preceded modern study; later 20th-century Eastern European research explored its role in strength, endurance, and recovery. Traditionally prepared as decoctions or tinctures, it remains valued for building capacity steadily rather than forcing output. Cultivated sources are preferred to protect wild populations.

---

## Core Herbal Category — Maral Root

**Primary Core: Adaptogens** herb with *(strength-building, recovery-oriented action that supports endocrine balance and physical adaptation to stress)*
**Secondary Cores:** Endurance & Physical Recovery · Hormonal Balance · Circulatory Activation · Stress Resilience

---

## How It Works

Maral Root supports adaptive responses to physical and metabolic stress. Its strengthening compounds assist muscular recovery and sustained energy output, while circulatory support enhances nutrient delivery and tissue repair after exertion. By stabilizing hormonal signaling during periods of demand, it promotes endurance, recovery, and stress resilience.

---

## Primary Uses

- Improves stamina, strength, and physical recovery
- Supports mental focus under fatigue or load
- Aids fertility and hormonal tone

- Speeds recovery after illness, training, or exhaustion

---

## 🧪 Scientific Backing

Maral Root contains phytoecdysteroids—most notably 20-hydroxyecdysone—associated with enhanced natural protein synthesis, improved muscle recovery and work capacity, better stress adaptation, and support for reproductive and endocrine balance. Effects are non-steroidal but may gently influence hormone metabolism.

---

## 🍵 Forms Available

- Powdered root (smoothies, capsules)
- Decoction or tea (traditional)
- Tincture or extract

---

## 🌿 How to Use — Maral Root

**Tea/Decoction:** Simmer 1 tsp dried root in 1 cup water for 15 minutes; drink 1× daily.
**Capsules/Powder:** 500–1,000 mg daily for strength, endurance, and focus.
**Tincture:** 1–2 mL, 1–2× daily as an adaptogenic tonic.
Most effective with consistent use over several weeks; commonly cycled 3–4 weeks on, 1–2 weeks off.

---

## ⚠️ Caution Level: 🟡 Caution (Moderate Awareness)

Potent, energizing, and hormone-influencing. Avoid or seek guidance with hypertension, cardiac arrhythmia, hormone-sensitive disorders, anxiety/overstimulation tendencies, or concurrent use of testosterone boosters, anabolic hormones, or stimulant supplements. Overuse may cause restlessness, insomnia, irritability, or mild blood-pressure elevation.
**Pregnancy & nursing: Avoid.**

---

## Gender-Specific Safety — Maral Root

**Men — Caution**
Supports stamina, endurance, libido, and recovery. Mild androgen-like effects possible. Avoid high doses if hypertensive or using stimulants; discontinue if headaches, rapid heartbeat, or irritability occur. Best for short-term performance, recovery, or convalescence.

**Women — Caution**
Supports energy, strength, recovery, and mood. High doses may cause acne, irritability, or cycle shifts. Avoid with PCOS, androgen-sensitive acne, or hormone-dominant conditions; do not combine with hormone-regulating medications unless supervised. Cyclic, moderate use is safest.

**Pregnancy & Nursing — Avoid**
Endocrine activity and lack of safety data.

---

## Expected Results

- Energy and focus: days
- Strength and stamina: several weeks
- Fertility/hormonal effects: weeks to months

---

## DIY Recipe — Maral Root Recovery Tea

Simmer 1 tsp dried Maral Root in 1 cup water for 20 minutes. Drink daily during recovery or training cycles.

---

## Same / Similar Results

Ginseng · Rhodiola · Maca Root

---

## Shelf Life / Potency After Preparation

- Dried root: 2–3 years (cool, dry, airtight)
- Powder: 1–2 years
- Capsules: 1–2 years

- Tincture: 4–5 years
- Prepared decoction: refrigerate; use within 48 hours

---

## 💭 Herbal Reflections — Maral Root

Maral Root represents earned momentum—each effort compounding rather than leaking away. It bridges exertion and recovery so progress holds. Its medicine is not heat, but hardiness: strength built gradually, stabilized through rest, nourishment, and patience.

---

## ⭐ Herbal Confidence Index 🌿 🌿 🌿 🌿 🌿 (5 / 5)

A powerful Siberian adaptogen valued for strength, stamina, hormonal resilience, and recovery. Maral Root builds capacity the steady way—transforming strain into durable strength.

# RED CLOVER

★★★★

*Trifolium pratense*

**Red Clover** is a gentle alterative and nutritive tonic—mineral-rich blossoms long used to support clear skin, calm dry coughs, and restore balance to overheated or stagnant systems. Herbalists value it for lymphatic movement and blood nourishment, helping the body "tidy from the inside out" through slow, steady support rather than force.

Its isoflavone-bearing flowers are a classic ally for perimenopausal balance, helping moderate hot flashes and cyclical fluctuations without stimulation. As a food-grade herb, Red Clover fits easily into daily routines—long infusions for minerals, syrups for throat comfort, and blends with Nettle or Calendula when skin and lymph benefit from consistent care.

Native to meadows across Europe and North America, Red Clover was praised by 19th-century Eclectic physicians as a premier alterative and favored in folk medicine for lingering coughs and convalescence. A soil-fixing plant that nourishes fields as well as people, it remains an emblem of reciprocity and gentle restoration.

---

## 🌿 Core Herbal Category — Red Clover

**Primary Core: Lymphatic & Skin Support** herb with *(phytoestrogenic, blood-cleansing action that supports hormonal balance and lymphatic circulation)*

**Secondary Cores:** Skin Health · Respiratory Comfort · Nutritive Mineral Tonic

---

## How It Works

Red Clover supports hormonal balance through plant-based estrogenic compounds that influence endocrine rhythm. Its lymphatic-moving action assists the clearance of metabolic congestion, supporting tissue renewal and skin clarity. Mineral nourishment strengthens blood quality and resilience, while soothing actions calm dry or irritated respiratory tissues. Together, these effects promote systemic balance and gentle restoration.

---

## 🌱 Primary Uses

- Women's wellness and cycle support
- Skin clarity and soothing care
- Gentle respiratory comfort for dry or irritated coughs

- Nutritive mineral and lymphatic support

---

## Scientific Backing

Red Clover blossoms contain isoflavones (including formononetin and biochanin A), studied for menopausal comfort, hot-flash modulation, and mild endocrine balance. Research also supports its anti-inflammatory and antioxidant actions. Traditional use emphasizes its mineral density and alterative role in lymphatic and skin health.

---

## Forms Available

- Dried blossoms (tea or long infusion)
- Tincture or liquid extract
- Capsules or tablets

---

## How to Use — Red Clover

**Tea/Infusion:** Steep 1–2 tsp dried blossoms in 1 cup hot water for 10 minutes; drink 1–2× daily.
**Capsules/Powder:** 400–800 mg daily for hormonal and circulatory support.
**Tincture:** 1–2 mL, 1–2× daily as a gentle lymphatic tonic.
Works best with regular, moderate daily use over several weeks.

---

## Caution Level: Caution (Moderate Awareness)

Generally well tolerated, but phytoestrogenic activity requires care.
Avoid or seek guidance with:

- Estrogen-sensitive cancers
- Endometriosis or fibroids
- Heavy menstrual bleeding
- Use of HRT, birth control, SERMs, or anticoagulants (e.g., warfarin)

Rare effects: mild headache or digestive upset at high doses.
**Pregnancy & nursing: Avoid.**

## Gender-Specific Safety — Red Clover

**Men — Caution**

Generally safe in tea or moderate supplement form. Use caution with anticoagulants; avoid long-term high dosing and discontinue before surgery.

**Women — Caution**

Commonly used for hot flashes, PMS tension, perimenopause, and skin support. Avoid excessive dosing with estrogen dominance, fibroids, endometriosis, or concurrent hormone therapy. Moderate, steady use is typically well tolerated.

**Pregnancy & Nursing — Avoid**

Hormone-modulating and mild blood-thinning properties; insufficient safety data.

## Expected Results

- Menopausal comfort: 2–6 weeks
- Skin and respiratory support: several weeks
- Nutritive and lymphatic effects: gradual, ongoing

## DIY Recipe — Red Clover Meadow Tea

Steep 1–2 tsp dried blossoms in 8 oz hot water for 10–15 minutes.
Sip 1–2 cups daily.

## Same / Similar Results

Nettle Leaf · Raspberry Leaf · Evening Primrose

## Shelf Life / Potency After Preparation

- Dried blossoms: 1–2 years (airtight, away from light)
- Capsules/powder: ~1 year
- Tincture: 4–5 years
- Prepared tea: refrigerate; use within 24–36 hours

## 💬 Herbal Reflections — Red Clover

Red Clover carries the warmth of a meadow afternoon—modest, generous, and quietly restorative. It loosens stagnation, cools overheated tissues, and moistens where dryness has taken hold. Its medicine works in soft increments: skin that settles, breath that eases, rhythms that smooth.
A companion herb rather than a corrective hammer, Red Clover teaches patience and routine. It reminds us that lasting renewal often comes not from dramatic intervention, but from steady nourishment that allows the body to remember its own balance.

---

## Herbal Confidence Index 🌿 🌿 🌿 🌿 (4 / 5)

A gentle alterative and hormonal balancer renowned for women's health, skin clarity, and respiratory ease. Red Clover offers mineral-rich, lymph-moving support through quiet strength and consistency.

# VALERIAN

★★★★

*Valeriana officinalis*

**Valerian** is a dependable nighttime nervine used to shorten sleep onset, ease anxious restlessness, and release muscle tension after demanding days. It supports GABA-mediated calm without "knockout" heaviness, making it useful for light sleepers, perimenopausal wake-ups, and wired-but-tired minds. Many find it softens jaw and shoulder tension while easing stress-related headaches. Practical pairings enhance its effects: Passionflower for racing thoughts, Lemon Balm for worry with digestive flutter, Hops for stubborn insomnia, and Magnesium for clenched muscles. Consistent evening use builds results over 1–2 weeks, though some individuals sleep better with lower doses than higher ones. A small minority experience stimulation rather than sedation—an indication to reduce dose or switch allies.

---

## Core Herbal Category — Valerian

**Primary Core: Nervous System Support (Nervines)** herb with (deeply calming, nervous-system–settling action that supports sleep onset and restorative rest)
**Secondary Cores:** Muscle Relaxation herb · Stress Relief herb · Migraine/Tension Support herb

### How It Works

Valerian quiets excessive nervous system activity while easing skeletal muscle tension. Its calming compounds reduce stress-driven nerve firing, allowing smoother transition into sleep and more restorative rest cycles. This settling effect also supports relief from tension-related discomfort, promoting physical relaxation alongside mental calm.

---

## Primary Uses

Supports sleep onset and quality
Calms nervous tension and mental restlessness
Relieves muscular tightness and tension headaches

## Scientific Backing

Valerian root contains valerenic acids and valepotriates that influence GABA activity, producing sedative, anxiolytic, and muscle-relaxing effects. Traditional records and clinical trials support its use for insomnia related to stress, nervous agitation, and anxiety-linked muscle tension.

## 🧴 Forms Available

- Dried root (tea or decoction)
- Tincture or liquid extract
- Capsules or tablets

---

## 🌿 How to Use — Valerian

**Tea:** Simmer 1 tsp dried root in 1 cup water for 10–15 minutes; drink 30–60 minutes before bed.
**Capsules/Powder:** 400–900 mg at bedtime.
**Tincture:** 1–3 mL in the evening.
Valerian may be used as needed, though some benefit from several consecutive evenings of use.

---

## ⚠ Caution Level: ▨ Caution (Moderate Awareness)

Use care if combining with sedatives, alcohol, benzodiazepines, opioids, or sleep aids. Avoid driving or operating machinery after use. Paradoxical stimulation (restlessness, vivid dreams, agitation) occurs in a minority. Long-term nightly use should be tapered to avoid rebound insomnia. Avoid during pregnancy or breastfeeding unless professionally supervised.
Possible side effects at higher doses include headache, emotional heaviness, dizziness, or next-day grogginess.

---

## 🚹 🚺 Gender-Specific Safety — Valerian Root

**Men — Caution:** Generally well tolerated for insomnia and tension. Use awareness with low blood pressure, sedating medications, or morning grogginess; discontinue if stimulation occurs.
**Women — Caution:** Helpful for stress-related insomnia and PMS tension. Use awareness with vivid dreams, next-day fogginess, sedatives, or hormonal migraines.
**Pregnancy — Professional Guidance Only:** Avoid medicinal dosing; avoid strong tinctures.
**Nursing — Caution:** May pass into breast milk; avoid heavy nightly use and monitor infant response.

---

## ⌛ Expected Results

- Calming effect: 30–90 minutes
- Improved sleep quality: after several nights
- Muscle/tension relief: progressive with steady evening use

## 🛠 DIY Recipe — Valerian Bedtime Steep

Simmer 1 tsp dried root in 8 oz water for 5 minutes, cover, and steep 10 minutes more. Drink 30–60 minutes before bed. Optional: blend with Lemon Balm or Chamomile.

## 🔄 Same / Similar Results

Chamomile · Lemon Balm · Passionflower Lavender

## Shelf Life / Potency After Preparation

- Dried root: 2 years
- Capsules/tablets: 1–2 years
- Tincture: 4–5 years
- Tea/decoction: 24–36 hours refrigerated

---

## 💬 Herbal Reflections — Valerian

Valerian is the exhale we forget to take. It loosens clenched muscles, quiets the overactive mind, and invites sleep by easing rather than forcing. Its medicine carries weight without heaviness—a grounding calm that teaches the body how to downshift again.

With Valerian, less is often more. The right dose acts like a dimmer, not a switch, reminding us that rest comes from release. When paired with evening ritual, it becomes a cue to let the day fall away. And when it stimulates instead of soothes, it offers guidance: listen, adjust, choose another ally.

---

## ★ Herbal Confidence Index

🌿 🌿 🌿 🌿 (4 / 5 — A time-honored nervine and sleep ally that calms an overactive mind, releases muscular tension, and supports natural sleep rhythms without dependency. Valerian remains one of herbal medicine's most reliable tools for restorative rest.)

# LADY'S MANTLE

★★★★

*Alchemilla vulgaris*

**Lady's Mantle** has long stood as a quiet guardian of womanhood. Native to the cool meadows and forest edges of Europe, this dew-catching herb has been treasured since the Middle Ages for its restorative influence on the female body. Medieval healers observed its ability to tone the uterus, regulate menstrual flow, and ease discomfort during menopause and postpartum recovery. The fan-shaped leaves, often holding morning dew once called "Heaven's Water," earned the plant sacred status among alchemists who viewed it as an embodiment of feminine balance.

Medicinally, Lady's Mantle offers astringent, anti-inflammatory, and tissue-strengthening properties. It supports reproductive tone, eases cramping, and encourages hormonal steadiness, acting as a grounding, stabilizing ally through life's reproductive transitions.

---

## Core Herbal Category — Lady's Mantle

**Primary Core: Reproductive & Women's Health Support** herb with (astringent, tissue-toning action that supports uterine stability and reproductive rhythm regulation)

**Secondary Cores:** Pelvic Toning herb · Tissue Repair herb · Hormonal Harmony herb

---

## How It Works

Lady's Mantle tones and strengthens pelvic and reproductive tissues, supporting structural integrity and balance. Its astringent compounds help moderate excessive tissue laxity and fluid loss, reinforcing uterine tone and stabilizing reproductive rhythms. The herb also supports gentle tissue repair following strain or imbalance, promoting pelvic resilience and hormonal harmony over time.

---

## Primary Uses

- Tones pelvic and uterine tissues; moderates heavy menstrual flow
- Eases menstrual cramps and supports cycle balance
- Supports postpartum recovery

- Mild digestive astringent for looseness

### 🧪 Scientific Backing

Rich in tannins and flavonoids, Lady's Mantle demonstrates astringent, anti-inflammatory, and antispasmodic actions. Traditional European medical texts consistently describe its use for menstrual regulation, postpartum healing, and pelvic tissue repair.

### Forms Available

- Dried aerial parts (infusion)
- Tincture or liquid extract
- Capsules or powdered herb

---

### How to Use — Lady's Mantle

**Tea:** Steep 1–2 tsp dried herb in 1 cup hot water for 10 minutes; drink 1–2× daily.
**Capsules/Powder:** 300–600 mg daily for women's health and tissue toning.
**Tincture:** 1–2 mL, 1–2× daily for cycle balance and mild inflammation relief.
Lady's Mantle works best with steady, month-long use rather than sporadic dosing.

---

### ⚠ Caution Level: Caution

Generally safe when used moderately. Use awareness if you take hormonal therapy or birth-control medications, if menstrual flow is already very light, or if you have kidney disease or use strong diuretics. Avoid during pregnancy unless under professional supervision due to uterine-toning effects.

---

### Gender-Specific Safety — Lady's Mantle

**Men — Safe:** Useful as a mild digestive astringent and anti-inflammatory. Helpful for loose stools, mouth or gum irritation (as a rinse), and minor tissue irritation. No hormonal effects documented. Overuse may cause dryness or mild constipation.
**Women — Safe:** A premier women's herb for heavy bleeding, PMS discomfort, postpartum recovery, pelvic tone, and emotional grounding during hormonal fluctuation. Use caution with very light flow, prescription blood thinners, or excessive long-term daily

use.

**Pregnancy — Avoid:** Astringent and uterine-toning effects may tighten uterine muscles. Avoid unless professionally guided.

**Nursing — Mild Caution:** Light, occasional tea may support postpartum tissue recovery. Avoid large doses, strong tinctures, or extended daily use, as excess astringency may reduce milk supply.

---

## Expected Results

- Cramp relief: within several doses
- Flow moderation / pelvic tone: 1–3 cycles
- Postpartum support: weeks of steady use

---

## DIY Recipe — Lady's Mantle Pelvic-Toning Tea

Steep 1–2 tsp dried herb in 8 oz hot water for 10–15 minutes. Drink 1–2 cups daily during the luteal phase or recovery periods. Optional: combine with Raspberry Leaf for deeper uterine support.

## Same / Similar Results

Raspberry Leaf · Vitex (Chaste Tree) · Shepherd's Purse

## Shelf Life / Potency After Preparation

- Dried herb: 1–2 years
- Tincture: 4–5 years
- Capsules/powder: 1–2 years
- Infusion: best within 24 hours refrigerated

---

## Herbal Reflections — Lady's Mantle

Lady's Mantle gathers what is scattered. Like dew resting in its pleated leaves, it helps the body remember form and rhythm when things feel loose or overextended. Its medicine is containment without rigidity — offering support that steadies rather than constricts.

Through cycles of change and recovery, it teaches composure: balance restored through quiet, faithful reinforcement. In this way, Lady's Mantle reminds us that strength can be soft, and structure can feel like care.

---

### ✿ Herbal Confidence Index

🌿 🌿 🌿 🌿 (4 / 5 — A revered women's tonic for uterine tone, menstrual regulation, and postpartum recovery. Lady's Mantle restores pelvic integrity, moderates excess bleeding, and supports hormonal equilibrium with gentle, stabilizing grace.)

# NETTLE SEED

★★★★★

*Urtica dioica*

**Nettle** is famed for its mineral-rich leaves, but the seeds hold a distinct place in Western herbalism as a tonic for stamina, kidney strength, and deep recovery. Harvested as tiny aromatic clusters, nettle seed is used to support renal resilience, lift depleted energy, and help the body adapt to prolonged stress without harsh stimulation.
Herbalists reach for nettle seed when recovery feels stalled or vitality has thinned after illness, burnout, or long demand. It is valued for sharpening mental focus, supporting healthy hair and scalp, and rebuilding reserves, often taken daily as a gentle nutritive ally. With a mild, nutty flavor, the seeds blend easily into food, offering steady support rather than a quick push.

---

### Core Herbal Category — Nettle Seed

**Primary Core: Endocrine & Hormonal Support** herb with (deeply restorative, nutritive action that supports renal resilience and adrenal recovery under stress)
**Secondary Cores:** Nervous System Rebuilding herb · Nutritive Tonic herb · Stress Resilience herb

---

### How It Works

Nettle Seed nourishes kidney and adrenal function depleted by prolonged stress or fatigue. Its concentrated nutritive profile supports cellular repair within endocrine and nervous system pathways. By restoring foundational energy reserves, it improves stress tolerance, mental clarity, and recovery capacity. This restorative action promotes long-term vitality without overstimulation.

---

### Primary Uses

- Supports kidney vitality and filtration
- Enhances stamina, energy, and stress resilience
- Aids post-illness recovery and mental clarity

- Encourages healthy hair and scalp through deep nourishment

### Scientific Backing

Traditional Western herbalism describes nettle seed as a trophorestorative for kidneys and vitality. The seeds contain fatty acids, sterols, antioxidants, and micronutrients consistent with adaptogenic-leaning and nutritive support.

---

### Forms Available

- Whole seed (sprinkled on food)
- Ground seed (powder or capsules)
- Tincture or liquid extract

---

### How to Use — Nettle Seed

**Tea:** Steep 1 tsp dried seed in 1 cup hot water for 10 minutes; drink 1× daily.
**Capsules/Powder:** 300–600 mg daily for energy, clarity, and kidney nourishment.
**Tincture:** 1–2 mL, 1–2× daily for steady restorative support.
Nettle Seed is mild enough for daily use and works gradually over weeks.

---

### ⚠ Caution Level: Safe

Generally safe for long-term use. Use mild awareness if taking blood-pressure or diabetes medications, or if highly stimulant-sensitive (may affect sleep at high doses). Individuals with advanced kidney disease should use only under supervision.

---

### Gender-Specific Safety — Nettle Seed

**Men — Safe:** Traditionally used for kidney nourishment, adrenal recovery, mental clarity, and vitality. Does **not** influence testosterone or DHT (unlike nettle root). Very high doses may cause mild restlessness; avoid strong dosing with advanced kidney disease.
**Women — Safe:** Helpful for fatigue, brain fog, post-illness weakness, kidney depletion patterns, and hair/scalp support. Does not affect estrogen or progesterone. High doses may feel overstimulating in sensitive individuals.
**Pregnancy — Caution (Limited Data):** Nettle leaf is common in pregnancy, but nettle

**seed** is more stimulating to kidneys and adrenals. Food-level use is likely safe; avoid medicinal doses unless supervised.
/ **Nursing — Mild Caution:** Often supportive for fatigued nursing mothers. Use light doses; avoid strong tinctures. Monitor infant for restlessness or digestive changes.

---

## ⌛ Expected Results

- Mental clarity and subtle lift: 3–7 days
- Stamina and recovery: 2–4 weeks
- Hair and scalp improvements: 4–8 weeks

---

## DIY Recipe — Nettle Seed Daily Sprinkle

Grind ½–1 tsp nettle seed and add to yogurt, oats, or smoothies. Optional: pair with citrus zest or cinnamon for a bright, steady tonic.

---

## Same / Similar Results

Nettles (leaf) · Ashwagandha · Schisandra

## Shelf Life / Potency After Preparation

- Whole seeds: 2–3 years
- Powdered seed: ~1 year
- Tincture: 4–5 years
- Infusion: best within 24 hours refrigerated

## Herbal Reflections — Nettle Seed

Nettle Seed is the spark inside the coal — quiet, durable energy that rebuilds rather than rushes. Where vitality has thinned after long strain, it restores steadiness and clear function. Its medicine is sustainability: endurance fed by nourishment, water, and rest, not forced momentum.
Taken in small, faithful doses, it becomes a daily practice — a sprinkle that keeps the lamp

trimmed, the mind focused, and resilience returning as a resource rather than a jolt.

---

🌟 **Herbal Confidence Index** 🌿 🌿 🌿 🌿 🌿 (5 / 5 — A deeply restorative tonic for kidneys, adrenals, and the nervous system. Nettle Seed rebuilds stamina, clarity, and resilience during exhaustion or chronic fatigue. Gentle yet profoundly strengthening, it supports renewal from the body's roots upward.)

# LEMON VERBENA

★★★★

*Aloysia citrodora*

**Lemon Verbena** is prized for its bright citrus aroma and gentle composure. Traditionally sipped after meals to settle the stomach and ease cramping, it also serves as an evening tea to quiet nervous tension and support natural sleep without heaviness. Even its fragrance lifts mood—sunlight in a cup.

Beyond digestion and nerves, Lemon Verbena appears in antioxidant tonics, blends for spasmodic coughs, and simple kitchen syrups that refresh the senses in busy seasons.

Carried from South America to European monastery and cottage gardens, its leaves became a favored after-supper cordial in the 18th–19th centuries—an old-world habit that still feels timely.

---

### Core Herbal Category — Lemon Verbena

**Primary Core: Nervous System Support (Nervines)** herb with (gently sedative, aromatic action that soothes nerve tension while relaxing digestive function)

**Secondary Cores:** Gentle Sedation herb · Mood Uplift herb · Respiratory Soothing herb

---

## How It Works

Lemon Verbena calms nervous system activity while easing digestive tension and spasms. Its aromatic compounds promote relaxation without heavy sedation, supporting emotional lightness and mental clarity. By soothing the gut–nerve connection, it reduces stress-related digestive discomfort and supports relaxed breathing.

---

### Primary Uses

- Calms digestive upset and eases cramping
- Soothes nervous tension and supports restful sleep
- Softens spasmodic coughs (adjunct use)

- Provides antioxidant refresh during demanding seasons

## 🧪 Scientific Backing

Rich in citral (neral/geranial), verbascoside, and flavonoids with carminative, antispasmodic, mild sedative, and antioxidant activity. Widely used as a digestive and calming tea in traditional practice.

---

## 🍵 Forms Available

- Dried or fresh leaf (tea, syrup)
- Tincture or liquid extract
- Culinary syrups or honey infusions
- Aromatic preparations (leaf/EO)

---

## 🌿 How to Use — Lemon Verbena

**Tea:** Steep 1–2 tsp dried leaf in 1 cup hot water for 10 minutes; drink 1–2× daily.
**Capsules/Powder:** 300–500 mg daily for calming or antioxidant support.
**Tincture:** 1–2 mL, 1–2× daily for stress relief or digestive comfort.
Well suited to gentle daily use.

---

## ⚠ Caution Level: ● Caution

Generally gentle. Large amounts may irritate sensitive digestion. Rare contact sensitivity—patch test infused oils. Limited data in pregnancy or lactation: use culinary/light tea amounts unless supervised.

---

## 🚹 🚺 Gender-Specific Safety — Lemon Verbena

● **Men — Safe:** Supports stress reduction, digestion, mild respiratory comfort, and sleep. Strong daytime doses may cause drowsiness in sensitive individuals.
● **Women — Safe (Mild Caution):** Helpful for anxiety, PMS irritability, sleep difficulty, and stress-related digestion. Very strong teas may aggravate sensitive digestion.
● **Pregnancy — Mild Caution:** Light tea generally acceptable for tension or mild nausea.

Avoid strong medicinal dosing (tinctures, capsules).
**Nursing — Mild Caution:** Mild tea usually well tolerated. Strong doses may slightly reduce milk supply or cause infant gas—observe and adjust.

---

## ⌛ Expected Results

- Post-meal comfort: 1–2 cups
- Calming/sleep support: same evening to 1–2 weeks
- Cough/spasm relief (in blends): several days

---

## DIY Recipe — Lemon Verbena Evening Tea

Steep 1–2 tsp dried (or 2–3 tsp fresh) leaf in 8 oz hot water for 7–10 minutes.
Sip after dinner or 30–60 minutes before bed. Optional: blend with Lemon Balm.

---

## Same / Similar Results

Lemon Balm · Chamomile · Passionflower

---

## Shelf Life / Potency After Preparation

- Dried leaf: 1–2 years
- Fresh leaf: 5–7 days refrigerated
- Tincture: 4–5 years
- Syrup: 2–3 weeks refrigerated
- Tea: best within 24 hours

---

## Herbal Reflections — Lemon Verbena

Lemon Verbena feels like opening a window—light, clarifying, and kind. It refreshes without rush, easing discomfort while inviting the mind to soften. Its lesson is brightness with boundaries: calm that remains vivid, and gentleness that still heals.

---

★ **Herbal Confidence Index** 🌿 🌿 🌿 🌿 (4 / 5 — A bright, aromatic nervine and digestive tonic that calms the mind, uplifts the spirit, and soothes the stomach. Lemon Verbena relieves tension, mild insomnia, and digestive unrest with graceful effectiveness.)

# PIPSISSEWA

★★★★

*Chimaphila umbellata*

**Pipsissewa** (Prince's Pine) is a small evergreen of pine forests, valued as a focused urinary remedy. Traditionally used to support bladder and kidney function, reduce urinary-tract irritation, and discourage microbial overgrowth, it is a classic "waterway" ally when comfort is needed most. Beyond the urinary system, its astringent toning can help ease lymphatic congestion and mild tissue swelling, and it has a long history of topical use for strains and irritated tissues. Its chemistry includes arbutin-type glycosides and tannins—constituents that, when used properly, provide measured cleansing and tissue tone rather than harsh purging.

---

**Core Herbal Category — Pipsissewa (Prince's Pine)**
**Primary Core: Kidney & Urinary Support** herb with (arbutin-rich, astringent principles that tone the urinary tract and support lymphatic clearing)
**Secondary Cores:** Lymphatic Clearing herb · Astringent Tissue Tone herb · Microbial Balance herb

---

## How It Works

Pipsissewa tones urinary tissues while supporting efficient kidney filtration and elimination. Its astringent properties help strengthen mucosal linings of the bladder and urinary tract, reducing irritation and excess discharge. By encouraging lymphatic clearing, it assists the body in resolving fluid stagnation and waste buildup. Its antimicrobial influence supports balanced urinary conditions without damaging tissue integrity. Together, these actions promote urinary clarity, tissue strength, and gentle detoxification.

---

**Primary Uses**

- Supports bladder and kidney comfort and function
- Eases urinary-tract irritation and discourages microbial overgrowth
- Provides astringent support for mild tissue swelling and lymphatic congestion

### Scientific Backing

Contains arbutin-like glycosides (which hydrolyze to urinary-antiseptic compounds under appropriate conditions) and tannins that contribute to tissue tone. Historical Eclectic and Indigenous sources describe its diuretic, tonic, and cleansing roles for lower-urinary-tract complaints.

---

### Forms Available

- Leaf / aerial parts (tea or cold maceration)
- Tincture or liquid extract
- Topical wash or soak

---

### How to Use — Pipsissewa

- **Tea:** Simmer 1 tsp dried leaf in 1 cup water for 10–15 minutes; drink 1× daily for urinary or lymphatic support
- **Capsules / Powder:** 300–500 mg daily for fluid balance and gentle cleansing
- **Tincture:** 1–2 mL, 1–2× daily for urinary tract tone and mild detoxification

Pipsissewa is best used **short-term** for targeted cleansing and support.

---

### Caution Level: *Caution*

Short courses preferred; avoid prolonged or high-dose use. Not for pregnancy or lactation without professional guidance. Ensure correct plant identification and favor cultivated sources to protect vulnerable wild populations.

---

### Gender-Specific Safety — Pipsissewa

#### Men — Caution

Traditionally used for:

- Urinary-tract discomfort
- Kidney congestion
- Prostate-related pelvic pressure
- Lymphatic stagnation with skin eruptions

Use awareness if you have kidney disease, take prescription diuretics, experience burning urination, or are prone to dehydration or electrolyte imbalance. Safe for **short-term therapeutic use only**.

**Women — Caution**

Helpful for:

- Urinary-tract irritation
- Pelvic congestion
- Lymphatic sluggishness
- Skin issues linked to poor elimination

Use extra caution with recurrent UTIs, interstitial cystitis, kidney sensitivity, or dehydration from heavy menstrual flow. Short-term use is appropriate; avoid long-term daily dosing.

**Pregnancy — Avoid**

Internal use should be avoided due to hydroquinone precursors, potential urinary irritation, and uterine sensitivity.

**Nursing — Mild Caution / Avoid**

Not ideal while breastfeeding, especially tinctures or strong teas. Hydroquinone compounds may pass into milk and infant kidneys are sensitive. If used at all, limit to very dilute, short-term preparations under guidance.

---

**Expected Results**

- Urinary comfort: 1–3 days (with adequate hydration)
- Tissue-tone and lymphatic support: 1–2 weeks
- Topical swelling relief: within days (adjunct use)

---

**DIY Recipe — Pipsissewa Cooling Rinse**

Steep 1 tbsp dried Pipsissewa in 10 oz warm (not boiling) water for 30 minutes.
Strain well.
Use as a gentle sitz rinse, or dilute 1:1 with cool water for external comfort 1–2× daily.

---

**Same / Similar Results**

- Corn Silk
- Uva Ursi *(use with caution)*
- Marshmallow Root

### Shelf Life / Potency After Preparation

- Dried herb: 1–2 years (airtight, dark storage)
- Powdered herb: 1 year
- Tincture: 4–6 years
- Cold infusion: 24–36 hours (refrigerated)
- Topical rinse: use within 24 hours

### Herbal Reflections — Pipsissewa

Pipsissewa is a quiet understory ally—low, evergreen, and persistent—teaching that true clearing happens slowly and with care. It does not force elimination; it tidies pathways and restores tone where irritation and stagnation have settled. When the bladder feels hot or fretful, or fluids linger too long in the tissues, this woodland plant suggests a cooler current and steadier flow. Historically carried by forest peoples for stubborn urinary and lymphatic complaints, Pipsissewa embodies modest strength: close to the ground, long-lived, and unhurried. Its medicine reminds us that some of the most effective remedies work without spectacle—patient, precise, and respectful of balance.

---

### Herbal Confidence Index

**(4 / 5 —** A traditional woodland urinary tonic long valued for kidney, bladder, and prostate support. Pipsissewa gently eases irritation, reduces water retention, and supports detoxification through astringent and antimicrobial action. Subtle, disciplined, and enduring—like the evergreen forest floor itself.)

# ANISE HYSSOP

★★★★

Agastache foeniculum

**Anise Hyssop** is a fragrant mint-family herb prized for its uplifting aroma and gentle healing qualities. **Native to North America, its leaves and lavender-blue blooms have long been brewed into teas that calm the nerves, ease coughs, and settle digestion.** It carries the sweet scent of anise and licorice yet has the soothing character of a mild mint — making it both comforting and refreshing.

**Traditionally used by Indigenous tribes and modern herbalists alike, Anise Hyssop supports the lungs, relaxes tension, and restores emotional balance during stress or fatigue.** It bridges the line between food and medicine: flavorful, aromatic, and healing to both body and spirit.

---

## Core Herbal Category — Anise Hyssop

**Primary Core: Nervous System Support (Nervines)** herb with *(gentle nervine, aromatic action that soothes emotional tension and supports relaxed mental states)*

**Secondary Cores:** Digestive Comfort herb · Respiratory Soothing herb · Mood & Spirit Uplift herb

---

## How It Works

Anise Hyssop works by gently calming nervous system activity while promoting emotional ease and lightness. Its aromatic compounds help relax tension without dulling mental clarity. By soothing the gut–nerve connection, it supports digestive comfort during stress. The herb also eases respiratory irritation through gentle relaxation of airway tissues. This combined action supports calm mood, open breathing, and emotional balance.

---

## Primary Uses

- Calms nervous tension and emotional fatigue
- Soothes coughs, sore throats, and mild respiratory irritation
- Aids digestion and reduces gas or bloating
- Supports immune resilience during seasonal changes
- Gently uplifts mood and promotes relaxation

---

## Scientific Backing

Studies show that Anise Hyssop contains flavonoids, phenolic acids, and essential oils (including methyl chavicol and limonene) that demonstrate antioxidant and antimicrobial activity. Early investigations suggest mild expectorant and relaxant actions, validating its historical use for colds, stress, and digestive discomfort.

---

## Forms Available

- Tea / infusion (classic use — soothing and aromatic)
- Tincture (concentrated extract for calming nerves or supporting digestion)
- Culinary use (fresh or dried leaves in salads, desserts, honey, and syrups)

---

## How to Use — Anise Hyssop

**Tea:** Use 1 Tbsp dried leaves/flowers (or 2–3 Tbsp fresh) per 8 oz boiling water. Steep 10–15 minutes, covered, then strain. Drink 1–3× daily for calm, respiratory comfort, or digestive ease.

**Tincture:** Take 1–2 mL (about 20–40 drops) up to 3× daily for nervous tension, mild coughs, or digestive upset.

**Culinary Use:** Sprinkle fresh or dried leaf into salads, desserts, syrups, or honey. Ideal as a gentle daily nervine–digestive support in food-level amounts.

Anise Hyssop is gentle enough for regular use; many people enjoy it most in the late afternoon or evening as a calming aromatic tea.

---

## Caution Level: Safe

- Generally considered very safe in tea and culinary amounts.
- Avoid excessive use of highly concentrated essential oil or extracts if sensitive to estragole-containing plants (e.g., tarragon, basil).

---

## Gender-Specific Safety — Anise Hyssop

**Men — Safe**

Anise Hyssop is safe for most men and supports:

- Nervous tension and mental fatigue
- Mild respiratory irritation and throat discomfort
- Digestive upset from stress or heavy meals

No known hormonal impact. Mild drowsiness may occur with strong evening teas.

**Women — Safe**

Women often use Anise Hyssop to:

- Ease anxiety and emotional overload
- Soothe PMS-related irritability and tension
- Support digestion and gentle sleep preparation

Non-hormonal and safe for routine use in moderate amounts.

**Pregnancy — Caution**
• Small culinary or light tea amounts are generally acceptable.
• Avoid strong tinctures and high-dose preparations due to limited safety data.
**Nursing — Mild Caution**
• Light teas are usually fine and may help relax both mother and baby.
• Avoid very strong teas or tinctures; monitor infant for gas, fussiness, or unusual sleepiness.

---

## Expected Results

• Calming and digestive relief: within ~30 minutes of tea or tincture
• Respiratory soothing and mood lift: within a few days of consistent use
• Overall stress reduction and improved clarity: 1–2 weeks of moderate intake

---

## DIY Recipe — Calming Anise Hyssop Tea

Use 1 Tbsp dried leaves or flowers per 8 oz boiling water.
Steep 10 minutes, strain, and sweeten lightly with honey.
Sip warm to ease stress, soothe throat irritation, or unwind in the evening.

---

## Shelf Life / Potency After Preparation

Dried leaf/flower: 1–2 years (airtight container, away from heat and light)
Tincture: 4–5 years (cool, dark storage)
Syrups and infused honey: 2–3 weeks refrigerated (discard if mold, off-smell, or fermentation appears)

Prepared tea: Best within 24 hours (refrigerated if not consumed immediately)

## Same/Similar Results

Lemon Balm — relaxing nervine, uplifts mood
Spearmint — refreshing digestive support
Holy Basil (Tulsi) — adaptogenic calm and clarity
Chamomile — gentle sedative for anxiety and rest

---

## Herbal Reflections of Anise Hyssop

Anise Hyssop reminds us that healing can be fragrant and gentle. It doesn't force calm; it invites it — through scent, taste, and quiet influence on the breath. Where stress, coughing, or scattered thoughts cloud the mind, this herb opens the chest and heart alike. Its soft anise–mint aroma embodies the meeting of sweetness and serenity, helping restore harmony from within.

---

## Herbal Confidence Index:

(4 / 5 — A pleasant, reliable, and safe respiratory–nervine herb offering balanced benefits for the mind and body when used consistently.)

# GARLIC

★★★★★

*Allium sativum*

**Garlic** is one of the world's most powerful and time-honored medicinal herbs—a cornerstone of traditional healing systems from Africa and Asia to the Mediterranean. Known for its profound cardiovascular, immune, and antimicrobial benefits, Garlic's sulfur-rich compounds (especially allicin) make it a natural defender against infection, inflammation, poor circulation, and metabolic imbalance.
For thousands of years, healers have relied on Garlic to open blood vessels, lower blood pressure, cleanse the blood, regulate cholesterol, support respiratory health, and strengthen overall vitality. Few herbs offer such broad protection with such an extensive history of proven usefulness.

---

🌿 **Core Herbal Category — Garlic**
**Primary Core: Cardiovascular System Support** herb with (circulatory-activating, sulfur-rich compounds that support healthy blood flow and metabolic efficiency)
**Secondary Cores:** Antimicrobial & Immune Defense herb · Respiratory Support herb · Digestive Warming & Detox herb

---

## How It Works

Garlic activates circulation and supports vascular flexibility, helping improve blood flow and metabolic signaling. Its sulfur compounds assist healthy lipid processing and cellular energy use while supporting immune defense against microbial threats. Garlic's warming action helps loosen respiratory mucus, stimulate digestion, and promote gentle detoxification through the liver and bloodstream.

---

🌱 **Primary Uses**

- Supports healthy blood pressure and circulation
- Helps regulate cholesterol and triglycerides
- Strengthens immune defense against bacteria, fungi, and viruses
- Assists respiratory clearing and congestion relief
- Supports liver detoxification and blood cleansing

- Aids digestion, gas reduction, and intestinal balance
- Supports blood sugar balance (adjunct use)

---

**Scientific Backing**

Garlic's allicin demonstrates strong antibacterial, antiviral, and antifungal activity. Clinical research shows consistent reductions in systolic and diastolic blood pressure, improvements in LDL cholesterol and triglycerides, and enhanced arterial flexibility. Studies also support Garlic's role in reducing cold frequency, severity, and recovery time, along with potent antioxidant and anti-inflammatory vascular protection.

---

**Forms Available**

- Fresh garlic cloves (raw or lightly cooked)
- Aged garlic extract
- Garlic oil or oil macerates
- Capsules or tablets (standardized allicin potential)
- Tincture or liquid extract
- Garlic-infused honey or syrups

---

**How to Use — Garlic**

- **Fresh clove:** 1 raw clove daily (crush and rest 10 minutes before consuming)
- **Capsules:** 300–600 mg standardized extract, 1–2× daily
- **Aged garlic extract:** 600–1200 mg daily
- **Tincture:** 1–2 mL, 2× daily
- **Respiratory honey:** ½–1 tsp during congestion

Use consistently for cardiovascular support; short courses for acute infections.

---

**Caution Level:** *Caution*

May thin blood—use caution with anticoagulants. Avoid very high doses before surgery. Raw garlic may irritate sensitive digestion or reflux. Strong odor and sweating may occur with heavy intake.

---

### 🚹 🚺 Gender-Specific Safety — Garlic

**Men — Safe**

Supports circulation, cholesterol balance, immune defense, respiratory health, and endurance.

**Women — Safe**

Supports blood pressure, antimicrobial protection, pelvic circulation, and inflammatory balance. Mild digestive sensitivity possible.

**Pregnancy — Caution**

Culinary use is safe. Avoid concentrated medicinal dosing unless guided.

**Nursing — Mild Caution**

Large amounts may alter milk flavor; monitor infant for gassiness.

---

### Expected Results

4. Immune response: 24–48 hours
5. Circulatory warmth: 5–7 days
6. Blood pressure & cholesterol support: 4–8 weeks

---

### DIY Recipe — Garlic Immune Honey

Crush 2–3 cloves and rest 10 minutes. Mix with 4 tbsp raw honey.
Take ½–1 tsp during colds or sluggish immunity.

---

### Same / Similar Results

- Ginger
- Onion
- Hawthorn
- Oregano Oil *(stronger antimicrobial)*
- Turmeric

---

### Shelf Life / Potency

- Fresh bulbs: 3–6 months
- Powder: 1–2 years
- Garlic oil: 1 year (refrigerated)
- Aged extract: 3–4 years

- Tincture: 3–5 years

---

💭 **Herbal Reflections — Garlic**

Garlic is the great equalizer—humble, fierce, and enduring. It cuts through stagnation, opens blocked pathways, and drives out what does not belong. Whether food or medicine, it protects life at its roots, reminding us that resilience often comes wrapped in simplicity.

---

🌟 **Herbal Confidence Index**

🌿 🌿 🌿 🌿 🌿 **(5 / 5 — A world-class cardiovascular and antimicrobial herb with unmatched historical validation and broad clinical support.)**

# BORAGE SEED

★★★★

*Borago officinalis* (Seed / Oil)

**Borage Seed**—best known through its oil—is one of nature's richest sources of gamma-linolenic acid (GLA), a rare omega-6 fatty acid used by the body to calm inflammation, restore skin integrity, and support hormonal balance. Historically valued across Europe, North Africa, and the Middle East, Borage has long been associated with courage, emotional uplift, and restorative moisture.

While the leaf soothes lungs and tissues, the **seed oil** is prized for repairing damaged skin barriers, easing eczema, balancing PMS and menopausal symptoms, calming inflammatory flare-ups, and restoring resilience to nerves and endocrine rhythms. Borage Seed is a true moisture restorer—quietly rebuilding where dryness and stress have worn the body thin.

---

**Core Herbal Category — Borage Seed**

**Primary Core: Reproductive & Women's Health Support** herb with (GLA-rich lipid support that restores tissue moisture and inflammatory balance)

**Secondary Cores:** Anti-Inflammatory Support herb · Nervous System Calm herb · Women's Wellness herb · Joint & Tissue Recovery herb

---

## How It Works

Borage Seed Oil delivers concentrated GLA, which the body converts into anti-inflammatory prostaglandins that calm irritated tissues and restore cellular moisture. This action supports skin barrier repair, hormonal steadiness, joint comfort, and nervous-system resilience during stress or depletion.

---

**Primary Uses**

- Restores damaged skin barrier (eczema, dermatitis, dryness)
- Reduces systemic inflammation
- Supports PMS and menopausal hormone balance
- Eases breast tenderness
- Supports joint and connective-tissue comfort
- Helps maintain skin, hair, and nail moisture

**Scientific Backing**

Borage Seed Oil contains 17–25% GLA—among the highest natural concentrations—along with linoleic and oleic acids and vitamin E compounds. Research shows improvements in eczema, inflammatory markers, skin hydration, hormonal discomfort, and immune regulation.

---

**Forms Available**

- Softgel capsules (borage oil)
- Liquid oil (internal or topical)
- Infused oils, creams, or balms

---

**How to Use — Borage Seed / Oil**

- **Capsules:** 500–1000 mg daily (up to 1500 mg short-term)
- **Liquid oil:** ½–1 tsp daily
- **Topical:** Apply thin layer to dry or irritated skin 1–2× daily

Best results occur with consistent use for 2–4 weeks.

---

**Caution Level:** *Moderate Caution*

Avoid during pregnancy. Use PA-free, purified oils only. Use caution with seizure disorders or anticoagulants. Mild GI upset possible at high doses.

---

**Gender-Specific Safety — Borage Seed**

**Men — Safe**

Supports skin, joints, inflammation balance, and stress-related hormone shifts.

**Women — Safe**

Supports PMS, menopausal dryness, eczema, hormonal skin issues and breast tenderness.

**Pregnancy — Avoid**

**Nursing — Mild Caution**

Small amounts likely safe if PA-free; monitor infant sensitivity.

---

**Expected Results**

- Skin hydration: 3–7 days
- Eczema improvement: 1–3 weeks
- Hormonal comfort: 2–4 weeks

🛠 **DIY Recipe — Borage Barrier-Repair Oil**
Mix 1 tsp borage oil with 1 tsp jojoba oil.
Optional: 1 drop lavender. Apply nightly to dry or irritated skin.

---

🔄 **Same / Similar Results**

4. Evening Primrose Oil
5. Black Currant Seed Oil
6. Flaxseed Oil
7. Chamomile
8. Comfrey *(topical, short-term only)*

---

🧪 **Shelf Life / Potency**

- Capsules: 1–2 years
- Liquid oil: 1 year (refrigerated after opening)
- Blended oils: 6–12 months

---

💬 **Herbal Reflections — Borage Seed**
Borage Seed restores what stress strips away. It returns softness, flexibility, and calm—not by force, but by nourishment. Its medicine is quiet renewal, rebuilding protective layers both physical and emotional, until resilience feels natural again.

---

⭐ **Herbal Confidence Index**
🌿 🌿 🌿 🌿 **(4 / 5 — A modern essential for skin repair, hormonal balance, and inflammatory support.)**

# PEPPERMINT

★★★★★

*Mentha × piperita*

Peppermint is one of the most widely used and instantly recognizable herbs in the world, valued for its cooling, relaxing, and clarifying effects on digestion, respiration, and the nervous system. Rich in menthol and aromatic oils, it quickly eases cramping, bloating, nausea, and tension while promoting smooth digestive flow. Its fresh, penetrating aroma also opens the sinuses and sharpens mental clarity.
Because of its broad usefulness and rapid action, Peppermint has long been considered a household cornerstone herb — effective, gentle, and reliable across many everyday discomforts.

---

### 🌿 Core Herbal Category — Peppermint

**Primary Core: Digestive System Support** herb (menthol-rich, smooth-muscle–relaxing action that eases digestive spasm and excess heat)
**Secondary Cores:** Respiratory Opening · Nervous System Calm · Anti-Spasmodic Support · Headache Relief

---

### 🌿 How It Works

Peppermint works by relaxing smooth muscle in the digestive tract, relieving cramping, gas, and tension while cooling irritated tissues. Its menthol content activates cold-sensing receptors that reduce discomfort, open respiratory passages, and ease headache pressure. By calming both gut and nerve tension, Peppermint restores comfort and clarity across multiple systems.

---

### 🌿 Primary Uses

- Relieves gas, bloating, indigestion, and cramping
- Eases nausea and motion sickness
- Opens sinuses and supports respiratory comfort
- Soothes tension headaches
- Calms stress-related digestive upset
- Cools hot, irritated tissues

---

### 🧪 Scientific Backing

Peppermint contains menthol, menthone, rosmarinic acid, flavonoids, and volatile oils with well-documented smooth-muscle–relaxing, analgesic, antimicrobial, and cooling effects. Clinical research strongly supports its use for IBS symptoms, functional indigestion, nausea, and tension headaches.

---

### How to Use (Dosage)

**Tea:** 1–2 tsp dried leaf per cup; steep 10 minutes; 1–3× daily
**Capsules:** 0.2–0.4 mL enteric-coated oil capsules, 2–3× daily (IBS support)
**Aromatherapy:** Steam inhalation or diffusion for sinus opening and mental clarity
**Topical (Diluted):** 1–2 drops essential oil per tsp carrier oil for temples or abdomen

---

### Caution Level — Moderate Awareness

Generally safe when used appropriately. Avoid undiluted essential oil on skin or near eyes. High-dose oil may worsen acid reflux. Use caution with infants and young children. Enteric-coated capsules may interact with antacids.

---

### Gender-Specific Safety

**Men:** Safe — supports digestion, respiration, and mental clarity
**Women:** Safe — helpful for PMS-related digestive upset and headaches
**Pregnancy:** Mild caution — tea is generally safe; avoid strong oil preparations
**Nursing:** Mild caution — excessive oil use may reduce milk supply

---

### Expected Results

- Digestive relief: 10–30 minutes
- Headache easing: 15–45 minutes
- Sinus opening: immediate to minutes
- IBS improvement: 1–2 weeks with capsules

---

### Same / Similar Results

Ginger · Lemon Balm · Chamomile · Spearmint · Fennel

---

### Shelf Life / Potency After Preparation

Dried leaf: 1–2 years · Tincture: 4–5 years · Essential oil: 2–3 years (cool, dark storage)

---

### Herbal Reflections of Peppermint

Peppermint brings movement where tension has settled. Cooling, clarifying, and gently stimulating, it lifts stagnation from the gut, the breath, and the mind. Its medicine reminds us that relief often comes not through force, but through restoring flow.

### Herbal Confidence Index

*(5/5 — A universally essential herb. Safe, effective, and remarkably versatile. A true household cornerstone.)*

# CEYLON CINNAMON

★★★★★

*Cinnamomum verum*

**Ceylon Cinnamon**—often called *true cinnamon*—is a prized warming spice and medicinal herb used for centuries to support circulation, digestion, metabolic balance, and immune resilience. Unlike Cassia cinnamon, Ceylon Cinnamon is gentler and naturally low in coumarin, making it suitable for regular, long-term use.

Its sweet warmth masks deep medicinal strength, helping steady blood sugar, improve circulation, calm digestive stagnation, and protect against microbial imbalance. Across traditional systems, it has been valued as a revitalizing herb that restores warmth, flow, and metabolic rhythm.

---

### Core Herbal Category — Ceylon Cinnamon

**Primary Core: Cardiovascular System Support** herb (warming, insulin-sensitizing compounds that support glucose regulation and healthy blood flow)
**Secondary Cores:** Digestive Strength · Immune Defense · Warming Anti-Inflammatory · Metabolic Balance

---

### How It Works

Ceylon Cinnamon supports insulin sensitivity and smoother blood-sugar response after meals. Its warming aromatic compounds stimulate circulation, improving nutrient delivery and metabolic efficiency. By strengthening digestion and moderating low-grade inflammation, it supports steady energy, circulation, and overall metabolic balance.

---

### Primary Uses

- Supports healthy blood-sugar regulation
- Improves circulation and peripheral warmth
- Relieves gas, bloating, and sluggish digestion
- Supports immune defense during cold seasons
- Helps reduce inflammation and oxidative stress
- Supports metabolic energy and lipid balance

---

### 🔬 Scientific Backing

Ceylon Cinnamon contains cinnamaldehyde, eugenol, flavonoids, and polyphenols shown to improve insulin receptor sensitivity, reduce post-meal blood-sugar spikes, promote circulation, and inhibit microbial growth. Clinical research supports its use in metabolic syndrome, type-2 diabetes support, mild digestive disturbances, and immune resilience.

---

### ☕ How to Use (Dosage)

Tea/Decoction:
Simmer 1 cinnamon stick or ½ tsp powder in 8–10 oz water for 10 minutes; drink 1–2× daily.
Capsules/Powder:
500–1,000 mg daily for metabolic or circulatory support.
Tincture:
1–2 mL, 1–2× daily for warming digestion or immune support.
Culinary:
Use regularly in teas, oatmeal, and warming foods.
*Always choose Ceylon Cinnamon—not Cassia—for ongoing use.*

---

### ⚠ Caution Level — 🟢 Safe (Mild Awareness)

Generally very safe in normal doses. May lower blood sugar—monitor if using diabetes medication. Avoid medicinal-level doses during pregnancy. Essential oil is highly concentrated and must be well diluted for topical use.

---

### 🚹 🚺 Gender-Specific Safety

**Men:** 🟢 **Safe** — supports circulation, metabolism, and digestive strength.
**Women:** 🟢 **Safe** — helpful for energy balance, circulation, and digestive comfort.
**Pregnancy:** 🟡 **Mild caution** — culinary use is safe; avoid strong medicinal doses.
Nursing: Mild caution — small amounts are well tolerated.

---

### ⏳ Expected Results

- Digestive warmth: immediate
- Circulatory improvement: several days
- Blood-sugar steadiness: 1–2 weeks
- Immune support: progressive with use

### 🔄 Same / Similar Results

Ginger · Fenugreek · Turmeric · Clove · Cardamom

### Shelf Life / Potency After Preparation

Powder: 1–2 years · Sticks: 2–3 years · Tincture: 4–5 years · Tea: best within 24 hours

### Herbal Reflections of Ceylon Cinnamon

True Cinnamon is warmth with restraint—stimulating without excess, strengthening without strain. It restores rhythm to digestion, circulation, and energy, reminding the body how to move sweetness and warmth where stagnation has taken hold.

### Herbal Confidence Index

🌿🌿🌿🌿🌿

*(5/5 — A foundational warming herb for metabolism, circulation, digestion, and immune defense. Safe, effective, and time-tested.)*

# SAGE

★★★★

Salvia officinalis

**Sage** is one of the oldest medicinal and culinary herbs known to humankind — a symbol of wisdom, longevity, and purification. **Its aromatic leaves have been used for thousands of years to strengthen digestion, clear the throat, sharpen the mind, cool excessive sweating, and restore balance during transitions of age or stress.** Few herbs carry such a blend of warmth, clarity, and cleansing power. **Sage steadies the nerves, dries what is too damp, warms what is too cold, and helps the body reorganize itself after depletion or overwhelm.**
**Its essential oils, tannins, and phenolic compounds give Sage broad-reaching influence across digestion, cognition, circulation, and hormone balance. Sage is particularly valued for easing menopausal night sweats, soothing sore throats, reducing gas and bloating, and improving memory and attention.** A bridge between kitchen and medicine chest, Sage stands as one of the true foundational herbs of European herbalism.

---

## 🌿 Core Herbal Category — Sage

**Primary Core: Nervous System Support (Nervines)** herb with *(aromatic, neurotonic action that supports mental clarity and endocrine rhythm regulation)*
**Secondary Cores:** Digestive Strengthening herb · Throat & Respiratory Support herb · Sweat Regulation herb

---

## How It Works

Sage works by toning nervous system signaling and supporting clear cognitive function, particularly during periods of mental fatigue or hormonal transition. Its aromatic compounds help regulate endocrine rhythms that influence mood, focus, and temperature control. By strengthening digestive function, it supports efficient assimilation and metabolic balance. The herb also soothes throat tissues and supports respiratory comfort. Its regulatory action helps normalize excessive sweating and promotes overall physiological balance.

---

## 🌱 Primary Uses

• Reduces excessive sweating and night sweats (especially menopausal)
• Enhances memory, clarity, and cognitive performance
• Soothes sore throat, laryngitis, and oral irritation
• Strengthens digestion; reduces gas, bloating, and sluggish metabolism
• Supports hormonal transitions (PMS, perimenopause, menopause)
• Helps regulate nervous tension and emotional fatigue
• Useful for mild respiratory congestion and post-viral weakness

---

## 🧪 Scientific Backing

Sage contains thujone, rosmarinic acid, cineole, and flavonoids with:
• Antioxidant and anti-inflammatory effects
• Acetylcholinesterase inhibition, improving memory and focus
• Antimicrobial activity against oral/throat pathogens
• Sweat-reducing actions via mild estrogenic and autonomic-modulating effects
Several human studies support its use for cognitive enhancement, menopausal symptoms, and throat inflammation.

---

## 🍵 Forms Available

• Dried leaf (tea or infusion)
• Tincture / liquid extract
• Lozenges or syrups for throat comfort
• Gargles and mouth rinses
• Capsules / powdered extract
• Culinary herb (fresh or dried)

---

## 🌿 How to Use — Sage

Tea: 1 tsp dried leaf per 8 oz hot water; steep 10 minutes.
• For digestion, throat, or cognitive clarity: 1–2 cups daily
• For night sweats: 1 cup before bed
Tincture: 1–2 mL, up to 3× daily
Gargle: Steep strong tea and gargle warm for sore throats or mouth irritation
Capsules: 300–500 mg, 1–2× daily for hormonal/cognitive support

---

⚠️ **Caution Level:** ⚪ **Caution**

• Avoid high doses during pregnancy (uterine-stimulating potential)
• Limit prolonged heavy use if prone to dry mouth or overheating
• Use caution with seizure disorders (thujone content)
• Essential oil should not be taken internally

---

**Gender-Specific Safety — Sage**

**Men — Safe**

Supports:
• Memory, cognition, clarity
• Digestion and bloating
• Sore throat and vocal strain
• Mild anxiety or nervous fatigue
Generally safe in moderate daily intake.

**Women — Mild Caution**

Helpful for:
• PMS mood shifts
• Hormone transition support
• Menopausal hot flashes and night sweats
Avoid large doses if very dry constitution or sensitive to warming herbs.

Pregnancy — Avoid

May stimulate uterine activity; avoid internal medicinal use.

Nursing — Mild Caution

Can reduce milk supply; light culinary use okay.

---

**Expected Results**

• Throat comfort: same day
• Digestive relief: 1–3 days
• Sweat reduction (night sweats): 3–7 days
• Cognitive clarity: 1–2 weeks
• Menopause symptom balancing: 2–4 weeks of consistent use

---

**DIY Recipe — Sage & Honey Throat Soothing Tea**

• 1 tbsp dried Sage

• 1 cup hot water
• Steep 10–12 minutes
• Add 1 tsp raw honey and lemon
Sip warm for throat irritation, coughing, or vocal strain.

---

### Same / Similar Results

- Lemon Balm — calming and cognitive support
- Rosemary — memory-enhancing circulatory tonic
- Black Cohosh — menopausal support
- Peppermint — digestive relief and mental clarity

---

### Shelf Life / Potency After Preparation

• Dried leaf: 1–2 years (airtight container)
• Tincture: 5+ years
• Tea (refrigerated): 24 hours
• Lozenges/syrups: follow manufacturer guidelines
• Powder: 1 year

---

### Herbal Reflections of Sage

Sage carries the medicine of remembrance — not only memory of the mind, but memory of balance, warmth, and inner composure. It acts like a gentle teacher, reminding the body of its own rhythms. Sage clears the fog from the thoughts, lifts the burden from the chest, and steadies the pulse when life becomes too damp, too heavy, or too uncertain. There is a quiet intelligence in Sage that moves through the mind and hormones alike, encouraging clarity where there is confusion and strength where there has been depletion.

To drink Sage is to reconnect with the part of yourself that knows when to release and when to hold firm. Its leaves have a way of drying what overwhelms, warming what has grown cold, and organizing what has scattered. Sage whispers the value of boundaries — physical, emotional, and energetic — and teaches that wisdom does not shout. It settles, clarifies, and restores, helping the body remember how to be whole again.

---

### Herbal Confidence Index:

(4 / 5 — A foundational herb of European tradition offering dependable benefits for cognition, digestion, throat support, and menopausal comfort.)

# ASH BARK

★★★★

*Fraxinus americana*

**Ash Bark** is a classic North American remedy for joints, connective tissue, and muscular stiffness. Traditionally used by Indigenous healers and Eclectic physicians, it supports mobility by easing inflammation, improving circulation to ligaments and tendons, and gently reducing swelling in overworked tissues. Its cooling, drying nature brings relief where heat, irritation, or stagnation have settled into muscles and joints.

Known as a subtle but reliable mover of the body's deeper fluids, Ash Bark also touches the lymphatic and digestive systems. Herbalists historically turned to it for sluggish bowels, lingering rheumatic discomfort, and muscular tightness following strain. It tones without tightening and moves without overstimulation, encouraging restoration of natural flow where tension has taken hold.

---

## 🌿 Core Herbal Category — Ash Bark

**Primary Core: Anti-Inflammatory & Pain Support** herb with (astringent, anti-inflammatory compounds that support tissue tone, flexibility, and structural resilience)
**Secondary Cores:** Anti-Inflammatory Relief herb · Lymphatic Movement herb · Muscular Recovery herb

---

## How It Works

Ash Bark tones connective tissues while supporting joint stability where strain or wear is present. Its anti-inflammatory constituents help reduce stiffness and discomfort associated with overuse. By encouraging lymphatic movement, it assists in clearing metabolic waste from tissues after exertion. Improved circulation to affected areas supports muscular recovery and long-term mobility. Together, these actions promote ease of movement, tissue integrity, and steady recovery.

---

## 🌱 Primary Uses

- Supports joint comfort, stiffness, and mild rheumatic aches
- Promotes mobility and ligament flexibility
- Reduces swelling in overworked or strained tissues
- Encourages healthy lymph flow and mild detoxification
- Gently supports sluggish digestion
- Useful for post-exertion soreness and chronic muscular tightness

---

## 🧪 Scientific Backing

Ash Bark contains coumarins, secoiridoids, flavonoids, and phenolic glycosides shown to:
- Reduce inflammation in connective tissue
- Provide mild analgesic support for rheumatic discomfort
- Enhance circulation and lymphatic movement
- Offer gentle digestive-toning effects

Traditional Eclectic literature describes Ash Bark as a dependable, cooling remedy for chronic joint and muscular stiffness, particularly where inflammation and stagnation coexist.

---

## Forms Available

- Dried bark (decoction)
- Capsules or powdered bark
- Tincture or liquid extract
- Topical preparations (often blended with warming herbs)

---

## How to Use — Ash Bark

**Decoction:**
Simmer 1 tsp bark in 12 oz water for 15 minutes. Drink 1–2 cups daily for joints, muscles, or swelling.
**Tincture:**
2–3 mL, up to 2× daily.
**Capsules:**
400–600 mg, 1–2× daily.
**Topical:**
Use as a warm compress or infused oil for stiff joints or muscles.

---

## ⚠ Caution Level: Safe / Mild Caution

Generally safe when used appropriately. Avoid very high or prolonged dosing if prone to dryness. Use mild caution with blood-thinning medications. Not recommended internally during pregnancy due to limited data. Large doses may cause mild digestive looseness.

---

## Gender-Specific Safety — Ash Bark

**Men — Safe**
Supports joint stiffness, overworked muscles, post-exercise recovery, and mild lymphatic stagnation.
**Women — Mild Caution**
Helpful for rheumatic discomfort and pelvic or lymphatic sluggishness. Avoid heavy daily use if experiencing dryness or low vitality.

🔴 **Pregnancy — Avoid**
Insufficient safety data for internal medicinal use.
⚪ **Nursing — Mild Caution**
Light, occasional use acceptable; avoid strong daily dosing.

---

## ⌛ Expected Results

- Joint or muscle relief: 3–7 days
- Improved mobility: 1–3 weeks
- Lymphatic support: gradual, 2–4 weeks
- Digestive improvement: 1–3 days

---

## 🛠 DIY Recipe — Ash Bark Mobility Decoction

- 1 tsp Ash Bark
- ½ tsp Ginger
- ½ tsp Meadowsweet

Simmer Ash Bark for 15 minutes. Remove from heat, add remaining herbs, steep 10 minutes. Sip daily for comfortable movement and joint ease.

---

## 🔄 Same / Similar Results

⚪ Meadowsweet · ⚪ Solomon's Seal · ⚪ Devil's Claw · ⚪ Willow Bark

---

## 🧪 Shelf Life / Potency After Preparation

- Dried bark: 2–3 years
- Tincture: 5+ years
- Decoction: 24–36 hours (refrigerated)
- Powder: 1 year

---

## 💬 Herbal Reflections — Ash Bark

Ash Bark carries the medicine of steadiness — cooling what is inflamed and loosening what has grown rigid through time or strain. Its action is slow, deliberate, and corrective, restoring ease rather than forcing release. Where joints feel tight and movement has become guarded, Ash invites the body back into quiet cooperation with itself.
Like the tree that bends without breaking, Ash teaches resilience through flexibility. Its strength lies not in force but in balance — encouraging the body to recover its natural rhythm, adapt to pressure, and move forward with renewed integrity.

---

★ **Herbal Confidence Index** 🌿 🌿 🌿 🌿

*(4 / 5 — A traditional connective-tissue ally offering cooling relief, improved mobility, and gentle anti-inflammatory support.)*

# *BLUE COHOSH*

★★

*Caulophyllum thalictroides*

**Blue Cohosh** is a woodland-rooted herb steeped in deep traditional use, known especially for its effects on the uterus, pelvic muscles, and subtle rhythms of reproductive health. Despite its strength, it is not a daily tonic herb — it is a **specialist**. Many herbalists describe Blue Cohosh as a "quiet strength": an herb that works beneath the surface, gradually influencing neuromuscular coordination within the reproductive system.

Because of its potency, this plant commands respect and knowledgeable guidance.

---

🌿 **Core Herbal Category — Blue Cohosh**

**Primary Core: Reproductive & Women's Health Support** herb with (uterine-directing, neuromuscular-modulating action that influences reproductive signaling and pelvic tone)

**Secondary Cores:** Musculoskeletal Support herb · Circulatory Toning herb · Hormonal Modulation herb

---

### *How It Works*

Blue Cohosh influences neuromuscular signaling within pelvic and uterine tissues, supporting coordinated muscular tone and rhythmic reproductive function. Its directing action encourages focused circulation to reproductive structures while supporting pelvic and lower-back stability. This combined effect promotes regulated reproductive movement and hormonal responsiveness rather than stimulation alone.

---

🌱 **Primary Uses**

- Supports menstrual comfort and uterine muscle coordination
- Traditionally used to ease menstrual cramping
- Historically used late-term only under supervision (not casual use)
- Supports female reproductive circulation
- Helps relieve tension in pelvic musculature

---

🧪 **Scientific Backing**

Contains caulosaponin, methylcytisine, and caulophyllosaponin — compounds shown to influence smooth muscle, particularly uterine tissue. Laboratory findings confirm uterotonic and neuromuscular activity.

⚠️ Modern literature emphasizes **dose sensitivity** and **cardiovascular caution**, requiring professional oversight.

---

### Forms Available

• Dried root (cut or powdered)
• Tincture (most common clinical form)
• Decoction (rare; strength-limited)
• Capsules (specialized professional use)

---

### ⚠️ Caution Level: ● Supervision Required

• **Not for casual or long-term use**
• Avoid during pregnancy unless guided by a trained professional
• Not recommended for heart conditions or hypertension
• Improper dosing may cause uterine or cardiovascular stress

---

### Gender-Specific Safety (GS)

**Men:** ● Caution — rarely indicated for male physiology

**Women:** ● Caution — appropriate only for guided menstrual or reproductive use

**Pregnancy / Nursing:** ● Avoid unless supervised by trained midwife or clinical herbalist

---

### Expected Results

• Menstrual comfort: 1–2 cycles
• Uterine toning effects: gradual, several weeks
• Pelvic tension relief: hours to days (dose-dependent)

---

### How to Use (Professional Context)

**Tincture:** 5–15 drops, 1–3× daily during acute menstrual discomfort (guided use only)
**Decoction:** Rarely used; if so, ½ tsp root simmered 10 minutes (professional oversight required)

This herb is **never** a daily tonic.

---

### Professional Blend Example (Reference Only)

Blue Cohosh · Black Cohosh · Chamomile · Cramp Bark
5–10 drops every 1–2 hours during acute discomfort; taper promptly

---

### Same / Similar Results

● Black Cohosh · ● Cramp Bark · ● Wild Yam · ● Dong Quai · ● Ginger

**Shelf Life**
• Tincture: ~5 years
• Dried root: 2–3 years
• Decoction: 24–48 hrs refrigerated

**Herbal Reflections — Blue Cohosh**

Blue Cohosh carries the presence of a forest elder — restrained, purposeful, and powerful when called upon. Its medicine speaks the language of timing and coordination rather than force. Historically trusted yet carefully respected, it reminds us that some plant allies are designed not for comfort, but for precision. When used with wisdom, it offers structure where imbalance once ruled.

**Herbal Confidence Index**

🌿 🌿 (2 / 5 — A potent but safety-limited uterine herb whose traditional strength is outweighed by narrow therapeutic margins and modern cardiovascular concerns.)

# *SHEA BARK*

★★★

*Vitellaria paradoxa*

**Shea Bark** comes from the same African tree renowned for its nourishing butter, yet the bark itself carries a distinct medicinal role. Across West Africa, it has long been used to calm muscular and menstrual spasms, support uterine tone, reduce inflammation, and strengthen circulation. Unlike Shea Butter's external emollience, Shea Bark works internally as a grounding, tonifying botanical with deep cultural roots.
It is valued for easing cramps, settling digestive tension, and restoring steadiness during periods of strain or congestion.

---

### 🌿 Core Herbal Category — Shea Bark

**Primary Core:** Anti-Inflammatory & Pain Support herb with (astringent, strengthening action that supports uterine tone and smooth-muscle stability)
**Secondary Cores:** Anti-Inflammatory Support herb · Circulatory Support herb · Digestive Calming herb

---

***How It Works***

Shea Bark tones smooth muscle tissue — particularly within the uterus — while reinforcing connective integrity. Its astringent action helps reduce excessive relaxation and strain, while anti-inflammatory compounds calm surrounding tissues. By supporting circulation, it aids nutrient delivery and recovery, while gently settling digestive spasm associated with muscular imbalance.

---

### 🌱 Primary Uses

- Relieves menstrual and muscular cramping
- Supports uterine tone and reproductive balance
- Provides gentle anti-inflammatory support
- Strengthens circulation and tissue vitality
- Reduces digestive spasms and abdominal tension

---

### 🧪 Scientific Backing

Contains triterpenes, catechins, saponins, and polyphenols with anti-inflammatory, antispasmodic, and antioxidant activity. While modern research emphasizes Shea

Butter, West African pharmacopeias document centuries of bark use for uterine support, bowel calming, and inflammatory conditions.

---

### Forms Available

- Dried bark (decoction)
- Powdered bark / capsules
- Tincture or liquid extract

---

### How to Use

**Decoction:** 1 tsp bark simmered in 8–10 oz water for 15–20 min; 1–2 cups daily
**Capsules:** 300–500 mg, 1–2× daily
**Tincture:** 2–3 mL, 1–2× daily

---

### ⚠ Caution Level: Use with Caution

- Avoid excessive or prolonged internal use
- Use caution with low blood pressure or circulatory weakness
- Possible mild interaction with blood-thinning medications
- Avoid during pregnancy due to uterine activity
- Tree-nut sensitivity possible (rare)

---

### ⚥ Gender-Specific Safety (GS)

**Men:** Safe

**Women:** Use with caution during reproductive years

**Pregnancy / Nursing:** Avoid internal medicinal use

---

### Expected Results

- Muscle & uterine calming: 1–3 days
- Digestive spasm relief: same day
- Cycle balance & tone: 2–4 weeks
- Inflammatory reduction: 1–2 weeks

---

### 🛠 DIY Decoction (Traditional)

Shea Bark · Ginger · Cramp Bark
Simmer 20 minutes; sip warm at onset of cramping.

---

### Same / Similar Results

Cramp Bark · Black Haw · Ginger · Turmeric · Dong Quai

### Shelf Life

- Dried bark: 2 years
- Powder: 1 year
- Decoction: 48 hrs refrigerated
- Tincture: 3–5 years

---

### Herbal Reflections — Shea Bark

Shea Bark carries a grounded, restorative presence — medicine that works through steadiness rather than force. It restores tone where slackness has crept in and calms where tension has taken hold. Rooted in African tradition, it bridges cultural wisdom and modern understanding, offering balance through quiet correction rather than dramatic effect.

---

### Herbal Confidence Index

(3 / 5 — A culturally significant uterine and muscular tonic with modest but reliable benefits and limited global standardization.)

# SAFFRON

★★★★

*Crocus sativus*

**Saffron** is one of the world's most treasured botanical substances — a vivid golden thread drawn from the delicate Crocus flower. For thousands of years it has been valued not only as a rare culinary spice, but as a therapeutic ally for uplifting mood, soothing the nerves, easing menstrual discomfort, and restoring emotional balance. Its active compounds, including crocin and safranal, support mental clarity, regulate stress responses, and gently brighten emotional tone during periods of heaviness or tension.

Across ancient Persia, Greece, Egypt, and India, saffron symbolized joy, vitality, and spiritual illumination. Despite its small size, each thread carries a potent legacy of comfort, resilience, and emotional restoration.

---

🌿 **Core Herbal Category — Saffron**

**Primary Core: Nervous System Support (Nervines)** herb with (neuroactive, emotionally balancing compounds that support mental clarity and emotional uplift)

**Secondary Cores:** Hormonal Modulation herb · Women's Wellness herb · Antioxidant Restoration herb

---

## *How It Works*

Saffron supports neurotransmitter balance associated with mood regulation and emotional well-being. Its active compounds help ease emotional heaviness, support stress adaptation, and promote mental clarity. By influencing hormonal signaling, it stabilizes mood during cyclical or transitional phases. Antioxidant activity protects neural and endocrine tissues from oxidative strain, contributing to emotional resilience and cognitive steadiness.

---

🌱 **Primary Uses**

- Supports emotional balance and uplifts low mood
- Helps ease occasional anxiety and nervous tension
- Supports menstrual comfort and cycle regularity
- Enhances cognitive clarity and memory
- Reduces oxidative stress system-wide
- May assist appetite balance and satiety

---

### Scientific Backing

Primary constituents — crocin, crocetin, safranal, and picrocrocin — are well studied for emotional, neurological, and metabolic effects.

Research indicates:

• Modulation of serotonin and dopamine pathways
• Mood support comparable to mild antidepressant classes in trials
• Neuroprotective and cognitive benefits
• PMS mood and discomfort reduction
• Strong antioxidant activity

Saffron is among the **most clinically validated herbs** for emotional and women's wellness.

---

### Forms Available

• Whole threads (highest potency)
• Powdered saffron
• Tincture or liquid extract
• Encapsulated extract
• Standardized crocin-safranal supplements

---

### Caution Level: Use Carefully

• Do **not** exceed recommended doses — high amounts may overstimulate or cause uterine contraction
• Avoid with known saffron allergy
• Excessive use may cause dizziness or agitation
• Use caution with antidepressant medications

---

### Gender-Specific Safety (GS)

**Men:** Safe at standard doses

**Women:** Helpful for PMS, mood, and emotional support

**Pregnancy:** Avoid high doses (uterine-active)

**Nursing:** Use cautiously — limited research

---

### Expected Results

• Mood uplift: 1–2 weeks
• Stress reduction: within days
• Menstrual comfort: 1 cycle
• Cognitive clarity: 2–4 weeks
• Appetite balance: 1–2 weeks

---

### How to Use

**Tea:** 3–5 threads steeped 8–10 minutes; 1–2× daily

**Capsules / Extract:** 15–30 mg/day standardized extract

**Culinary (therapeutic):** 3–6 threads added to food or warm milk

Saffron is potent — small amounts are sufficient.

### DIY Recipe — Saffron Golden Milk

5–7 saffron threads · 1 cup warm almond or oat milk · ½ tsp turmeric · honey & cinnamon optional

Drink in the evening for calm, mood support, and comfort.

### Same / Similar Results

Turmeric · St. John's Wort · Lemon Balm · Holy Basil · Rhodiola

### Shelf Life

- Whole threads: 3–4 years (airtight, dark)
- Powder: 1–2 years
- Tincture: 4–5 years
- Prepared tea: 24 hrs refrigerated

Whole threads retain potency best.

### Herbal Reflections — Saffron

Saffron is the medicine of light — subtle, radiant, and precise. Within its fine threads lies a warmth that lifts heaviness without force and restores harmony without excess. Long used in healing, ceremony, and nourishment, it teaches that power need not be loud. Sometimes the smallest dose carries the greatest illumination, reminding the spirit how to brighten gently from within.

### Herbal Confidence Index

(4 / 5 — A radiant mood and emotional wellness herb with strong scientific support, gentle action at proper doses, and broad historical validation, limited primarily by cost and potency sensitivity.)

# *MULLEIN ROOT*

★★★★

*Verbascum thapsus (Radix)*

**Mullein root** is one of herbalism's quiet structural allies — far less known than the leaf or flower, yet uniquely valuable for deep musculoskeletal and urinary support. While the leaf tends the lungs and the flower calms the nerves, the root works at the foundation: strengthening bladder tone, supporting pelvic floor integrity, easing sciatic tension, and helping the spine settle into steadier alignment. Traditional healers valued it for its grounding, stabilizing influence — medicine that helps the body hold itself together. Used by Native American and Appalachian herbalists, Mullein root became known for supporting recovery after strain, pelvic imbalance, or chronic weakness. It teaches the principle of structure: that healing often begins by restoring strength to the body's deepest framework.

---

🌿 **Core Herbal Category — Mullein Root**
**Primary Core: Anti-Inflammatory & Pain Support** herb with (deeply grounding, nerve- and connective-tissue–supportive action that stabilizes structural alignment and spinal integrity)
**Secondary Cores:** Urinary Tone & Pelvic Floor Strength herb · Nerve Stabilization herb · Anti-Inflammatory Support herb

---

### *How It Works*

Mullein root supports structural tissues of the spine, hips, and lower back, helping restore stability where weakness or misalignment contributes to discomfort. Its grounding action supports nerve signaling when compression or irritation affects strength or coordination. By toning pelvic and urinary tissues, it reinforces foundational muscular support in the lower body. Anti-inflammatory activity helps calm stressed joints and connective tissue, promoting steadiness and resilience.

---

🌱 **Primary Uses**

- Supports bladder tone and urinary control
- Strengthens pelvic floor musculature
- Helps relieve sciatic and nerve-related discomfort
- Supports spinal alignment and vertebral stability
- Reduces inflammation in musculoskeletal tissues

• Useful post-strain or during pelvic / low-back recovery

---

### Scientific Backing

Contains aucubin, verbascoside, tannins, and glycosides associated with anti-inflammatory, nerve-stabilizing, and tissue-toning effects.

Traditional and ethnobotanical sources document its use for sciatic discomfort and urinary weakness.

Constituent research indicates:

• Anti-inflammatory action in nerve-rich tissues
• Modulation of pelvic and spinal tension
• Tonifying effect on smooth muscle, including bladder tissue
• Mild analgesic properties

While modern trials are limited, historical consistency across traditions is strong.

---

### Forms Available

• Dried root (cut or powdered)
• Tincture (most effective)
• Decoction
• Root-infused oil (topical nerve support)

---

### Caution Level: Use Responsibly

• Avoid during acute urinary tract infection
• Not recommended in early pregnancy without supervision
• Mildly drying — pair with moistening herbs if constitution is dry
• Those with kidney inflammation should seek guidance

---

### Gender-Specific Safety (GS)

**Men:** Safe; supports pelvic tone and sciatic relief

**Women:** Safe; traditionally used postpartum for pelvic strengthening

**Pregnancy:** Avoid unless professionally guided

**Nursing:** Generally safe

**Seniors:** Start low; bladder response varies

---

### Expected Results

• Sciatic relief: hours to days (cause-dependent)
• Inflammation reduction: 2–7 days
• Spinal tension relief: 1–2 weeks
• Pelvic floor support: 1–3 weeks
• Bladder tone improvement: 3–6 weeks

### How to Use

**Tincture (preferred):** 10–30 drops, 1–3× daily
**Decoction:** 1 Tbsp root simmered in 16 oz water for 20 minutes; 1–2 cups daily
**Topical:** Apply root-infused oil or salve to affected area 1–2× daily

### DIY — Mullein Root Pelvic-Tone Tincture

Fresh or dried root · 40–50% alcohol · Infuse 4–6 weeks
Use 10–20 drops daily for pelvic or bladder strengthening.

### Same / Similar Results

Horse Chestnut · Black Cohosh · Solomon's Seal · Marshmallow Root · Ash Bark

### Shelf Life

- Dried root: 2–3 years
- Tincture: 5–7 years (most stable)
- Decoction: 24–36 hours refrigerated
- Oil infusion: 6–12 months

Tincture retains potency best.

### Herbal Reflections — Mullein Root

Mullein root is the pillar of the Mullein family — steady, grounding, and quietly strong. Its medicine moves downward, into bones, nerves, and the deep structures that hold us upright. It restores balance not by force, but by reinforcing foundation. In easing sciatic tension, strengthening the bladder, or supporting spinal alignment, it reminds the body how to support itself from within. This is resilience medicine — calm, enduring, and structural.

### Herbal Confidence Index

(4 / 5 — A deeply supportive structural herb offering rare benefits for bladder tone, nerve relief, and musculoskeletal stability.)

# *IRISH MOSS / SEA MOSS*

★★★★1/2

*Chondrus crispus / Eucheuma spp.*

**Irish Moss,** also known as Sea Moss, is a mineral-rich sea vegetable long cherished across coastal cultures for its deep nourishment and soothing, mucilaginous properties. Packed with iodine, calcium, magnesium, silica, sulfur, and trace minerals, it functions almost like a "liquid multivitamin" for depleted systems—fortifying tissues, supporting thyroid balance, calming digestive irritation, and restoring foundational vitality.
Used traditionally in Ireland, the Caribbean, and West Africa, Irish Moss is both food and medicine: gentle enough for daily restoration yet powerful enough to assist recovery from chronic fatigue, poor nutrition, respiratory congestion, and digestive distress. Its action is rebuilding rather than stimulating, making it ideal for long-term nourishment and resilience.

---

### *Core Herbal Category — Irish Moss*

**Primary Core: Nutritional & Tonic Support** herb with (mineral-dense, mucilaginous nourishment that supports cellular repair and foundational rebuilding)
**Secondary Cores:** Thyroid & Metabolic Support herb · Digestive Soothing herb · Respiratory Support herb · Skin & Beauty Support herb

---

### *How It Works*

Irish Moss supplies highly absorbable minerals and soothing mucilage that nourish cells and support tissue repair. Its demulcent compounds coat and protect the digestive tract, improving comfort and nutrient absorption. By contributing iodine and trace minerals, it supports healthy thyroid signaling and metabolic balance. The same mucilaginous action soothes respiratory tissues and supports healthy mucus regulation. Together, these effects promote systemic rebuilding, hydration, and long-term resilience.

---

### *Primary Uses*

- Supports thyroid function and metabolic balance (natural iodine source)
- Soothes acid reflux, gastritis, ulcers, and digestive irritation
- Provides deep mineral nourishment for depleted diets or chronic fatigue
- Supports healthy respiratory and gastrointestinal mucous membranes

• Promotes skin hydration, joint comfort, and post-illness recovery
• Aids overall vitality, immune resilience, and rebuilding strength

---

## 🧪 Scientific Backing

Studies on Chondrus crispus and Eucheuma cottonii demonstrate:
• High iodine content supporting thyroid hormone production
• Sulfated polysaccharides (carrageenans) with demulcent, prebiotic, and immune-modulating effects
• Antiviral and antibacterial activity in vitro
• Significant mineral density beneficial in malnutrition, anemia, and chronic fatigue
• GI-soothing mucilage shown to calm inflamed digestive tissues

---

## *Forms Available*

• Raw dried sea moss
• Sea moss gel (homemade or prepared)
• Powders (smoothies or capsules)
• Extracts or tinctures
• Topical gels for skin hydration

---

## ⚠ Caution Level: Caution

Generally safe for most individuals.
• Avoid excessive intake with hyperthyroidism or while on thyroid medication
• Source carefully—sea moss can accumulate heavy metals in polluted waters
• Start with small amounts to prevent digestive upset

---

## Gender-Specific Safety (GS)

**Men:** Generally safe; supports vitality and metabolic balance

**Women:** Safe; supportive for nutrition, skin, and recovery

**Pregnancy / Nursing:** Likely safe in food amounts only; avoid high or concentrated doses and use clean, verified sources

---

## *Expected Results*

• Digestive soothing & hydration: 1–3 days
• Respiratory comfort & skin softness: 1–2 weeks
• Energy, mineral repletion & thyroid support: 3–6 weeks

• Long-term use: deeper vitality, immunity, and digestive stability

---

## 🛠 DIY Recipe — Simple Sea Moss Gel

• Rinse 1 cup dried Irish Moss three times
• Soak in clean water 12–24 hours (do not boil)
• Blend with fresh spring water until smooth
• Refrigerate to set
**Use:** 1–2 tablespoons daily in smoothies, juice, tea, or food

---

## 🔄 *Same / Similar Results*

• Bladderwrack — thyroid & mineral support
• Nettle Leaf — mineral restoration
• Marshmallow Root — digestive soothing
• Aloe Vera — mucosal healing
• Slippery Elm — gut & respiratory demulcent support

---

## 🧪 Shelf Life / Potency After Preparation

• Dried sea moss: 1–2 years (airtight, cool storage)
• Sea moss gel: 2–3 weeks refrigerated; up to 6 months frozen
• Powder: 18–24 months if kept dry and sealed

---

## 💬 Herbal Reflections of Irish Moss

Irish Moss is the quiet nourisher of herbal medicine—steady, patient, and deeply restorative. Where other herbs stimulate or purge, Sea Moss replenishes, reminding the body of what abundance feels like again. Its mucilaginous nature softens irritation, restores moisture, and rebuilds strength worn thin by stress, illness, or deprivation.
It carries the memory of the sea itself: mineral-rich, sustaining, and enduring. Irish Moss teaches that resilience is often rebuilt slowly, layer by layer, from the most fundamental supports of life.

---

## ★ Herbal Confidence Index – Irish Moss

🌿🌿🌿🌿½ (4.5 / 5 — Exceptionally nourishing and restorative, Irish Moss excels as a long-term rebuilding and mineral-support herb for digestion, skin, respiratory tissues, and metabolic balance. Its action is foundational rather than fast, placing it just below a full five.)

# *BALA*

★★★

*Sida cordifolia*

**Bala,** meaning "strength" in Sanskrit, is a classic Ayurvedic rejuvenative valued for rebuilding vitality, calming the nervous system, and restoring physical resilience after fatigue or strain. Rather than stimulating energy, it nourishes depleted tissues, supports healthy circulation, and steadies systems worn thin by stress, illness, or overexertion. Its grounding nature makes it especially useful when weakness or irritation reflects loss of internal reserve rather than excess.

Traditionally used across India, Bala was regarded as a tonic for joints, respiration, and muscular endurance, as well as a restorative for the nervous system. Though gentle in its long-term effects, the plant contains naturally occurring ephedrine-related alkaloids, requiring respectful dosing and informed use consistent with its historical lineage.

---

🌿 **Core Herbal Category — Bala**

**Primary Core: Nutritional & Tonic Support** herb with (deeply nourishing, tissue-restorative action that supports nerve integrity and systemic vitality)

**Secondary Cores:** Musculoskeletal Support herb · Respiratory Balance herb · Vitality & Strength herb

---

### *How It Works*

Bala restores strength by nourishing depleted nerve and connective tissues while supporting coordinated circulation and repair. Its rejuvenative action stabilizes weakened systems without overstimulation, easing inflammatory stress in muscles and joints while gently supporting respiratory ease and endurance. With consistent use, Bala promotes steadiness, resilience, and sustainable vitality.

---

🌱 **Primary Uses**

- Supports nervous system calm and recovery from fatigue
- *Restores energy without stimulation*
- Soothes joints, muscles, and connective tissue strain

- Supports respiratory comfort and overall vitality

---

### 🧪 Scientific Profile & Forms

Bala contains alkaloids (including vasicinone and trace ephedrine-related compounds), flavonoids, sterols, and glycosides associated with:

- Mild bronchodilating respiratory support
- Nervine-restorative and tissue-nourishing effects
- Anti-inflammatory and antioxidant activity
- *Circulatory and musculoskeletal support*

**Forms:** dried root (preferred), dried leaf, powder (churna), tincture, external oil.

---

### ⚠ Caution Level: ● Use Carefully

- Avoid high doses due to alkaloid content
- Use caution with high blood pressure, heart rhythm issues, or anxiety
- *Do not combine with stimulants*
- Not for long-term continuous use without guidance

---

### Gender-Specific Safety (GS)

- **Men:** ● Generally safe at moderate doses
- **Women:** ● Use cautiously if stimulant-sensitive
- ***Pregnancy:*** ● *Avoid*
- ***Nursing:*** ● *Use only with guidance*

---

### 🧪 How to Use

- ***Powder:*** *¼–½ tsp, 1–2× daily*

- ***Tincture:*** *10–20 drops, 1–2× daily*

- **External oil:** massage into joints or muscles
  Start low and increase slowly.

---

**Same / Similar Results**
Ashwagandha · Gotu Kola · Licorice Root · Ginseng · Guduchi

---

**Shelf Life**
Root/leaf: 2–3 yrs · Powder: 1–2 yrs · Tincture: 4–5 yrs · Oil: 6–12 mos

---

**Herbal Reflections of Bala**
Bala embodies quiet strength—the kind that rebuilds rather than excites. Its medicine restores endurance by nourishing what has been worn down, offering steadiness instead of force. In Ayurvedic tradition, Bala teaches that true resilience comes not from stimulation, but from restoration patiently rebuilt and carefully held.

---

**Herbal Confidence Index**

(3 / 5 — A respected Ayurvedic rejuvenative offering steady strength and nervous-system support, tempered by dosing sensitivity.)

# *NEEM*

★★★★★

*Azadirachta indica*

**Neem** is one of the most powerful and respected cleansing herbs in traditional medicine, **prized for its ability to purify the blood, support skin health, and combat harmful microbes. It has been used for centuries to address acne, eczema, fungal infections, digestive imbalance, and oral health issues.** Neem's bitter compounds help cool excess heat in the body, making it especially useful for inflammatory and infection-related conditions.

*Often called the* ***"Village Pharmacy"*** *in India, Neem has served entire communities as a single, multi-purpose medicinal plant. From leaves and bark to oil and twigs, nearly every part of the tree has been used for healing. Modern research continues to confirm Neem's broad antimicrobial, antifungal, antiparasitic, and immune-modulating properties.*

---

**Core Herbal Category — Neem Primary Core: Antimicrobial Support** herb with (bitter, cleansing compounds that support systemic purification and microbial balance)
**Secondary Cores:** Skin & Immune Support herb · Antiparasitic Support herb · Oral & Dental Health herb · Inflammatory Cooling herb

***How It Works*** *Neem works by supporting systemic cleansing through its bitter compounds that help reduce internal heat and microbial overload. Its antimicrobial action assists the body in maintaining balanced internal and external ecosystems. By purifying the blood and calming inflammatory stress, it supports clearer skin and immune resilience. The herb also supports oral and dental tissues by discouraging microbial imbalance. This cooling, cleansing action promotes long-term internal clarity and tissue health.*

---

### 🌱 *Primary Uses*

- Clears acne, eczema, boils, and skin eruptions
- Supports blood purification and detoxification
- Helps combat bacterial, fungal, and parasitic infections
- Supports oral health (gums, plaque, breath)
- Assists liver function and immune balance

---

### 🧪 Scientific Backing

*Neem contains limonoids (including azadirachtin), flavonoids, and polyphenols with well-documented antibacterial, antifungal, antiviral, and antiparasitic effects. Studies show Neem extracts inhibit acne-causing bacteria, support wound healing, and demonstrate immune-regulating activity. Neem has also been researched for its role in managing blood sugar and reducing inflammatory markers.*

---

### 💊 Forms Available

- *Dried leaf (tea or capsules)*
- *Powdered leaf*
- *Tincture or liquid extract*
- *Neem oil (external use only)*
- *Dental sticks / oral powders*

---

### ● How to Use (Dosage & Methods)

- ***Tea:*** *Steep ½–1 tsp dried Neem leaf in hot water for 10 minutes; drink 1× daily (very bitter).*
- **Capsules/Powder:** 300–500 mg once or twice daily for blood and skin support.
- ***Tincture:*** *1–2 mL, up to 2× daily.*

- ***Topical:*** *Dilute Neem oil heavily in carrier oil and apply to fungal or irritated skin.*
- ***Oral Rinse:*** *Weak Neem tea used as a mouth rinse for gum health.*

---

### ⚠ Caution Level — Caution

- Extremely bitter; may cause nausea if taken on an empty stomach.
- Avoid during pregnancy due to potential effects on fertility and uterine tone.
- Use cautiously in individuals with very low blood sugar.
- *Neem oil should **never** be taken internally.*

---

### ♀ ♂ Gender-Specific Safety (GS)

**Men:** Generally safe in moderate doses. Supports skin clarity, immune balance, and microbial defense. Avoid excessive long-term use without breaks.

**Women:** Helpful for acne, skin flare-ups, and inflammatory heat conditions. Avoid during pregnancy; moderate use otherwise.

**Pregnancy / Nursing:** Avoid internal use during pregnancy. External use only with professional guidance.

---

### Expected Results

- *Skin improvement: 7–14 days*
- Reduced infections or fungal issues: 5–10 days
- *Blood-cleansing effects: 14–30 days*
- *Oral health improvement: 3–7 days*

---

### Same / Similar Results

Pau D'Arco · Burdock Root · Goldenseal · Cleavers · Yellow Dock

---

### Shelf Life / Potency After Preparation

- ***Dried leaf:*** *1–2 years airtight*

- ***Powder:*** *6–12 months*
- ***Tincture:*** *3–5 years*
- **Prepared tea:** Best within 24 hours refrigerated
- ***Neem oil:*** *1–2 years (cool, dark storage)*

---

**💉 DIY Recipe — Neem Skin-Clearing Wash**
*Steep 1 tsp dried Neem leaf in 1 cup hot water for 15 minutes. Cool, strain, and use as a facial or skin wash once daily for acne or fungal irritation.*

---

**💬 Herbal Reflections of Neem**
*Neem is not a gentle whisper of medicine — it is a firm instruction. It teaches the body how to say no to what does not belong: excess microbes, inflammation, and internal heat. Bitter by nature, Neem reminds us that healing is not always sweet, but it is honest and effective.*

*Used wisely, Neem restores clarity — to the skin, the blood, and the internal terrain — helping the body reclaim balance through purification rather than suppression.*

⭐ **Herbal Confidence Index:** 🌿 🌿 🌿 🌿 🌿
(5/5 green stars — a globally revered cleansing and antimicrobial herb; powerful, time-tested, and highly effective when used with respect and moderation.)

# *KUDZU ROOT*

★★★★

*Pueraria lobata*

**Kudzu Root** is a powerful yet often overlooked medicinal root traditionally used to calm tension, reduce cravings, relax muscles, and support vascular and nervous system balance. Long valued in East Asian medicine, it is especially known for easing alcohol cravings, headaches, neck and shoulder tension, and stress-related hypertension. Rather than stimulating or sedating, Kudzu works by releasing constraint—softening tight muscles, calming overactive nerve signaling, and improving blood flow to the brain and upper body. This makes it uniquely effective for addiction support, tension headaches, and neurovascular stress patterns.

---

### Core Herbal Category — Kudzu Root

**Primary Core: Cardiovascular System Support** herb (relaxes constricted muscles and blood vessels while calming nervous overactivity)
**Secondary Cores:** Addiction Support · Musculoskeletal Relaxant · Cardiovascular Support · Stress Modulation

---

### How It Works

Kudzu Root contains isoflavones (notably puerarin) that relax smooth muscle and improve cerebral and peripheral blood flow. This reduces pressure-related headaches, eases muscle tension, and stabilizes stress-driven cravings. Its balancing effect on dopamine and vascular tone helps interrupt compulsive patterns without overstimulation.

---

### Primary Uses

- Reduces alcohol and sugar cravings
- Eases tension headaches and neck stiffness
- Supports blood-pressure balance
- Relieves muscle tightness and stress-related pain
- Calms nervous agitation without sedation
- Supports recovery from addiction-related fatigue

---

### Scientific Backing

Research shows Kudzu's isoflavones improve cerebral circulation, reduce alcohol intake behavior, relax vascular smooth muscle, and modulate neurotransmitter activity. Clinical and traditional use supports its role in addiction support, headache relief, and cardiovascular stress patterns.

---

### How to Use (Dosage)

**Decoction:**
Simmer 1–2 tsp dried root in water for 20 minutes; drink 1–2× daily.
**Tincture:**
1–3 mL, up to 3× daily.
**Capsules:**
500–1,500 mg daily, divided doses.

---

### Caution Level — Safe

Very well tolerated. Use caution with hormone-sensitive conditions due to mild phytoestrogen content. Avoid excessive doses during pregnancy.

---

### Gender-Specific Safety

**Men:** Safe — supports addiction recovery, circulation, and tension relief.
**Women:** Safe — supports stress-related headaches and nervous balance.
**Pregnancy/Nursing:** Mild caution — avoid concentrated extracts.

---

### Expected Results

- Headache relief: 30–60 minutes
- Muscle relaxation: several hours
- Craving reduction: days to weeks with consistent use

---

### Same / Similar Results

Skullcap · Valerian · Passionflower · Lobelia (low dose)

---

### Shelf Life / Potency After Preparation

Dried root: 2–3 years · Tincture: 4–5 years · Decoction: 24 hours refrigerated

---

### Herbal Reflection s of Kudzu Root

Kudzu teaches release. Where tension grips the body or habits bind the mind, it loosens the hold—quietly, steadily, without force. Its medicine is freedom through relaxation, restoring ease where pressure once ruled.

### Herbal Confidence Index

(4/5 — A highly valuable neurovascular and addiction-support herb with unique tension-releasing properties.)

# BAMBOO SILICA

★★★★★

*Bambusa arundinacea*

**Bamboo Silica** is a concentrated mineral-rich preparation derived from bamboo, prized for its exceptional ability to strengthen connective tissue, fascia, bones, hair, skin, and nails. Unlike diuretic silica sources, Bamboo delivers structural support *without draining fluids*, making it ideal for long-term rebuilding and repair.

It is especially valuable in recovery from injury, degeneration, aging, and structural weakness where integrity—not inflammation—is the core issue.

---

**Core Herbal Category — Bamboo SilicaPrimary Core: Immune System Support** (highly bioavailable silica for tissue integrity and regeneration)**Secondary Cores:** Musculoskeletal Support · Skin & Hair Health · Anti-Aging Support

---

**How It Works**Silica is essential for collagen synthesis and connective tissue strength. Bamboo Silica provides one of the richest, most absorbable plant-based silica sources available, supporting fascia resilience, bone mineralization, tendon elasticity, and skin structure without stimulating elimination.

---

**Primary Uses**

- Strengthens joints, ligaments, and tendons
- Supports bone density and skeletal integrity
- Improves hair, skin, and nail strength
- Aids recovery after injury or surgery
- Supports aging connective tissue
- Enhances fascia resilience

---

**Scientific Backing**Silica is a critical cofactor in collagen and elastin formation. Studies associate adequate silica intake with improved bone density, connective tissue repair, and skin elasticity. Bamboo-based silica offers superior concentration without the diuretic action seen in horsetail.

---

**How to Use (Dosage)**
**Capsules/Powder:**

300–1,000 mg daily.
**Liquid Extract:**
Follow manufacturer dosing; typically 10–30 drops daily.

---

### ⚠ Caution Level — Safe

Very safe and non-stimulating. Suitable for long-term use. Ensure product purity and standardized silica content.

---

### Gender-Specific Safety

**Men:** Safe — supports joints, recovery, and structural strength.
**Women:** Safe — supports skin, hair, bones, and fascia.
**Pregnancy/Nursing:** Safe at nutritional doses.

---

### Expected Results

- Nail and hair strength: 2–4 weeks
- Joint and fascia support: 4–8 weeks
- Bone support: long-term, cumulative

---

### Same / Similar Results

Horsetail · Nettle Seed · Oatstraw

---

### Shelf Life / Potency After Preparation

Capsules/Powder: 2–3 years · Liquid extract: 2 years

---

**Herbal Reflections of Bamboo Silica**Bamboo bends without breaking. Its medicine rebuilds the body's scaffolding—quietly strengthening what holds us upright, flexible, and whole. It restores form where time or injury has worn the frame thin.

---

### Herbal Confidence Index

*(4/5 — An exceptional structural tonic for connective tissue, fascia, and skeletal resilience.)*

# ELDERBERRY

★★★★★

***Sambucus nigra fructus***

**Elderberry** is one of the most widely respected traditional immune-support herbs, known for its deep, nourishing relationship with the body's natural defense systems. For centuries, it has been used across European, African, and Indigenous traditions to support the body during seasonal challenges—particularly those involving cold, flu, and respiratory stress. The dark purple berries are rich in anthocyanins and antioxidants, giving Elderberry its reputation as both a protector and a restorative tonic.

Unlike the elder leaf, which requires caution, properly prepared elderberries are considered safe and effective when used correctly. Elderberry works not by overpowering the body, but by supporting its natural immune response, helping the body recognize, respond to, and recover from external stressors more efficiently. It is especially valued for shortening the duration and severity of seasonal illness when taken early.

Elderberry is best understood as a foundational immune ally—a bridge between traditional wisdom and modern herbal science.

---

**Core Herbal Category — Elderberry**
**Primary Core: Immune System Support** herb with (antiviral and immune-modulating action that helps the body respond to and recover from seasonal illness)
**Secondary Cores:** Respiratory Support herb · Antioxidant Support herb · Circulatory Support herb

---

## How It Works

Elderberry supports immune function by enhancing cytokine activity and helping regulate the body's inflammatory response during infection. Its high anthocyanin content provides strong antioxidant protection, while its antiviral properties have been shown to interfere with viral replication and entry into cells. Elderberry also supports the respiratory system by helping to reduce mucus buildup and soothe inflamed airways. Rather than acting as a direct suppressant, it strengthens the body's natural defense coordination—making it especially effective when taken at the early onset of symptoms.

---

## 🌱 Primary Uses

- Supports immune response during cold and flu
- Helps reduce duration and severity of viral illness
- Supports respiratory health and mucus clearance
- Provides antioxidant protection for cellular health
- Supports recovery during seasonal immune stress

---

## 🔬 Scientific Backing

Elderberry has been studied for its antiviral effects, particularly against influenza viruses. Research suggests that elderberry extracts may reduce symptom duration and severity when taken early in infection. Its anthocyanins provide strong antioxidant support, while immune-modulating effects help regulate inflammatory responses. Clinical studies support its role as a complementary immune-support agent rather than a replacement for medical treatment.

---

## 💊 Forms Available

🟢 Syrup (most common and effective)
🟢 Capsules / extracts
🟢 Tea (dried berries)
🟢 Lozenges / gummies
🔴 Raw berries (not recommended; must be cooked)

---

## 📏 How to Use (Dosage)

- Syrup: 1–2 teaspoons daily (preventive); up to 3–4× daily during acute use
- Tea: 1–2 teaspoons dried berries simmered 10–15 minutes
- Capsules/extract: follow standardized product directions

⚠️ Always use properly prepared (cooked or processed) elderberries

---

## ⚠️ Caution Level: 🟡 Moderate Use

- Raw or unripe berries can cause nausea—must be properly prepared
- Use cautiously in individuals with autoimmune conditions (immune stimulation)
- Not a substitute for medical treatment in serious infection
- Avoid combining with strong immune-stimulating protocols without guidance

---

## Gender-Specific Safety (GS)

Men: Safe when properly prepared; supports immune resilience

Women: Safe when properly prepared; supportive during seasonal illness

Pregnancy / Nursing: Use with guidance; moderate intake generally considered acceptable in food-level forms (e.g., syrup)

---

## Expected Results

- Immune response support: 24–48 hours
- Symptom reduction (if taken early): 2–4 days
- Recovery support: 3–7 days

---

## DIY Recipe — Elderberry Immune Syrup

1 cup dried elderberries
3 cups water
1 cinnamon stick
1 tsp ginger
½ cup honey (after cooling)

Simmer berries and herbs for 30–45 minutes, strain, cool, then add honey. Store refrigerated.

---

## Same / Similar Results

Echinacea — immune activation + infection response

Andrographis — antiviral + immune modulation

Astragalus — long-term immune strengthening

Garlic — antimicrobial + immune support

Rose Hips — vitamin C + antioxidant support

---

## Shelf Life / Potency After Preparation

- Dried berries: 1–2 years (cool, dark, airtight)
- Syrup: 2–3 months refrigerated
- Tincture/extract: 2–3 years
- Tea (prepared): use within 24 hours

### 💭 Herbal Reflections of Elderberry

Elderberry stands as one of nature's most trusted guardians—quietly strengthening the body's defenses while allowing the immune system to act with clarity and precision. It does not overwhelm or force action; instead, it supports readiness. In this way, Elderberry represents preparedness rather than reaction—a steady ally in times of seasonal challenge.

---

### 🌟 Herbal Confidence Index: 🌿 🌿 🌿 🌿 🌿 (5/5 green stars)

Reasoning: Widely supported by both traditional use and modern research, Elderberry is one of the most effective and accessible immune-support herbs available. Its strong antiviral properties, safety (when properly prepared), and consistent results make it a cornerstone herb in immune health systems.

# GENTIAN

★★★★★

*Gentiana lutea*

**Gentian** is a classical bitter tonic traditionally used to stimulate digestive function and strengthen the body's appetite and assimilation processes. Derived from the bright yellow root of *Gentiana lutea*, this intensely bitter herb has been a cornerstone of European herbal medicine for centuries. It is widely recognized for supporting gastric secretions, bile flow, and overall digestive vitality through its powerful bitter compounds.

Unlike warming digestive herbs such as Ginger or carminatives like Peppermint, Gentian works primarily through its profound bitter principle. Its action stimulates the body's natural digestive reflexes, enhancing stomach acid production and preparing the gastrointestinal tract for efficient breakdown and absorption of nutrients. Gentian is not soothing — it is activating and strengthening, making it particularly valuable in cases of sluggish digestion and weak appetite.

---

## 🌿 Core Herbal Category — Gentian

**Primary Core: Digestive System Support herb** (true bitter tonic that stimulates gastric secretion, bile flow, and digestive readiness)

**Secondary Cores:** Liver & Detoxification herb · Circulatory stimulant (mild) · Immune resilience support (via digestive strengthening)

---

## 🌿 How It Works

Gentian contains secoiridoid glycosides, including gentiopicroside and amarogentin — among the most bitter compounds known in herbal medicine. These compounds activate bitter receptors in the mouth and digestive tract, triggering a reflex increase in saliva, gastric acid, pancreatic enzymes, and bile secretion. This cascade enhances nutrient breakdown and absorption while stimulating healthy digestive motility.

By improving digestive efficiency, Gentian indirectly supports immune function and systemic vitality, as proper assimilation of nutrients is foundational to overall health.

---

## 🌱 Primary Uses

- Low appetite or weak digestion
- Sluggish gastric secretions
- Occasional bloating due to insufficient stomach acid

• Digestive fatigue patterns
• Bitter tonic before meals to enhance assimilation

---

### Scientific Backing

Research confirms that Gentian's bitter glycosides stimulate gastric secretion and digestive enzyme activity. Studies show activation of bitter taste receptors (T2Rs) leading to enhanced digestive reflex responses. Clinical use supports its role in dyspepsia, reduced appetite, and digestive insufficiency. Its compounds also demonstrate mild anti-inflammatory and cholagogue (bile-stimulating) effects.

---

### Forms Available

• Dried root (decoction)
• Tincture (most common form)
• Digestive bitters formulas
• Capsules (standardized extract)

---

### How to Use (Dosage)

Tincture: 1–2 mL taken 10–15 minutes before meals
Decoction: ½–1 teaspoon root simmered 10–15 minutes, taken before meals
Capsules: 300–600 mg before meals
Best used short-term or intermittently before meals rather than continuously.

---

### Caution Level: Caution

Avoid in active gastric or duodenal ulcers.
May aggravate excessive stomach acid conditions.
Use cautiously in individuals with reflux associated with high acidity.
Pregnancy/Nursing: Avoid strong preparations unless supervised.

---

### Gender-Specific Safety

Men:
Helpful for sluggish digestion and appetite recovery. Avoid if prone to hyperacidity or ulcer history.

Women:
Supports digestive vitality and nutrient assimilation. Use cautiously if experiencing reflux with burning.

**Pregnancy/Nursing:**
Avoid strong bitters unless guided by a qualified practitioner.

---

### ⏳ Expected Results

- Increased appetite: Immediate to 3 days
- Reduced bloating from weak digestion: 1–2 weeks
- Improved assimilation patterns: 2–4 weeks

---

### 🛠 DIY Recipe — Classic Digestive Bitter Tonic

Add 1 teaspoon Gentian root to 1 cup water.
Simmer gently for 10 minutes.
Strain and take ¼ cup 10–15 minutes before meals.
Alternatively, add 1 mL tincture to a small amount of water before meals.

---

### 🔄 Same / Similar Results

- Dandelion Root
- Yellow Dock
- Artichoke Leaf
- Wormwood
- Goldenseal

---

### Shelf Life / Potency After Preparation

- Dried root: 2–3 years (airtight, cool, dark)
- Tincture: 3–5 years
- Decoction: Use within 24 hours refrigerated

---

### 💬 Herbal Reflections of Gentian

Gentian represents clarity through intensity. Its bitterness awakens the digestive fire and reminds us that strength often begins with activation. It does not comfort — it corrects. In teaching the body to prepare and respond, Gentian reflects the principle that vitality depends upon proper assimilation and readiness before nourishment can truly be received.

---

### ⭐ Herbal Confidence Index: 🌿🌿🌿🌿🌿

(5/5 — cornerstone bitter tonic; essential for teaching digestive physiology and strengthening foundational assimilation processes.)

# CATNIP

★★★★

*Nepeta cataria*

**Catnip** is a gentle nervine and digestive-support herb traditionally used to calm nervous tension while easing mild digestive discomfort. Though widely known for its effect on cats, Catnip has a long history of medicinal use in European and North American herbal traditions. It is particularly valued for its soothing influence on the nervous system and its ability to relax spasmodic patterns in the digestive tract.

Catnip acts as a mild carminative and calming herb, making it especially helpful for children and individuals sensitive to stronger nervines. Its warming yet non-stimulating nature allows it to settle restlessness, relieve mild tension headaches, and ease digestive unease associated with stress. Unlike stronger sedatives, Catnip supports calm alertness rather than drowsiness.

---

### 🌿 Core Herbal Category — Catnip

**Primary Core: Nervous System Support (Nervines)** herb (gentle calming herb that relaxes nervous tension and stress-related digestive patterns)
**Secondary Cores:** Digestive & Gut Support herb · Mild Diaphoretic herb · Pediatric support herb

---

### 🌿 How It Works

Catnip contains nepetalactone and volatile oils that act on the nervous system to promote relaxation and reduce mild anxiety-related tension. Its antispasmodic properties help ease smooth muscle contractions within the digestive tract, reducing bloating and cramping. As a mild diaphoretic, it can also support the body during early stages of fever by gently encouraging peripheral circulation and mild perspiration.

Its dual action on the nervous and digestive systems makes it especially useful when emotional tension manifests as stomach discomfort.

---

### 🌱 Primary Uses

- Mild nervous tension and restlessness
- Stress-related digestive discomfort
- Occasional bloating or cramping
- Gentle pediatric calming support
- Early-stage mild fever support (combined formulas)

---

### Scientific Backing

Studies confirm Catnip's mild sedative and antispasmodic properties, attributed to nepetalactone and related volatile oils. Research demonstrates central nervous system calming effects and smooth muscle relaxation activity. While not heavily studied in large clinical trials, its long-standing traditional use supports its role as a safe, mild nervine and digestive relaxant.

---

### Forms Available

• Dried leaf and flowering tops (tea)
• Tincture
• Capsules (less common)
• Fresh herb preparations

---

### How to Use (Dosage)

Tea: 1–2 teaspoons dried herb per 8 oz hot water, steep 10–15 minutes, up to 2–3× daily
Tincture: 1–2 mL, up to 3× daily
Children (tea): ¼–½ cup mild infusion as needed
Best used short-term or as needed for calming and digestive support.

---

### Caution Level: Safe

Generally safe for adults and children in tea form.

Large doses may cause mild sedation.

Pregnancy: Use mild tea only; avoid concentrated extracts without guidance.

---

### Gender-Specific Safety

Men:
Supports stress-related digestive tension and mild nervous restlessness. Suitable for regular tea use.

Women:
Helpful during periods of mild tension, stress, or digestive upset. Safe as tea; avoid excessive use during pregnancy.

Pregnancy/Nursing:
Mild tea considered generally safe in moderation; avoid strong extracts unless supervised.

---

### Expected Results

• Reduced nervous tension: 15–30 minutes

- Relief of mild digestive cramping: 30–60 minutes
- Calming support before sleep: Same day

---

🛠️ **DIY Recipe — Gentle Calming Tea**

Combine 1 teaspoon Catnip with 1 teaspoon Chamomile.
Pour 1 cup hot water over herbs and steep 10–15 minutes.
Strain and sip in the evening or during periods of mild tension.

---

🔄 **Same / Similar Results**

🟢 Lemon Balm
🟢 Chamomile
🔵 Skullcap
🟣 Passionflower
🟡 Fennel

---

💉 **Shelf Life / Potency After Preparation**

🧴 ✨ Dried herb: 1–2 years (airtight, cool, dark)
🧴 ✨ Tincture: 3–5 years
🧴 ✨ Prepared tea: Use within 24 hours refrigerated

---

💬 **Herbal Reflections of Catnip**

Catnip represents gentleness in medicine. It does not overpower or suppress; it reassures and relaxes. Its quiet strength lies in its ability to calm both the mind and the stomach without heaviness. In teaching the nervous system to soften, Catnip reflects the wisdom that restoration often begins with simple, steady ease.

---

⭐ **Herbal Confidence Index:** 🌿 🌿 🌿 🌿

(4/5 — reliable and gentle nervine/digestive crossover herb; excellent for pediatric and stress-related patterns with strong safety profile.)

# UVA URSI

★★★★

***Arctostaphylos uva-ursi***

**Uva Ursi,** traditionally known as Bearberry, is a classic urinary-support herb long used to promote bladder integrity and healthy urinary tract balance. Rich in arbutin and tannins, it supports antimicrobial action within the urinary system while also providing astringent toning effects that help tighten and soothe mucosal tissues. Historically used by Indigenous North American and European herbal traditions, Uva Ursi has been valued for its targeted support during acute urinary discomfort.

Unlike broad-spectrum immune tonics, Uva Ursi is considered a focused and situational herb. It is most effective when used short-term and appropriately prepared. Its action is both antimicrobial and tissue-toning, making it particularly suited for urinary irritation patterns associated with mild infection or inflammation.

---

🌿 **Core Herbal Category — Uva Ursi**
**Primary Core: Kidney & Urinary Support herb** (urinary antiseptic and mucosal astringent that supports bladder integrity and fluid balance)
**Secondary Cores:** Antimicrobial herb · Astringent herb · Digestive astringent support (mild)

---

## 🌿 How It Works

Uva Ursi contains arbutin, which converts in the body to hydroquinone compounds that exert antimicrobial activity within the urinary tract. Its tannins provide astringent action that tones and tightens irritated mucosal tissues, helping reduce excessive discharge or inflammation. This dual mechanism supports both microbial balance and tissue integrity, particularly in the bladder and lower urinary system.

Uva Ursi works best in alkaline urinary environments, which is why it has traditionally been paired with alkalizing dietary strategies during short-term use.

---

## 🌱 Primary Uses

- Mild urinary tract discomfort
- Bladder irritation patterns
- Occasional urinary frequency associated with irritation

• Short-term antimicrobial urinary support
• Situational urinary toning support

---

## Scientific Backing

Research supports Uva Ursi's antimicrobial properties through arbutin-derived hydroquinone compounds active in the urinary tract. Clinical and laboratory studies demonstrate its ability to inhibit bacterial growth commonly associated with urinary tract infections. Tannins contribute additional astringent effects that support tissue integrity. Its use is generally recommended short-term due to potency and hydroquinone metabolism considerations.

---

## Forms Available

• Dried leaf (decoction or infusion)
• Tincture
• Capsules (standardized leaf extract)

---

## How to Use (Dosage)

Tea (decoction): 1 teaspoon dried leaf per 8 oz water, simmer 10–15 minutes, up to 2× daily
Tincture: 1–2 mL, 2–3× daily (short-term use only)
Capsules: 400–800 mg extract, up to 3× daily
Best used for no more than 5–7 consecutive days unless supervised.

---

## Caution Level: Caution

Intended for short-term use only.
Avoid in pregnancy and nursing.
Avoid in children under 12 unless supervised.
Not recommended for individuals with kidney disease.
Do not use continuously beyond 1 week without practitioner guidance.

---

## Gender-Specific Safety

Men:
Helpful for short-term bladder support. Avoid prolonged use or combination with kidney-compromising medications.

Women:
Commonly used for occasional urinary discomfort. Limit to short-term use and ensure adequate hydration.

● Pregnancy/Nursing:
Avoid use due to hydroquinone metabolites.

---

## ⏳ Expected Results

• Reduction in urinary discomfort: 1–3 days
• Improved bladder tone: 3–5 days
• Symptom stabilization: Within 1 week (short-term use)

---

## 🛠 DIY Recipe — Uva Ursi Short-Term Bladder Decoction

Simmer 1 teaspoon dried Uva Ursi leaf in 1 cup water for 10–15 minutes.
Strain and allow to cool slightly.
Drink up to twice daily for no more than 5 days.
Pair with adequate hydration.

---

## 🔄 Same / Similar Results

● Corn Silk
● Goldenrod
● Gravel Root
● Juniper Berry
● Cranberry

---

## Shelf Life / Potency After Preparation

Dried leaf: 1–2 years (airtight, cool, dark)
Tincture: 3–5 years
Prepared decoction: Use within 24 hours refrigerated

---

## 💬 Herbal Reflections of Uva Ursi

Uva Ursi reflects the principle of precision in herbal practice. It does not nourish broadly like tonics nor calm gently like nervines — it acts with purpose and restraint. It teaches the value of short, targeted intervention when imbalance arises. Strong yet disciplined, it reminds us that some medicines are not for constant use but for careful, intentional application.

---

## ⭐ Herbal Confidence Index: 🌿 🌿 🌿 🌿

(4/5 — powerful and reliable short-term urinary support herb; highly effective when properly used but requires mindful dosing and duration awareness.)

# LAVENDER

★★★★

***Lavandula angustifolia***

**Lavender** is a gentle yet highly effective calming nervine known for its ability to ease anxiety, promote restful sleep, and soothe the nervous system without heavy sedation. Its aromatic compounds help relax both the mind and body, making it one of the most widely used herbs for stress, tension, and emotional imbalance. Lavender offers a light, uplifting calm—reducing nervous agitation while maintaining clarity and ease.
Traditionally used across European, Mediterranean, and Middle Eastern herbal systems, Lavender has long been valued for both its medicinal and aromatic qualities. Whether used as a tea, essential oil, or topical preparation, it supports relaxation, reduces mild pain, and enhances mood stability. Its versatility allows it to be used both during the day for stress relief and at night for sleep support, making it one of the most accessible and dependable calming herbs.

---

**Core Herbal Category — Lavender**
**Primary Core: Nervous System Support (Nervines)** (Nervous System Support) herb with (gentle calming, anxiolytic action that relaxes the mind and body without heavy sedation)
Secondary Cores: Sleep Support herb · Digestive Support herb · Skin & Tissue Repair herb

---

**How It Works**
Lavender works through its volatile aromatic compounds, particularly linalool and linalyl acetate, which interact with the nervous system to reduce excitability and promote relaxation. It helps regulate stress-response pathways, calming overactive neural signaling and supporting parasympathetic (rest-and-digest) activation. Lavender also exhibits mild antispasmodic and analgesic effects, which contribute to its ability to relieve tension headaches, digestive discomfort, and muscular tightness. Through both internal and aromatic use, it provides a balanced calming effect that soothes without impairing mental clarity. Overall, it functions as a gentle nervine that restores calm, improves mood, and supports natural sleep rhythms.

---

### 🌱 Primary Uses

- Anxiety, stress, mild depression, emotional tension
- Insomnia, restlessness, difficulty falling asleep
- Headaches, mild digestive discomfort, and skin irritation

---

### Scientific Backing

• Clinical studies show lavender essential oil significantly reduces anxiety and improves sleep quality.
• Demonstrates anxiolytic effects comparable to mild pharmaceutical agents in some trials.
• Exhibits anti-inflammatory, antimicrobial, and mild analgesic properties.
• Supports traditional use for stress, insomnia, and nervous-system regulation.

---

### Forms Available

- Essential oil (aromatherapy or diluted topical use)
- Dried flowers (tea or infusion)
- Capsules or tinctures

---

### How to Use

Tea: 1–2 tsp dried flowers steeped 10 minutes; 1–2 times daily
Essential oil: 2–4 drops in diffuser or diluted in carrier oil for topical use
Capsules: Follow standardized extract dosage (commonly 80–160 mg daily)

---

### ⏱ Expected Results

Calming effect: 15–30 minutes (aromatic use)
Sleep support: same night to several days
Mood stabilization: 1–2 weeks

---

### ⚠ Caution Level: Generally Safe / Gentle

• May cause mild drowsiness in sensitive individuals
• Use caution with sedatives or anti-anxiety medications
• Essential oil must be diluted before skin application
• Rare allergic reactions possible—patch test recommended

---

### Gender-Specific Safety — Lavender

**Men — Safe:**
Supports stress reduction, relaxation, and sleep. Occasional use preferred if concerned about long-term hormonal sensitivity (rare and debated).

**Women — Safe:**
Helpful for anxiety, sleep, and hormonal-related mood tension. Gentle and well-tolerated.

**Pregnancy / Nursing — Caution:**
Light tea or mild aromatherapy generally considered safe, but avoid concentrated essential oil use unless approved by a professional.

---

### Same / Similar Results

Chamomile · Lemon Balm · Passionflower · Valerian · Holy Basil

---

### Shelf Life & Potency After Preparation

- Dried flowers: 1–2 years
- Capsules/extracts: 1–2 years
- Essential oil: 3–5 years
- Tea/infusion: Use within 24 hours

---

### DIY Recipe — Lavender Sleep Tea

1–2 tsp dried Lavender flowers
1 cup hot water
Steep for 10 minutes; drink 30–60 minutes before bed.

---

### Herbal Reflections of Lavender

Lavender carries a quiet intelligence—soft, floral, and reassuring. It does not force the body into rest but gently invites it there, easing tension layer by layer until calm naturally returns. Where stress tightens, Lavender loosens; where the mind races, it slows the pace just enough to restore balance.
It reminds us that healing does not always come through strength—sometimes it comes through softness, through breath, through allowing the body to settle into peace.

**Herbal Confidence Index:** ½
(4.5/5 — a highly reliable, versatile nervine that excels in calming the mind, improving sleep, and supporting emotional balance with gentle effectiveness.)

# ZEDOARY

★★★★

*(Curcuma zedoaria)*

**Zedoary** is a pungent, camphor-bright rhizome used to cut through sluggish digestion and reduce inflammatory stagnation. Compared with turmeric, it is sharper and more aromatic, traditionally used for post-meal bloating and topical support for irritated tissues. Rooted in Ayurvedic, Chinese, and Southeast Asian traditions, it traveled spice routes into kitchens and apothecaries alike—medicine carried by aroma and bitterness.

---

## Core Herbal Category — Zedoary

**Primary Core: Digestive System Support** herb with (warming, aromatic action that stimulates digestion and clears stagnation)

**Secondary Cores:** Liver & Detoxification herb · Women's Health herb · Skin & Tissue Repair herb

---

## How It Works

**Zedoary** supports digestion by stimulating gastric and biliary secretions and improving digestive "flow," which can ease bloating and heaviness after meals. Its aromatic constituents support circulation into congested tissues, helping reduce inflammatory tightness and promoting recovery. In traditional women's health use, it is classified as a **blood-moving** herb—helpful for pelvic stagnation patterns, but **not appropriate** when bleeding is heavy or when pregnancy is possible. Topically, its warming circulation support can aid comfort in irritated or tense areas.

---

## Primary Uses

- Post-meal bloating, gas, sluggish digestion
- Digestive stagnation with heaviness
- Support for liver/gallbladder "sluggishness" patterns
- Topical support for irritated tissues
- Menstrual discomfort linked to stagnation patterns (non-pregnant adults only)

---

## Scientific Backing

Zedoary contains curcuminoids and sesquiterpenes (including aromatic oils) associated with anti-inflammatory, antioxidant, antimicrobial, and digestive-support actions. Research is still developing; traditional use is strongest for digestive stagnation and topical support.

## 📦 Forms Available

- Dried root powder
- Fresh rhizome
- Capsules/tablets
- Tincture
- Essential oil (**external only**)

## How to Use / Dosage

- **Powder:** 1–2 g daily in warm water/tea (start low)
- **Tincture:** 1–2 mL, 1–3× daily
- **Food use:** thin slices or small amounts (potent)
- **Topical:** infused oil or paste to affected area 1–2× daily

**Essential oil:** external use only, diluted.

## ⌛ Expected Results

- Digestive ease: 3–5 days
- Inflammation balance/support: 2–3 weeks
- Tissue comfort/topical support: several days to 2 weeks

## ⚠ Caution Level: Caution

- **Avoid in pregnancy and breastfeeding** (traditional blood-moving/emmenagogue use)
- Avoid with **active ulcers** or severe GERD/acid sensitivity
- Use cautiously with **gallstones or bile-duct obstruction** unless supervised
- Use cautiously with **blood thinners / antiplatelet drugs**
- High doses may irritate the stomach or increase warmth/loose stools
- Essential oil is **topical only** and must be diluted

Stop if nausea, burning, or cramping occurs.

## 🧬 Gender-Specific Safety (GS)

**Men — Safe**

Appropriate for short-term digestive support at standard doses.

**Women — Caution**

May increase pelvic circulation; **avoid if heavy bleeding** or if cramping worsens. Use short-term only.

**Pregnancy / Nursing — Avoid**

Not appropriate due to traditional emmenagogue/blood-moving actions and limited safety data.

---

## 🔄 Same / Similar Results

- Ginger
- Turmeric

---

## 📦 Shelf Life / Potency After Preparation

- Whole dried root: 3–4 years (cool, dark, airtight)
- Powder: 1–1.5 years (aroma fades fastest)
- Capsules: ~1–2 years sealed
- Tincture: 5–7 years
- Prepared paste/decoction: 24 hours refrigerated

---

## 🛠 DIY Recipe — Zedoary Digestive Tonic

½–1 tsp zedoary powder in warm water or tea (start low).
Use **as needed** for heaviness/bloating; avoid daily long-term use.

---

## 💬 Herbal Reflections of Zedoary

Zedoary is the clarifier of the rhizome family—precise, aromatic, and movement-restoring. Where digestion feels "stuck," it brings direction and flow without heaviness. Its teaching is moderation: a small amount can restore rhythm, while excess can irritate. Used respectfully, it supports clearer digestion, steadier circulation, and cleaner tissue recovery.

---

## ★ Herbal Confidence Index

🌿🌿🌿🌿 (4/5 green stars — a strong digestive mover with reliable traditional value and supportive research signals; best for short, intentional use due to its stimulating, blood-moving nature.)

# MEDICAL CHARTS 1 THROUGH 33

The following section contains thirty-three organized Medical Charts designed to help readers quickly identify which herbs have traditionally been associated with supporting specific areas of wellness. Each chart focuses on a single medical or natural condition, presenting the herbs in a clear, ranked format for ease of study and reference.

These charts do not diagnose or prescribe. Instead, they serve as an educational guide—summarizing long-standing herbal uses, providing a structured overview of supportive herbs, and offering readers a way to navigate the wide range of plant remedies discussed throughout this book. In addition, the charts are designed to assist readers in recognizing how herbs may be combined, allowing them to observe natural pairings and develop a clearer understanding of well-balanced and synergistic herbal mixtures.

Readers may use these charts to:

- Identify herbs commonly linked with various wellness categories
- Compare which herbs are considered most supportive for each condition
- Recognize how herbs can be combined based on their roles and complementary actions
- Locate full herb pages by using the page numbers listed on each chart
- Deepen their study of the 15 Core Herbal Categories and the broader Herbal Resurrection system

Together, these charts create a concise visual guide to the herbal traditions represented in this volume, offering a practical starting point for further reading, structured understanding, and personal exploration.

## MEDICAL HERBAL SUPPORT CHARTS — PAGE NUMBERS

### CORE SYSTEMS

I. Cardiovascular Herbal Support Chart ............................ 908
II. Nervous System Herbal Support Chart ......................... 910
III. Immune System Herbal Support Chart ........................ 912
IV. Digestive System Herbal Support Chart ...................... 914
V. Respiratory System Herbal Support Chart .................... 916
VI. Urinary System Herbal Support Chart ........................ 918
VII. Liver & Detox Herbal Support Chart ........................ 920
VIII. Endocrine & Hormonal System Herbal Support Chart... 922

### GENDER HEALTH

IX. Women's Health Herbal Support Chart ....................... 924
X. Men's Health Herbal Support Chart ............................ 926

### INFLAMMATION / STRUCTURE

XI. Anti-Inflammatory Herbal Support Chart .................... 928
XII. Musculoskeletal & Joint Support Herbal Chart ........... 930
XIII. Bone, Connective Tissue & Structural Support Chart ..932

### ENERGY / STRESS / SLEEP

XIV. Energy & Vitality Herbal Support Chart .................... 934
XV. Stress & Adrenal Support Herbal Support Chart ..........936
XVI. Sleep & Circadian Rhythm Herbal Support Chart ....... 938

### METABOLIC / ENDOCRINE

XVII. Blood Sugar & Metabolic Balance Herbal Chart ........ 940
XVIII. Weight & Appetite Regulation Herbal Chart ........... 942
XIX. Thyroid & Endocrine Support Herbal Chart ............... 945

### BLOOD / LYMPH

XX. Lymphatic System Herbal Support Chart ................... 947
XXI. Blood Building & Circulation Herbal Support Chart ..... 950

### SKIN / EXTERNAL

XXII. Skin Health & Repair Herbal Support Chart ............ 953
XXIII. Hair, Nails & Integumentary Support Chart ............ 956

### DIGESTIVE SPECIALIZATION

XXIV. Gut Lining & Mucosal Support Herbal Chart ........... 959
XXV. Bile Flow & Fat Digestion Herbal Support Chart ...... 962

### 🌿 BRAIN / SENSORY

XXVI. Cognitive Function & Memory Herbal Chart ............ 965
XXVII. Eye & Vision Herbal Support Chart ...................... 967

---

### 🌿 IMMUNE / RECOVERY

XXVIII. Seasonal & Acute Immune Support Chart ............. 970
XXIX. Recovery, Healing & Tissue Repair Chart ............... 973

---

### 🌿 NUTRITION / LONGEVITY

XXX. Mineral & Nutritive Tonics Herbal Support Chart ..... 976
XXXI. Longevity & Cellular Protection Herbal Chart .......... 979
XXXII. Gentle Daily Tonics & Nervine Support Chart ........ 982

---

### ⚠ SPECIAL CATEGORY

XXXIII. Strong / High-Caution Herbs (Educational Chart) .... 985

# I. The Cardiovascular Herbal Support Chart

This chart highlights the herbs most trusted for supporting heart strength, healthy circulation, and balanced blood pressure. Use it to quickly identify leading cardiovascular herbs and refer to their full entries for detailed usage guidance, cautions, and supporting insights.

I. **Cardiovascular Herbal Support Chart**
(Enhanced Clinical Format)
**Purpose:**
Herbs used to support heart strength, circulation quality, vascular tone, and balanced blood pressure.

---

### PRIMARY HEART TONICS

Support cardiac strength and long-term heart function

Rank Herb Rating Page Primary Role

1 **Hawthorn Berry** ★★★★★ 314
Premier cardiac tonic supporting heart strength, rhythm balance, and coronary circulation

2 **Motherwort** ★★★★ 116
Supports heart tone and calming of stress-related cardiac tension

---

### CIRCULATION & VASCULAR SUPPORT

Promote healthy blood flow and vascular integrity

Rank Herb Rating Page Primary Role

3 **Ginkgo Biloba** ★★★★ 279
Supports peripheral circulation and oxygen delivery

4 **Cayenne Pepper** ★★★★ 53
Stimulates circulation and supports vascular movement

---

### BLOOD PRESSURE & CARDIAC BALANCE

Support vascular tone and pressure balance

Rank Herb Rating Page Primary Role

5 **Garlic** ★★★★ 841
Supports cholesterol balance, circulation, and vascular health

6 **Olive Leaf** ★★★★ 351
Supports vascular tone and balanced blood pressure

---

### How to Use This Chart

- General heart support: **Hawthorn Berry** + **Motherwort**
- Circulation & blood flow: **Ginkgo Biloba** + **Cayenne Pepper**
- Blood pressure balance: **Garlic** + **Olive Leaf**

Consult each herb's full entry for safety considerations, contraindications, and appropriate context before use.

# II. The Nervous System Herbal Support Chart

This chart highlights herbs traditionally used to support the nervous system, promote calm, and help the body respond more smoothly to stress and tension. Use it to quickly identify nervine and supportive herbs, then refer to their full entries for proper use, cautions, and deeper context.

## II. The Nervous System Herbal Support Chart

### PRIMARY NERVOUS TONICS

Rank Herb Rating Page Primary Role

1 **Oatstraw** ★★★★★ 591

Deep nervous-system nourishment and long-term resilience

2 **Skullcap** ★★★★★ 668

Restores nerve tone and calms overstimulation

### CALMING & ANXIETY SUPPORT

Rank Herb Rating Page Primary Role

3 **Lemon Balm** ★★★★ 299

Lifts mood and eases nervous tension

4 **Passionflower** ★★★★ 95

Calms racing thoughts and supports relaxation

5 **Lavender** ★★★★ 900

Fast-acting calming nervine that reduces anxiety and supports emotional balance, especially through aromatic use

6 **Roman Chamomile** ★★★★ 56

Gentle calming herb for stress and irritability

### SLEEP & DEEP REST SUPPORT

Rank Herb Rating Page Primary Role

7 **Valerian** ★★★★ 819

Supports deep sleep and nervous reset

8 **California Poppy** ★★★★ 50

Relaxes the nervous system and aids sleep onset

### How to Use This Chart

- Long-term nerve support: **Oatstraw + Skullcap**
- Daytime calm: **Lemon Balm + Passionflower**
- Gentle relaxation: **Roman Chamomile + Lavender**
- Sleep support: **Valerian + California Poppy**

# III. The Immune Herbal Support Chart

This chart highlights herbs commonly used to support immune resilience, seasonal wellness, and the body's natural defense responses. Use it to quickly identify immune-supportive herbs and refer to their full entries for appropriate use, cautions, and supporting insights.

## III. Immune System Herbal Support Chart

### PRIMARY IMMUNE TONICS

Rank Herb Rating Page Primary Role

1 **Astragalus** ★★★★★ 25

Deep immune tonic that strengthens long-term resistance

2 **Reishi** ★★★★★ 691

Immune modulator and resilience builder

3 **Elderberry** ★★★★ 887

Supports immune defense and recovery

### ANTIVIRAL & ACUTE SUPPORT

Rank Herb Rating Page Primary Role

4 **Andrographis** ★★★★ 104

Acute immune activation and infection support

5 **Garlic** ★★★★ 841

Antimicrobial and immune stimulant

6 **Olive Leaf** ★★★★ 351

Broad immune and antimicrobial support

### IMMUNE–INFLAMMATION BALANCE

Rank Herb Rating Page Primary Role

7 **Turmeric** ★★★★ 514

Anti-inflammatory immune regulation

8 **Echinacea** ★★★★ 746

Stimulates immune response in early infection

### How to Use This Chart

- Long-term immune strengthening: **Astragalus + Reishi**
- Early illness response: **Echinacea + Elderberry**
- Viral/infection pressure: **Garlic + Olive Leaf**
- Immune–inflammation balance: **Turmeric**

# IV. The Digestive Herbal Support Chart

This chart highlights herbs traditionally used to support digestion, ease bloating and discomfort, and promote healthy stomach and intestinal function. Use it to quickly identify digestive allies and refer to their full entries for preparation methods, cautions, and supportive details.

## IV. Digestive System Herbal Support Chart

---

### PRIMARY DIGESTIVE TONICS

Rank Herb Rating Page Primary Role

1 **Ginger Root** ★★★★★ 339
Core digestive stimulant and circulation activator

2 **Dandelion Root** ★★★★ 80
Supports bile flow and digestive function

3 **Peppermint** ★★★★ 635
Relieves gas, bloating, and digestive tension

---

### GAS, BLOATING & CRAMPING

Rank Herb Rating Page Primary Role

4 **Fennel Seed** ★★★★ 771
Reduces gas and intestinal cramping

5 **Roman Chamomile** ★★★★ 56
Calms digestive irritation and spasms

---

### GUT LINING & SOOTHING SUPPORT

Rank Herb Rating Page Primary Role

6 **Slippery Elm** ★★★★ 295
Soothes and protects digestive lining

7 **Marshmallow Root** ★★★★ 629
Coats and repairs inflamed gut tissue

---

### How to Use This Chart

- Weak digestion: **Ginger Root + Dandelion Root**
- Gas & bloating: **Peppermint + Fennel Seed**
- Irritated gut lining: **Slippery Elm + Marshmallow Root**
- Stress digestion: **Roman Chamomile**

# V. The Respiratory Herbal Support Chart

This chart highlights herbs traditionally used to support healthy lung function, clear the airways, and promote comfortable breathing. Use it to quickly identify respiratory-supportive herbs and refer to their full entries for preparation methods, cautions, and supportive guidance.

**V. Respiratory System Herbal Support Chart**

---

### PRIMARY LUNG TONICS

Rank Herb Rating Page Primary Role

1 **Mullein Leaf** ★★★★★ 310
Core lung tonic that strengthens and restores respiratory tissue

2 **Elecampane** ★★★★ 266
Deep lung restorative and expectorant

3 **Black Horehound** ★★★★ 225
Clears mucus and supports bronchial function

---

### EXPECTORANT & CONGESTION RELIEF

Rank Herb Rating Page Primary Role

4 **Thyme** ★★★★ 372
Clears mucus and supports antimicrobial defense

5 **Plantain Leaf** ★★★★ 210
Soothes inflamed airways and supports lung repair

6 **Eucalyptus** ★★★★ 624
Opens airways and supports clear breathing

---

### SOOTHING & LUNG LINING SUPPORT

Rank Herb Rating Page Primary Role

7 **Marshmallow Root** ★★★★ 629
Soothes irritated respiratory tissue

8 **Licorice Root** ★★★★ 687
Moistens lungs and reduces inflammation

---

### How to Use This Chart

- Chronic lung weakness: Mullein Leaf + Elecampane
- Thick mucus & congestion: Black Horehound + Thyme

- Irritated airways: Plantain Leaf + Marshmallow Root
- Dry inflamed lungs: Licorice Root + Marshmallow Root

# VI. The Urinary & Kidney Herbal Support Chart

This chart highlights herbs traditionally used to support kidney function, urinary tract health, and healthy fluid balance. Use it to quickly identify urinary-supportive herbs and refer to their full entries for preparation guidance, cautions, and supportive context.

## VI. Urinary System Herbal Support Chart

### PRIMARY URINARY TONICS

| Rank | Herb | Rating | Page | Primary Role |
|---|---|---|---|---|
| 1 | **Goldenrod** | ★★★★★ | 129 | Supports urinary tract cleansing and infection control |
| 2 | **Corn Silk** | ★★★★ | 74 | Soothes urinary irritation and supports fluid balance |
| 3 | **Horsetail** | ★★★★ | 433 | Strengthens urinary tissues and supports kidney function |

### DIURETIC & FLUSHING SUPPORT

| Rank | Herb | Rating | Page | Primary Role |
|---|---|---|---|---|
| 4 | **Dandelion Leaf** | ★★★★ | 86 | Gentle diuretic that supports kidney filtration |
| 5 | **Cleavers** | ★★★★ | 775 | Supports urinary and lymphatic drainage |
| 6 | **Parsley** | ★★★ | 213 | Mild diuretic that supports urinary flushing |

### SOOTHING & LINING SUPPORT

| Rank | Herb | Rating | Page | Primary Role |
|---|---|---|---|---|
| 7 | **Marshmallow Root** | ★★★★ | 629 | Soothes urinary tract lining and reduces irritation |
| 8 | **Plantain Leaf** | ★★★★ | 210 | Supports tissue repair and urinary tract soothing |

### How to Use This Chart

- Urinary irritation: Corn Silk + Marshmallow Root
- Fluid retention: Dandelion Leaf + Parsley
- Urinary cleansing: Goldenrod + Cleavers
- Tissue repair: Plantain Leaf + Marshmallow Root

### CONSISTENCY NOTES

✓ Converted all ratings to ★ **system (uniform across all charts)**

✓ Standardized herb naming in “How to Use” section

✓ Cleaned spacing for **better print readability**

# VII. The Liver & Detox Herbal Support Chart

This chart highlights herbs traditionally used to support liver function, assist natural detoxification processes, and promote healthy metabolic balance. Use it to quickly identify liver-supportive herbs and refer to their full entries for preparation guidance, cautions, and supportive details.

**VII. Liver & Detox Herbal Support Chart *(Enhanced Clinical Format)***

**Purpose:**

Herbs used to support liver function, assist natural detoxification processes, promote bile flow, and maintain healthy metabolic balance.

---

### PRIMARY LIVER TONICS

(Support liver regeneration, detox capacity, and long-term function)

Rank Herb Rating Page Primary Role

1 **Milk Thistle** ★★★★★ 31

Premier liver-protective herb supporting regeneration and detoxification

2 **Dandelion Root** ★★★★ 80

Supports bile flow and liver detox pathways

3 **Schisandra** ★★★★ 219

Enhances liver resilience and detox efficiency

---

### DETOXIFICATION & METABOLIC SUPPORT

(Assist toxin processing, metabolic balance, and systemic cleansing)

Rank Herb Rating Page Primary Role

4 **Burdock Root** ★★★★ 44

Supports blood purification and liver detox pathways

5 **Yellow Dock** ★★★★ 147

Supports elimination and liver cleansing

6 **Turmeric** ★★★★ 514

Supports liver function and anti-inflammatory detox balance

---

### BILE FLOW & DIGESTIVE DETOX SUPPORT

(Promote bile movement and digestive-based detoxification)

Rank Herb Rating Page Primary Role

7 **Artichoke Leaf** ★★★★ 19

Stimulates bile production and supports liver digestion

8 **Ginger Root** ★★★★ 339

Enhances circulation and supports digestive detox pathways

---

### How to Use This Chart

- Liver regeneration & protection: **Milk Thistle + Schisandra**
- Daily detox support: **Dandelion Root + Burdock Root**
- Bile flow & digestion: **Artichoke Leaf + Ginger Root**
- Deep detox support: **Turmeric + Yellow Dock**

# VIII. The Endocrine & Hormonal System Herbal Support Chart

This chart highlights herbs traditionally used to support reproductive health, hormonal balance, and overall vitality for both men and women. Use it to quickly identify reproductive-supportive herbs and refer to their full entries for appropriate use, cautions, and supportive insight.

## VIII. Endocrine & Hormonal System Herbal Support Chart

### 🔘 PRIMARY ADAPTOGENIC TONICS

Rank Herb Rating Page Primary Role

1 🌿 **Ashwagandha** ★★★★★ 22

Stabilizes stress hormones and supports adrenal–thyroid balance

2 🌿 **Rhodiola** ★★★★ 711

Improves endocrine resilience and stress tolerance

3 🌿 **Eleuthero** ★★★★ 651

Supports adrenal endurance and hormonal stability

### 🔘 GLANDULAR & THYROID SUPPORT

Rank Herb Rating Page Primary Role

4 🌿 **Bladderwrack** ★★★★ 113

Supports thyroid function and iodine balance

5 🌿 **Irish Moss / Sea Moss** ★★★★ 873

Mineral-rich thyroid and endocrine support

6 🌿 **Schisandra** ★★★★ 219

Supports endocrine balance and adrenal regulation

### 🔘 HORMONAL BALANCE & CYCLE SUPPORT

Rank Herb Rating Page Primary Role

7 🌿 **Vitex** ★★★★ 153

Supports reproductive hormone balance

8 🌿 **Maca Root** ★★★★ 803

Enhances endocrine vitality and hormonal resilience

### How to Use This Chart

- Adrenal fatigue: **Ashwagandha + Rhodiola**
- Thyroid support: **Bladderwrack + Sea Moss**
- Hormonal balance**: Vitex + Maca**
- Endocrine resilience: **Schisandra + Eleuthero**

# IX. The Women's Health Herbal Support Chart

This chart highlights herbs traditionally used to support women's health across different life stages, including hormonal balance, menstrual comfort, reproductive tissue support, and overall vitality. It is designed to help readers quickly identify women's health–supportive herbs and understand how they are commonly grouped by function within herbal practice.

Use this chart as a reference guide to locate herbs associated with women's wellness needs, then consult each herb's full entry for detailed information on traditional use, safety considerations, cautions, and appropriate supportive context.

**IX. Women's Health Herbal Support Chart (Enhanced Clinical Format)**
**Purpose:**
Herbs used to support women's health across life stages, including hormonal balance, menstrual comfort, reproductive tissue tone, and overall vitality.

---

### PRIMARY HORMONAL & CYCLE REGULATION

(Support endocrine rhythm and menstrual balance)

Rank Herb Rating Page Primary Role

1 **Vitex (Chaste Tree Berry)** ★★★★★ 153
Regulates hormonal signaling and supports healthy menstrual rhythm

2 **Shatavari** ★★★★ 795
Deeply nourishing female tonic that supports hormonal balance and reproductive tissue vitality

---

### REPRODUCTIVE TISSUE & UTERINE TONE

(Strengthen pelvic tissues and reproductive resilience)

Rank Herb Rating Page Primary Role

3 **Red Raspberry Leaf** ★★★★ 414
Tones uterine and pelvic tissues and supports reproductive strength

4 **Dong Quai** ★★★★ 98
Traditional female tonic that supports pelvic circulation and cycle balance

---

### VITALITY & ADAPTIVE SUPPORT

(Support energy, fertility potential, and stress resilience)

Rank Herb Rating Page Primary Role

5 **Maca Root** ★★★★ 803
Adaptogenic root that supports vitality, stamina, and reproductive energy

---

### How to Use This Chart

- Hormonal rhythm & menstrual balance: **Vitex + Shatavari**
- Uterine tone & reproductive support: **Red Raspberry Leaf + Dong Quai**
- Vitality & resilience: **Maca Root**

# X. The Men's Health Herbal Support Chart

This chart highlights herbs traditionally used to support men's health, vitality, hormonal balance, reproductive function, and age-related wellness concerns. It is intended to help readers quickly identify herbs commonly associated with men's physiological support needs within herbal practice.

Use this chart as a reference guide to locate men's health–supportive herbs, then refer to each herb's full entry for detailed information on traditional use, safety considerations, cautions, and appropriate supportive context.

## X. Men's Health Herbal Support Chart *(Enhanced Clinical Format)*

**Purpose:**

Herbs used to support men's vitality, hormonal balance, reproductive health, prostate function, urinary comfort, and overall strength.

---

### 🔘 PRIMARY PROSTATE & URINARY SUPPORT

(Support prostate tissue health and urinary flow)

Rank Herb Rating Page Primary Role

1 🌿 **Saw Palmetto** ★★★★★ 257

Foundational prostate herb supporting urinary flow and hormonal balance

2 🌿 **Pumpkin Seed** ★★★★★ 242

Nutritive prostate tonic supporting urinary comfort and tissue strength

---

### 🔘 HORMONAL & REPRODUCTIVE VITALITY

(Support libido, reproductive function, and endocrine balance)

Rank Herb Rating Page Primary Role

3 🌿 **Maca Root** ★★★★ 803

Supports stamina, fertility, and overall male vitality

4 🌿 **Tribulus** ★★★★ 320

Supports reproductive vitality, libido, and physical strength

---

### 🔘 URINARY & AGE-RELATED SUPPORT

(Support comfort, flow, and long-term male wellness)

Rank Herb Rating Page Primary Role

5 🌿 **Pygeum** ★★★★ 727

Supports prostate comfort and healthy urinary function

6 🌿 **Tongkat Ali** ★★★★ 13

Supports healthy testosterone balance and stress resilience *(cycled use)*

---

### 🧭 How to Use This Chart

- Prostate & urinary support: **Saw Palmetto + Pumpkin Seed**
- Vitality & reproductive strength: **Maca Root + Tribulus**
- Age-related hormonal support: **Pygeum + Tongkat Ali**

# XI. The Anti-Inflammatory Herbal Support Chart

This chart highlights herbs traditionally used to help moderate inflammation, support tissue comfort, and promote healthy recovery responses throughout the body. It is designed to give readers a clear, system-based view of herbs commonly associated with inflammatory balance within herbal practice.

Use this chart as a reference guide to identify inflammation-supportive herbs and understand how they are functionally grouped, then consult each herb's full entry for detailed information on traditional use, safety considerations, cautions, and appropriate supportive context.

**XI. Anti-Inflammatory Herbal Support Chart** ***(Enhanced Clinical Format)***

**Purpose:**
Herbs used to help moderate inflammation, support tissue comfort, and promote healthy recovery responses throughout the body.

---

### PRIMARY SYSTEMIC INFLAMMATION MODULATORS

(Support balanced inflammatory signaling and tissue protection)

Rank Herb Rating Page Primary Role

1 **Turmeric** ★★★★★ 514
Core anti-inflammatory herb that supports systemic balance and antioxidant defense

2 **Boswellia** ★★★★★ 719
Supports joint comfort and healthy inflammatory response, especially in connective tissues

---

### CIRCULATORY & INFLAMMATORY TENSION RELIEF

(Reduce inflammatory stiffness and improve tissue circulation)

Rank Herb Rating Page Primary Role

3 **Ginger Root** ★★★★ 339
Helps moderate inflammatory processes while supporting circulation and comfort

4 **Cayenne Pepper** ★★★★ 53
Improves blood flow to inflamed tissues and provides warming relief

---

### MUSCULOSKELETAL & JOINT COMFORT SUPPORT

(Support mobility and recovery in muscles and joints)

Rank Herb Rating Page Primary Role

5 **Devil's Claw** ★★★★ 101
Supports mobility and recovery in joints and muscles

6 **Willow Bark** ★★★★ 489
Traditional support for inflammation-related discomfort

---

### How to Use This Chart

- Systemic inflammation balance: **Turmeric + Boswellia**
- Stiffness with poor circulation: **Ginger + Cayenne**
- Joint or muscle discomfort: **Devil's Claw + Willow Bark**

## XII. The Musculoskeletal & Joint Support Herbal Support Chart

This chart highlights herbs traditionally used to support muscles, joints, connective tissue, and overall structural comfort. It is designed to help readers quickly identify herbs commonly associated with mobility support, joint resilience, and physical recovery within herbal practice.

Use this chart as a reference guide to locate musculoskeletal-supportive herbs and understand how they are functionally grouped, then refer to each herb's full entry for detailed information on traditional use, safety considerations, cautions, and appropriate supportive context.

**XII. Musculoskeletal & Joint Support Herbal Support Chart *(Enhanced Clinical Format)***

**Purpose:**

Herbs used to support muscles, joints, connective tissue, mobility, and physical recovery.

---

### ⚪ PRIMARY JOINT & CONNECTIVE TISSUE SUPPORT

(Promote joint comfort, cartilage resilience, and healthy inflammatory balance)

Rank Herb Rating Page Primary Role

1 🌿 **Boswellia** ★★★★★ 719

Foundational joint-support herb that promotes comfort and healthy inflammatory response

2 🌿 **Turmeric** ★★★★★ 514

Supports connective tissue integrity and balances inflammation affecting joints

---

### ⚪ MOBILITY & MUSCLE COMFORT SUPPORT

(Ease stiffness, soreness, and movement-related discomfort)

Rank Herb Rating Page Primary Role

3 🌿 **Devil's Claw** ★★★★ 101

Supports joint mobility and muscular recovery

4 🌿 **Willow Bark** ★★★★ 489

Traditional support for musculoskeletal discomfort and recovery

---

### ⚪ CIRCULATION & TISSUE NOURISHMENT

(Improve blood flow to tissues and support structural resilience)

Rank Herb Rating Page Primary Role

5 🌿 **Cayenne Pepper** ★★★★ 53

Enhances circulation to muscles and joints, supporting warmth and comfort

6 🌿 **Horsetail** ★★★★ 433

Silica-rich herb supporting connective tissue strength and structural integrity

---

### How to Use This Chart

- Joint inflammation & stiffness: **Boswellia + Turmeric**
- Mobility & recovery support: **Devil's Claw + Willow Bark**
- Structural strength & circulation: **Horsetail + Cayenne**

# XIII. The Bone, Connective Tissue & Structural Support Herbal Support Chart

This chart highlights herbs traditionally used to support bone strength, connective tissue integrity, mineral balance, and long-term structural resilience. It is intended to help readers quickly identify herbs commonly associated with skeletal support, tissue repair, and foundational physical strength within herbal practice.

Use this chart as a reference guide to locate structure-supportive herbs and understand how they are functionally grouped, then consult each herb's full entry for detailed information on traditional use, safety considerations, cautions, and appropriate supportive context.

## XIII. Bone, Connective Tissue & Structural Support Herbal Support Chart

*(Enhanced Clinical Format)*

**Purpose:**

Herbs used to support bone strength, connective tissue integrity, mineral balance, and long-term structural resilience.

---

### PRIMARY STRUCTURAL & MINERAL TONICS

(Build and maintain bone density and connective tissue strength)

| Rank | Herb | Rating | Page | Primary Role |
|---|---|---|---|---|
| 1 | **Oatstraw** | ★★★★★ | 591 | Premier nutritive tonic rich in minerals that supports bones, nerves, and connective tissue |
| 2 | **Horsetail** | ★★★★ | 433 | Silica-rich herb that strengthens connective tissue, cartilage, hair, and nails |

---

### NUTRITIVE SUPPORT FOR TISSUE REPAIR

(Provide minerals and nourishment for structural maintenance)

| Rank | Herb | Rating | Page | Primary Role |
|---|---|---|---|---|
| 3 | **Nettle Leaf** | ★★★★ | 132 | Mineral-dense tonic supporting bone health, tissue repair, and long-term resilience |
| 4 | **Red Clover** | ★★★ | 815 | Traditional nutritive and lymph-supportive herb aiding tissue health and mineral balance |

---

### CIRCULATION & METABOLIC SUPPORT FOR STRUCTURE

(Support nutrient delivery and waste removal from tissues)

| Rank | Herb | Rating | Page | Primary Role |
|---|---|---|---|---|
| 5 | **Dandelion Leaf** | ★★★★ | 86 | Nutritive diuretic that supports mineral balance and tissue nourishment |
| 6 | **Burdock Root** | ★★★★ | 44 | Supports connective tissue health through detox and metabolic support |

### How to Use This Chart

- Bone density & long-term strength: **Oatstraw + Nettle Leaf**
- Connective tissue & cartilage support: **Horsetail + Oatstraw**
- Structural repair & nourishment: **Nettle Leaf + Burdock Root**

## XIV. Energy & Vitality Herbal Support Chart

This chart highlights herbs traditionally used to support physical energy, mental stamina, resilience, and overall vitality without overstimulation. It is designed to help readers quickly identify herbs commonly associated with sustained energy, adaptive strength, and recovery support within herbal practice.

Use this chart as a reference guide to locate energy- and vitality-supportive herbs and understand how they are functionally grouped. Each grouping reflects a specific role in supporting endurance, stress balance, or long-term vitality. Readers are encouraged to consult each herb's full entry for detailed information on traditional use, safety considerations, cautions, and appropriate supportive context.

**XIV. Energy & Vitality Herbal Support Chart**
**Purpose:**
Herbs used to support physical energy, mental stamina, resilience, and overall vitality without overstimulation.

---

### PRIMARY ADAPTOGENIC ENERGY TONICS

Support sustained energy, mental clarity, and vitality

Rank | Herb | Rating | Page | Primary Role
1 | **Ginseng (Panax / American) | ★★★★★** | 639 | Foundational adaptogen that supports sustained energy, mental clarity, and vitality
2 | **Rhodiola | ★★★★★** | 711 | Enhances stamina, reduces fatigue, and supports stress resilience

---

### LONG-TERM VITALITY & STRESS BALANCE

Support balanced energy and long-term resilience

Rank | Herb | Rating | Page | Primary Role
3 | **Ashwagandha | ★★★★★** | 22 | Builds long-term vitality and supports balanced energy under stress
4 | **Eleuthero | ★★★★** | 651 | Promotes steady energy, immune resilience, and adaptability

---

### ENDURANCE & OXYGEN UTILIZATION SUPPORT

Support stamina, oxygen use, and physical performance

Rank | Herb | Rating | Page | Primary Role
5 | **Cordyceps | ★★★★** | 71 | Supports oxygen utilization, endurance, and physical performance
6 | **Schisandra | ★★★★** | 219 | Supports stamina, liver–energy efficiency, and recovery

---

### How to Use This Chart

- Sustained energy & resilience: **Ginseng (Panax / American) + Rhodiola**
- Stress-balanced vitality: **Ashwagandha + Eleuthero**
- Physical endurance & recovery: **Cordyceps + Schisandra**

# XV. The Stress & Adrenal Support Herbal Support Chart

This chart highlights herbs traditionally used to support the body's response to stress, promote adrenal balance, and protect against physical and mental exhaustion. It is intended to help readers quickly identify herbs commonly associated with stress resilience, nervous–endocrine support, and recovery from prolonged strain within herbal practice.
Use this chart as a reference guide to locate stress- and adrenal-supportive herbs and understand how they are functionally grouped, then consult each herb's full entry for detailed information on traditional use, safety considerations, cautions, and appropriate supportive context.

**XV. Stress & Adrenal Support Herbal Support Chart**
**Purpose:**
Herbs used to support the body's stress response, promote adrenal balance, and protect against physical and mental exhaustion.

---

### 🔘 PRIMARY ADRENAL & STRESS-RESPONSE TONICS

Build resilience and regulate the stress–endocrine axis

Rank | Herb | Rating | Page | Primary Role
1 | 🌿 Ashwagandha | ★★★★★ | 22 | Foundational adaptogen that supports adrenal recovery and balances stress hormones
2 | 🌿 Rhodiola | ★★★★★ | 711 | Enhances stress tolerance, reduces fatigue, and supports mental stamina

---

### 🔘 ADAPTIVE ENERGY & RESILIENCE SUPPORT

Improve endurance and resistance to prolonged stress

Rank | Herb | Rating | Page | Primary Role
3 | 🌿 Eleuthero | ★★★★ | 651 | Supports steady energy output and long-term stress resilience
4 | 🌿 Schisandra | ★★★★ | 219 | Adaptogenic tonic that supports endurance, recovery, and stress adaptation

---

### 🔘 HORMONAL & NERVOUS SYSTEM BALANCE

Support adrenal–nervous system coordination

Rank | Herb | Rating | Page | Primary Role
5 | 🌿 Licorice Root | ★★★★ | 687 | Supports adrenal hormone balance and stress-related fatigue (use with guidance)
6 | 🌿 Maca Root | ★★★★ | 803 | Supports vitality, stamina, and adaptive energy under stress

---

### How to Use This Chart

- Chronic stress & burnout: Ashwagandha + Eleuthero
- Mental fatigue & pressure: Rhodiola + Schisandra
- Low stamina under stress: Maca Root + Ashwagandha
- Adrenal hormone support: Licorice Root (context-dependent)

# XVI. The Sleep & Circadian Rhythm Herbal Support Chart

This chart highlights herbs traditionally used to support healthy sleep patterns, nervous system relaxation, and the body's natural circadian rhythm. It is designed to help readers quickly identify herbs commonly associated with sleep readiness, nighttime calm, and restorative rest within herbal practice.

Use this chart as a reference guide to locate sleep-supportive herbs and understand how they are functionally grouped, then consult each herb's full entry for detailed information on traditional use, safety considerations, cautions, and appropriate supportive context.

**XVI. Sleep & Circadian Rhythm Herbal Support Chart**
**Purpose:**
Herbs used to support healthy sleep patterns, nervous system relaxation, and alignment of the body's natural circadian rhythm.

---

**PRIMARY SLEEP-INITIATION & RELAXATION SUPPORT**

Calm the nervous system and support the transition into sleep

Rank | Herb | Rating | Page | Primary Role

1 | Valerian Root | ★★★★ | 819 | Strong nervine relaxant that supports sleep onset and deep relaxation

2 | Passionflower | ★★★★ | 95 | Calms overactive thoughts and supports sleep readiness

---

**NIGHTTIME CALM & NERVOUS SYSTEM SOOTHING**

Reduce restlessness and promote gentle nighttime calm

Rank | Herb | Rating | Page | Primary Role

3 | Roman Chamomile | ★★★★ | 56 | Gently soothes the nervous system and supports relaxation before sleep

4 | Lavender | ★★★★ | 900 | Fast-acting calming nervine that supports relaxation and sleep onset, especially through aromatic use

5 | Lemon Balm | ★★★★★ | 299 | Calms nervous tension and supports circadian ease without heavy sedation

---

**DEEP REST & SLEEP QUALITY SUPPORT**

Support sustained, restorative sleep

Rank | Herb | Rating | Page | Primary Role

6 | Hops | ★★★ | 260 | Supports deep relaxation and improves sleep continuity

7 | Skullcap | ★★★★ | 668 | Restorative nervine that supports nervous system recovery during sleep

---

**How to Use This Chart**

- Difficulty falling asleep: Valerian Root + Passionflower
- Nighttime restlessness: Roman Chamomile + Lavender
- Light or broken sleep: Hops + Skullcap

## XVII. The Blood Sugar & Metabolic Balance Herbal Support Chart

This chart highlights herbs traditionally used to support healthy blood sugar regulation, metabolic balance, and efficient energy use within the body. It is designed to help readers quickly identify herbs commonly associated with glucose balance, insulin sensitivity support, and metabolic resilience within herbal practice.

Use this chart as a reference guide to locate metabolic-supportive herbs and understand how they are functionally grouped, then consult each herb's full entry for detailed information on traditional use, safety considerations, cautions, and appropriate supportive context.

## XVII. Blood Sugar & Metabolic Balance Herbal Support Chart

**Purpose:**

Herbs used to support healthy blood sugar regulation, metabolic balance, and efficient energy utilization.

---

### ● PRIMARY GLUCOSE & METABOLIC REGULATORS

Support balanced blood sugar handling and metabolic efficiency

Rank | Herb | Rating | Page | Primary Role

1 | 🌿 **Bitter Melon** | ★★★★ | 272 | Supports healthy glucose balance and moderates excessive sugar response

2 | 🌿 **Fenugreek** | ★★★★ | 263 | Supports glucose metabolism and post-meal blood sugar balance

---

### ● INSULIN SENSITIVITY & METABOLIC FLOW

Improve metabolic responsiveness and nutrient handling

Rank | Herb | Rating | Page | Primary Role

3 | 🌿 **Cinnamon** | ★★★★ | 850 | Supports insulin sensitivity and healthy glucose utilization

4 | 🌿 **Nettle Leaf** | ★★★★ | 132 | Nutritive tonic supporting metabolic balance and insulin responsiveness

---

### ● DIGESTIVE–METABOLIC SUPPORT

Support metabolism through digestive and hepatic pathways

Rank | Herb | Rating | Page | Primary Role

5 | 🌿 **Ginger Root** | ★★★★ | 339 | Supports metabolic circulation and healthy post-meal glucose response

6 | 🌿 **Dandelion Root** | ★★★★ | 80 | Supports liver-mediated glucose regulation and metabolic cleansing

---

### 🧭 How to Use This Chart

- Blood sugar balance support: **Bitter Melon + Fenugreek**
- Insulin sensitivity & metabolic efficiency: **Cinnamon + Nettle Leaf**
- Digestive–metabolic support: **Ginger Root + Dandelion Root**

## XVIII. The Weight & Appetite Regulation Herbal Support Chart

This chart highlights herbs traditionally used to support healthy appetite regulation, metabolic efficiency, and balanced weight management. It is designed to help readers quickly identify herbs commonly associated with satiety support, digestive efficiency, and metabolic balance within herbal practice.
Use this chart as a reference guide to locate weight- and appetite-supportive herbs and understand how they are functionally grouped, then consult each herb's full entry for detailed information on traditional use, safety considerations, cautions, and appropriate supportive context.

**XVIII. Weight & Appetite Regulation Herbal Support Chart**
**Purpose:**
Herbs used to support healthy appetite regulation, metabolic efficiency, satiety signaling, and balanced weight management.

---

🟢 **PRIMARY APPETITE & SATIETY REGULATORS**
Support appetite awareness and reduce excessive cravings

Rank | Herb | Rating | Page | Primary Role
1 | 🌿 **Cinnamon | ★★★★** | 850 | Supports satiety signaling and stabilizes appetite through glucose balance
2 | 🌿 **Bitter Melon | ★★★★** | 272 | Supports appetite control and moderates sugar-driven cravings

---

🟢 **METABOLIC EFFICIENCY & FAT UTILIZATION**
Support metabolic rate and energy use

Rank | Herb | Rating | Page | Primary Role
3 | 🌿 **Green Tea | ★★★★** | 441 | Supports metabolic efficiency and fat utilization
4 | 🌿 **Ginger Root | ★★★★** | 339 | Enhances metabolic circulation and digestive efficiency

---

🟢 **DIGESTIVE & APPETITE BALANCE SUPPORT**
Promote balanced digestion and nutrient signaling

Rank | Herb | Rating | Page | Primary Role
5 | 🌿 **Fenugreek | ★★★★** | 263 | Supports satiety and post-meal appetite regulation
6 | 🌿 **Dandelion Root | ★★★★** | 80 | Supports liver–digestive pathways influencing metabolic balance

---

🧭 **How to Use This Chart**
• Appetite control & cravings**: Cinnamon + Fenugreek**
• Metabolic efficiency & fat use: **Green Tea + Ginger Root**
• Digestive–metabolic support: **Dandelion Root + Bitter Melon**

# XIX. The Thyroid & Endocrine Support Herbal Support Chart

This chart highlights herbs traditionally used to support thyroid function, endocrine balance, and hormonal regulation throughout the body. It is designed to help readers quickly identify herbs commonly associated with metabolic signaling, energy regulation, and endocrine system support within herbal practice.

Use this chart as a reference guide to locate thyroid- and endocrine-supportive herbs and understand how they are functionally grouped, then consult each herb's full entry for detailed information on traditional use, safety considerations, cautions, and appropriate supportive context.

**XIX. Thyroid & Endocrine Support Herbal Support Chart**
**Purpose:**
Herbs used to support thyroid function, endocrine balance, metabolic signaling, and healthy hormonal regulation throughout the body.

---

🔘 **PRIMARY ENDOCRINE & THYROID-AXIS TONICS**
Support hormonal signaling and metabolic regulation
Rank | Herb | Rating | Page | Primary Role

1 | 🌿 **Ashwagandha |** ★★★★★ | 22 | Adaptogenic endocrine tonic supporting thyroid balance, stress modulation, and hormonal stability

2 | 🌿 **Schisandra |** ★★★★ | 219 | Supports endocrine resilience, metabolic signaling, and stress–hormone regulation

---

🔘 **ADAPTIVE METABOLIC & HORMONAL SUPPORT**
Promote balanced energy use and endocrine adaptability
Rank | Herb | Rating | Page | Primary Role

3 | 🌿 **Ginseng (American) |** ★★★★ | 639 | Supports endocrine vitality, metabolic signaling, and energy regulation

4 | 🌿 **Rhodiola |** ★★★★ | 711 | Enhances endocrine stress tolerance and supports metabolic balance

---

🔘 **ADRENAL–THYROID COORDINATION SUPPORT**
Supports hormone balance influenced by stress and fatigue
Rank | Herb | Rating | Page | Primary Role

5 | 🌿 **Licorice Root |** ★★★★ | 687 | Supports adrenal–endocrine coordination and hormonal endurance (context-dependent use)

6 | 🌿 **Lemon Balm |** ★★★★ | 299 | Gently calms endocrine overstimulation and supports hormonal balance through nervous-system modulation

---

🧭 **How to Use This Chart**
- Stress-related thyroid imbalance: **Ashwagandha + Schisandra**
- Low metabolic drive or fatigue: **Ginseng (American) + Rhodiola**
- Endocrine strain under stress: **Licorice Root + Ashwagandha**
- Overstimulation or tension: **Lemon Balm**

# XX. The Lymphatic System Herbal Support Chart

This chart highlights herbs traditionally used to support lymphatic circulation, fluid movement, immune waste clearance, and overall cleansing of the body's internal transport system. It is designed to help readers quickly identify herbs commonly associated with lymph flow, tissue drainage, and detox-supportive processes within herbal practice.

Use this chart as a reference guide to locate lymphatic-supportive herbs and understand how they are functionally grouped, then consult each herb's full entry for detailed information on traditional use, safety considerations, cautions, and appropriate supportive context.

**XX. Lymphatic System Herbal Support Chart**
**Purpose:**
Herbs used to support lymphatic circulation, fluid movement, immune waste clearance, and healthy tissue drainage.

---

● **PRIMARY LYMPHATIC MOVERS & CLEANSERS**
Stimulate lymph flow and assist waste transport

Rank | Herb | Rating | Page | Primary Role
1 | 🌿 **Cleavers | ★★★★★** | 775 | Premier lymphatic tonic that promotes gentle lymph flow and tissue drainage
2 | 🌿 **Red Clover | ★★★★** | 815 | Supports lymphatic cleansing and healthy tissue filtration

---

● **FLUID MOVEMENT & TISSUE DRAINAGE SUPPORT**
Encourage circulation of lymph and interstitial fluids

Rank | Herb | Rating | Page | Primary Role
3 | 🌿 **Dandelion Leaf | ★★★★** | 86 | Supports fluid balance and lymph-associated elimination pathways
4 | 🌿 **Parsley | ★★★** | 213 | Mild diuretic supporting fluid movement and tissue drainage

---

● **LYMPH–SKIN & IMMUNE INTERFACE SUPPORT**
Support external elimination and immune-related lymph function

Rank | Herb | Rating | Page | Primary Role
5 | 🌿 **Burdock Root | ★★★★** | 44 | Supports lymphatic detox through blood and skin-clearing pathways
6 | 🌿 **Yellow Dock | ★★★★** | 147 | Supports lymph-linked elimination and metabolic waste clearance

---

**How to Use This Chart**
• Sluggish lymph flow or congestion: **Cleavers + Red Clover**
• Fluid retention & tissue heaviness: **Dandelion Leaf + Parsley**
• Skin-related lymph imbalance: **Burdock Root + Yellow Dock**

# XXI. The Blood Building & Circulation Support Herbal Support Chart

This chart highlights herbs traditionally used to support healthy blood formation, circulation quality, and nutrient delivery throughout the body. It is designed to help readers quickly identify herbs commonly associated with blood nourishment, oxygen transport, and circulatory support within herbal practice, distinct from direct cardiac support.

Use this chart as a reference guide to locate blood-building and circulation-supportive herbs and understand how they are functionally grouped, then consult each herb's full entry for detailed information on traditional use, safety considerations, cautions, and appropriate supportive context.

**XXI. Blood Building & Circulation Support Herbal Support Chart**
**Purpose:**
Herbs used to support healthy blood formation, circulation quality, oxygen delivery, and nutrient transport throughout the body, distinct from direct cardiac support.

---

### ● PRIMARY BLOOD NOURISHING & BUILDING TONICS

Support red blood cell production and overall blood quality

Rank | Herb | Rating | Page | Primary Role
1 | 🌿 Nettle Leaf | ★★★★★ | 132 | Mineral-rich blood tonic that supports red blood cell formation and overall blood nourishment
2 | 🌿 Yellow Dock | ★★★★ | 147 | Supports iron utilization and healthy blood building through improved assimilation

---

### ● CIRCULATION & OXYGEN DELIVERY SUPPORT

Improve blood movement and tissue oxygenation

Rank | Herb | Rating | Page | Primary Role
3 | 🌿 Ginkgo Biloba | ★★★★ | 279 | Enhances peripheral circulation and supports oxygen delivery to tissues
4 | 🌿 Cayenne | ★★★★ | 53 | Stimulates circulation and improves blood flow to extremities

---

### ● BLOOD CLEANSING & QUALITY MAINTENANCE

Support detoxification and blood purity

Rank | Herb | Rating | Page | Primary Role
5 | 🌿 Burdock Root | ★★★★ | 44 | Supports blood cleansing and metabolic waste removal
6 | 🌿 Red Clover | ★★★ | 815 | Traditional blood-cleansing and lymph-supportive tonic aiding circulation quality

---

### How to Use This Chart

- Blood nourishment & rebuilding: Nettle Leaf + Yellow Dock
- Poor circulation or cold extremities: Ginkgo + Cayenne
- Blood cleansing & quality support: Burdock Root + Red Clover

## XXII. The Skin Health & Repair Herbal Support Chart

This chart highlights herbs traditionally used to support skin integrity, repair, and overall dermatological health. It is designed to help readers quickly identify herbs commonly associated with tissue repair, inflammation balance, detox-through-skin pathways, and protection of the body's outer barrier within herbal practice.

Use this chart as a reference guide to locate skin-supportive herbs and understand how they are functionally grouped, then consult each herb's full entry for detailed information on traditional use, safety considerations, cautions, and appropriate supportive context.

## XXII. Skin Health & Repair Herbal Support Chart

**Purpose:**

Herbs used to support skin integrity, tissue repair, inflammation balance, and healthy elimination through the skin.

---

### 🔘 PRIMARY SKIN HEALING & REPAIR TONICS

Promote tissue repair and strengthen the skin barrier

Rank | Herb | Rating | Page | Primary Role

1 | 🌿 Calendula | ★★★★★ | 47 | Premier skin-repair herb supporting wound healing, tissue regeneration, and barrier integrity

2 | 🌿 Aloe Vera | ★★★★★ | 1 | Soothes irritated skin, supports tissue hydration, and promotes repair

---

### 🔘 INFLAMMATION & IRRITATION BALANCE

Calm redness, irritation, and inflammatory skin responses

Rank | Herb | Rating | Page | Primary Role

3 | 🌿 Chamomile (German) | ★★★★ | 396 | Gently soothes inflamed or irritated skin and supports calming repair

4 | 🌿 Plantain Leaf | ★★★★ | 210 | Draws out irritation and supports tissue soothing and repair

---

### 🔘 DETOX & SKIN–LYMPH INTERFACE SUPPORT

Support skin health through internal cleansing pathways

Rank | Herb | Rating | Page | Primary Role

5 | 🌿 Burdock Root | ★★★★ | 44 | Supports skin clarity through blood and lymphatic cleansing

6 | 🌿 Red Clover | ★★★★ | 815 | Supports skin health through lymphatic and detoxification pathways

---

### How to Use This Chart

- Wounds, cuts, or tissue repair: Calendula + Aloe Vera
- Inflamed or irritated skin: Chamomile + Plantain Leaf
- Chronic skin imbalance: Burdock Root + Red Clover

## XXIII. The Hair, Nails & Integumentary Support Herbal Support Chart

This chart highlights herbs traditionally used to support hair strength, nail integrity, skin appendages, and the overall health of the integumentary system. It is designed to help readers quickly identify herbs commonly associated with structural nourishment, mineral support, and long-term tissue resilience within herbal practice.

Use this chart as a reference guide to locate hair-, nail-, and integument-supportive herbs and understand how they are functionally grouped, then consult each herb's full entry for detailed information on traditional use, safety considerations, cautions, and appropriate supportive context.

**XXIII. Hair, Nails & Integumentary Support Herbal Support Chart**

**Purpose:**

Herbs used to support hair strength, nail integrity, mineral nourishment, and long-term health of the integumentary system.

---

### PRIMARY MINERAL & STRUCTURAL TONICS

Provide foundational minerals and structural support

Rank | Herb | Rating | Page | Primary Role

1 | Oatstraw | ★★★★★ | 591 | Mineral-rich nutritive tonic supporting hair strength, nail integrity, and connective tissue

2 | Horsetail | ★★★★ | 433 | Silica-dense herb that strengthens hair, nails, and structural tissues

---

### NUTRITIVE & GROWTH SUPPORT

Support healthy growth and tissue nourishment

Rank | Herb | Rating | Page | Primary Role

3 | Nettle Leaf | ★★★★ | 132 | Provides minerals that support hair growth, nail strength, and tissue resilience

4 | Gotu Kola | ★★★★ | 162 | Supports connective tissue repair, scalp circulation, and structural integrity of skin and hair

---

### CIRCULATION & SCALP SUPPORT

Enhance nutrient delivery to hair follicles

Rank | Herb | Rating | Page | Primary Role

5 | Rosemary | ★★★★ | 369 | Supports scalp circulation and hair follicle nourishment

6 | Burdock Root | ★★★★ | 44 | Supports hair and nail health through blood and detox pathways

---

### How to Use This Chart

- Hair thinning or brittleness: Oatstraw + Nettle Leaf
- Weak nails & structural support: Horsetail + Oatstraw
- Scalp health & circulation: Rosemary + Gotu Kola

# XXIV. The Gut Lining & Mucosal Support Herbal Support Chart

This chart highlights herbs traditionally used to support the integrity of the gut lining, soothe mucosal tissues, and protect the digestive tract from irritation and imbalance. It is designed to help readers quickly identify herbs commonly associated with mucosal repair, barrier protection, and digestive tissue resilience within herbal practice.

Use this chart as a reference guide to locate gut-lining–supportive herbs and understand how they are functionally grouped, then consult each herb's full entry for detailed information on traditional use, safety considerations, cautions, and appropriate supportive context.

**XXIV. Gut Lining & Mucosal Support Herbal Support Chart**
**Purpose:**
Herbs used to support gut lining integrity, soothe mucosal tissues, and protect the digestive tract from irritation and imbalance.

---

### 🔘 PRIMARY MUCOSAL SOOTHING & BARRIER SUPPORT

Protect and repair irritated digestive lining

Rank | Herb | Rating | Page | Primary Role
1 | 🌿 Slippery Elm | ★★★★★ | 295 | Premier demulcent that coats, soothes, and protects the gut lining
2 | 🌿 Marshmallow Root | ★★★★★ | 629 | Deeply soothing mucilage herb supporting mucosal repair and barrier integrity

---

### 🔘 INFLAMMATION & IRRITATION MODULATION

Calm digestive inflammation and sensitivity

Rank | Herb | Rating | Page | Primary Role
3 | 🌿 Licorice Root | ★★★★ | 687 | Supports mucosal healing and reduces inflammatory irritation (context-dependent use)
4 | 🌿 Chamomile (German) | ★★★★ | 396 | Gently calms digestive irritation and supports mucosal comfort

---

### 🔘 MUCOSAL RESILIENCE & DIGESTIVE SUPPORT

Support long-term digestive tissue health

Rank | Herb | Rating | Page | Primary Role
5 | 🌿 Plantain Leaf | ★★★★ | 210 | Draws irritation from mucosal tissues and supports tissue repair
6 | 🌿 Aloe Vera | ★★★★ | 1 | Soothes and hydrates digestive lining while supporting tissue recovery

---

### 🧭 How to Use This Chart

- Irritated or sensitive gut lining: Slippery Elm + Marshmallow Root
- Inflammatory digestive discomfort: Licorice Root + Chamomile
- Barrier repair & resilience: Plantain Leaf + Aloe Vera

## XXV. The Bile Flow & Fat Digestion Herbal Support Chart

This chart highlights herbs traditionally used to support healthy bile production, bile flow, and efficient fat digestion. It is designed to help readers quickly identify herbs commonly associated with liver–digestive coordination, fat metabolism, and digestive comfort within herbal practice.

Use this chart as a reference guide to locate bile- and fat-digestion–supportive herbs and understand how they are functionally grouped, then consult each herb's full entry for detailed information on traditional use, safety considerations, cautions, and appropriate supportive context.

**XXV. Bile Flow & Fat Digestion Herbal Support Chart**
**Purpose:**
Herbs used to support healthy bile production, bile flow, efficient fat digestion, and coordination between the liver and digestive system.

---

### ● PRIMARY BITTER & BILE-STIMULATING TONICS
Stimulate bile flow and improve fat digestion

Rank | Herb | Rating | Page | Primary Role
1 | 🌿 Dandelion Root | ★★★★★ | 80 | Foundational bitter that stimulates bile flow and supports fat digestion
2 | 🌿 Gentian Root | ★★★★★ | 578 | Powerful bitter that stimulates bile flow and digestive secretions, enhancing fat digestion and overall digestive efficiency

---

### ● LIVER–DIGESTIVE AXIS SUPPORT
Enhance liver function related to digestion

Rank | Herb | Rating | Page | Primary Role
3 | 🌿 Artichoke Leaf | ★★★★ | 19 | Promotes bile production and supports fat metabolism
4 | 🌿 Yellow Dock | ★★★★ | 147 | Supports bile movement and elimination of metabolic waste

---

### ● DIGESTIVE COMFORT & FAT UTILIZATION
Support digestion of fats without irritation

Rank | Herb | Rating | Page | Primary Role
5 | 🌿 Ginger | ★★★★ | 339 | Enhances digestive circulation and supports fat utilization
6 | 🌿 Turmeric | ★★★★ | 514 | Supports bile flow while balancing digestive inflammation

---

### 🧭 How to Use This Chart
- Poor fat digestion or heaviness after meals: Dandelion Root + Gentian Root
- Sluggish bile or gallbladder support: Artichoke Leaf + Yellow Dock
- Digestive discomfort with fats: Ginger + Turmeric

# XXVI. The Cognitive Function & Memory Herbal Support Chart

This chart highlights herbs traditionally used to support cognitive clarity, memory retention, focus, and healthy brain function. It is designed to help readers quickly identify herbs commonly associated with mental performance, neurological resilience, and long-term cognitive support within herbal practice.

Use this chart as a reference guide to locate cognitive-supportive herbs and understand how they are functionally grouped, then consult each herb's full entry for detailed information on traditional use, safety considerations, cautions, and appropriate supportive context.

**XXVI. Cognitive Function & Memory Herbal Support Chart**
**Purpose:**
Herbs used to support cognitive clarity, memory retention, focus, neurological resilience, and long-term brain health.

---

🔘 **PRIMARY COGNITIVE & MEMORY TONICS**
Enhance memory formation, recall, and mental clarity

Rank | Herb | Rating | Page | Primary Role
1 | 🌿 Ginkgo Biloba | ★★★★★ | 279 | Improves cerebral circulation and supports memory, focus, and mental clarity
2 | 🌿 Bacopa | ★★★★ | 107 | Traditional nootropic supporting memory consolidation and cognitive resilience

---

🔘 **NEUROPROTECTIVE & STRESS-COGNITION SUPPORT**
Protect brain tissue and reduce stress-related cognitive decline

Rank | Herb | Rating | Page | Primary Role
3 | 🌿 Rhodiola | ★★★★ | 711 | Supports mental stamina, focus, and cognitive performance under stress
4 | 🌿 Lion's Mane | ★★★★ | 695 | Supports nerve growth, cognitive clarity, and long-term brain health

---

🔘 **FOCUS, ALERTNESS & MENTAL ENERGY**
Support attention, alertness, and sustained mental energy

Rank | Herb | Rating | Page | Primary Role
5 | 🌿 Rosemary | ★★★★ | 369 | Enhances mental alertness and supports memory through circulatory stimulation
6 | 🌿 Gotu Kola | ★★★★ | 162 | Supports cognitive calm, focus, and nervous system–brain integration

**How to Use This Chart**
• Memory & long-term cognitive support: Ginkgo Biloba + Bacopa
• Mental fatigue or stress-related decline: Rhodiola + Lion's Mane
• Focus, alertness, and clarity: Rosemary + Gotu Kola

## XXVII. The Eye & Vision Herbal Support Chart

This chart highlights herbs traditionally used to support eye health, visual clarity, circulation to ocular tissues, and long-term vision protection. It is designed to help readers quickly identify herbs commonly associated with retinal support, eye strain relief, and visual system nourishment within herbal practice.

Use this chart as a reference guide to locate eye- and vision-supportive herbs and understand how they are functionally grouped, then consult each herb's full entry for detailed information on traditional use, safety considerations, cautions, and appropriate supportive context.

**XXVII. Eye & Vision Herbal Support Chart**
**Purpose:**
Herbs used to support eye health, visual clarity, circulation to ocular tissues, and long-term protection of vision.

---

### 🔘 PRIMARY RETINAL & VISION TONICS

Support retinal integrity and visual acuity

Rank | Herb | Rating | Page | Primary Role
1 | 🌿 Bilberry | ★★★★★ | 726 | Premier vision herb supporting retinal health, night vision, and capillary strength
2 | 🌿 Eyebright | ★★★★ | 276 | Traditional ocular tonic supporting eye comfort and visual clarity

---

### 🔘 OCULAR CIRCULATION & OXYGEN DELIVERY

Improve blood flow to eye tissues

Rank | Herb | Rating | Page | Primary Role
3 | 🌿 Ginkgo Biloba | ★★★★ | 279 | Enhances circulation to ocular tissues and supports oxygen delivery
4 | 🌿 Cayenne | ★★★★ | 53 | Stimulates circulation, supporting nutrient delivery to the eyes

---

### 🔘 ANTIOXIDANT & CELLULAR PROTECTION

Protect eye tissues from oxidative stress

Rank | Herb | Rating | Page | Primary Role
5 | 🌿 Turmeric | ★★★★ | 514 | Supports ocular tissue protection through anti-inflammatory and antioxidant action
6 | 🌿 Schisandra | ★★★★ | 219 | Supports cellular protection and microcirculation relevant to eye health

---

### How to Use This Chart

- Retinal support & visual acuity: Bilberry + Eyebright
- Poor ocular circulation or eye strain: Ginkgo + Cayenne
- Oxidative or inflammatory eye stress: Turmeric + Schisandra
- Consult each herb's full entry for safety considerations, cautions, and appropriate context

# XXVIII. The Seasonal & Acute Immune Support Herbal Support Chart

This chart highlights herbs traditionally used to support the body during short-term immune challenges, seasonal stressors, and periods of increased immune demand. It is designed to help readers quickly identify herbs commonly associated with acute immune readiness, early-response support, and recovery during temporary immune strain within herbal practice.

Use this chart as a reference guide to locate seasonal and acute immune–supportive herbs and understand how they are functionally grouped, then consult each herb's full entry for detailed information on traditional use, safety considerations, cautions, and appropriate supportive context.

**XXVIII. Seasonal & Acute Immune Support Herbal Support Chart**
**Purpose:**
Herbs used to support the body during short-term immune challenges, seasonal stressors, and periods of increased immune demand.

---

### ● RAPID IMMUNE RESPONSE
Activate the body's defenses at the first sign of illness

Rank | Herb | Rating | Page | Primary Role
1 | 🌿 Echinacea | ★★★★★ | 746 | Activates immune response and shortens the course of early-stage illness
2 | 🌿 Elderberry | ★★★★★ | 887 | Antiviral support that reduces duration and severity of seasonal illness

---

### ● FEVER & ACUTE SYMPTOM SUPPORT
Ease fever, aches, and acute febrile discomfort

Rank | Herb | Rating | Page | Primary Role
3 | 🌿 Yarrow | ★★★★★ | 122 | Traditional fever-management herb that promotes healthy sweating and early symptom relief
4 | 🌿 Boneset | ★★★★ | 37 | Classic acute-fever and flu-onset herb, traditionally used for body aches

---

### ● ANTIMICROBIAL DEFENSE
Support the body's resistance to seasonal pathogens

Rank | Herb | Rating | Page | Primary Role
5 | 🌿 Garlic | ★★★★ | 841 | Broad-spectrum antimicrobial support during cold and flu season
6 | 🌿 Oregano Oil | ★★★★ | 291 | Potent antimicrobial oil for acute seasonal infections

---

### How to Use This Chart
- Early illness response: Echinacea + Elderberry
- Fever and body aches: Yarrow + Boneset
- Antimicrobial defense: Garlic + Oregano Oil

## XXIX. The Recovery, Healing & Tissue Repair Herbal Support Chart

This chart highlights herbs traditionally used to support the body's natural healing processes, tissue repair, and recovery following physical strain, injury, or prolonged stress. It is designed to help readers quickly identify herbs commonly associated with regeneration, restorative support, and strengthening of healing pathways within herbal practice.

Use this chart as a reference guide to locate recovery- and repair-supportive herbs and understand how they are functionally grouped, then consult each herb's full entry for detailed information on traditional use, safety considerations, cautions, and appropriate supportive context.

**XXIX. Recovery, Healing & Tissue Repair Herbal Support Chart**
**Purpose:**
Herbs used to support tissue repair, recovery from physical strain or injury, and the body's natural healing processes.

---

### 🔘 PRIMARY TISSUE HEALING & REGENERATION SUPPORT

Promote repair, regeneration, and recovery

Rank | Herb | Rating | Page | Primary Role

1 | 🌿 Comfrey (external use) | ★★★★★ | 68 | Traditionally used to support tissue repair and regeneration (external use only)

2 | 🌿 Calendula | ★★★★★ | 47 | Supports wound healing, tissue regeneration, and recovery of damaged skin

---

### 🔘 INFLAMMATION & RECOVERY MODULATION

Support healing by moderating inflammation

Rank | Herb | Rating | Page | Primary Role

3 | 🌿 Turmeric | ★★★★ | 514 | Supports tissue repair by balancing inflammation and oxidative stress

4 | 🌿 Boswellia | ★★★★ | 719 | Supports recovery and comfort in healing tissues and joints

---

### 🔘 CIRCULATION & NUTRIENT DELIVERY

Enhance blood flow to healing tissues

Rank | Herb | Rating | Page | Primary Role

5 | 🌿 Cayenne | ★★★★ | 53 | Improves circulation to injured tissues, supporting healing processes

6 | 🌿 Gotu Kola | ★★★★ | 162 | Supports connective tissue repair and microcirculation during recovery

---

### How to Use This Chart

- Wound or tissue repair: Calendula + Comfrey (external)
- Inflammation during recovery: Turmeric + Boswellia
- Circulation to healing tissues: Cayenne + Gotu Kola

# XXX. The Mineral & Nutritive Tonics Herbal Support Chart

This chart highlights herbs traditionally used to provide foundational nourishment, mineral replenishment, and long-term support for overall vitality. It is designed to help readers quickly identify herbs commonly associated with nutritive support, tissue nourishment, and rebuilding strength through gentle, food-like herbal tonics within herbal practice.

Use this chart as a reference guide to locate mineral- and nutritive-supportive herbs and understand how they are functionally grouped, then consult each herb's full entry for detailed information on traditional use, safety considerations, cautions, and appropriate supportive context.

## XXX. Mineral & Nutritive Tonics Herbal Support Chart

**Purpose:**
Herbs used to provide foundational nourishment, mineral replenishment, and long-term support for tissue strength, vitality, and rebuilding.

---

### PRIMARY MINERAL & NUTRITIVE TONICS

Deliver broad-spectrum minerals and food-like nourishment

| Rank | Herb | Rating | Page | Primary Role |
|---|---|---|---|---|
| 1 | Oatstraw | ★★★★★ | 591 | Premier nutritive tonic rich in minerals that support bones, nerves, and connective tissue |
| 2 | Nettle Leaf | ★★★★★ | 132 | Mineral-dense tonic supporting blood, bones, and long-term tissue nourishment |

---

### CONNECTIVE TISSUE & STRUCTURAL NOURISHMENT

Support cartilage, skin, hair, nails, and structural resilience

| Rank | Herb | Rating | Page | Primary Role |
|---|---|---|---|---|
| 3 | Horsetail | ★★★★ | 433 | Silica-rich herb supporting connective tissue strength and integrity |
| 4 | Red Clover | ★★★★ | 815 | Nutritive and lymph-supportive tonic aiding tissue nourishment and balance |

---

### DIGESTIVE & ASSIMILATION SUPPORT

Improve nutrient uptake and metabolic utilization

| Rank | Herb | Rating | Page | Primary Role |
|---|---|---|---|---|
| 5 | Dandelion Leaf | ★★★★ | 86 | Supports mineral assimilation and nutritive balance through gentle elimination |
| 6 | Alfalfa | ★★★★ | 7 | Deeply nutritive herb supporting vitamin and mineral replenishment |

---

### How to Use This Chart

- General nourishment & rebuilding: Oatstraw + Nettle Leaf
- Connective tissue & mineral support: Horsetail + Red Clover
- Improved nutrient assimilation: Dandelion Leaf + Alfalfa

## XXXI. The Longevity & Cellular Protection Herbal Support Chart

This chart highlights herbs traditionally used to support cellular health, resilience against oxidative stress, and long-term vitality associated with healthy aging. It is designed to help readers quickly identify herbs commonly associated with cellular protection, antioxidant support, and preservation of functional capacity over time within herbal practice.

Use this chart as a reference guide to locate longevity- and cellular-supportive herbs and understand how they are functionally grouped, then consult each herb's full entry for detailed information on traditional use, safety considerations, cautions, and appropriate supportive context.

## XXXI. Longevity & Cellular Protection Herbal Support Chart

**Purpose**
Herbs used to support cellular health, protect against oxidative stress, and promote long-term vitality associated with healthy aging.

---

### PRIMARY CELLULAR PROTECTION & ANTIOXIDANT TONICS

Protect cells from oxidative damage and support longevity pathways

| Rank | Herb | Rating | Page | Primary Role |
|---|---|---|---|---|
| 1 | **Milk Thistle** | ★★★★★ | 31 | Protects liver cells, supports detoxification, and enhances cellular resilience |
| 2 | **Turmeric** | ★★★★★ | 514 | Supports antioxidant defense and cellular inflammation balance |

---

### ADAPTOGENIC & STRESS-RESILIENCE SUPPORT

Support cellular adaptation and long-term vitality under stress

| Rank | Herb | Rating | Page | Primary Role |
|---|---|---|---|---|
| 3 | **Schisandra** | ★★★★ | 219 | Adaptogenic tonic supporting cellular endurance and detox efficiency |
| 4 | **Rhodiola** | ★★★★ | 711 | Supports cellular energy balance and resilience to stress-related aging |

---

### CIRCULATORY & MITOCHONDRIAL SUPPORT

Support nutrient delivery and cellular energy production

| Rank | Herb | Rating | Page | Primary Role |
|---|---|---|---|---|
| 5 | **Ginkgo Biloba** | ★★★★ | 279 | Enhances microcirculation and oxygen delivery to cells |
| 6 | **Cordyceps** | ★★★★ | 71 | Supports mitochondrial efficiency and cellular energy production |

---

### How to Use This Chart

- Cellular protection & detox support: **Milk Thistle + Turmeric**
- Stress resilience & longevity: **Schisandra + Rhodiola**
- Cellular energy & circulation: **Cordyceps + Ginkgo**

Consult each herb's full entry for safety considerations, cautions, and appropriate context.

# XXXII. The Gentle Daily Tonics & Nervine Support Herbal Support Chart

This chart highlights herbs traditionally used for gentle, ongoing support of overall vitality, emotional steadiness, and nervous system balance. It is designed to help readers identify herbs commonly regarded as suitable for regular use that nourish the body, support resilience to daily stress, and promote calm, steady well-being without excessive stimulation or heavy sedation.

Use this chart as a reference guide to locate gentle tonic, nutritive, nervine, and adaptogenic-supportive herbs and to understand how they are functionally grouped. Then consult each herb's full entry for detailed information on traditional use, safety considerations, cautions, and appropriate supportive context.

## XXXII. Gentle Daily Tonics & Nervine Support Herbal Support Chart

**Purpose:**
Herbs used for gentle, ongoing daily support of nourishment, emotional steadiness, nervous system balance, and resilience without overstimulation.

---

### ● PRIMARY DAILY NOURISHING TONICS

| Rank | Herb | Rating | Page | Primary Role |
|---|---|---|---|---|
| 1 | 🌿 Oatstraw | ★★★★★ | 591 | Deep nutritive tonic supporting nerves and long-term vitality |
| 2 | 🌿 Nettle Leaf | ★★★★★ | 132 | Mineral-rich tonic supporting blood, tissues, and steady nourishment |

---

### ● CALMING NERVINE SUPPORT

| Rank | Herb | Rating | Page | Primary Role |
|---|---|---|---|---|
| 3 | 🌿 Lemon Balm | ★★★★ | 299 | Gentle nervine supporting mood balance and calm resilience |
| 4 | 🌿 Chamomile (Roman) | ★★★★ | 56 | Calms nervous tension and supports daily emotional balance |

---

### ● ADAPTIVE DAILY RESILIENCE

| Rank | Herb | Rating | Page | Primary Role |
|---|---|---|---|---|
| 5 | 🌿 Skullcap | ★★★★ | 668 | Restorative nervine supporting nervous system repair |
| 6 | 🌿 Holy Basil (Tulsi) | ★★★★ | 715 | Adaptogenic tonic supporting steady daily stress balance |

---

### How to Use This Chart

- Daily nourishment: Oatstraw + Nettle
- Gentle calm: Lemon Balm + Chamomile

- **Nervous system restoration: Skullcap**
- **Daily stress balance: Holy Basil**

**Consult full herb entries for safety and context.**

## XXXIII. The Strong / High-Caution Herbs (Educational Reference Chart)

This chart highlights herbs traditionally regarded as **powerful, fast-acting, or requiring heightened caution** due to their potency, narrow safety margins, or context-dependent use. It is intended strictly as an **educational reference**, not as a recommendation for casual or unsupervised use.

Use this chart to understand which herbs are considered high-impact within herbal practice, why additional care is required, and where professional guidance, dosage awareness, and individual health considerations are essential. Always consult each herb's full entry for detailed safety information, contraindications, and proper context of use.

## XXXIII. Strong / High-Caution Herbs (Educational Reference Chart)

### *(Enhanced Clinical Format — EDUCATIONAL USE ONLY)*

**Purpose:**
Herbs recognized for strong physiological effects that require heightened caution, precise dosing, context awareness, or professional guidance. This chart is not a recommendation list; it exists solely to educate readers about potency and risk.

---

● **CARDIOVASCULAR & NEUROACTIVE STIMULANTS**
Powerful effects on circulation, nerves, or cardiac output

| Rank | Herb | Rating | Page | Primary Role |
|---|---|---|---|---|
| 1 | 🌿 **Yohimbe** | ★★★ | 417 | Potent circulatory and neuroactive stimulant; narrow safety margin |
| 2 | 🌿 **Cayenne** | ★★★ | 53 | Strong circulatory stimulant affecting blood flow and heat regulation |

---

● **HORMONAL & ENDOCRINE-ACTIVE HERBS**
Strong effects on hormonal signaling; context-dependent use

| Rank | Herb | Rating | Page | Primary Role |
|---|---|---|---|---|
| 3 | 🌿 **Tongkat Ali** | ★★★★ | 13 | Potent endocrine modulator supporting testosterone balance (cycled use) |
| 4 | 🌿 **Licorice Root** | ★★★★ | 687 | Influences adrenal hormones and electrolyte balance (dose-dependent use) |

---

● **NEUROSEDATIVE & CNS-ACTIVE HERBS**
Strong effects on the central nervous system

| Rank | Herb | Rating | Page | Primary Role |
|---|---|---|---|---|
| 5 | 🌿 **Valerian Root** | ★★★ | 819 | Strong nervine sedative affecting sleep and CNS tone |
| 6 | 🌿 **Skullcap** | ★★★ | 668 | Deep CNS-active nervine requiring proper context and dosing |

---

### 🔘 TOXICITY-SENSITIVE / RESTRICTED-USE HERBS

Require strict context, preparation, or avoidance

| Rank | Herb | Rating | Page | Primary Role |
|---|---|---|---|---|
| 7 | 🌿 **Comfrey (internal use restricted)** | ★★★ | 68 | Tissue-repair herb with hepatotoxic risk when used internally |
| 8 | 🌿 **Nightshade (*Atropa belladonna*)** | ★★ | 450 | Highly toxic anticholinergic herb — historical use only |

---

### 🧭 How to Use This Chart

**This chart is provided strictly for educational and safety awareness purposes.**
**It is not a recommendation list and is not intended to guide casual, unsupervised, or self-directed use.**

**The herbs included here are recognized for their potency, narrow safety margins, or context-dependent effects. Because of this, their casual or uninformed use is not recommended. Their presence in this chart is intended only to help readers recognize herbs traditionally regarded as high-impact and requiring greater caution within herbal practice.**

# How to Use the Symptoms Index

The Symptoms Index in this section is designed as a reference tool to help readers explore common symptoms and locate herbs within this book that have traditionally been used to support the body systems involved.
These charts are not diagnostic. A single symptom may arise from many underlying causes and may appear in more than one chart. For this reason, the Symptoms Index is intended to guide you in your studies, not to identify conditions or prescribe treatment.

Using the Index

- Locate the symptom you wish to explore
- Note the herbs listed alongside it
- Turn to the referenced herb pages for full details, including safety guidance
- Cross-reference charts when symptoms overlap

The Symptoms Index works best when used alongside the Herbal Support Charts and individual herb entries, allowing the reader to understand both the system involved and the nature of the herbal support.

**Important Note:**

**Persistent or severe symptoms should always be evaluated by a qualified healthcare provider. Herbs should be used with care, respect, and attention to individual response.**

# EXPANDED SYMPTOM INDEX

*The Herbal Resurrection • A Quick Reference Guide for Finding the Right Herbs*

*Look up your symptom or concern, find the herbs traditionally associated with it, then turn to each herb's full page for safety notes, dosage, and complete guidance. This index is not a diagnostic tool — it is a directional reference only.*

## A — *15 symptoms*


**Acid Reflux** — *Slippery Elm* (297) · *Marshmallow* (654) · *Licorice Root* (700)
**Acidic Body (pH Balance Support)** — *Barley Grass* (334) · *Alfalfa* (7) · *Lemon Balm* (301)
**Acne** — *Burdock Root* (43) · *Neem* (890) · *Yellow Dock* (146)
**Acne (Hormonal)** — *Chaste Tree* (152) · *Burdock Root* (43) · *Neem* (890)
**Adrenal Fatigue** — *Ashwagandha* (22) · *Rhodiola* (724) · *Eleuthero* (665)
**Adrenal Stress** — *Ashwagandha* (22) · *Rhodiola* (724) · *Eleuthero* (665)
**Aging (General Vitality)** — *Gynostemma* (668) · *Reishi* (704) · *Ashwagandha* (22)
**Alcohol Recovery Support** — *Milk Thistle* (31) · *Kudzu Root* (894) · *Dandelion Root* (79)
**Allergies (Seasonal)** — *Nettle Leaf* (131) · *Eyebright* (277) · *Turmeric* (515)
**Anemia** — *Nettle Leaf* (131) · *Yellow Dock* (146) · *Dandelion Root* (79)
**Anxiety / Nervous Tension** — *Passion Flower* (94) · *Lemon Balm* (301) · *Skullcap* (682) · *Lavender* (911)
**Appetite Loss** — *Dandelion Root* (79) · *Fennel Seed* (783)
**Arthritis / Joint Pain** — *Turmeric* (515) · *Boswellia* (732) · *Ginger Root* (341)
**Asthma** — *Mullein Leaf* (312) · *Elecampane* (267) · *Licorice Root* (700)
**Athlete's Foot (Fungal)** — *Tea Tree* (521) · *Garlic* (853) · *Pau d'Arco* (675)


## B — *10 symptoms*


**Back Pain (General)** — *Willow Bark* (491) · *Turmeric* (515) · *Ginger Root* (341)
**Bloating / Gas** — *Fennel Seed* (783) · *Peppermint* (860) · *Ginger Root* (341)
**Blood Circulation (Poor)** — *Ginkgo Biloba* (281) · *Cayenne Pepper* (52) · *Hawthorn Berry* (316)
**Blood Cleansing** — *Burdock Root* (43) · *Yellow Dock* (146) · *Red Clover* (827)
**Blood Pressure (High)** — *Hawthorn Berry* (316) · *Olive Leaf* (353) · *Garlic* (853)
**Blood Sugar (High / Diabetes Support)** — *Bitter Melon* (273) · *Ceylon Cinnamon* (862) · *Fenugreek* (264)
**Brain Fog** — *Bacopa* (106) · *Ginkgo Biloba* (281) · *Lion's Mane* (1011)
**Bronchitis / Chest Congestion** — *Mullein Leaf* (312) · *Elecampane* (267) · *Thyme* (374)
**Bruises / Swelling** — *Arnica* (16) · *Calendula* (46) · *Comfrey* (67)
**Burns (Minor)** — *Aloe Vera* (1) · *Calendula* (46)


## C — *9 symptoms*

**Candida / Yeast Overgrowth** — *Pau d'Arco* (675) · *Oregano Oil* (293) · *Garlic* (853)
**Chronic Fatigue** — *Rhodiola* (724) · *Ashwagandha* (22) · *American Ginseng* (652)
**Chronic Pain** — *Turmeric* (515) · *Willow Bark* (491) · *Corydalis* (404)
**Cognitive Decline (Support)** — *Bacopa* (106) · *Ginkgo Biloba* (281) · *Lion's Mane* (1011)
**Cold Hands & Feet** — *Ginger Root* (341) · *Cayenne Pepper* (52) · *Ginkgo Biloba* (281)
**Cold Sores** — *Lemon Balm* (301) · *Licorice Root* (700) · *Echinacea* (758)
**Constipation** — *Slippery Elm* (297) · *Senna Leaf* (641) · *Aloe Vera* (1)
**Constipation (Chronic)** — *Slippery Elm* (297) · *Marshmallow Root* (671) · *Senna Leaf* (641)
**Cuts / Wounds** — *Calendula* (46) · *Plantain Leaf* (210) · *Comfrey* (67)

## D — *6 symptoms*

**Dandruff / Scalp Issues** — *Neem* (890) · *Rosemary* (371) · *Tea Tree* (521)
**Depression (Mild Support)** — *St. John's Wort* (377) · *Rhodiola* (724) · *Ashwagandha* (22)
**Detox (General Support)** — *Milk Thistle* (31) · *Burdock Root* (43) · *Dandelion Root* (79)
**Diarrhea** — *Slippery Elm* (297) · *Red Raspberry Leaf* (416)
**Digestive Weakness** — *Ginger Root* (341) · *Dandelion Root* (79)
**Dry Skin** — *Sea Buckthorn* (697) · *Aloe Vera* (1) · *Borage Seed* (857)

## E — *5 symptoms*

**Ear Infections** — *Garlic* (853) · *Mullein Leaf* (312) · *Echinacea* (758)
**Eczema** — *Chickweed* (58) · *Calendula* (46) · *Burdock Root* (43)
**Edema (Fluid Retention)** — *Dandelion Leaf* (85) · *Parsley* (214) · *Cleavers* (787)
**Energy (Low)** — *Rhodiola* (724) · *Eleuthero* (665) · *Maca Root* (815)
**Eye Fatigue / Strain** — *Bilberry* (766) · *Eyebright* (277) · *Goji Berry* (621)

## F — *6 symptoms*

**Fatigue (General)** — *American Ginseng* (652) · *Ashwagandha* (22) · *Rhodiola* (724)
**Fever** — *Yarrow* (121) · *Willow Bark* (491)
**Fibromyalgia** — *Ashwagandha* (22) · *Rhodiola* (724) · *Turmeric* (515)
**Flatulence (Chronic)** — *Fennel Seed* (783) · *Caraway Seed* (389) · *Ginger Root* (341)
**Fungal Infections (Internal)** — *Pau d'Arco* (675) · *Oregano Oil* (293) · *Garlic* (853)
**Fungal Infections (Skin)** — *Tea Tree* (521) · *Neem* (890) · *Garlic* (853)

## G — *6 symptoms*

**Gallbladder Support** — *Dandelion Root* (79) · *Turmeric* (515) · *Artichoke Leaf* (19)
**Gastric Ulcers** — *Slippery Elm* (297) · *Licorice Root* (700) · *Aloe Vera* (1)
**Gastritis (Stomach Inflammation)** — *Roman Chamomile* (55) · *Licorice Root* (700) · *Marshmallow Root* (671)
**Gout** — *Nettle Leaf* (131) · *Turmeric* (515)
**Gums (Inflamed / Bleeding)** — *Myrrh* (237) · *Sage* (865)
**Gut Healing** — *Slippery Elm* (297) · *Marshmallow Root* (671) · *Licorice Root* (700)

## H — *6 symptoms*

**Hair Loss / Thinning** — *Rosemary* (371) · *Nettle Leaf* (131) · *Horsetail* (435)
**Headaches (General)** — *Peppermint* (860) · *Willow Bark* (491) · *Lavender* (911)
**Heart Health (General Tonic)** — *Hawthorn Berry* (316) · *Motherwort* (115) · *Garlic* (853)
**Hemorrhoids** — *Witch Hazel* (182) · *Horse Chestnut* (736) · *Butcher's Broom* (383)
**High Cholesterol** — *Garlic* (853) · *Artichoke Leaf* (19)
**Hormonal Imbalance (General)** — *Maca Root* (815) · *Chaste Tree* (152) · *Dong Quai* (97)

## I — *6 symptoms*

**Immune Defense (Preventative)** — *Astragalus* (25) · *Reishi* (704) · *Elderberry* (898)
**Immune Weakness** — *Astragalus* (25) · *Reishi* (704) · *Elderberry* (898)
**Indigestion** — *Ginger Root* (341) · *Peppermint* (860) · *Fennel Seed* (783)
**Inflammation (Chronic)** — *Turmeric* (515) · *Boswellia* (732) · *Ginger Root* (341)
**Insomnia / Sleep Trouble** — *Valerian* (831) · *Passion Flower* (94) · *Lemon Balm* (301) · *Lavender* (911)
**Irritable Bowel (IBS)** — *Peppermint* (860) · *Roman Chamomile* (55) · *Slippery Elm* (297)

## J — *2 symptoms*

**Joint Inflammation** — *Turmeric* (515) · *Boswellia* (732) · *Devil's Claw* (100)
**Joint Stiffness (Morning)** — *Turmeric* (515) · *Ginger Root* (341) · *Boswellia* (732)

## K — *3 symptoms*

**Kidney Inflammation** — *Corn Silk* (73) · *Couch Grass* (185) · *Nettle Leaf* (131)
**Kidney Stones (Support)** — *Chanca Piedra* (149) · *Corn Silk* (73) · *Goldenrod* (128)
**Kidney Support / Cleanse** — *Nettle Leaf* (131) · *Parsley* (214) · *Corn Silk* (73) · *Juniper Berry* (506)

## L — *7 symptoms*

**Leaky Gut** — *Slippery Elm* (297) · *Marshmallow Root* (671) · *Licorice Root* (700)
**Libido (Low)** — *Maca Root* (815) · *Tongkat Ali* (13) · *Damiana* (82)
**Liver Health / Detox** — *Milk Thistle* (31) · *Dandelion Root* (79) · *Burdock Root* (43)
**Low Immunity (Chronic)** — *Astragalus* (25) · *Reishi* (704) · *Echinacea* (758)
**Low Testosterone** — *Tongkat Ali* (13) · *Tribulus* (322) · *Ashwagandha* (22)
**Lung Support (General)** — *Mullein Leaf* (312) · *Elecampane* (267) · *Licorice Root* (700)
**Lymphatic Congestion** — *Cleavers* (787) · *Red Clover* (827) · *Burdock Root* (43)

## M — *7 symptoms*

**Memory / Focus Support** — *Ginkgo Biloba* (281) · *Bacopa* (106) · *Rosemary* (371)
**Menopause (Hot Flashes)** — *Black Cohosh* (799) · *Sage* (865) · *Red Clover* (827)
**Menstrual Cramps** — *Cramp Bark* (76) · *Ginger Root* (341) · *Roman Chamomile* (55)
**Migraine Headaches** — *Feverfew* (61) · *Peppermint* (860)
**Mood Support** — *St. John's Wort* (377) · *Rhodiola* (724)

**Muscle Cramps** — *Cramp Bark* (76) · *Oatstraw* (593) · *Valerian* (831)
**Muscle Soreness (Post-Exercise)** — *Arnica* (16) · *Turmeric* (515) · *Ginger Root* (341)

## N — *6 symptoms*

**Nail Fungus** — *Tea Tree* (521) · *Pau d'Arco* (675) · *Garlic* (853)
**Nausea (General)** — *Ginger Root* (341) · *Peppermint* (860) · *Fennel Seed* (783)
**Nerve Pain** — *St. John's Wort* (377) · *Corydalis* (404) · *Skullcap* (682)
**Neuropathy (Peripheral)** — *St. John's Wort* (377) · *Corydalis* (404) · *Ginkgo Biloba* (281)
**Night Sweats** — *Sage* (865) · *Black Cohosh* (799) · *Motherwort* (115)
**Numbness / Tingling** — *Ginkgo Biloba* (281) · *Cayenne Pepper* (52) · *St. John's Wort* (377)

## O — *4 symptoms*

**Obesity / Weight Management** — *Green Tea* (443) · *Yerba Maté* (669)
**Oedema (Ankles / Legs)** — *Dandelion Leaf* (85) · *Horse Chestnut* (736) · *Cleavers* (787)
**Oral Health (General)** — *Myrrh* (237) · *Sage* (865) · *Peppermint* (860)
**Osteoarthritis** — *Boswellia* (732) · *Turmeric* (515) · *Devil's Claw* (100)

## P — *6 symptoms*

**Pain (General)** — *Willow Bark* (491) · *Turmeric* (515) · *Ginger Root* (341)
**Panic Attacks** — *Passion Flower* (94) · *Valerian* (831) · *Lemon Balm* (301) · *Lavender* (911)
**Parasites (Intestinal)** — *Wormwood* (429) · *Black Walnut Hull* (289) · *Clove Basil* (350)
**PMS (Premenstrual Syndrome)** — *Chaste Tree Berry* (152) · *Cramp Bark* (76) · *Lemon Balm* (301)
**Poor Circulation** — *Ginkgo Biloba* (281) · *Cayenne Pepper* (52) · *Hawthorn Berry* (316)
**Prostate Health (BPH)** — *Saw Palmetto* (258) · *Pygeum* (740) · *Nettle Leaf* (131)

## R — *4 symptoms*

**Respiratory Infections (Colds / Flu)** — *Echinacea* (758) · *Garlic* (853)
**Restlessness / Hyperactivity** — *Lemon Balm* (301) · *Passion Flower* (94) · *Skullcap* (682) · *Lavender* (911)
**Rheumatism** — *Nettle Leaf* (131) · *Turmeric* (515) · *Devil's Claw* (100)
**Rosacea** — *Calendula* (46) · *Chickweed* (58) · *Burdock Root* (43)

## S — *7 symptoms*

**Sciatica** — *Corydalis* (404) · *Devil's Claw* (100) · *Willow Bark* (491)
**Sinus Congestion** — *Eucalyptus* (633) · *Peppermint* (860)
**Skin Healing** — *Calendula* (46) · *Comfrey* (67) · *Aloe Vera* (1)
**Skin Irritations / Rashes** — *Calendula* (46) · *Roman Chamomile* (55) · *Aloe Vera* (1)
**Stress (Chronic)** — *Ashwagandha* (22) · *Rhodiola* (724) · *Holy Basil* (728)
**Sunburn Relief** — *Aloe Vera* (1) · *Calendula* (46) · *Lavender* (911)
**Swollen Lymph Nodes** — *Cleavers* (787) · *Echinacea* (758) · *Red Clover* (827)

## T — *5 symptoms*

**Tendonitis** — *Turmeric* (515) · *Boswellia* (732) · *Ginger Root* (341)

**Tension Headaches** — *Peppermint* (860) · *Lavender* (911) · *Willow Bark* (491)

**Thyroid Support (General)** — *Bladderwrack* (112) · *Ashwagandha* (22)

**Tinnitus (Ringing Ears)** — *Ginkgo Biloba* (281) · *Hawthorn Berry* (316)

**Tonsillitis** — *Echinacea* (758) · *Goldenseal* (779) · *Myrrh* (237)

## U — *4 symptoms*

**Ulcers (Stomach)** — *Licorice Root* (700) · *Slippery Elm* (297) · *Marshmallow Root* (671)

**Urinary Infections (Recurrent)** — *Uva Ursi* (908) · *Cranberry* (217) · *Corn Silk* (73)

**Urinary Tract Health** — *Cranberry* (217) · *Corn Silk* (73) · *Parsley* (214)

**Uterine Fibroids (Support)** — *Chaste Tree Berry* (152) · *Red Clover* (827) · *Dong Quai* (97)

## V — *4 symptoms*

**Varicose Veins** — *Horse Chestnut* (736) · *Butcher's Broom* (383) · *Witch Hazel* (182)

**Vertigo / Dizziness** — *Ginkgo Biloba* (281) · *Ginger Root* (341)

**Viral Infections (General)** — *Elderberry* (898) · *Echinacea* (758) · *Olive Leaf* (353)

**Vision Support** — *Bilberry* (766) · *Goji Berry* (621) · *Ginkgo Biloba* (281)

## W — *6 symptoms*

**Water Retention** — *Dandelion Leaf* (85) · *Parsley* (214) · *Cleavers* (787)

**Weak Digestion (Elderly)** — *Ginger Root* (341) · *Gentian* (902) · *Cardamom* (410)

**Weak Immune System (Children)** — *Echinacea* (758) · *Elderberry* (898) · *Astragalus* (25)

**Weight Gain (Hormonal)** — *Maca Root* (815) · *Chaste Tree Berry* (152) · *Ashwagandha* (22)

**Wound Healing** — *Calendula* (46) · *Comfrey* (67) · *Plantain Leaf* (210)

**Wounds (Slow Healing)** — *Comfrey* (67) · *Calendula* (46) · *Aloe Vera* (1)

## Y — *2 symptoms*

**Yeast Infections (Vaginal)** — *Pau d'Arco* (675) · *Oregano Oil* (293) · *Calendula* (46)

**Yeast Overgrowth (Systemic)** — *Pau d'Arco* (675) · *Garlic* (853) · *Usnea* (587)

---

*Always consult each herb's full entry for complete safety information, caution levels, dosage guidance, and contraindications before use.*

# Glossary

A–Z terms, including general wellness concepts so new readers aren't left guessing.

**Adaptogen** — A class of herbs that help the body adapt to physical, mental, and emotional stress while promoting balance and resilience.
**Adrenal Glands** — Small glands that produce stress hormones like cortisol and adrenaline, crucial for energy, focus, and recovery.
**Aloe Vera** — A cooling, soothing plant used topically for burns and internally for digestive comfort and gut lining support.
**Analgesic** — A substance that helps reduce the perception of pain.
**Antimicrobial** — An agent that fights microbes such as bacteria, viruses, and fungi.
**Anti-inflammatory** — A substance that reduces redness, heat, swelling, and pain associated with inflammation.
**Antioxidant** — A compound that protects cells from damage by neutralizing free radicals.
**Astringent** — An herb or compound that tightens and tones tissues, helping reduce secretions and minor bleeding.
**Bitter** — A taste quality that stimulates digestive juices, appetite, and bile flow.
**Bioavailability** — How well a nutrient or compound is absorbed and used by the body.
**Botanical Name** — The Latin scientific name of a plant, used for clarity across regions and languages.
**Carminative** — An herb that relieves gas, bloating, and cramping by relaxing intestinal muscles.
**Cardiovascular System** — The heart and blood vessels that circulate blood, oxygen, and nutrients throughout the body.

**Chamomile** — A gentle herb that calms the nerves and soothes digestion; helpful for sleep and stress.
**Decoction** — A preparation method where tougher plant parts (roots, barks) are simmered to extract their constituents.
**Demulcent** — An herb rich in soothing mucilage that coats and protects irritated tissues, especially in the throat and gut.
**Diaphoretic** — A substance that promotes sweating to support fever management and detoxification.
**Digestion** — The breakdown of food into nutrients the body can absorb and use for energy and repair.
**Diuretic** — A substance that increases urination and supports kidney and bladder function.
**Dose / Dosage** — The amount of an herb or medicine to take, along with frequency of use.
**Echinacea** — A classic immune herb used at first sign of a cold to support the body's defenses.
**Edema** — Swelling caused by excess fluid trapped in tissues.
**Electrolytes** — Minerals like sodium and potassium that support hydration, nerves, and muscle function.

**Elecampane** — A lung-supporting herb that helps loosen and clear mucus while soothing the airways.
**Essential Oils** — Concentrated aromatic oils distilled from plants; potent and typically used externally or in tiny internal amounts with guidance.
**Feverfew** — An herb traditionally used to help prevent migraines and reduce fever, inflammation, and menstrual discomfort.
**Flavonoids** — Plant-based compounds with antioxidant and anti-inflammatory properties, abundant in fruits, vegetables, and many herbs.
**Free Radicals** — Unstable molecules that can damage cells and tissues, linked to aging and chronic disease.
**Fungicidal** — A substance that destroys or inhibits the growth of fungi.
**Gallbladder** — A small organ beneath the liver that stores bile to aid fat digestion.

**Gastrointestinal Tract (GI Tract)** — The path from stomach through intestines where food is broken down and absorbed.
**Ginger** — A warming herb known for easing nausea, improving circulation, and reducing inflammation.
**Ginseng** — An adaptogenic herb that supports energy, immune function, and cognitive performance.
**Hemostatic** — A substance that helps stop bleeding by promoting clotting or tissue contraction.
**Herbalism** — The study and practice of using plants for healing, prevention, and wellness.
**Homeopathy** — A system of alternative medicine using very small doses of natural substances to stimulate healing.
**Hormones** — Chemical messengers that regulate growth, mood, metabolism, and reproduction.
**Immune System** — The body's defense network that protects against infections and harmful substances.
**Inflammation** — The body's natural response to injury or infection, often marked by redness, heat, and swelling.
**Infusion** — A tea-like preparation made by steeping leaves or flowers in hot water.
**Insomnia** — Difficulty falling asleep or staying asleep.
**Joints** — Where bones meet, enabling movement and flexibility.
**Juniper Berry** — A diuretic, cleansing herb traditionally used for urinary tract health and digestion.
**Kidneys** — Organs that filter waste from blood and regulate fluid, electrolytes, and blood pressure.
**Kombucha** — A fermented tea drink containing probiotics and organic acids that support gut health.
**Laxative** — A substance that promotes bowel movements and relieves constipation.
**Lemon Balm** — A calming herb that supports sleep, reduces anxiety, and soothes digestion.
**Liver** — A vital organ that detoxifies the body and produces bile for digestion.

**Lymphatic System** — A network that clears waste, maintains fluid balance, and supports immunity.

**Macronutrients** — Carbohydrates, proteins, and fats — the main nutrients the body needs in large amounts.
**Magnesium** — A mineral essential for muscle function, nerve health, and relaxation.
**Menopause** — The natural life stage when menstruation ceases, marked by hormonal shifts.
**Minerals** — Natural elements (like calcium, zinc, iron) required for body functions.
**Nervine** — An herb that calms, nourishes, and strengthens the nervous system.
**Neurotransmitters** — Brain chemicals that influence mood, memory, and body functions.
**Nutrients** — Substances from food and herbs necessary for energy, growth, and repair.
**Nutrition** — The process of consuming and utilizing food for health and vitality.
**Ointment** — A topical preparation of herbs in oils/waxes used on skin.
**Oxidative Stress** — Cellular damage caused by an imbalance between free radicals and antioxidants.
**Oxygenation** — Supplying oxygen to blood and tissues.
**Palpitations** — The sensation of irregular, rapid, or strong heartbeat.
**Phytochemicals** — Natural plant compounds that confer health benefits.
**Poultice** — A soft moist herbal mass applied to the skin to soothe inflammation or infection.
**Probiotic** — Beneficial microorganisms that support gut health and immunity.
**Purgative** — A strong laxative that cleanses the digestive tract.
**Qi (Chi)** — In Traditional Chinese Medicine, the body's vital energy or life force.
**Quercetin** — A flavonoid with antioxidant and anti-inflammatory actions.
**Respiratory System** — Organs involved in breathing: lungs, airways, sinuses.
**Restorative** — An herb that rebuilds strength and vitality after stress or illness.
**Rosemary** — A stimulating herb supporting memory, circulation, and digestion.
**Salve** — An herbal ointment applied to skin for cuts, burns, or irritation.
**Secondary Descriptor** — A clarifying term used with a Core Herbal Category to explain *how* a particular herb works within that category and *when* it is best used.
**Sedative** — A substance that calms the nervous system and promotes sleep.
**Stimulant** — A substance that increases alertness and activity.
**Stress** — The body's response to pressure; often eased by adaptogens and nervines.
**Tannins** — Astringent plant compounds that tone tissues and reduce inflammation.
**Tea (Herbal Infusion)** — A beverage made by steeping herbs in hot water to extract actives.
**Tincture** — A concentrated liquid extract made with alcohol or glycerin.
**Tonic** — An herb that nourishes and strengthens long-term body function.
**Turmeric** — A golden spice with notable anti-inflammatory and antioxidant properties.
**Urinary Tract** — The kidneys, bladder, and urethra system that removes urine.
**Uterine Tonic** — An herb that supports the uterus and female reproductive health.
**Valerian** — A calming herb often used for insomnia and nervous tension.
**Vitamins** — Organic compounds essential for body functions and health.
**Volatile Oils** — Aromatic components of herbs responsible for scent and many effects.
**Wellness** — A state of overall health and balance in body, mind, and spirit.
**Willow Bark** — An herb traditionally used for pain relief and reducing inflammation.
**Xerostomia** — The medical term for dry mouth.
**Yellow Dock** — A liver-supporting herb and gentle laxative.
**Ylang-Ylang** — A fragrant flower used to reduce stress and uplift mood.

**Zinc** — A trace mineral essential for immune health and wound healing.
**Zingiberaceae** — The botanical family that includes ginger, turmeric, and cardamom.

# HERB INDEX

*The Herbal Resurrection • All 282 Herbs Listed Alphabetically with Page References*

*Page numbers refer to the first page of each herb's entry in the main reference.*

## A — *20 herbs*


| Herb | Page | Herb | Page | Herb | Page |
|---|---|---|---|---|---|
| Acorus / Sweet Flag | 252 | Agrimony | 4 | Ajwain | 633 |
| Alfalfa | 7 | Alkanet | 680 | Allspice | 636 |
| Aloe Vera | 1 | American Ginseng | 639 | Andrographis | 104 |
| Angelica Root | 10 | Anise Hyssop | 838 | Annatto | 89 |
| Arjuna | 642 | Arnica | 16 | Artichoke Leaf | 19 |
| Ash Bark | 857 | Ashitaba | 791 | Ashwagandha | 22 |
| Astragalus | 25 | Atractylodes | 344 | | |


## B — *31 herbs*


| Herb | Page | Herb | Page | Herb | Page |
|---|---|---|---|---|---|
| Bacopa | 107 | Bala | 876 | Balloon Flower | 204 |
| Balsam Fir | 573 | Bamboo Silica | 885 | Baobab | 799 |
| Barley Grass | 332 | Bayberry | 138 | Bee Balm | 156 |
| Beet Root | 192 | Betel Leaf | 571 | Betony | 110 |
| Bilberry | 726 | Bitter Melon | 272 | Black Cardamom | 566 |
| Black Cardoon | 576 | Black Cohosh | 787 | Black Horehound | 225 |
| Black Seed | 201 | Black Walnut Hull | 287 | Bladderwrack | 113 |
| Blessed Thistle | 28 | Blue Cohosh | 861 | Blue Vervain | 34 |
| Blueberry | 563 | Boneset | 37 | Borage | 40 |
| Borage Seed | 845 | Boswellia | 719 | Burdock Root | 44 |
| Butcher's Broom | 381 | | | | |

## C — *46 herbs*


| Herb | Page | Herb | Page | Herb | Page |
|---|---|---|---|---|---|
| Calaguala | 326 | Calendula | 47 | California Poppy | 50 |
| Camu Camu | 384 | Canary Seed | 556 | Caraway Seed | 387 |
| Cardamom | 408 | Cascara Sagrada | 627 | Cassia Bark | 195 |
| Catnip | 894 | Cat's Claw | 119 | Catuaba Bark | 703 |
| Cayenne Pepper | 53 | Celandine | 207 | Ceylon Cinnamon | 850 |
| Chaga | 390 | Chanca Piedra | 150 | Chaste Tree Berry | 153 |
| Chickpea | 222 | Chickweed | 59 | Chicory Root | 228 |
| Chinese Skullcap | 603 | Chrysanthemum | 323 | Chuchuhuasi | 646 |
| Cilantro | 171 | Cissus Quadrangularis | 606 | Cistanche Tubulosa | 597 |
| Cistus Incanus | 306 | Cleavers | 775 | Cleome | 600 |
| Clove Basil | 348 | Coleus Forskohlii | 763 | Coltsfoot | 65 |
| Comfrey | 68 | Coptis Root | 250 | Cordyceps | 71 |
| Coriander | 283 | Corn Silk | 74 | Cornflower | 189 |
| Corydalis | 402 | Costus Root | 126 | Couch Grass | 186 |
| Cowslip | 474 | Cramp Bark | 77 | Cranberry | 216 |
| Cranesbill | 269 | | | | |


## D — *9 herbs*


| Herb | Page | Herb | Page | Herb | Page |
|---|---|---|---|---|---|
| Damiana | 83 | Dandelion Leaf | 86 | Dandelion Root | 80 |
| Danshen | 621 | Devil's Claw | 101 | Devil's Club | 477 |
| Dodder | 329 | Dong Quai | 98 | Dulse | 649 |


## E — *9 herbs*


| Herb | Page | Herb | Page | Herb | Page |
|---|---|---|---|---|---|
| Echinacea | 746 | Eclipta Alba | 471 | Elder Leaf | 405 |
| Elderberry | 887 | Elecampane | 266 | Eleuthero | 651 |
| Eucalyptus | 624 | European Mistletoe | 302 | Eyebright | 276 |

## F — *8 herbs*


| | | | | | |
|---|---|---|---|---|---|
| False Unicorn Root | 462 | Fennel Seed | 771 | Fenugreek | 263 |
| Fever Tree | 354 | Feverfew | 62 | Fig Leaf | 245 |
| Figwort | 399 | Fo-Ti | 411 | | |


## G — *21 herbs*


| | | | | | |
|---|---|---|---|---|---|
| Galangal Root | 393 | Gambir | 231 | Garlic | 841 |
| Gentian | 578 | German Chamomile | 396 | Giant Hyssop | 248 |
| Ginger Root | 339 | Ginkgo Biloba | 279 | Goji Berry | 615 |
| Goldenrod | 129 | Goldenseal | 767 | Gotu Kola | 162 |
| Grape Seed | 739 | Grapefruit Seed | 439 | Gravel Root | 480 |
| Green Tea | 441 | Ground Ivy | 483 | Guaraná | 174 |
| Guava Leaf | 436 | Guduchi | 731 | Gynostemma | 654 |


## H — *9 herbs*


| | | | | | |
|---|---|---|---|---|---|
| Haritaki | 517 | Hawthorn Berry | 314 | Heartsease | 363 |
| Hibiscus | 378 | Holy Basil | 715 | Hops | 260 |
| Horse Chestnut | 723 | Horsetail | 433 | Houttuynia | 552 |


## I — *3 herbs*


| | | | | | |
|---|---|---|---|---|---|
| Indian Gooseberry | 177 | Irish Moss / Sea Moss | 873 | Isatis | 357 |


## J — *2 herbs*


| | | | | | |
|---|---|---|---|---|---|
| Jujube | 447 | Juniper Berry | 504 | | |


## K — *2 herbs*


| | | | | | |
|---|---|---|---|---|---|
| Kanna | 757 | Kudzu Root | 883 | | |


## L — *10 herbs*

| | | | | | |
|---|---|---|---|---|---|
| Labrador Tea | 366 | Lady's Mantle | 822 | Lamb's Ear | 135 |
| Lavender | 900 | Lemon Balm | 299 | Lemon Verbena | 830 |
| Lemongrass | 676 | Licorice Root | 687 | Linden Flower | 141 |
| Lion's Mane | 695 | | | | |


## M — *16 herbs*


| | | | | | |
|---|---|---|---|---|---|
| Maca Root | 803 | Magnolia | 560 | Maitake | 699 |
| Maral Root | 811 | Marshmallow Root | 629 | Meadowsweet | 144 |
| Milk Thistle | 31 | Moringa Leaf | 612 | Motherwort | 116 |
| Mugwort | 779 | Muira Puama | 609 | Mullein Flower | 783 |
| Mullein Leaf | 310 | Mullein Root | 870 | Mulungu | 760 |
| Myrrh | 236 | | | | |


## N — *4 herbs*


| | | | | | |
|---|---|---|---|---|---|
| Neem | 879 | Nettle Leaf | 132 | Nettle Seed | 826 |
| Nightshade | 450 | | | | |


## O — *4 herbs*


| | | | | | |
|---|---|---|---|---|---|
| Oak Bark | 233 | Oatstraw | 591 | Olive Leaf | 351 |
| Oregano Oil | 291 | | | | |


## P — *14 herbs*


| | | | | | |
|---|---|---|---|---|---|
| Parsley | 213 | Pasque Flower | 360 | Passion Flower | 95 |
| Pau d'Arco | 660 | Peppermint | 635 | Pine Bark | 743 |
| Pipsissewa | 834 | Plantain Leaf | 210 | Pleurisy Root | 735 |
| Prickly Ash Bark | 468 | Pumpkin Seed | 242 | Purple Dead Nettle | 594 |
| Purslane | 569 | Pygeum | 727 | | |


## R — *8 herbs*

| | | | | | |
|---|---|---|---|---|---|
| Red Clover | 815 | Red Raspberry Leaf | 414 | Red Root | 465 |
| Reishi | 691 | Rhodiola | 711 | Roman Chamomile | 56 |
| Rosemary | 369 | Rue | 430 | | |


## S — *30 herbs*


| | | | | | |
|---|---|---|---|---|---|
| Saffron | 867 | Sage | 853 | Sarsaparilla | 254 |
| Saw Palmetto | 257 | Schisandra | 219 | Sea Buckthorn | 684 |
| Senna Leaf | 630 | | | Shatavari | 795 |
| Shea Bark | 864 | Shepherd's Purse | 444 | Shilajit | 664 |
| Skullcap | 668 | Skunk Cabbage | 548 | Slippery Elm | 295 |
| Snowberry | 544 | Soapwort | 540 | Solomon's Seal | 750 |
| Soursop | 536 | Speedwell | 532 | Spikenard | 529 |
| Spilanthes | 239 | St. John's Wort | 375 | Suma Root | 807 |
| Sumac | 526 | Swedish Bitters | 523 | Sweet Annie | 198 |
| Sweet Cicely | 92 | Sweet Violet | 168 | Sweet Woodruff | 159 |


## T — *10 herbs*


| | | | | | |
|---|---|---|---|---|---|
| Tamarind | 335 | Tansy | 317 | Tea Tree | 520 |
| Teasel Root | 579 | Thyme | 372 | Tongkat Ali | 13 |
| Tribulus | 320 | Turkey Rhubarb | 582 | Turkey Tail | 707 |
| Turmeric | 514 | | | | |


## U — *2 herbs*


| | | | | | |
|---|---|---|---|---|---|
| Usnea | 585 | Uva Ursi | 897 | | |


## V — *4 herbs*


| | | | | | |
|---|---|---|---|---|---|
| Valerian | 819 | Velvet Bean | 510 | Verbena | 507 |
| Vidanga | 588 | | | | |

## W — *12 herbs*


| | | | | | |
|---|---|---|---|---|---|
| Watercress | 165 | Western Red Cedar | 501 | White Oak Bark | 454 |
| White Peony | 424 | White Spruce | 618 | Wild Indigo | 495 |
| Wild Lettuce | 180 | Wild Yam | 492 | Willow Bark | 489 |
| Wintergreen | 498 | Witch Hazel | 183 | Wormwood | 427 |


## Y — *7 herbs*


| | | | | | |
|---|---|---|---|---|---|
| Yarrow | 122 | Yellow Dock | 147 | Yellow Jasmine | 486 |
| Yerba Mansa | 421 | Yerba Maté | 672 | Yohimbe | 417 |
| Yucca Root | 458 | | | | |


## Z — *1 herb*


| | | | | | |
|---|---|---|---|---|---|
| Zedoary | 903 | | | | |

# CORE HERBAL CATEGORY INDEX

*The Herbal Resurrection • All 282 Herbs Organized by Primary Core Category*

*Each herb is listed under its single Primary Core Herbal Category, alphabetically within each group, with its page number and Herbal Confidence Index (★ = 1 star through ★★★★★ = 5 stars).*

## I. ADAPTOGENS — *13 herbs*


| Herb | Page | Herb | Page |
|---|---|---|---|
| **Ashwagandha** ★★★★★ | 22 | **Astragalus** ★★★★★ | 25 |
| **Cordyceps** ★★★★★ | 71 | **Devil's Club** ★★★ | 477 |
| **Eleuthero** ★★★★★ | 651 | **Gynostemma** ★★★★★ | 654 |
| **Holy Basil** ★★★★ | 715 | **Maral Root** ★★★★★ | 811 |
| **Rhodiola** ★★★★★ | 711 | **Schisandra** ★★★★★ | 219 |
| **Shilajit** ★★★★★ | 664 | **Suma Root** ★★★★ | 807 |
| **Tongkat Ali** ★★★★ | 13 | | |


## II. NERVOUS SYSTEM SUPPORT — *44 herbs*


| Herb | Page | Herb | Page |
|---|---|---|---|
| **Anise Hyssop** ★★★★ | 838 | **Bacopa** ★★★★ | 107 |
| **Betony** ★★★★ | 110 | **Black Horehound** ★★ | 225 |
| **Blue Vervain** ★★★★★ | 34 | **California Poppy** ★★★★ | 50 |
| **Catnip** ★★★★ | 894 | **Catuaba Bark** ★★★★ | 703 |
| **Damiana** ★★★★ | 83 | **German Chamomile** ★★★★★ | 396 |
| **Giant Hyssop** ★★★★ | 248 | **Guaraná** ★★★★ | 174 |
| **Hops** ★★★★ | 260 | **Jujube** ★★★★★ | 447 |
| **Kanna** ★★★★ | 757 | **Lavender** ★★★★ | 900 |
| **Lemon Balm** ★★★★ | 299 | **Lemon Verbena** ★★★★ | 830 |

| Herb | Page | | Herb | Page |
|---|---|---|---|---|
| Linden Flower ★★★★ | 141 | | Lion's Mane ★★★★★ | 695 |
| Magnolia ★★★★ | 560 | | Motherwort ★★★★ | 116 |
| Mugwort ★★★★ | 779 | | Muira Puama ★★★★ | 609 |
| Nightshade ★★ | 450 | | Oatstraw ★★★★ | 591 |
| Pasque Flower ★★ | 360 | | Passion Flower ★★★★★ | 95 |
| Roman Chamomile ★★★★ | 56 | | Saffron ★★★★ | 867 |
| Sage ★★★★ | 853 | | Skullcap ★★★★★ | 668 |
| Skunk Cabbage ★★★ | 548 | | Soursop ★★★★ | 536 |
| Spikenard ★★★★ | 529 | | St. John's Wort ★★★★ | 375 |
| Sweet Woodruff ★★★ | 159 | | Valerian ★★★★ | 819 |
| Velvet Bean ★★★★ | 510 | | Verbena ★★★ | 507 |
| Wild Lettuce ★★★ | 180 | | Yellow Jasmine ★★ | 486 |
| Yerba Maté ★★★★ | 672 | | Mulungu ★★★★ | 760 |


## III. DIGESTIVE SYSTEM SUPPORT — *38 herbs*


| Herb | Page | | Herb | Page |
|---|---|---|---|---|
| Acorus / Sweet Flag ★★ | 252 | | Agrimony ★★★★ | 4 |
| Ajwain ★★★★ | 633 | | Allspice ★★★★ | 636 |
| Aloe Vera ★★★★★ | 1 | | Atractylodes ★★★★★ | 344 |
| Bayberry ★★★★ | 138 | | Bee Balm ★★★★ | 156 |
| Betel Leaf ★★★ | 571 | | Blessed Thistle ★★★★ | 28 |
| Caraway Seed ★★★★ | 387 | | Cardamom ★★★★★ | 408 |
| Cascara Sagrada ★★★ | 627 | | Cassia Bark ★★★★ | 195 |
| Chicory Root ★★★★ | 228 | | Coptis Root ★★★★ | 250 |
| Coriander ★★★ | 283 | | Costus Root ★★★ | 126 |

| Cranesbill ★★★★ | 269 | Fennel Seed ★★★★★ | 771 |
|---|---|---|---|
| Galangal Root ★★★★ | 393 | Gentian ★★★★★ | 578 |
| Ginger Root ★★★★★ | 339 | Guava Leaf ★★★★ | 436 |
| Haritaki ★★★★★ | 517 | Lemongrass ★★★★ | 676 |
| Licorice Root ★★★★★ | 687 | Marshmallow Root ★★★★ | 629 |
| Peppermint ★★★★★ | 635 | Senna Leaf ★★★ | 630 |
| Slippery Elm ★★★★★ | 295 | Swedish Bitters ★★★★ | 523 |
| Sweet Cicely ★★★★ | 92 | Tamarind ★★★★ | 335 |
| Turkey Rhubarb ★★★★ | 582 | Vidanga ★★★★ | 588 |
| Wormwood ★★★ | 427 | Zedoary ★★★★ | 903 |


## IV. IMMUNE SYSTEM SUPPORT — *28 herbs*


| Andrographis ★★★★ | 104 | Bamboo Silica ★★★★★ | 885 |
|---|---|---|---|
| Black Seed ★★★★★ | 201 | Boneset ★★★★★ | 37 |
| Calaguala ★★★★ | 326 | Camu Camu ★★★★★ | 384 |
| Cat's Claw ★★★★ | 119 | Chaga ★★★★★ | 390 |
| Cistus Incanus ★★★★ | 306 | Clove Basil ★★★★ | 348 |
| Elderberry ★★★★★ | 887 | Fever Tree ★★ | 354 |
| Grapefruit Seed ★★★ | 439 | Guduchi ★★★★★ | 731 |
| Isatis ★★★ | 357 | Maitake ★★★★★ | 699 |
| Olive Leaf ★★★★★ | 351 | Oregano Oil ★★★★ | 291 |
| Purple Dead Nettle ★★★ | 594 | Reishi ★★★★★ | 691 |
| Spilanthes ★★★★★ | 239 | Sweet Annie ★★★★★ | 198 |
| Tansy ★★ | 317 | Turkey Tail ★★★★★ | 707 |

| | | | | |
|---|---|---|---|---|
| Usnea ★★★★ | 585 | | Wild Indigo ★★★ | 495 |
| Yarrow ★★★★★ | 122 | | Echinacea ★★★★★ | 746 |

## V. RESPIRATORY SYSTEM SUPPORT — *20 herbs*

| | | | | |
|---|---|---|---|---|
| Balloon Flower ★★★★ | 204 | | Balsam Fir ★★★★ | 573 |
| Black Cardamom ★★★★ | 566 | | Chinese Skullcap ★★★★★ | 603 |
| Coltsfoot ★★★ | 65 | | Cowslip ★★★★ | 474 |
| Elecampane ★★★★ | 266 | | Eucalyptus ★★★★ | 624 |
| Eyebright ★★★★★ | 276 | | Ground Ivy ★★★★ | 483 |
| Houttuynia ★★★ | 552 | | Labrador Tea ★★ | 366 |
| Mullein Leaf ★★★★★ | 310 | | Pleurisy Root ★★★★ | 735 |
| Soapwort ★★★ | 540 | | Speedwell ★★★★ | 532 |
| Thyme ★★★★★ | 372 | | Western Red Cedar ★★ | 501 |
| White Spruce ★★★★ | 618 | | Yerba Mansa ★★★★ | 421 |

## VI. CARDIOVASCULAR SYSTEM SUPPORT — *27 herbs*

| | | | | |
|---|---|---|---|---|
| Angelica Root ★★★★ | 10 | | Arjuna ★★★★ | 642 |
| Beet Root ★★★★ | 192 | | Bilberry ★★★★ | 726 |
| Blueberry ★★★★★ | 563 | | Butcher's Broom ★★★★ | 381 |
| Cayenne Pepper ★★★★★ | 53 | | Ceylon Cinnamon ★★★★★ | 850 |
| Chrysanthemum ★★★★ | 323 | | Coleus Forskohlii ★★★★ | 763 |
| Danshen ★★★★ | 621 | | European Mistletoe ★★★ | 302 |
| Garlic ★★★★★ | 841 | | Ginkgo Biloba ★★★★★ | 279 |
| Gotu Kola ★★★★★ | 162 | | Grape Seed ★★★ | 739 |
| Green Tea ★★★★★ | 441 | | Hawthorn Berry ★★★★★ | 314 |

| | | | |
|---|---|---|---|
| Hibiscus ★★★★★ | 378 | Horse Chestnut ★★★★ | 723 |
| Kudzu Root ★★★★ | 883 | | |
| Pine Bark ★★★★ | 743 | Prickly Ash Bark ★★★★ | 468 |
| Rosemary ★★★★★ | 369 | Rue ★★ | 430 |
| Shepherd's Purse ★★★★ | 444 | Yohimbe ★★ | 417 |

## VII. ANTI-INFLAMMATORY & PAIN SUPPORT — *18 herbs*

| | | | |
|---|---|---|---|
| Arnica ★★★★ | 16 | Ash Bark ★★★★ | 857 |
| Boswellia ★★★★★ | 719 | Chuchuhuasi ★★★★ | 646 |
| Cissus Quadrangularis ★★★★ | 606 | Corydalis ★★★★ | 402 |
| Devil's Claw ★★★★ | 101 | | |
| Feverfew ★★★★ | 62 | Meadowsweet ★★★★ | 144 |
| Mullein Flower ★★★★ | 783 | Mullein Root ★★★★ | 870 |
| Shea Bark ★★★ | 864 | Solomon's Seal ★★★★★ | 750 |
| Teasel Root ★★★★ | 579 | Turmeric ★★★★★ | 514 |
| Willow Bark ★★★★ | 489 | Wintergreen ★★★ | 498 |
| Yucca Root ★★★★ | 458 | | |

## VIII. LIVER & DETOX SUPPORT — *12 herbs*

| | | | |
|---|---|---|---|
| Artichoke Leaf ★★★★ | 19 | Black Cardoon ★★★★ | 576 |
| Burdock Root ★★★★★ | 44 | Celandine ★★★ | 207 |
| Cilantro ★★★★ | 171 | Dandelion Root ★★★★★ | 80 |
| Eclipta Alba ★★★★★ | 471 | Indian Gooseberry ★★★★★ | 177 |
| Milk Thistle ★★★★★ | 31 | Sarsaparilla ★★★★ | 254 |
| Watercress ★★★★ | 165 | Yellow Dock ★★★★ | 147 |

## IX. KIDNEY & URINARY SUPPORT — *12 herbs*

| Herb | Page | Herb | Page |
|---|---|---|---|
| Chanca Piedra ★★★★ | 150 | Corn Silk ★★★★ | 74 |
| Couch Grass ★★★★ | 186 | Cranberry ★★★★ | 216 |
| Goldenrod ★★★★★ | 129 | Gravel Root ★★★★ | 480 |
| Juniper Berry ★★★★ | 504 | Parsley ★★★★ | 213 |
| Pipsissewa ★★★★ | 834 | Pygeum ★★★★ | 727 |
| Saw Palmetto ★★★★★ | 257 | Uva Ursi ★★★★ | 897 |

## X. ENDOCRINE & HORMONAL SUPPORT — *10 herbs*

| Herb | Page | Herb | Page |
|---|---|---|---|
| Bitter Melon ★★★★ | 272 | Canary Seed ★★★ | 556 |
| Chaste Tree Berry ★★★★ | 153 | Dodder ★★★ | 329 |
| Fenugreek ★★★★ | 263 | Fig Leaf ★★★★ | 245 |
| Maca Root ★★★★★ | 803 | Nettle Seed ★★★★★ | 826 |
| Tribulus ★★★★ | 320 | White Peony ★★★★★ | 424 |

## XI. LYMPHATIC & SKIN SUPPORT — *23 herbs*

| Herb | Page | Herb | Page |
|---|---|---|---|
| Alkanet ★★★ | 680 | Annatto ★★★ | 89 |
| Calendula ★★★★★ | 47 | Chickweed ★★★★ | 59 |
| Cleavers ★★★★ | 775 | Comfrey ★★★ | 68 |
| Cornflower ★★★ | 189 | Elder Leaf ★★★ | 405 |
| Figwort ★★★★ | 399 | Gambir ★★★ | 231 |
| Heartsease ★★★★ | 363 | Lamb's Ear ★★★★ | 135 |
| Oak Bark ★★★★ | 233 | Plantain Leaf ★★★★★ | 210 |
| Red Clover ★★★★ | 815 | Red Root ★★★★ | 465 |
| Sea Buckthorn ★★★★★ | 684 | Snowberry ★★ | 544 |

| Herb | Page | Herb | Page |
|---|---|---|---|
| Sumac ★★★★ | 526 | Sweet Violet ★★★★★ | 168 |
| Tea Tree ★★★★ | 520 | White Oak Bark ★★★★ | 454 |
| Witch Hazel ★★★★ | 183 | | |


## XII. ANTIMICROBIAL SUPPORT — *5 herbs*


| Herb | Page | Herb | Page |
|---|---|---|---|
| Black Walnut Hull ★★★★ | 287 | Goldenseal ★★★★ | 767 |
| Myrrh ★★★★★ | 236 | Neem ★★★★★ | 879 |
| Pau d'Arco ★★★★ | 660 | | |


## XIII. REPRODUCTIVE & WOMEN'S HEALTH SUPPORT — *11 herbs*


| Herb | Page | Herb | Page |
|---|---|---|---|
| Black Cohosh ★★★★ | 787 | Blue Cohosh ★★ | 861 |
| Borage Seed ★★★★ | 845 | Cramp Bark ★★★★ | 77 |
| Dong Quai ★★★★ | 98 | False Unicorn Root ★★★★ | 462 |
| Lady's Mantle ★★★★ | 822 | Pumpkin Seed ★★★★★ | 242 |
| Red Raspberry Leaf ★★★★★ | 414 | Shatavari ★★★★★ | 795 |
| Wild Yam ★★★★★ | 492 | | |


## XIV. NUTRITIONAL & TONIC SUPPORT — *20 herbs*


| Herb | Page | Herb | Page |
|---|---|---|---|
| Alfalfa ★★★★★ | 7 | American Ginseng ★★★★★ | 639 |
| Ashitaba ★★★★★ | 791 | Bala ★★★ | 876 |
| Baobab ★★★★★ | 799 | Barley Grass ★★★★★ | 332 |
| Bladderwrack ★★★★ | 113 | Borage ★★★★ | 40 |
| Chickpea ★★★★ | 222 | Cistanche Tubulosa ★★★★★ | 597 |
| Cleome ★★★ | 600 | Dandelion Leaf ★★★★★ | 86 |
| Dulse ★★★★ | 649 | Fo-Ti ★★★★ | 411 |
| Goji Berry ★★★★★ | 615 | Horsetail ★★★★ | 433 |

| | | | | |
|---|---|---|---|---|
| **Irish Moss / Sea Moss** ★★★★ | 873 | | **Moringa Leaf** ★★★★★ | 612 |
| **Nettle Leaf** ★★★★★ | 132 | | **Purslane** ★★★★★ | 569 |

## XV. FOUNDATIONAL / SYSTEMIC SUPPORT — *0 herbs*

*Most, if not all, herbs broad enough to be considered Foundational or Systemic in nature also carry a Primary Core function within one of the other 14 categories — the specific area where their action is most concentrated. For this reason, no herb in this reference currently carries Foundational / Systemic Support as a Primary Core.*

*It does, however, appear as a Secondary Core on the following herb pages: Agrimony, Angelica Root, Nettle Leaf, Sarsaparilla, Sea Buckthorn, and Yarrow — each selected for genuine, independent support across multiple systems without any single system clearly dominating.*

---

*Each herb is placed under its single Primary Core Herbal Category as designated in this reference. Secondary Core designations are noted on each individual herb page.*

# BONUS MATERIALS

Three Special Gifts for Your Herbal Journey

As a thank-you for choosing *The Herbal Resurrection*, the following pages include three bonus reference guides created to support your wellness goals. These bonuses are designed to give you quick, practical starting points using some of the most trusted herbs in the book.

### Bonus #1 — Immune-Boosting Herbal Guide

A focused list of herbs traditionally used to strengthen natural defenses, support recovery, and promote overall resilience during seasonal challenges.

### Bonus #2 — Mind & Mood Support Guide

A gentle guide to herbs that help calm the mind, ease tension, support rest, and promote emotional balance in daily life.

### Bonus #3 — My Herbal Cabinet

A simple, helpful checklist of essential herbs many people like to keep on hand at home for everyday needs, minor discomforts, and general family wellness.
These bonuses are meant to be easy to read, easy to use, and easy to return to—whenever you want quick direction or inspiration on your herbal path.

# Bonus #1 – Immune Boosting

Strengthening the immune system is one of the most important steps you can take to protect your health. This chart highlights ten of the most powerful immune-boosting herbs, each chosen for their ability to fortify your body's natural defenses against colds, flu, and other common infections.

Use this chart as a quick-reference for daily wellness, seasonal tonics, or recovery. Many of these herbs work well together, and blending them often produces even greater results.

✨ **Author's Choice for Best Immune-Boosting Recipe** ✨

To prepare it, just combine equal parts of Echinacea, Elderberry, Astragalus, and Ginger. Add some Licorice Root — about one half part — for soothing balance. You can make extra, seal it in a jar, and keep it handy on your shelf whenever you need it.

Whenever you're ready for it, just steep 1 tablespoon of this blend in 2 cups of hot water for 15 minutes, strain, and sip warm.

## ✨ IMMUNE BOOSTING ✨

### IMMUNE-BOOSTING HERBAL SUPPORT — BONUS CHART

| Rank | Herb | HCI ★ | Page | Key Benefits |
|---|---|---|---|---|
| 1 | *Echinacea* | ★★★★★ | 743 | Activates immune defense |
| 2 | *Elderberry* | ★★★★★ | 884 | Antiviral — shortens colds |
| 3 | *Garlic* | ★★★★★ | 838 | Antibacterial, antifungal |
| 4 | *Astragalus* | ★★★★★ | 25 | Restores vitality & energy |
| 5 | *Olive Leaf* | ★★★★★ | 348 | Fights infections broadly |
| 6 | *Ginger Root* | ★★★★★ | 336 | Warming — clears congestion |
| 7 | *Turmeric* | ★★★★★ | 510 | Anti-inflammatory support |
| 8 | *Reishi* | ★★★★★ | 688 | Immune tonic — adaptogen |
| 9 | *Licorice Root* | ★★★★★ | 684 | Soothes lungs & throat |

| Rank | Herb | HCI ★ | Page | Key Benefits |
|---|---|---|---|---|
| 10 | ***Andrographis*** | ★★★★ | 103 | Potent antiviral & bitter |

# Bonus #2 – Mind & Mood

Herbal medicine has long been used to balance the mind and restore emotional well-being. This chart highlights reliable herbs for calming stress, lifting low moods, and promoting restful sleep. Use it any time you feel tense, overwhelmed, or emotionally drained. Whether you're seeking a calming tea, a mood-lifting tonic, or gentle sleep support, these herbs offer trusted allies.

**Author's Choice for Best Mood & Mind Recipe**

To prepare it, just combine equal parts of Lemon Balm, Passionflower, and Chamomile. Add some Skullcap — about one half part — for extra calming support. It works well to prepare a larger blend in advance and tuck it away in a jar, ready for when the moment calls.
Whenever you're ready for it, just steep 1 tablespoon of this blend in 2 cups of hot water for 10–15 minutes, strain, and sip slowly.

## HERBAL MIND & MOOD SUPPORT — BONUS CHART

| Rank | Herb | HCI ★ | Page | Key Benefits |
|---|---|---|---|---|
| 1 | *Lemon Balm* | ★★★★★ | 296 | Calms nerves — uplifts mood |
| 2 | *Passionflower* | ★★★★★ | 94 | Relieves anxiety — aids sleep |
| 3 | *Roman Chamomile* | ★★★★ | 55 | Soothes stress & digestion |
| 4 | *Valerian* | ★★★★ | 816 | Promotes deep sleep |
| 5 | *Skullcap* | ★★★★★ | 665 | Relieves nervous tension |
| 6 | *Ashwagandha* | ★★★★★ | 22 | Adaptogen — stress balance |
| 7 | *Holy Basil* | ★★★★ | 712 | Lifts mood — reduces fatigue |
| 8 | *St. John's Wort* | ★★★★ | 372 | Traditional herb for low mood |
| 9 | *Lavender* | ★★★★ | 897 | Calms anxiety — eases restlessness |
| 10 | *Oatstraw* | ★★★★★ | 588 | Nourishes nerves — gentle tonic |

# Bonus #3 – Herbal Cabinet

Every home should have a small collection of reliable herbs ready for everyday use. This chart highlights essentials that are versatile, effective, and easy to keep on hand.
Think of this chart as your starter kit. Build a dependable home supply that covers common needs; expand later with specialized herbs as you grow.

✨ **Author's Choice for Best Everyday Herbal Blend** ✨

To prepare it, just combine equal parts of Chamomile, Peppermint, and Ginger. Add some Echinacea — about one half part — for immune support. Mixing a bigger batch and storing it in a container makes it easy to grab and brew anytime.
Whenever you're ready for it, just steep 1 tablespoon of this blend in 2 cups of hot water for 10–15 minutes, strain, and sip.

## ✨ FOUNDATIONAL HERBAL CABINET ✨

### FOUNDATIONAL HERBAL CABINET — BONUS CHART

| Rank | Herb | HCI ★ | Page | Key Benefits |
|---|---|---|---|---|
| 1 | *Roman Chamomile* | ★★★★ | 55 | Calms nerves — soothes digestion |
| 2 | *Peppermint* | ★★★★★ | 845 | Relieves gas — clears head |
| 3 | *Ginger Root* | ★★★★★ | 336 | Aids digestion — eases nausea |
| 4 | *Echinacea* | ★★★★★ | 743 | Supports immune defenses |
| 5 | *Garlic* | ★★★★★ | 838 | Antimicrobial — heart health |
| 6 | *Lavender* | ★★★★ | 897 | Eases stress — promotes rest |
| 7 | *Turmeric* | ★★★★★ | 510 | Anti-inflammatory — joint support |
| 8 | *Lemon Balm* | ★★★★★ | 296 | Relieves anxiety — uplifts mood |
| 9 | *Nettle Leaf* | ★★★★ | 131 | Nutritive tonic — energy support |
| 10 | *Calendula* | ★★★★★ | 46 | Soothes skin — supports healing |

And here's One '1' more for you because I appreciate you and your support!

# Bonus #4 – Nutritive Survival

In times of need or when nourishing food is scarce, certain herbs offer both medicine and sustenance. This chart highlights nutrient-dense herbs that supply minerals, vitamins, and steady energy.

Use this as a quick-reference for preparedness, travel, or outdoor living. Many of these herbs are 'food-like,' designed to sustain and fortify over time.

✨ **Author's Choice for Best Nutritive Survival Blend** ✨

To prepare it, just combine equal parts of Nettle, Alfalfa, and Oatstraw. Add some Dandelion Leaf — about one half part — for added minerals and cleansing support. This mixture can be blended ahead of time, stored dry in a jar, and kept shelf-stable for whenever nourishment is needed most.

Whenever you're ready for it, just steep 1 tablespoon of this blend in 2 cups of hot water for 15 minutes, strain, and drink warm.

---

## ✨ Nutritive Herbs Survival Guide ✨

---

### NUTRITIVE HERB SUPPORT — BONUS CHART

| Rank | Herb | HCI ★ | Page | Key Benefits |
|---|---|---|---|---|
| 1 | ***Nettle Leaf*** | ★★★★ | 131 | Rich in iron — energy tonic |
| 2 | ***Alfalfa*** | ★★★★★ | 7 | Packed with vitamins & minerals |
| 3 | ***Oatstraw*** | ★★★★★ | 588 | Nervine — strengthens bones |
| 4 | ***Dandelion Leaf*** | ★★★★ | 85 | Mineral-rich — supports liver |
| 5 | ***Irish Moss / Sea Moss*** | ★★★★ | 870 | Mineral-dense — thyroid support |
| 6 | ***Barley Grass*** | ★★★★★ | 329 | Chlorophyll-rich — alkalizing |
| 7 | ***Red Clover*** | ★★★★ | 812 | Mineral tonic — cleanses blood |

| Rank | Herb | HCI ★ | Page | Key Benefits |
|---|---|---|---|---|
| 8 | ***Moringa Leaf*** | ★★★★★ | 609 | Nutrient-dense superfood |
| 9 | ***Cleavers*** | ★★★★ | 772 | Lymphatic nutritive tonic |
| 10 | ***Nettle Seed*** | ★★★★ | 823 | Restorative adrenal tonic |

# Obtaining Herbs Safely and Responsibly

For many readers, the journey into herbal study begins with a simple question:

"Where do I obtain the herbs?"

Today, herbs can be obtained in several safe and responsible ways. While herbs have been gathered from the wild for centuries, modern beginners usually obtain them through reputable herb growers, herbal retailers, or cultivated gardens.

Understanding how herbs are obtained will help you approach herbal study with both confidence and respect for nature.

---

### Purchasing Herbs

Many medicinal herbs are now widely available through:

- herbal apothecaries
- herb farms
- health food stores
- reputable online herbal businesses

These suppliers specialize in growing, harvesting, drying, and storing herbs properly. Purchasing herbs from knowledgeable herbal businesses is often the safest and most convenient option for beginners, as the plants have already been correctly identified and prepared.

When selecting herbs, look for signs of freshness such as natural color, pleasant aroma, and proper storage in sealed containers.

---

### Growing Your Own Herbs

Another excellent way to become familiar with medicinal plants is to grow them yourself.

Many herbs discussed in this book can be cultivated in:

- home gardens
- backyard plots
- community gardens
- potted containers

Growing herbs allows students to observe the plant's appearance, scent, and seasonal growth, which deepens familiarity and appreciation for the plant itself.

---

### A Note on Wildcrafting

Wildcrafting refers to harvesting herbs directly from their natural environment.

While this practice has a long historical tradition, it requires experience and careful plant identification. Some plants have toxic look-alikes, and harvesting from the wrong location can introduce contamination or environmental harm.

For this reason, beginners are encouraged to avoid wild harvesting unless they have received proper training in plant identification and responsible harvesting methods.

Herbal practice should always respect both human safety and the natural environment.

---

### Quality and Care

Whether herbs are purchased or grown, their quality depends on freshness and proper storage.

**Herbs should generally be kept:**

- in sealed containers
- away from direct sunlight
- in a cool, dry environment

Proper storage helps preserve the plant's natural qualities and ensures the herb remains suitable for study and responsible use.

---

### 🌿 Responsible Herbal Practice Reminder

Herbal study is a journey of learning and respect for the natural world. Beginners are encouraged to obtain herbs through trusted herbal suppliers or cultivated gardens rather than harvesting unknown plants in the wild.

Correct plant identification, responsible harvesting practices, and environmental awareness are essential parts of traditional herbal knowledge. When approached with patience and care, herbal study becomes both educational and meaningful.

---

Readers interested in working with herbs are encouraged to begin with small quantities and become familiar with each plant gradually. **Those seeking to purchase herbs or learn more about reputable herbal producers and wholesalers may also visit the**

**Resources section of the Herbal Resurrection website at *herbalresurrection.com* for assistance.**

# The End

# Thank You

I want to thank you for choosing The Herbal Resurrection. I truly appreciate you. In a world where so many have become disconnected from the gifts of nature, your choice to explore the healing power of herbs is an act of courage, wisdom, and self-care. I 'salute' you.

This book was written to be more than just a guide — it is meant to be a companion on your journey to better health, balance, and wellness. My hope is that the pages you've read will not only continue to provide knowledge to you for some years to come- but will also inspire you to take practical steps toward natural healing, renewed energy, and lasting vitality for yourself and others.

By opening this book, you have also become a part of something greater — the living tradition of herbal wisdom that has been passed down through generations. Every time you use an herb for healing, you help to keep this knowledge alive and ensure that it is never lost to time. In this way, you are not just a reader, but a guardian of a legacy that belongs to all people.

May the wisdom of the herbs bless your path, restore your spirit, and empower you to share these gifts with others.

With gratitude,
**Fred Vincent Jenkins**
Author, *The Herbal Resurrection*
Creator of the Ja'hem — Jenkins Herbal Education Method

# APPENDIX A

***Selected Scientific Literature for Further Study***

---

CORE HERBAL CATEGORY I

## ADAPTOGENS

### Scientific Perspective

Adaptogens are a class of medicinal plants and fungi studied for their potential to support the body's capacity to respond to physical, psychological, and environmental stress while maintaining physiological balance. The modern adaptogen concept developed partly from research in the former Soviet Union, while many plants now discussed as adaptogens also have long histories of use in Ayurveda, Traditional Chinese Medicine, and other traditional medical systems. Contemporary research has examined effects on stress-response signaling, neuroendocrine regulation, fatigue, cognition, immune function, physical performance, recovery, and processes associated with healthy aging, with Ashwagandha and Rhodiola carrying the most substantial human evidence in the group. Individual species differ substantially in chemistry, preparation, dosage, and depth of evidence, so the literature supports herb-specific interpretation rather than treating adaptogens as a single uniform effect.

### Representative Herbs

- Ashwagandha (*Withania somnifera*)
- Rhodiola (*Rhodiola rosea*)
- Eleuthero (*Eleutherococcus senticosus*)
- Schisandra (*Schisandra chinensis*)
- Reishi (*Ganoderma lucidum*)
- Cordyceps (*Cordyceps militaris / Ophiocordyceps sinensis*)
- Tulsi (*Ocimum tenuiflorum*)

### Major Areas of Scientific Investigation

- Adaptation to physical and psychological stress
- Hypothalamic-pituitary-adrenal (HPA) axis and stress-response signaling
- Mental and physical fatigue
- Attention, cognition, and work performance under stress
- Exercise performance, endurance, and recovery
- Immune and inflammatory regulation
- Neuroprotective and cellular stress-response mechanisms
- Resilience and processes associated with healthy aging

### Selected Scientific Literature


1. **Panossian AG, Efferth T, Shikov AN, et al.** Evolution of the adaptogenic concept from traditional use to medical systems: pharmacology of stress- and aging-related diseases. *Medicinal Research Reviews.* 2021;41(1):630-703. doi:10.1002/med.21743.

2. **Panossian A.** Understanding adaptogenic activity: specificity of the pharmacological action of adaptogens and other phytochemicals. *Annals of the New York Academy of Sciences.* 2017;1401(1):49-64. doi:10.1111/nyas.13399.

3. **Panossian A, Wikman G.** Evidence-based efficacy of adaptogens in fatigue, and molecular mechanisms related to their stress-protective activity. *Current Clinical Pharmacology.* 2009;4(3):198-219. doi:10.2174/157488409789375311.

4. **Panossian A, Wikman G.** Effects of adaptogens on the central nervous system and the molecular mechanisms associated with their stress-protective activity. *Pharmaceuticals (Basel).* 2010;3(1):188-224. doi:10.3390/ph3010188.

5. **Wagner H, Nörr H, Winterhoff H.** Plant adaptogens. *Phytomedicine.* 1994;1(1):63-76. doi:10.1016/S0944-7113(11)80025-5.

6. **Panossian A, Wikman G, Wagner H.** Plant adaptogens III: earlier and more recent aspects and concepts on their mode of action. *Phytomedicine.* 1999;6(4):287-300. doi:10.1016/S0944-7113(99)80023-3.

## Authoritative Scientific Resources

- World Health Organization (WHO), Monographs on Selected Medicinal Plants
- European Medicines Agency (EMA), European Union herbal monographs and assessment reports
- European Scientific Cooperative on Phytotherapy (ESCOP), ESCOP Monographs
- National Center for Complementary and Integrative Health (NCCIH)
- PubMed, U.S. National Library of Medicine

## Clinical Consideration

Adaptogens should not be assumed automatically safe for everyone, and product quality, species identity, and extract standardization vary considerably across the market. Ashwagandha should be used cautiously in pregnancy, autoimmune thyroid disease, and alongside sedative or thyroid medications, and has been associated with rare reports of liver-related effects. Rhodiola may cause overstimulation or interfere with sleep in sensitive individuals and should be used cautiously with antidepressants or stimulant medications. Eleuthero and Schisandra may affect blood pressure, blood sugar, or the metabolism of certain drugs, including some prescribed for anxiety, blood clotting, or seizure control. Reishi may increase bleeding risk and should be used cautiously with anticoagulant or antiplatelet medications, or before surgery. Cordyceps and Tulsi may also affect blood sugar or bleeding. Persistent fatigue, unexplained weight change, or symptoms suggesting thyroid, adrenal, or autoimmune disease should be evaluated by a healthcare professional rather than managed with adaptogens alone.

## Research Snapshot

Ashwagandha and Rhodiola have the most substantial bodies of human research in this category, with multiple controlled trials reporting benefits for stress, fatigue, and related outcomes, even as study quality, extract standardization, and sample size vary. Eleuthero, Schisandra, Reishi, Cordyceps, and Tulsi have also been investigated in laboratory, animal, and human research, with evidence that is real but less extensive than for Ashwagandha or

Rhodiola. Taken together, the adaptogen literature is active and expanding, and several of these herbs have genuine research support for specific outcomes—best interpreted herb by herb and preparation by preparation rather than as proof of one effect shared by the whole category.

# APPENDIX A

***Selected Scientific Literature for Further Study***

CORE HERBAL CATEGORY II

## NERVOUS SYSTEM SUPPORT (NERVINES)

### Scientific Perspective

Nervines are a traditional functional grouping of medicinal herbs used to support nervous system balance, emotional steadiness, relaxation, restorative sleep, and recovery during periods of strain. The term does not describe a single pharmacological class; it spans botanicals with different constituents and proposed actions, from gently calming herbs to sleep-supportive agents to herbs studied for mood-related effects. St. John's Wort has one of the largest clinical evidence bases in this category, with a substantial body of trials supporting its use for mild-to-moderate depressive disorders, alongside clinically important drug-interaction concerns that require attention. Chamomile, Passionflower, and Lemon Balm have encouraging clinical evidence for anxiety, stress, and sleep-related outcomes, and Valerian and American Skullcap have been studied for similar purposes, though results are less consistent. California Poppy and Catnip remain supported more by traditional use and preclinical research than by extensive human trials. Because nervous system complaints may reflect medical, psychiatric, medication-related, or situational causes, findings from one preparation should not be generalized to all products bearing the same common name.

### Representative Herbs

- Skullcap (*Scutellaria lateriflora*)
- Chamomile (*Matricaria chamomilla / Chamaemelum nobile*)
- Lemon Balm (*Melissa officinalis*)
- Passionflower (*Passiflora incarnata*)
- Valerian (*Valeriana officinalis*)
- St. John's Wort (*Hypericum perforatum*)
- California Poppy (*Eschscholzia californica*)
- Catnip (*Nepeta cataria*)

### Major Areas of Scientific Investigation

- Anxiety, nervous tension, and perceived stress
- Sleep onset, sleep quality, and insomnia-related symptoms
- Mood regulation and mild-to-moderate depressive disorders
- GABAergic and other neurotransmitter-related mechanisms
- Cognitive performance and psychophysiological responses under stress
- Sedative, anxiolytic, and neuroprotective activity
- Safety, tolerability, extract standardization, and herb-drug interactions
- Differences between traditional preparations and standardized extracts

## Selected Scientific Literature


1. **Sarris J, Panossian A, Schweitzer I, Stough C, Scholey A.** Herbal medicine for depression, anxiety and insomnia: a review of psychopharmacology and clinical evidence. *European Neuropsychopharmacology.* 2011;21(12):841-860. doi:10.1016/j.euroneuro.2011.04.002.
2. **Savage K, Firth J, Stough C, Sarris J.** GABA-modulating phytomedicines for anxiety: a systematic review of preclinical and clinical evidence. *Phytotherapy Research.* 2018;32(1):3-18. doi:10.1002/ptr.5940.
3. **Hieu TH, Dibas M, Surya Dila KA, et al.** Therapeutic efficacy and safety of chamomile for state anxiety, generalized anxiety disorder, insomnia, and sleep quality: a systematic review and meta-analysis of randomized trials and quasi-randomized trials. *Phytotherapy Research.* 2019;33(6):1604-1615. doi:10.1002/ptr.6349.
4. **Ghazizadeh J, Sadigh-Eteghad S, Marx W, et al.** The effects of lemon balm (Melissa officinalis L.) on depression and anxiety in clinical trials: a systematic review and meta-analysis. *Phytotherapy Research.* 2021;35(12):6690-6705. doi:10.1002/ptr.7252.
5. **Brock C, Whitehouse J, Tewfik I, Towell T.** American Skullcap (Scutellaria lateriflora): a randomised, double-blind placebo-controlled crossover study of its effects on mood in healthy volunteers. *Phytotherapy Research.* 2014;28(5):692-698. doi:10.1002/ptr.5044.
6. **Linde K, Berner MM, Kriston L.** St John's wort for major depression. *Cochrane Database of Systematic Reviews.* 2008;(4):CD000448. doi:10.1002/14651858.CD000448.pub3.
7. **Valente V, Machado D, Jorge S, Drake CL, Marques DR.** Does valerian work for insomnia? An umbrella review of the evidence. *European Neuropsychopharmacology.* 2024;82:6-28. doi:10.1016/j.euroneuro.2024.01.008.


## Authoritative Scientific Resources

- World Health Organization (WHO), Monographs on Selected Medicinal Plants
- European Medicines Agency (EMA), European Union herbal monographs and assessment reports
- European Scientific Cooperative on Phytotherapy (ESCOP), ESCOP Monographs
- National Center for Complementary and Integrative Health (NCCIH)
- PubMed, U.S. National Library of Medicine

## Clinical Consideration

St. John's Wort carries the most significant interaction profile in this category: it induces liver enzymes that can reduce the effectiveness of hormonal contraceptives, anticoagulants such as warfarin, certain anticonvulsants, immunosuppressants, and some HIV and cancer medications, and it may cause serotonin syndrome when combined with SSRIs, SNRIs, MAOIs, or other serotonergic drugs. It should not be started or stopped without medical guidance in anyone taking prescription medication. Valerian, Passionflower, Chamomile, Lemon Balm, and California Poppy may cause additive sedation when combined with alcohol, benzodiazepines, opioids, or other sedating medications, and should be used cautiously before driving or operating machinery. Chamomile may trigger allergic reactions in people sensitive to the Asteraceae family, including ragweed. American Skullcap products have occasionally been associated with liver-related concerns linked to species misidentification or adulteration, so product sourcing matters. Persistent depression, anxiety, insomnia, or mood changes—particularly with thoughts of self-harm—require prompt evaluation by a qualified healthcare professional rather than self-treatment with nervines alone.

### Research Snapshot

The evidence base within Nervous System Support is genuinely substantial for several individual herbs. St. John's Wort has comparatively strong systematic-review evidence for mild-to-moderate major depression, making it one of the better-supported herbs in this book, though its interaction profile requires particular caution. Chamomile and Passionflower have encouraging clinical evidence for anxiety-related outcomes, and Lemon Balm has shown promising findings for anxiety, mood, and stress. Valerian has been studied extensively for sleep, with mixed results across modern reviews. American Skullcap has limited but suggestive human trial evidence for mood or anxiety benefit, while California Poppy and Catnip rest on smaller evidence bases. Overall, several nervines have real, trial-supported roles for specific outcomes, best applied by distinguishing traditional use from clinically established effects on a herb-by-herb basis.

# APPENDIX A

***Selected Scientific Literature for Further Study***

CORE HERBAL CATEGORY III

# DIGESTIVE SYSTEM SUPPORT

## Scientific Perspective

Digestive-support herbs are traditionally selected to influence distinct aspects of gastrointestinal function, including appetite, gastric comfort, intestinal motility, smooth-muscle tension, gas, nausea, bowel regularity, and protection of irritated tissues. Ginger has a substantial clinical literature for nausea and vomiting, especially pregnancy-associated and postoperative nausea, and enteric-coated Peppermint oil has one of the stronger evidence bases among digestive botanicals, with controlled trials supporting short-term relief of global symptoms and abdominal pain in irritable bowel syndrome. Fennel has pharmacological and clinical evidence related to smooth-muscle relaxation, gas, cramping, and colic, and research on bitter substances and Gentian supports real physiologic effects on taste receptors, gastric signaling, and appetite. Slippery Elm is widely used as a demulcent to soothe irritated mucosal tissue. Evidence from an essential oil, standardized extract, tea, powdered bark, or multi-herb formula should not automatically be generalized to every preparation of the same plant.

Persistent pain, bleeding, unexplained weight loss, progressive swallowing difficulty, recurrent vomiting, or major changes in bowel habits require medical evaluation rather than self-treatment with herbs alone.

## Representative Herbs

Ginger Root (Zingiber officinale)

Peppermint (Mentha x piperita)

Fennel Seed (Foeniculum vulgare)

Slippery Elm (Ulmus rubra)

Gentian (Gentiana lutea)

## Major Areas of Scientific Investigation

Nausea and vomiting, including pregnancy-associated and postoperative nausea

Irritable bowel syndrome, abdominal pain, bloating, and intestinal spasm

Functional dyspepsia and upper gastrointestinal discomfort

Carminative activity, gas, cramping, and smooth-muscle relaxation

Appetite, bitter-taste receptors, gastric signaling, and digestive reflexes

Mucosal soothing, demulcent activity, and protection of irritated tissues

Bowel regularity, motility, and stool consistency

Preparation-specific efficacy, dosage, safety, and herb-drug interactions

## Selected Scientific Literature

1. **Viljoen E, Visser J, Koen N, Musekiwa A.** A systematic review and meta-analysis of the effect and safety of ginger in the treatment of pregnancy-associated nausea and vomiting. *Nutrition Journal.* 2014;13:20. doi:10.1186/1475-2891-13-20. PMID: 24642205.
2. **Alammar N, Wang L, Saberi B, Nanavati J, Holtmann G, Shinohara RT, Mullin GE.** The impact of peppermint oil on the irritable bowel syndrome: a meta-analysis of the pooled clinical data. *BMC Complementary and Alternative Medicine.* 2019;19(1):21. doi:10.1186/s12906-018-2409-0. PMID: 30654773.
3. **European Medicines Agency, Committee on Herbal Medicinal Products.** European Union herbal monograph on *Foeniculum vulgare Miller subsp. vulgare var. dulce (Mill.) Batt. & Trab., fructus (Sweet Fennel Fruit). Revision 1.* EMEA/HMPC/372839/2016. Adopted 31 January 2024.
4. **European Medicines Agency, Committee on Herbal Medicinal Products.** European Union herbal monograph on *Gentiana lutea L., radix (Gentian Root).* EMA/HMPC/607861/2017. Adopted 20 November 2018.

## Authoritative Scientific Resources

- European Medicines Agency (EMA) herbal monographs and assessment reports
- PubMed, U.S. National Library of Medicine
- Cochrane Library
- National Center for Complementary and Integrative Health (NCCIH)
- World Health Organization (WHO) medicinal-plant monographs
- European Scientific Cooperative on Phytotherapy (ESCOP) monographs

## Clinical Consideration

Ginger, Peppermint, Fennel, Gentian, and Slippery Elm are not substitutes for diagnosis or treatment of gastrointestinal disease. Peppermint oil should be used cautiously by people with gastroesophageal reflux disease, since it can relax the lower esophageal sphincter and worsen heartburn, and enteric-coated capsules should not be crushed or taken with antacids. Fennel and Gentian may stimulate gastric acid and are best avoided in active peptic ulcer disease or significant reflux; Gentian, as a bitter, should also be avoided in gastritis. Slippery Elm's mucilage may slow or reduce the absorption of oral medications taken at the same time and should be spaced apart from other drugs. Ginger may increase bleeding risk at high doses and should be used cautiously with anticoagulant or antiplatelet medications.

## Research Snapshot

Ginger has the most substantial clinical evidence in this category, with systematic review and meta-analysis data supporting its use for pregnancy-associated and other forms of nausea, an area where safety during pregnancy is also relatively well characterized. Peppermint oil, particularly in enteric-coated form, has real trial-supported benefit for global IBS symptoms and abdominal pain, making it one of the better-evidenced digestive herbs in this book. Fennel and Gentian are recognized in European herbal monographs for traditional digestive use, supported by pharmacological and phytochemical research, though with a smaller body of controlled human trials than Ginger or Peppermint. Slippery Elm remains supported principally by its long-standing traditional use as a demulcent rather than by controlled clinical trials. This category therefore includes at least two herbs—Ginger and Peppermint—with genuinely strong, symptom-specific evidence, alongside others whose support rests more on traditional and pharmacological grounds.

# APPENDIX A

***Selected Scientific Literature for Further Study***

---

CORE HERBAL CATEGORY IV

# IMMUNE SYSTEM SUPPORT

## Scientific Perspective

Immune-support herbs are used to influence host defense, inflammatory signaling, recovery, and resistance to seasonal or recurrent illness. The category is not pharmacologically uniform: some preparations are studied mainly for short-term use during upper respiratory infections, while others are investigated for broader immunomodulatory effects. Echinacea has been examined extensively for prevention and early treatment of the common cold, with several trials reporting reduced symptom duration, though findings vary by species, plant part, and product composition. Elderberry has shown benefit for reducing upper respiratory symptom duration in a number of studies, and Reishi beta-glucan preparations have demonstrated measurable immune-marker changes in controlled research. Astragalus has substantial laboratory and traditional support for immune regulation, with more limited Western clinical trial evidence for routine self-care. Because product identity, dose, timing, health status, and concurrent medication use materially affect both safety and outcome, the literature supports a herb-specific rather than a one-size-fits-all approach to immune support.

## Representative Herbs

- Echinacea (*Echinacea purpurea*)
- Astragalus (*Astragalus membranaceus*)
- Reishi (*Ganoderma lucidum*)
- Elderberry (*Sambucus nigra*)
- Yarrow (*Achillea millefolium*)
- Olive Leaf (*Olea europaea*)

## Major Areas of Scientific Investigation

Prevention and early treatment of upper respiratory tract infections

Duration and severity of cold- and influenza-like symptoms

Innate immune activity, including macrophage and natural killer cell function

Adaptive immune markers, including T-lymphocyte populations and immunoglobulins

Cytokine regulation and inflammatory signaling

Antiviral and antimicrobial activity in laboratory models

Immune recovery during chronic stress, fatigue, or conventional treatment

Preparation-specific efficacy, safety, allergy risk, and medication interactions

## Selected Scientific Literature

1. **Karsch-Volk M, Barrett B, Kiefer D, Bauer R, Ardjomand-Woelkart K, Linde K.** Echinacea for preventing and treating the common cold. *Cochrane Database of Systematic Reviews.* 2014;(2):CD000530. doi:10.1002/14651858.CD000530.pub3.
2. **Schapowal A, Klein P, Johnston SL.** Echinacea reduces the risk of recurrent respiratory tract infections and complications: a meta-analysis of randomized controlled trials. *Advances in Therapy.* 2015;32(3):187-200. doi:10.1007/s12325-015-0194-4.
3. **Hawkins J, Baker C, Cherry L, Dunne E.** Black elderberry (Sambucus nigra) supplementation effectively treats upper respiratory symptoms: a meta-analysis of randomized, controlled clinical trials. *Complementary Therapies in Medicine.* 2019;42:361-365. doi:10.1016/j.ctim.2018.12.004.
4. **Wieland LS, Piechotta V, Feinberg T, Ludeman E, Hutton B, Kanji S, Seely D, Garritty C.** Elderberry for prevention and treatment of viral respiratory illnesses: a systematic review. *BMC Complementary Medicine and Therapies.* 2021;21(1):112. doi:10.1186/s12906-021-03283-5.
5. **Block KI, Mead MN.** Immune system effects of echinacea, ginseng, and astragalus: a review. *Integrative Cancer Therapies.* 2003;2(3):247-267. doi:10.1177/1534735403256419.
6. **Chen SN, Nan FH, Liu MW, Yang MF, Chang YC, Chen S.** Evaluation of immune modulation by beta-1,3; 1,6 D-glucan derived from Ganoderma lucidum in healthy adult volunteers: a randomized controlled trial. *Foods.* 2023;12(3):659. doi:10.3390/foods12030659.

## Authoritative Scientific Resources

- World Health Organization (WHO), Monographs on Selected Medicinal Plants
- European Medicines Agency (EMA), European Union herbal monographs and assessment reports
- European Scientific Cooperative on Phytotherapy (ESCOP), ESCOP Monographs
- National Center for Complementary and Integrative Health (NCCIH)
- Cochrane Library
- PubMed, U.S. National Library of Medicine

## Clinical Consideration

Immune-support herbs are not substitutes for vaccination, diagnostic testing, antimicrobial treatment when indicated, or urgent medical care. Persistent high fever, difficulty breathing, chest pain, confusion, dehydration, rapidly worsening symptoms, or illness in a medically vulnerable person requires prompt professional evaluation. People with autoimmune disease, organ transplants, cancer treatment, or immunosuppressive therapy should obtain clinical guidance before using immune-active herbs.

## Research Snapshot

Echinacea has the largest body of clinical literature in this category, with a number of trials reporting reduced cold symptom duration or severity, though results depend strongly on the exact preparation studied. Elderberry has real, if still-developing, evidence for reducing the duration or severity of upper respiratory symptoms. Reishi beta-glucan has shown measurable immune-marker changes in controlled research, and Astragalus is well supported by mechanistic and traditional literature, with adjunctive-treatment studies adding further support. Yarrow and Olive Leaf carry meaningful traditional and laboratory backing. This category therefore includes several herbs with genuine, trial-supported roles in immune support—best understood as a collection of distinct immune-modulating herbs rather than a single class of universal immune stimulants.

# APPENDIX A

***Selected Scientific Literature for Further Study***

CORE HERBAL CATEGORY V

## RESPIRATORY SYSTEM SUPPORT

### Scientific Perspective

Respiratory-support herbs have long been used in traditional Western herbal medicine to soothe irritated respiratory tissues, support normal mucus clearance, promote productive expectoration, and assist recovery from common respiratory illnesses. Standardized thyme-containing combination products have the strongest evidence in this category, with randomized controlled trials supporting their use for acute bronchitis. Mullein has extensive traditional respiratory use and relevant preclinical findings, and Elecampane and Speedwell have pharmacological findings relevant to antimicrobial activity and inflammatory signaling. Pleurisy Root is supported principally by traditional herbal literature. In modern evidence-informed practice, these botanicals are best regarded as complementary measures that support respiratory comfort and normal airway function alongside, rather than in place of, appropriate diagnosis and medical treatment.

### Representative Herbs

- Mullein Leaf (*Verbascum thapsus*)
- Thyme (*Thymus vulgaris*)
- Elecampane (*Inula helenium*)
- Pleurisy Root (*Asclepias tuberosa*)
- Speedwell (*Veronica officinalis*)

### Major Areas of Scientific Investigation

Acute cough and uncomplicated bronchitis

Productive cough associated with colds

Bronchial secretions and expectoration

Airway inflammation and bronchial irritation

Demulcent support of irritated mucous membranes

Antimicrobial and antiviral activity

Antispasmodic effects

Oxidative stress in respiratory tissues

Traditional respiratory applications

### Selected Scientific Literature


1. **Kemmerich B.** Evaluation of efficacy and tolerability of a fixed combination of dry extracts of thyme herb and primrose root in adults suffering from acute bronchitis with productive cough:

a prospective, double-blind, placebo-controlled multicentre clinical trial. *Arzneimittelforschung.* 2007;57(9):607–615. doi:10.1055/s-0031-1296656.

2. **Kemmerich B, Eberhardt R, Stammer H.** Efficacy and tolerability of a fluid extract combination of thyme herb and ivy leaves and matched placebo in adults suffering from acute bronchitis with productive cough: a prospective, double-blind, placebo-controlled clinical trial. *Arzneimittelforschung.* 2006;56(9):652–660. doi:10.1055/s-0031-1296767.
3. **Turker AU, Camper ND.** Biological activity of common mullein, a medicinal plant. *Journal of Ethnopharmacology.* 2002;82(2–3):117–125. doi:10.1016/S0378-8741(02)00186-1.
4. **Turker AU, Gurel E.** Common mullein (Verbascum thapsus L.): recent advances in research. *Phytotherapy Research.* 2005;19(9):733–739. doi:10.1002/ptr.1653.
5. **Seca AML, Grigore A, Pinto DCGA, Silva AMS.** The genus Inula and their metabolites: from ethnopharmacological to medicinal uses. *Journal of Ethnopharmacology.* 2014;154(2):286–310. doi:10.1016/j.jep.2014.04.010.
6. **Kenny C-R, Stojakowska A, Furey A, Lucey B.** From monographs to chromatograms: the antimicrobial potential of Inula helenium L. (Elecampane) naturalised in Ireland. *Molecules.* 2022;27(4):1406. doi:10.3390/molecules27041406.
7. **Gründemann C, Garcia-Käufer M, Sauer B, et al.** Traditionally used Veronica officinalis inhibits proinflammatory mediators via the NF-κB signalling pathway in a human lung cell line. *Journal of Ethnopharmacology.* 2013;145(1):118–126. doi:10.1016/j.jep.2012.10.039.

## Authoritative Scientific Resources

European Medicines Agency (EMA) herbal monographs and assessment reports

World Health Organization (WHO) monographs on selected medicinal plants

ESCOP monographs

- National Center for Complementary and Integrative Health (NCCIH)
- Cochrane Library
- PubMed

**Regulatory distinction:** EMA recognition of thyme for productive cough is based principally on long-standing traditional use. The EMA mullein monograph applies to mullein flower (Verbasci flos), not specifically to Mullein Leaf.

## Clinical Consideration

Respiratory herbs should not delay evaluation of potentially serious illness. Significant shortness of breath, coughing blood, chest pain, bluish discoloration, confusion, high or persistent fever, rapidly worsening symptoms, or unexplained weight loss require prompt medical assessment. Individuals with asthma, chronic obstructive pulmonary disease (COPD), interstitial lung disease, or other chronic pulmonary conditions should use herbal products as complementary measures within an appropriately supervised treatment plan.

## Research Snapshot

Clinical evidence within this category is strongest for standardized thyme-containing combination preparations, with randomized trials supporting their use for uncomplicated acute bronchitis and productive cough—a genuine strength, though those results apply specifically to the tested combination products rather than thyme tea or thyme alone. Mullein has extensive traditional respiratory use and relevant preclinical findings, with regulatory recognition applying most specifically to mullein flower. Elecampane and Speedwell have pharmacological findings relevant to antimicrobial activity and inflammatory signaling, and Pleurisy Root remains supported principally by traditional herbal literature. Together, these herbs offer real complementary support for respiratory comfort, appropriately scaled to the strength of evidence behind each preparation.

# APPENDIX A

***Selected Scientific Literature for Further Study***

CORE HERBAL CATEGORY VI

# CARDIOVASCULAR SYSTEM SUPPORT

## Scientific Perspective

Cardiovascular-support herbs have traditionally been used to promote healthy cardiac function, vascular integrity, circulation, and peripheral blood flow. Hawthorn has one of the strongest bodies of clinical evidence in this entire book, with multiple trials supporting its use for chronic heart failure and long-term cardiac support. Garlic has been extensively investigated for blood pressure regulation, with clinical studies reporting modest blood-pressure-lowering effects. Ginkgo has substantial research support for peripheral circulation and vascular cognitive disorders, and Cayenne has pharmacologic evidence related to vascular responses and circulation. Motherwort is supported principally by traditional herbal literature, phytochemical investigation, and limited clinical research. These herbs are not pharmacologically identical, and the literature supports evaluating each individually rather than assuming equivalent cardiovascular effects across the category.

## Representative Herbs

- Hawthorn (*Crataegus* spp.)
- Garlic (*Allium sativum*)
- Ginkgo (*Ginkgo biloba*)
- Cayenne (*Capsicum annuum*)
- Motherwort (*Leonurus cardiaca*)

## Major Areas of Scientific Investigation

- Chronic heart failure
- Cardiac contractility
- Coronary circulation
- Peripheral vascular circulation
- Blood pressure regulation
- Endothelial function
- Lipid metabolism
- Platelet aggregation
- Oxidative stress and vascular inflammation
- Long-term cardiovascular risk reduction

## Selected Scientific Literature


1. **Pittler MH, Guo R, Ernst E.** Hawthorn extract for treating chronic heart failure. *Cochrane Database of Systematic Reviews.* 2008;(1):CD005312. doi:10.1002/14651858.CD005312.pub2.

2. **Walker AF, Marakis G, Morris AP, Robinson PA.** Promising hypotensive effect of hawthorn extract: a randomized double-blind pilot study of mild, essential hypertension. *Phytotherapy Research.* 2002;16(1):48-54. doi:10.1002/ptr.947.
3. **Tassell MC, Kingston R, Gilroy D, Lehane M, Furey A.** Hawthorn (Crataegus spp.) in the treatment of cardiovascular disease. *Pharmacognosy Reviews.* 2010;4(7):32-41. doi:10.4103/0973-7847.65324.
4. **Stabler SN, Tejani AM, Huynh F, Fowkes C.** Garlic for the prevention of cardiovascular morbidity and mortality in hypertensive patients. *Cochrane Database of Systematic Reviews.* 2012;(8):CD007653. doi:10.1002/14651858.CD007653.pub2.
5. **Xiong XJ, Wang PQ, Li SJ, Li XK, Zhang YQ, Wang J.** Garlic for hypertension: a systematic review and meta-analysis of randomized controlled trials. *Phytomedicine.* 2015;22(3):352-361. doi:10.1016/j.phymed.2014.12.013.
6. **Diamond BJ, Bailey MR.** Ginkgo biloba: indications, mechanisms, and safety. *Psychiatric Clinics of North America.* 2013;36(1):73-83. doi:10.1016/j.psc.2012.12.006.
7. **European Medicines Agency, Committee on Herbal Medicinal Products (HMPC).** European Union herbal monograph on *Ginkgo biloba* L., folium. EMA/HMPC/321097/2012. London: 28 January 2015.

## Authoritative Scientific Resources

- World Health Organization (WHO)
- European Medicines Agency (EMA)
- ESCOP Monographs
- Cochrane Library
- National Center for Complementary and Integrative Health (NCCIH)
- PubMed

## Clinical Consideration

Cardiovascular-support herbs should not replace evidence-based treatment for heart disease, hypertension, arrhythmias, heart failure, or acute cardiovascular emergencies. Garlic, Ginkgo, Hawthorn, and Cayenne may interact with anticoagulants, antiplatelet agents, antihypertensive medications, or other cardiovascular drugs.

## Research Snapshot

Hawthorn has one of the strongest evidence bases among all traditional cardiovascular herbs, with a substantial body of clinical trials supporting its use for chronic heart failure and cardiac function, though outcomes vary by extract and patient population. Garlic has demonstrated modest, real blood-pressure-lowering effects in clinical studies. Ginkgo is well supported for peripheral circulation and vascular cognitive conditions. Cayenne and Motherwort derive meaningful support from traditional use and pharmacologic investigation, with a smaller body of controlled clinical evidence than Hawthorn or Garlic. This is a category where the strongest herbs have genuine, well-documented cardiovascular research behind them.

# APPENDIX A

***Selected Scientific Literature for Further Study***

CORE HERBAL CATEGORY VII

# LIVER & DETOX SUPPORT

## Scientific Perspective

Liver- and detox-support herbs have traditionally been used to promote normal hepatic function, support digestion and bile-related processes, and protect tissues from physiological stress. Artichoke Leaf has controlled clinical evidence for functional dyspepsia and is recognized in European herbal monographs for traditional relief of digestive complaints. Milk Thistle has the largest experimental and clinical literature in this category, with an extensive body of research examining its hepatoprotective properties, although human trial results for established liver disease are mixed. Dandelion Root is supported by long-standing traditional use for mild digestive symptoms and temporary appetite loss, and Burdock Root and Yellow Dock are grounded in traditional practice and phytochemical research. The literature supports evaluating each herb according to plant part, preparation, dose, and clinical context rather than treating all liver-support herbs as interchangeable.

## Representative Herbs

- Milk Thistle (*Silybum marianum*)
- Dandelion Root (*Taraxacum officinale*)
- Burdock Root (*Arctium lappa*)
- Yellow Dock (*Rumex crispus*)
- Artichoke Leaf (*Cynara cardunculus* syn. *Cynara scolymus*)

## Major Areas of Scientific Investigation

- Hepatocellular protection and liver-related biomarkers
- Oxidative stress and antioxidant activity
- Inflammatory signaling
- Bile-associated digestive function
- Functional dyspepsia and slow digestion
- Lipid and metabolic regulation
- Drug- and toxin-induced liver-injury models
- Phytochemistry and pharmacologic mechanisms
- Product standardization and extract-specific effects
- Safety, contraindications, and herb-drug interactions

## Selected Scientific Literature


1. **Saller R, Meier R, Brignoli R.** The use of silymarin in the treatment of liver diseases. *Drugs.* 2001;61(14):2035-2063. doi:10.2165/00003495-200161140-00003.
2. **Loguercio C, Festi D.** Silybin and the liver: from basic research to clinical practice. *World Journal of Gastroenterology.* 2011;17(18):2288-2301. doi:10.3748/wjg.v17.i18.2288.

3. **Holtmann G, Adam B, Haag S, Collet W, Grünewald E, Windeck T.** Efficacy of artichoke leaf extract in the treatment of patients with functional dyspepsia: a six-week placebo-controlled, double-blind, multicentre trial. *Alimentary Pharmacology & Therapeutics.* 2003;18(11-12):1099-1105. doi:10.1046/j.1365-2036.2003.01767.x.
4. **European Medicines Agency, Committee on Herbal Medicinal Products.** European Union herbal monograph on *Cynara cardunculus L. (syn. Cynara scolymus L.), folium.* EMA/HMPC/194014/2017. London: 27 March 2018.
5. **European Medicines Agency, Committee on Herbal Medicinal Products.** European Union herbal monograph on *Taraxacum officinale F.H. Wigg., radix.* EMA/HMPC/475726/2020. Adopted 24 November 2021.
6. **Chan YS, Cheng LN, Wu JH, Chan E, Kwan YW, Lee SMY, Leung GPH, Yu PHF, Chan SW.** A review of the pharmacological effects of Arctium lappa (burdock). *Inflammopharmacology.* 2011;19(5):245-254. doi:10.1007/s10787-010-0062-4.
7. **Qian H, Jia Y, Zheng K, Li C, Shao J, Wang J, Xu H, Zhou X.** Rumex crispus L.: a comprehensive review on botany, traditional uses, phytochemistry, pharmacology, and safety. *International Immunopharmacology.* 2024;143:113569. doi:10.1016/j.intimp.2024.113569.

## Authoritative Scientific Resources

- European Medicines Agency (EMA) herbal monographs and assessment reports
- National Center for Complementary and Integrative Health (NCCIH)
- PubMed, U.S. National Library of Medicine
- Cochrane Library
- World Health Organization (WHO) medicinal-plant monographs
- European Scientific Cooperative on Phytotherapy (ESCOP) monographs

## Clinical Consideration

Liver-support herbs should not replace medical evaluation or evidence-based treatment for hepatitis, cirrhosis, fatty liver disease, gallbladder disease, biliary obstruction, or suspected drug-induced liver injury. Jaundice, dark urine, pale stools, persistent right-upper-abdominal pain, vomiting blood, confusion, abdominal swelling, or markedly abnormal liver tests require prompt medical assessment.

Dandelion Root and Artichoke Leaf may stimulate bile-related digestive activity and are not appropriate for every person with gallstones, bile-duct obstruction, cholangitis, or other biliary disease. Individuals using prescription medications, especially those with chronic liver disease or complex medication regimens, should consult a qualified healthcare professional before use. Safety and effectiveness may also vary with species identification, plant part, extraction method, dose, and product quality.

## Research Snapshot

Artichoke Leaf has comparatively clear human evidence for functional dyspepsia and is well recognized for traditional digestive use. Milk Thistle has the largest research base in this category by far, with an extensive body of experimental and clinical literature, though controlled human evidence for established liver disease specifically remains inconsistent, and authoritative reviews stop short of definite conclusions there. Dandelion Root is well recognized for traditional use in mild digestive complaints and temporary appetite loss. Burdock Root and Yellow Dock have a growing pharmacologic and phytochemical literature supporting their traditional roles, with fewer large human trials to date. This category's strongest evidence supports specific digestive applications for Artichoke Leaf and Milk Thistle, distinct from broader detoxification or liver-disease-treatment claims.

# APPENDIX A

***Selected Scientific Literature for Further Study***

---

CORE HERBAL CATEGORY VIII

## ANTI-INFLAMMATORY & PAIN SUPPORT

### Scientific Perspective

Anti-inflammatory and pain-support herbs have traditionally been used to ease musculoskeletal discomfort, joint stiffness, swelling, soreness, and pain associated with overuse or minor injury. Modern research evaluates these herbs through specific outcomes such as pain intensity, physical function, joint stiffness, inflammatory signaling, local circulation, and the need for conventional pain medication.

The evidence is strongest for particular standardized preparations rather than for every form of the whole herb. Turmeric and curcumin formulations have been studied extensively for osteoarthritis symptoms, with several systematic reviews reporting real improvements in pain and function, though formulations differ greatly in curcuminoid content and absorption. Boswellia extracts also have controlled clinical evidence for knee osteoarthritis. Ginger has clinical and mechanistic evidence relevant to inflammatory pain and muscle soreness, Arnica has an established topical role for bruising and localized swelling, and Willow Bark and Devil's Claw are recognized in European herbal monographs for traditional relief of minor joint or musculoskeletal pain.

Used this way, several of these herbs have a genuinely solid evidence base—Turmeric and Boswellia in particular are among the better-studied natural options for osteoarthritis symptom relief. That said, the literature is specific about what they do: they support symptom management rather than reversing structural joint disease, and persistent, severe, or unexplained pain still calls for medical evaluation.

### Representative Herbs

- Turmeric (*Curcuma longa*)
- Willow Bark (*Salix* species)
- Boswellia (*Boswellia serrata*)
- Ginger Root (*Zingiber officinale*)
- Arnica (*Arnica montana*) – topical use
- Devil's Claw (*Harpagophytum procumbens* and/or *H. zeyheri*)
- Meadowsweet (*Filipendula ulmaria*)

### Major Areas of Scientific Investigation

- Osteoarthritis pain and stiffness
- Joint mobility and physical function
- Low-back and minor musculoskeletal pain
- Exercise-related muscle soreness
- Inflammatory signaling and oxidative stress

- Topical relief of bruising, swelling, and localized pain
- Analgesic and antipyretic traditional uses
- Extract standardization and bioavailability
- Comparisons with conventional pain medication
- Safety, gastrointestinal effects, bleeding risk, and herb-drug interactions

## Selected Scientific Literature


1. **Daily JW, Yang M, Park S.** Efficacy of turmeric extracts and curcumin for alleviating the symptoms of joint arthritis: a systematic review and meta-analysis of randomized clinical trials. *Journal of Medicinal Food.* 2016;19(8):717-729. PMID: 27533649.
2. **Bannuru RR, Osani MC, Al-Eid F, Wang C.** Efficacy of curcumin and Boswellia for knee osteoarthritis: systematic review and meta-analysis. *Seminars in Arthritis and Rheumatism.* 2018;48(3):416-429. PMID: 29622343.
3. **Kimmatkar N, Thawani V, Hingorani L, Khiyani R.** Efficacy and tolerability of Boswellia serrata extract in treatment of osteoarthritis of knee: a randomized double-blind placebo-controlled trial. *Phytomedicine.* 2003;10(1):3-7. PMID: 12622457.
4. **Sengupta K, Alluri KV, Satish AR, Mishra S, Golakoti T, Sarma KVS, Dey D, Raychaudhuri SP.** A double-blind, randomized, placebo-controlled study of the efficacy and safety of 5-Loxin for treatment of osteoarthritis of the knee. *Arthritis Research & Therapy.* 2008;10(4):R85. PMID: 18667054.
5. **European Medicines Agency, Committee on Herbal Medicinal Products.** European Union herbal monograph on *Salix species, cortex (Willow Bark).* EMA/HMPC/80630/2016. Adopted 31 January 2017.
6. **European Medicines Agency, Committee on Herbal Medicinal Products.** European Union herbal monograph on *Harpagophytum procumbens DC. and/or Harpagophytum zeyheri Decne., radix (Devil's Claw Root).* EMA/HMPC/627057/2015. Adopted 12 July 2016.
7. **Shep D, Khanwelkar C, Gade P, Karad S.** Safety and efficacy of curcumin versus diclofenac in knee osteoarthritis: a randomized open-label parallel-arm study. *Trials.* 2019;20:214. PMID: 30975196.


## Authoritative Scientific Resources

- European Medicines Agency (EMA) herbal monographs and assessment reports
- PubMed, U.S. National Library of Medicine
- Cochrane Library
- National Center for Complementary and Integrative Health (NCCIH)
- World Health Organization (WHO) medicinal-plant monographs
- European Scientific Cooperative on Phytotherapy (ESCOP) monographs

## Clinical Consideration

Pain accompanied by major swelling, redness, fever, deformity, inability to bear weight, sudden weakness or numbness, chest pain, severe headache, or pain following significant trauma requires medical assessment. Persistent pain may reflect arthritis, infection, fracture, nerve compression, vascular disease, or another condition that should not be managed solely with herbal products.

Willow Bark and Meadowsweet contain salicylate-related constituents and may be unsuitable for people with aspirin or salicylate sensitivity, active peptic ulcer disease, bleeding disorders, or anticoagulant therapy. Willow Bark should not be given to children or adolescents with viral illness. Turmeric, Ginger, and Boswellia may also affect bleeding or digestive tolerance in susceptible individuals. Arnica whole-herb preparations should not be taken internally and should not be applied to broken skin unless a specifically authorized product states otherwise. Devil's Claw may cause gastrointestinal effects and requires caution in people with gallstones or significant digestive disease.

### Research Snapshot

Turmeric/curcumin and Boswellia have the most substantial controlled human evidence in this category. Multiple randomized trials have reported improvements in knee osteoarthritis pain, stiffness, and function with these extracts, and systematic reviews describe the findings as encouraging, though certainty is limited by small trial sizes, variable product composition, and differences in bioavailability. Ginger has clinical and mechanistic evidence relevant to inflammatory and exercise-related pain, and Arnica has an established traditional role as a topical treatment for bruising and localized swelling. Willow Bark and Devil's Claw are recognized in European herbal monographs for traditional use in minor joint and musculoskeletal pain, supported by a smaller body of controlled trial evidence than Turmeric or Boswellia. Across this category, the research base supports these herbs as adjunctive options for symptom management—a meaningful role, though distinct from treating, curing, or reversing arthritis or replacing standard medical care.

# APPENDIX A

***Selected Scientific Literature for Further Study***

CORE HERBAL CATEGORY IX

# KIDNEY & URINARY SUPPORT

## Scientific Perspective

Kidney- and urinary-support herbs have traditionally been used to promote normal urine flow, soothe irritated urinary tissues, support bladder comfort, and assist the body's fluid-elimination processes. Cranberry has the strongest modern evidence in this category, with a substantial body of trials and reviews supporting its use for reducing the risk of recurrent urinary tract infections in selected populations—a genuinely well-established preventive role, distinct from treatment of an active infection. Uva Ursi has been studied for uncomplicated cystitis, with trials showing it can reduce antibiotic use, alongside some tradeoffs in symptom burden. Goldenrod, Nettle Herb, and related diuretic preparations are recognized in European herbal monographs for traditional use in minor urinary complaints. Nettle Root has been studied for male lower-urinary-tract symptoms, and Corn Silk is supported by traditional use and phytochemical investigation. This evidence supports careful distinction between urinary prevention, symptom support, and the treatment of infection or kidney disease.

## Representative Herbs

- Nettle (*Urtica dioica* and/or *Urtica urens*; herb or root according to use)
- Corn Silk (*Zea mays*, stigma)
- Uva Ursi / Bearberry Leaf (*Arctostaphylos uva-ursi*)
- Cranberry (*Vaccinium macrocarpon*)
- Goldenrod (*Solidago virgaurea*)
- Saw Palmetto (*Serenoa repens*)
- Pipsissewa (*Chimaphila umbellata*)

## Major Areas of Scientific Investigation

- Prevention of recurrent urinary tract infection
- Bacterial anti-adhesion within the urinary tract
- Uncomplicated cystitis and reduction of antibiotic use
- Urine flow and traditional diuretic use
- Bladder and lower-urinary-tract comfort
- Male lower-urinary-tract symptoms associated with benign prostatic enlargement
- Arbutin metabolism and urinary excretion
- Kidney-stone and urinary-mineral research
- Phytochemistry and preclinical renal or metabolic effects
- Safety, duration limits, hydration, and herb-drug interactions

## Selected Scientific Literature

1. **Williams G, Stothart CI, Hahn D, Stephens JH, Craig JC, Hodson EM.** Cranberries for preventing urinary tract infections. *Cochrane Database of Systematic Reviews.* 2023;11(11):CD001321. doi:10.1002/14651858.CD001321.pub7. PMID: 37947276.
2. **Moore M, Trill J, Simpson C, et al.** Uva-ursi extract and ibuprofen as alternative treatments for uncomplicated urinary tract infection in women: a factorial randomized trial. *Clinical Microbiology and Infection.* 2019;25(8):973-980. doi:10.1016/j.cmi.2019.01.011. PMID: 30685500.
3. **Gágyor I, Hummers E, Schmiemann G, Friede T, Pfeiffer S, Afshar K, Bleidorn J.** Herbal treatment with uva ursi extract versus fosfomycin in women with uncomplicated urinary tract infection: a randomized controlled trial. *Clinical Microbiology and Infection.* 2021;27(10):1441-1447. doi:10.1016/j.cmi.2021.05.032. PMID: 34111592.
4. **Schindler G, Patzak U, Brinkhaus B, et al.** Urinary excretion and metabolism of arbutin after oral administration of Arctostaphylos uva-ursi extract. *Journal of Clinical Pharmacology.* 2002;42(8):920-927. doi:10.1177/009127002401102740. PMID: 12162475.
5. **Fursenco C, Calalb T, Uncu L, Dinu M, Ancuceanu R.** Solidago virgaurea L.: a review of its ethnomedicinal uses, phytochemistry, and pharmacological activities. *Biomolecules.* 2020;10(12):1619. doi:10.3390/biom10121619. PMID: 33266185.
6. **Wang Y, Mao J, Zhang M, et al.** An umbrella insight into the phytochemistry features and biological activities of Corn Silk: a narrative review. *Molecules.* 2024;29(4):891. doi:10.3390/molecules29040891. PMID: 38398644.
7. **Franco JVA, Trivisonno L, Sgarbossa NJ, Alvez GA, Fieiras C, Escobar Liquitay CM, Jung JH.** Serenoa repens for the treatment of lower urinary tract symptoms due to benign prostatic enlargement. *Cochrane Database of Systematic Reviews.* 2023;6:CD001423. doi:10.1002/14651858.CD001423.pub4. PMID: 37345871.
8. **European Medicines Agency, Committee on Herbal Medicinal Products.** European Union herbal monograph on *Solidago virgaurea L., herba (European Goldenrod).* EMEA/HMPC/285758/2007. Adopted 4 September 2008.
9. **European Medicines Agency, Committee on Herbal Medicinal Products.** European Union herbal monograph on *Urtica dioica L. and Urtica urens L., herba (Nettle Herb, Revision 1) and Urtica dioica L. and Urtica urens L., radix (Nettle Root, Revision 1).* EMA/HMPC/261302/2022 (herba) and EMA/HMPC/322646/2023 (radix). Both published 14 June 2024.

## Authoritative Scientific Resources

- European Medicines Agency (EMA) herbal monographs and assessment reports
- Cochrane Library
- PubMed, U.S. National Library of Medicine
- National Center for Complementary and Integrative Health (NCCIH)
- World Health Organization (WHO) medicinal-plant monographs
- European Scientific Cooperative on Phytotherapy (ESCOP) monographs

## Clinical Consideration

Burning urination, urgency, frequency, blood in the urine, fever, chills, flank or back pain, vomiting, inability to urinate, new confusion, or symptoms during pregnancy require medical evaluation. Cranberry is not a treatment for an active urinary tract infection, and delaying appropriate antibiotics may allow progression to kidney infection or sepsis. Recurrent urinary symptoms may reflect infection, stones, prostate enlargement, pelvic-floor dysfunction, medication effects, diabetes, or another condition requiring diagnosis.

Uva Ursi contains arbutin-derived constituents and should be reserved for short-term, appropriately selected use; prolonged or repeated courses are not advisable. Diuretic herbs such as Goldenrod, Nettle Herb, Corn Silk, or Pipsissewa may alter fluid balance and may be unsuitable in significant kidney disease, heart failure, edema caused by organ disease, or alongside prescription diuretics without professional guidance. Saw Palmetto should not be relied upon to exclude prostate cancer or urinary obstruction. People taking anticoagulants, diuretics, lithium, blood-pressure medicines, diabetes medicines, or drugs affected by kidney function should consult a qualified healthcare professional before use.

### Research Snapshot

Cranberry has the clearest, best-established evidence in this category: a substantial body of research supports its use for prevention of recurrent urinary tract infection in some populations, making it one of the more solidly evidenced herbs in this book, though benefit varies by formulation and patient group. Uva Ursi has measurable urinary pharmacology and real trial support for uncomplicated cystitis, used short-term. Goldenrod and Nettle preparations carry established traditional-use monographs for minor urinary complaints, and Corn Silk and Pipsissewa are supported by traditional and preclinical evidence. Saw Palmetto has a long history of traditional use for male urinary symptoms, though contemporary systematic reviews find little added benefit from the herb alone for benign prostatic enlargement. Overall, this category includes at least one herb—Cranberry—with genuinely strong preventive evidence, alongside others whose roles are best understood as traditional symptom support rather than treatment of infection or kidney disease.

# APPENDIX A

***Selected Scientific Literature for Further Study***

CORE HERBAL CATEGORY X

# ENDOCRINE & HORMONAL SUPPORT

## Scientific Perspective

Endocrine- and hormonal-support herbs are used in traditional herbal practice to influence menstrual symptoms, reproductive function, sexual health, stress-related vitality, glucose regulation, and other processes governed by hormonal signaling. Chaste Tree Berry has the clearest clinical evidence in this category, with multiple trials supporting its use for premenstrual syndrome and related cyclical symptoms. Fenugreek has promising trial evidence for improving glycemic measures, and Maca has suggestive evidence for sexual function and menopausal complaints. Bitter Melon and Tribulus have been studied for metabolic and sexual-function outcomes with more variable results. Canary Seed, Dodder, Fig Leaf, Nettle Seed, and White Peony are supported mainly by traditional use and preclinical investigation. Each of these herbs must be evaluated according to the specific endocrine pathway, symptom pattern, and clinical outcome studied, rather than treated as interchangeable hormone balancers.

## Representative Herbs

- Bitter Melon (*Momordica charantia*)
- Canary Seed (*Phalaris canariensis*)
- Chaste Tree Berry / Vitex (*Vitex agnus-castus*)
- Dodder (*Cuscuta* species)
- Fenugreek (*Trigonella foenum-graecum*)
- Fig Leaf (*Ficus carica*)
- Maca Root (*Lepidium meyenii*)
- Nettle Seed (*Urtica dioica*)
- Tribulus (*Tribulus terrestris*)
- White Peony (*Paeonia lactiflora*)

## Major Areas of Scientific Investigation

- Premenstrual syndrome and cyclical breast discomfort
- Menstrual regularity and pituitary-related signaling
- Sexual desire and sexual function
- Menopausal symptoms
- Male reproductive parameters
- Glucose regulation and insulin sensitivity
- Metabolic and lipid-related outcomes
- Stress-related vitality and fatigue
- Phytochemical mechanisms affecting endocrine pathways
- Safety, pregnancy precautions, and herb-drug interactions

## Selected Scientific Literature


1. **European Medicines Agency, Committee on Herbal Medicinal Products.** European Union herbal monograph on *Vitex agnus-castus L., fructus. Revision 1.* EMA/HMPC/606742/2017. Adopted 27 March 2018.
2. **Schellenberg R.** Treatment for the premenstrual syndrome with agnus castus fruit extract: prospective, randomised, placebo controlled study. *BMJ.* 2001;322(7279):134-137. doi:10.1136/bmj.322.7279.134. PMID: 11159568.
3. **Shin BC, Lee MS, Yang EJ, Lim HS, Ernst E.** Maca (L. meyenii) for improving sexual function: a systematic review. *BMC Complementary and Alternative Medicine.* 2010;10:44. doi:10.1186/1472-6882-10-44. PMID: 20691074.
4. **Brooks NA, Wilcox G, Walker KZ, Ashton JF, Cox MB, Stojanovska L.** Beneficial effects of Lepidium meyenii (Maca) on psychological symptoms and measures of sexual dysfunction in postmenopausal women are not related to estrogen or androgen content. *Menopause.* 2008;15(6):1157-1162. doi:10.1097/gme.0b013e3181732953. PMID: 18784609.
5. **Neelakantan N, Narayanan M, de Souza RJ, van Dam RM.** Effect of fenugreek (Trigonella foenum-graecum L.) intake on glycemia: a meta-analysis of clinical trials. *Nutrition Journal.* 2014;13:7. doi:10.1186/1475-2891-13-7. PMID: 24438170.
6. **Yin RV, Lee NC, Hirpara H, Phung OJ.** The effect of bitter melon (Momordica charantia) in patients with diabetes mellitus: a systematic review and meta-analysis. *Nutrition & Diabetes.* 2014;4:e145. doi:10.1038/nutd.2014.42. PMID: 25504465.
7. **Qureshi A, Naughton DP, Petroczi A.** A systematic review on the herbal extract Tribulus terrestris and the roots of its putative aphrodisiac and performance-enhancing effect. *Journal of Dietary Supplements.* 2014;11(1):64-79. doi:10.3109/19390211.2014.887602. PMID: 24559105.
8. **Ulloa del Carpio N, Alvarado-Corella D, Quiñones-Laveriano DM, Araya-Sibaja A, Vega-Baudrit J, Monagas-Juan M, Navarro-Hoyos M, Villar-López M.** Exploring the chemical and pharmacological variability of Lepidium meyenii: a comprehensive review of the effects of maca. *Frontiers in Pharmacology.* 2024;15:1360422. doi:10.3389/fphar.2024.1360422. PMID: 38440178.


## Authoritative Scientific Resources

- European Medicines Agency (EMA) herbal monographs and assessment reports
- PubMed, U.S. National Library of Medicine
- Cochrane Library
- National Center for Complementary and Integrative Health (NCCIH)
- World Health Organization (WHO) medicinal-plant monographs
- European Scientific Cooperative on Phytotherapy (ESCOP) monographs

## Clinical Consideration

Endocrine symptoms may reflect thyroid disease, diabetes, pituitary disorders, medication effects, pregnancy, menopause, polycystic ovary syndrome, infertility, or other conditions requiring diagnosis. Unexplained menstrual changes, persistent fatigue, rapid weight change, excessive thirst or urination, recurrent low blood sugar, abnormal bleeding, breast discharge, or symptoms of pregnancy should receive appropriate medical evaluation.

Chaste Tree may affect dopaminergic and hormonal signaling and should be used cautiously with dopamine-active medicines, hormonal contraceptives, fertility treatment, pregnancy, or a history of pituitary disease. Bitter Melon and Fenugreek may lower blood glucose and can increase the risk of hypoglycemia when combined with diabetes medication. Fenugreek may cause gastrointestinal effects or allergic reactions, particularly in individuals sensitive to legumes. Evidence for Maca, Tribulus, White Peony, Dodder, Nettle Seed, Canary Seed, and Fig Leaf is insufficient to assume safety during pregnancy, breastfeeding, hormone-sensitive illness, or complex endocrine treatment.

### Research Snapshot

Chaste Tree Berry has the most clearly defined and well-supported clinical role in this category, with trial evidence specifically for premenstrual syndrome and related cyclical symptoms. Fenugreek has genuinely promising evidence for improving glycemic measures, though preparation and study quality vary. Maca has suggestive evidence for sexual function and menopausal complaints, without measurable changes in circulating sex hormones. Bitter Melon research shows modest glucose-lowering effects in some trials, with mixed results overall, and Tribulus remains inconclusive for testosterone enhancement specifically. For Canary Seed, Dodder, Fig Leaf, Nettle Seed, and White Peony, evidence remains at the traditional-use and preclinical stage. Chaste Tree Berry and Fenugreek stand out in this category as having real, outcome-specific trial support.

# APPENDIX A

***Selected Scientific Literature for Further Study***

CORE HERBAL CATEGORY XI

# LYMPHATIC & SKIN SUPPORT

## Scientific Perspective

Lymphatic- and skin-support herbs are used in traditional herbal practice to promote tissue drainage, support the skin barrier, soothe irritation, assist minor wound repair, and address patterns historically described as lymphatic or cutaneous congestion. Topical Comfrey preparations have controlled clinical evidence for selected sprains, strains, back pain, and joint complaints. Tea Tree oil has clinical evidence supporting its use for acne and some superficial fungal conditions. Calendula has clinical and preclinical research related to wound healing, and Witch Hazel is recognized in European herbal monographs for minor skin inflammation and superficial wounds. For herbs traditionally described as lymphatic movers or alteratives—Cleavers, Red Root, Figwort, Chickweed, Sweet Violet, Elder Leaf, and Red Clover—the evidence rests mainly on traditional herbal classification rather than controlled human studies of lymphatic flow.

## Representative Herbs

- Annatto (*Bixa orellana*)
- Calendula (*Calendula officinalis*)
- Chickweed (*Stellaria media*)
- Cleavers (*Galium aparine*)
- Comfrey (*Symphytum officinale*) – topical use
- Cornflower (*Centaurea cyanus*)
- Elder Leaf (*Sambucus nigra*)
- Figwort (*Scrophularia nodosa*)
- Gambir (*Uncaria gambir*)
- Heartsease (*Viola tricolor*)
- Lamb's Ear (*Stachys byzantina*)
- Oak Bark (*Quercus* species)
- Plantain Leaf (*Plantago major* and/or *Plantago lanceolata*)
- Red Clover (*Trifolium pratense*)
- Red Root (*Ceanothus americanus*)
- Sea Buckthorn (*Hippophae rhamnoides*)
- Snowberry (*Symphoricarpos* species)
- Sumac (*Rhus* species)
- Sweet Violet (*Viola odorata*)
- Tea Tree (*Melaleuca alternifolia*) – topical essential oil
- White Oak Bark (*Quercus alba*)
- Witch Hazel (*Hamamelis virginiana*)

- Alkanet (*Alkanna tinctoria*)

## Major Areas of Scientific Investigation

- Minor wound healing and re-epithelialization
- Skin-barrier repair and tissue regeneration
- Inflammation, itching, and irritation
- Bruising, swelling, sprains, and localized pain
- Acne and superficial microbial skin conditions
- Astringent effects on minor skin and mucosal irritation
- Antioxidant and photoprotective activity
- Traditional lymphatic drainage and alterative use
- Topical product standardization and sensitization risk
- Safety limitations, including pyrrolizidine alkaloids and essential-oil toxicity

## Selected Scientific Literature


1. **Leach MJ.** Calendula officinalis and wound healing: a systematic review. *Wounds.* 2008;20(8):236-243. PMID: 25941793.
2. **Givol O, Kornhaber R, Visentin D, Cleary M, Haik J, Harats M.** A systematic review of Calendula officinalis extract for wound healing. *Wound Repair and Regeneration.* 2019;27(5):548-561. doi:10.1111/wrr.12737. PMID: 31145533.
3. **Giostri GS, Novak EM, Buzzi M, Guarita-Souza LC.** Treatment of acute wounds in hand with Calendula officinalis L.: a randomized trial. *Tissue Barriers.* 2022;10(3):1994822. doi:10.1080/21688370.2021.1994822. PMID: 34674610.
4. **Frost R, MacPherson H, O'Meara S.** A critical scoping review of external uses of comfrey (Symphytum spp.). *Complementary Therapies in Medicine.* 2013;21(6):724-745. doi:10.1016/j.ctim.2013.09.009. PMID: 24280482.
5. **Staiger C.** Comfrey: a clinical overview. *Phytotherapy Research.* 2012;26(10):1441-1448. doi:10.1002/ptr.4612. PMID: 22359388.
6. **European Medicines Agency, Committee on Herbal Medicinal Products.** European Union herbal monograph on *Hamamelis virginiana L., cortex (Witch Hazel Bark).* EMA/HMPC/114583/2008. Adopted 12 November 2009.
7. **Kairey L, Agnew T, Bowles EJ, Barkla BJ, Wardle J, Lauche R.** Efficacy and safety of Melaleuca alternifolia (tea tree) oil for human health: a systematic review of randomized controlled trials. *Frontiers in Pharmacology.* 2023;14:1116077. doi:10.3389/fphar.2023.1116077. PMID: 37033604.
8. **Bassett IB, Pannowitz DL, Barnetson RSC.** A comparative study of tea-tree oil versus benzoyl peroxide in the treatment of acne. *Medical Journal of Australia.* 1990;153(8):455-458. PMID: 2145499.


## Authoritative Scientific Resources

- European Medicines Agency (EMA) herbal monographs and assessment reports
- PubMed, U.S. National Library of Medicine
- Cochrane Library

- National Center for Complementary and Integrative Health (NCCIH)
- World Health Organization (WHO) medicinal-plant monographs
- European Scientific Cooperative on Phytotherapy (ESCOP) monographs

### Clinical Consideration

Persistent or unexplained swollen lymph nodes, rapidly spreading redness, fever, pus, severe pain, skin necrosis, nonhealing wounds, suspicious moles, or swelling of an arm or leg require medical evaluation. Lymphedema, cellulitis, venous disease, autoimmune skin disorders, and skin cancer should not be managed solely with herbal products.

Comfrey should not be taken internally because pyrrolizidine alkaloids can cause serious liver injury. Topical Comfrey should be limited to intact skin and appropriately manufactured products. Tea Tree oil should never be swallowed and must be properly diluted for topical use; allergic contact dermatitis and irritation are possible. Oak Bark, White Oak Bark, Witch Hazel, and Gambir are strongly astringent and may aggravate very dry, cracked, or sensitive tissue. Plants such as Calendula, Chickweed, Cornflower, Heartsease, and others may trigger allergic reactions in susceptible users.

### Research Snapshot

Topical Comfrey and Tea Tree oil have the most directly relevant modern clinical evidence within this category, supporting real, if narrow, uses: Comfrey for selected painful musculoskeletal conditions, and Tea Tree oil for acne and certain superficial microbial conditions. Calendula research supports possible benefit for wound healing, and Witch Hazel is well recognized for traditional topical use in minor inflammation and superficial skin complaints. For the remaining herbs, modern clinical research is limited, so their traditional lymphatic and skin-support roles are best presented as historical and practice-based. This category's clearest strength lies in topical, symptom-specific applications rather than broad claims of treating lymphatic disease.

# APPENDIX A

***Selected Scientific Literature for Further Study***

CORE HERBAL CATEGORY XII

# ANTIMICROBIAL SUPPORT

## Scientific Perspective

Antimicrobial-support herbs are traditionally used to help the body resist or limit bacterial, fungal, parasitic, and other microbial challenges. Myrrh has authoritative European recognition for traditional topical use in minor mouth ulcers, oral inflammation, and small superficial wounds. Neem has real, if still-limited, human clinical research supporting oral-health preparations evaluated for dental plaque and gingival inflammation. Goldenseal contains alkaloids, including berberine, with well-documented antimicrobial activity in laboratory models. Black Walnut Hull and Pau d'Arco have antimicrobial, antifungal, or antiparasitic activity demonstrated in laboratory and preclinical research. Because a plant extract inhibiting microorganisms in a laboratory does not automatically translate to effective concentrations in human tissue, these herbs are best understood through the specific outcomes studied—dental plaque, gingival inflammation, or minor wound care—rather than as broad-spectrum replacements for antibiotics or antifungal treatment.

## Representative Herbs

- Black Walnut Hull (*Juglans nigra*)
- Goldenseal (*Hydrastis canadensis*)
- Myrrh (*Commiphora myrrha* and/or *Commiphora molmol*)
- Neem (*Azadirachta indica*)
- Pau d'Arco (*Handroanthus impetiginosus*; synonym *Tabebuia impetiginosa*)

## Major Areas of Scientific Investigation

- Antibacterial and antifungal activity in laboratory models
- Antibiofilm activity and interference with microbial adhesion
- Oral bacteria, dental plaque, and gingival inflammation
- Minor mouth ulcers and localized oral inflammation
- Topical cleansing of minor superficial wounds
- Antiparasitic and anthelmintic activity
- Activity of berberine, hydrastine, juglone, lapachol, β-lapachone, terpenoids, limonoids, and related plant constituents
- Extract composition, preparation standardization, and dose variability
- Herb–drug interactions and effects on drug-metabolizing enzymes
- Reproductive, hepatic, renal, gastrointestinal, and neurologic safety
- The difference between laboratory antimicrobial activity and clinically demonstrated treatment efficacy

## Selected Scientific Literature

1. **Batiha GES, Wasef L, Teibo JO, Shaheen HM, Zakariya AM, Akinfe OA, Teibo TKA, Al-kuraishy HM, Al-Garbee AI, Alexiou A, Papadakis M.** Commiphora myrrh: a phytochemical and pharmacological update. *Naunyn-Schmiedeberg's Archives of Pharmacology.* 2023;396(3):405-420. doi:10.1007/s00210-022-02325-0. PMID: 36399185.
2. **European Medicines Agency, Committee on Herbal Medicinal Products.** European Union herbal monograph on *Commiphora molmol Engler, gummi-resina.* EMA/HMPC/96911/2010. Adopted 12 July 2011.
3. **Ho KV, Lei Z, Sumner LW, Coggeshall MV, Hsieh HY, Stewart GC, Lin CH.** Identifying antibacterial compounds in black walnuts (Juglans nigra) using a metabolomics approach. *Metabolites.* 2018;8(4):58. doi:10.3390/metabo8040058. PMID: 30274312.
4. **Zhang J, Hunto ST, Yang Y, Lee J, Cho JY.** Tabebuia impetiginosa: a comprehensive review on traditional uses, phytochemistry, and immunopharmacological properties. *Molecules.* 2020;25(18):4294. doi:10.3390/molecules25184294. PMID: 32962180.
5. **Gómez Castellanos JR, Prieto JM, Heinrich M.** Red Lapacho (Tabebuia impetiginosa)—a global ethnopharmacological commodity? *Journal of Ethnopharmacology.* 2009;121(1):1-13. doi:10.1016/j.jep.2008.10.004. PMID: 18992801.
6. **Mandal SK, Maji AK, Mishra SK, Ishfaq PM, Devkota HP, Silva AS, Das N.** Goldenseal (Hydrastis canadensis L.) and its active constituents: a critical review of their efficacy and toxicological issues. *Pharmacological Research.* 2020;160:105085. doi:10.1016/j.phrs.2020.105085. PMID: 32683037.
7. **Ettefagh KA, Burns JT, Junio HA, Kaatz GW, Cech NB.** Goldenseal extracts synergistically enhance the antibacterial activity of berberine via efflux-pump inhibition. *Planta Medica.* 2011;77(8):835-840. PMID: 21157683.
8. **Lakshmi T, Krishnan V, Rajendran R, Madhusudhanan N.** Azadirachta indica: a herbal panacea in dentistry—an update. *Pharmacognosy Reviews.* 2015;9(17):41-44. doi:10.4103/0973-7847.156337. PMID: 26009692.
9. **Chatterjee A, Saluja M, Singh N, Kandwal A.** To evaluate the antigingivitis and antiplaque effect of an Azadirachta indica mouthrinse on plaque-induced gingivitis: a double-blind, randomized, controlled trial. *Journal of Indian Society of Periodontology.* 2011;15(4):398-401. doi:10.4103/0972-124X.92578. PMID: 22368367.
10. **Dhingra K, Vandana KL.** Effectiveness of Azadirachta indica (neem) mouthrinse in plaque and gingivitis control: a systematic review. *International Journal of Dental Hygiene.* 2017;15(1):4-15. doi:10.1111/idh.12191. PMID: 26876277.
11. **Wylie MR, Merrell DS.** The antimicrobial potential of the neem tree Azadirachta indica. *Frontiers in Pharmacology.* 2022;13:891535. doi:10.3389/fphar.2022.891535. PMID: 35712721.
12. **McClure C, Bollen M, Buttolph L, Stack E, Langley BO, Hanes D, Wright KM, Tibbitts D, Bradley R.** Safety and tolerability of Pau d' Arco (Tabebuia avellanedae) for primary dysmenorrhea: a single-arm, open-label trial on adults ages 18–45. *Advances in Integrative Medicine.* 2022;9(3):159-166. doi:10.1016/j.aimed.2022.04.003. PMID: 36960315.

## Authoritative Scientific Resources

- European Medicines Agency herbal monographs and assessment reports
- PubMed, U.S. National Library of Medicine
- National Center for Complementary and Integrative Health
- World Health Organization medicinal-plant monographs
- Cochrane Library
- European Scientific Cooperative on Phytotherapy monographs
- Peer-reviewed systematic reviews and controlled clinical studies
- Pharmacovigilance and herb–drug-interaction literature

## Clinical Consideration

Suspected bacterial, fungal, parasitic, or systemic infection should not be managed solely with herbal products. High fever, confusion, breathing difficulty, severe weakness, rapidly spreading redness, red streaking, pus, tissue discoloration, persistent vomiting or diarrhea, dehydration, severe abdominal pain, an infected wound, blood in urine or stool, or symptoms in an infant, frail older adult, pregnant individual, or immunocompromised person require prompt medical evaluation.

Herbal products should not be substituted for prescribed antibiotics, antifungal agents, antiparasitic medicines, vaccination, surgical drainage, wound debridement, or other clinically necessary treatment. Inappropriate antimicrobial self-treatment can delay diagnosis, allow infection to spread, and contribute indirectly to poor outcomes.

Goldenseal has limited high-quality evidence for treating human infection and may affect drug-metabolizing enzymes and transport proteins. It should be avoided during pregnancy and breastfeeding and should not be given to newborns or infants because berberine exposure may worsen neonatal jaundice. NCCIH also cautions that Goldenseal may alter the effects or toxicity of commonly used medicines.

Black Walnut Hull lacks reliable human clinical evidence for eradicating intestinal parasites, Candida infection, or systemic fungal disease. Its juglone and tannin content, product variability, allergy potential, and uncertain long-term safety support only cautious, short-duration use. It should not be used as a substitute for laboratory diagnosis and approved antiparasitic or antifungal treatment.

Pau d'Arco contains naphthoquinones such as lapachol and β-lapachone that show biological activity in preclinical research. However, clinically effective antimicrobial dosing has not been established. Concentrated preparations may cause gastrointestinal upset and may present bleeding, reproductive, hepatic, or renal concerns. Avoid during pregnancy and breastfeeding and use cautiously with anticoagulant or antiplatelet medicines.

Neem preparations vary greatly according to the plant part and extraction method. Neem oil should not be swallowed; serious poisoning, particularly in children, has been reported in the medical literature. Internal use during pregnancy should be avoided because reproductive safety has not been established. Human evidence is most relevant to specific oral-care products and should not be generalized to systemic infection treatment.

Myrrh is best supported for limited, traditional topical use involving minor oral inflammation, small mouth ulcers, and minor superficial wounds. Concentrated preparations may irritate mucous membranes, and internal use may cause gastrointestinal effects. It should be avoided during pregnancy because of traditional uterine-stimulating concerns and insufficient reproductive-safety data.

### Research Snapshot

Myrrh has the clearest authoritative recognition in this category, supported by European herbal monographs for narrow, traditional topical applications in minor oral inflammation, mouth ulcers, and superficial wounds. Neem has real human clinical evidence in preparation-specific oral-health products, particularly for dental plaque and gingival inflammation. Goldenseal has well-documented in-vitro antibacterial activity associated with berberine and other constituents, and Black Walnut and Pau d'Arco show antibacterial and antiparasitic activity in laboratory studies, with human trials still developing. This category is scientifically strongest for its localized, preparation-specific applications—genuine antimicrobial potential and documented traditional anti-infective use—distinct from broader claims that these herbs independently cure bacterial, viral, fungal, or parasitic disease.

# APPENDIX A

***Selected Scientific Literature for Further Study***

---

CORE HERBAL CATEGORY XIII

# REPRODUCTIVE & WOMEN'S HEALTH SUPPORT

## Scientific Perspective

Reproductive- and women's-health herbs are traditionally used to support menstrual comfort, reproductive-tissue tone, menopausal transition, postpartum recovery, lactation, and general reproductive vitality. Black Cohosh has the most developed regulatory and clinical literature in this category: the European Medicines Agency recognizes certain preparations for relief of menopausal complaints such as hot flashes and sweating, supported by a substantial body of clinical trials, alongside possible liver-related adverse effects that require attention. Shatavari has emerging small controlled trials for menopausal symptoms. Red Raspberry Leaf has a long history of pregnancy and childbirth use, though modern reviews find the evidence for shortening labor weak. Dong Quai, Lady's Mantle, Cramp Bark, and False Unicorn Root are supported chiefly by traditional practice. Blue Cohosh requires particular caution: despite historical use near childbirth, safety reviews identify possible uterine-stimulating, cardiovascular, and developmental risks, and it should not be treated as a routine pregnancy or labor herb.

## Representative Herbs

- Black Cohosh (*Actaea racemosa*; synonym *Cimicifuga racemosa*)
- Blue Cohosh (*Caulophyllum thalictroides*)
- Cramp Bark (*Viburnum opulus*)
- Dong Quai (*Angelica sinensis*)
- False Unicorn Root (*Chamaelirium luteum*)
- Lady's Mantle (*Alchemilla vulgaris*)
- Red Raspberry Leaf (*Rubus idaeus*)
- Shatavari (*Asparagus racemosus*)
- Wild Yam (*Dioscorea villosa*)

## Major Areas of Scientific Investigation

- Menopausal vasomotor, sleep, mood, and quality-of-life outcomes
- Menstrual pain, pelvic cramping, and smooth-muscle activity
- Premenstrual and cyclical symptoms
- Uterine contractility and reproductive-tissue responses
- Pregnancy, labor duration, birth outcomes, and maternal safety
- Postpartum recovery and lactation
- Estrogenic, serotonergic, dopaminergic, and other signaling mechanisms
- Phytoestrogenic constituents and steroidal saponins
- Product identity, extract standardization, and adulteration

- Hepatic, cardiovascular, reproductive, fetal, and neonatal safety

## Selected Scientific Literature


1. **European Medicines Agency, Committee on Herbal Medicinal Products.** European Union herbal monograph on *Cimicifuga racemosa (L.) Nutt., rhizoma. Revision 1.* EMA/HMPC/48745/2017. Adopted 27 March 2018.
2. **Leach MJ, Moore V.** Black cohosh (Cimicifuga spp.) for menopausal symptoms. *Cochrane Database of Systematic Reviews.* 2012;(9):CD007244. doi:10.1002/14651858.CD007244.pub2. PMID: 22972105.
3. **Sadahiro R, Matsuoka LN, Zeng BS, et al.** Black cohosh extracts in women with menopausal symptoms: an updated pairwise meta-analysis. *Menopause.* 2023;30(7):766-773. doi:10.1097/GME.0000000000002196. PMID: 37192826.
4. **Bowman R, Taylor J, Muggleton S, Davis D.** Biophysical effects, safety and efficacy of raspberry leaf use in pregnancy: a systematic integrative review. *BMC Complementary Medicine and Therapies.* 2021;21(1):56. doi:10.1186/s12906-021-03230-4. PMID: 33563275.
5. **Simpson M, Parsons M, Greenwood J, Wade K.** Raspberry leaf in pregnancy: its safety and efficacy in labor. *Journal of Midwifery & Women's Health.* 2001;46(2):51-59. PMID: 11370690.
6. **Gudise VS, Dasari MP, Kuricheti SSK.** Efficacy and safety of Shatavari root extract for the management of menopausal symptoms: a double-blind, multicenter, randomized controlled trial. *Cureus.* 2024;16(4):e57879. doi:10.7759/cureus.57879. PMID: 38725785.
7. **Komesaroff PA, Black CV, Cable V, Sudhir K.** Effects of wild yam extract on menopausal symptoms, lipids and sex hormones in healthy menopausal women. *Climacteric.* 2001;4(2):144-150. doi:10.1080/713605087. PMID: 11428178.
8. **Hirata JD, Swiersz LM, Zell B, Small R, Ettinger B.** Does Dong Quai have estrogenic effects in postmenopausal women? A double-blind, placebo-controlled trial. *Fertility and Sterility.* 1997;68(6):981-986. PMID: 9418683.
9. **Dugoua JJ, Perri D, Seely D, Mills E, Koren G.** Safety and efficacy of Blue Cohosh (Caulophyllum thalictroides) during pregnancy and lactation. *Canadian Journal of Clinical Pharmacology.* 2008;15(1):e66-e73. PMID: 18204101.
10. **Kronenberg F, Fugh-Berman A.** Complementary and alternative medicine for menopausal symptoms: a review of randomized, controlled trials. *Annals of Internal Medicine.* 2002;137(10):805-813. PMID: 12435217.


## Authoritative Scientific Resources

- European Medicines Agency (EMA) herbal monographs and assessment reports
- PubMed, U.S. National Library of Medicine
- Cochrane Library
- National Center for Complementary and Integrative Health (NCCIH)
- World Health Organization (WHO) medicinal-plant monographs
- European Scientific Cooperative on Phytotherapy (ESCOP) monographs

## Clinical Consideration

Abnormal uterine bleeding, bleeding after menopause, severe pelvic pain, fever, suspected pregnancy complications, a pelvic mass, recurrent pregnancy loss, infertility, breast changes, or rapidly worsening menopausal symptoms require medical evaluation. Herbal products should not be used to delay diagnosis of ectopic pregnancy, miscarriage, endometriosis, fibroids, or reproductive cancer, and no herb in this category should be assumed safe in pregnancy merely because it has a history of midwifery use.

Black Cohosh is intended for menopausal complaints, not pregnancy or labor; discontinue and seek care if jaundice, dark urine, or upper-abdominal pain develops. Red Raspberry Leaf has insufficient evidence to support routine claims of shortening labor and should be discussed with a maternity-care provider, particularly in high-risk pregnancy. Blue Cohosh should never be used for self-directed labor induction; reviews describe uterine-stimulating, cardiovascular, and developmental risks, including reports of serious neonatal complications. Dong Quai may affect bleeding and should not be assumed to act as estrogen replacement. Wild Yam should not be described as natural progesterone, since diosgenin does not convert to human hormones in the body. Shatavari, Lady's Mantle, Cramp Bark, and False Unicorn Root have limited controlled human evidence; their traditional use for uterine tone, cramping, or reproductive weakness should be identified as traditional practice rather than established treatment.

### Research Snapshot

Black Cohosh has the strongest formal clinical and regulatory support in this category: a substantial trial literature, including a later meta-analysis reporting improvement in overall menopausal symptoms and hot flashes, backs its EMA-recognized use for menopausal complaints, though findings vary by extract and product. Shatavari shows promising, preliminary trial results for menopausal symptoms. Red Raspberry Leaf remains a prominent traditional pregnancy herb, though available trials do not establish reliable shortening of labor. Blue Cohosh is scientifically important here as a safety example: historical reproductive use does not establish modern obstetric safety. Cramp Bark, Lady's Mantle, and False Unicorn Root remain largely traditional herbs with limited direct clinical research. Black Cohosh stands out in this category as genuinely well-supported for a specific, defined use—menopausal symptom relief—distinct from claims of treating infertility, miscarriage prevention, or pregnancy complications.

CORE HERBAL CATEGORY XIV

# NUTRITIONAL & TONIC SUPPORT

## Scientific Perspective

Nutritional- and tonic-support herbs are used to provide food-like nourishment—minerals, vitamins, amino acids, fatty acids, and polysaccharides associated with tissue maintenance and gradual restoration. Moringa Leaf, Nettle Leaf, Purslane, and Goji Berry have substantial, well-documented compositional evidence: real proteins, minerals, carotenoids, and fatty acids, genuinely supporting their use as nourishing, food-like botanicals, even though composition varies with soil, climate, and processing. The marine plants Bladderwrack, Dulse, and Irish Moss (Sea Moss) supply iodine and trace minerals, though content varies enormously among species and products, making dose awareness important. American Ginseng and Bala are traditional restorative tonics with medication-relevant effects. Fo-Ti and Horsetail require the most caution: Fo-Ti is strongly associated with herb-induced liver injury despite its traditional restorative reputation, and Horsetail's structural claims exceed what controlled trials support.

## Representative Herbs

- American Ginseng (*Panax quinquefolius*)
- Bala (*Sida cordifolia*)
- Bladderwrack (*Fucus vesiculosus*)
- Borage (*Borago officinalis*)
- Dulse (*Palmaria palmata*)
- Fo-Ti / He Shou Wu (*Polygonum multiflorum*; accepted name *Reynoutria multiflora*)
- Goji Berry (*Lycium barbarum* and/or *Lycium chinense*)
- Horsetail (*Equisetum arvense*)
- Irish Moss / Sea Moss (*Chondrus crispus* and related commercial seaweeds)
- Moringa Leaf (*Moringa oleifera*)
- Nettle Leaf (*Urtica dioica*)
- Purslane (*Portulaca oleracea*)

The reference book's full Core Herbal Category Index assigns 20 herbs to Nutritional & Tonic Support; the 12 listed above carry the category's direct scientific and safety evidence. The remaining herbs—including Alfalfa, Ashitaba, Baobab, Barley Grass, Chickpea, Cistanche, Cleome, and Dandelion Leaf—are best understood as food-like botanicals whose value depends on preparation, serving size, and overall diet.

## Major Areas of Scientific Investigation

- Protein, vitamin, mineral, and fatty-acid composition
- Nutrient density and contribution to dietary adequacy
- Alpha-linolenic acid and other plant-derived fatty acids
- Antioxidant capacity and polyphenol content

- Iodine content and thyroid effects of sea vegetables
- Metabolic, lipid, glucose, and inflammatory outcomes
- Fatigue, physical performance, and perceived well-being
- Variability caused by species, soil, harvesting, and processing
- Antinutrients, allergens, and heavy-metal exposure
- Hepatotoxicity and other safety concerns associated with concentrated tonic herbs

## Selected Scientific Literature


1. **Pareek A, Pant M, Gupta MM, Kashania P, Ratan Y, Jain V, Pareek A, Chuturgoon AA.** Moringa oleifera: an updated comprehensive review of its pharmacological activities, ethnomedicinal, phytopharmaceutical formulation, clinical, phytochemical, and toxicological aspects. *International Journal of Molecular Sciences.* 2023;24(3):2098. doi:10.3390/ijms24032098. PMID: 36768420.
2. **Devkota HP, Paudel KR, Khanal S, et al.** Stinging Nettle (Urtica dioica L.): nutritional composition, bioactive compounds, and food functional properties. *Molecules.* 2022;27(16):5219. doi:10.3390/molecules27165219. PMID: 36014458.
3. **Kumar A, Sreedharan S, Kashyap AK, Singh P, Ramchiary N.** A review on bioactive phytochemicals and ethnopharmacological potential of Purslane (Portulaca oleracea L.). *Heliyon.* 2022;8(1):e08669. doi:10.1016/j.heliyon.2021.e08669. PMID: 35028454.
4. **Petropoulos SA, Fernandes Â, Dias MI, Vasilakoglou IB, Petrotos K, Barros L, Ferreira ICFR.** Nutritional value, chemical composition and cytotoxic properties of common Purslane in relation to harvesting stage and plant part. *Antioxidants.* 2019;8(8):293. doi:10.3390/antiox8080293. PMID: 31398846.
5. **Teas J, Pino S, Critchley A, Braverman LE.** Variability of iodine content in common commercially available edible seaweeds. *Thyroid.* 2004;14(10):836-841. doi:10.1089/thy.2004.14.836. PMID: 15588380.
6. **Smyth PPA.** Iodine, seaweed, and the thyroid. *European Thyroid Journal.* 2021;10(2):101-108. doi:10.1159/000512971. PMID: 33981614.
7. **Teixeira F, Silva AM, Delerue-Matos C, Rodrigues F.** Lycium barbarum berries (Solanaceae) as source of bioactive compounds for healthy purposes: a review. *International Journal of Molecular Sciences.* 2023;24(5):4777. doi:10.3390/ijms24054777. PMID: 36902206.
8. **Rao T, Liu YT, Zeng XC, Li CP, Ou-Yang DS.** The hepatotoxicity of Polygonum multiflorum: the emerging role of immune-mediated liver injury. *Acta Pharmacologica Sinica.* 2021;42(1):27-35. doi:10.1038/s41401-020-0360-3. PMID: 32123300.
9. **Liu Y, Wang Q, Yang JB, et al.** Polygonum multiflorum Thunb.: a review on chemical analysis, processing mechanism, quality evaluation, and hepatotoxicity. *Frontiers in Pharmacology.* 2018;9:364. PMID: 29713283.
10. **National Institute of Diabetes and Digestive and Kidney Diseases.** Horsetail. *LiverTox: Clinical and Research Information on Drug-Induced Liver Injury.* Updated 25 July 2022. Bookshelf ID: NBK583202. PMID: 35998247.


## Authoritative Scientific Resources

- PubMed, U.S. National Library of Medicine
- National Center for Complementary and Integrative Health (NCCIH)
- National Institutes of Health Office of Dietary Supplements
- LiverTox, National Institute of Diabetes and Digestive and Kidney Diseases
- World Health Organization (WHO) nutrition and medicinal-plant resources
- European Scientific Cooperative on Phytotherapy (ESCOP) monographs

## Clinical Consideration

Nutritional herbs should not be used to self-diagnose or independently treat anemia, malnutrition, vitamin or mineral deficiency, thyroid disease, unexplained weight loss, or malabsorption; persistent weakness, fainting, swelling, or laboratory evidence of deficiency requires medical evaluation. A capsule of powdered leaf may contain measurable nutrients but still provide far less protein, iron, or vitamins than an ordinary food serving, so label claims such as "superfood" or "complete nutrition" should be evaluated against tested serving size, not descriptive language.

Bladderwrack, Dulse, and Irish Moss may contain widely variable iodine and can aggravate hyperthyroidism, hypothyroidism, or autoimmune thyroid disease; people with thyroid disease, kidney disease, or pregnancy should seek professional guidance before concentrated use. Fo-Ti should not be regarded as a routine daily tonic—both raw and processed products have been associated with liver injury, and jaundice, dark urine, or right-upper-abdominal discomfort requires immediate discontinuation and medical assessment. Bala may contain ephedrine-related alkaloids and requires caution with hypertension, arrhythmia, or stimulant-medication use. American Ginseng may affect blood glucose, sleep, and anticoagulant response. Borage seed oil and leaf or aerial-part preparations are not interchangeable, since the latter may contain unsaturated pyrrolizidine alkaloids. Horsetail's traditional claims for bone, hair, or connective tissue are not established by controlled trials, and LiverTox advises against high-dose, long-term use in people with existing liver disease.

## Research Snapshot

The strongest scientific foundation for this category is compositional, and it is genuinely solid: Moringa Leaf, Nettle Leaf, Purslane, and Goji Berry contain well-documented proteins, minerals, vitamins, and fatty acids that support describing them as nourishing, food-like botanicals. The marine plants' variability is itself an important finding—iodine exposure from Bladderwrack, Dulse, or Irish Moss can range from modest to excessive depending on species and product, so dose awareness matters more than broad thyroid-nourishment claims. American Ginseng and Bala are well-established traditional restorative tonics with real, medication-relevant effects. Fo-Ti carries the strongest warning in this category, given its documented association with liver injury, and Horsetail's traditional structural and urinary uses exceed current clinical evidence. This category spans a genuine spectrum, from well-documented nutrient-containing foods to traditional tonics that require real safety awareness.

CORE HERBAL CATEGORY XV

# FOUNDATIONAL / SYSTEMIC SUPPORT

## Scientific Perspective

Foundational / Systemic Support is the broadest and most conceptual of the 15 Core Herbal Categories, describing herbs that support several physiological systems rather than acting narrowly within one organ or symptom pattern. The Core Herbal Category Index assigns no herb here as a Primary Core; herbs broad enough to be considered foundational still have a more concentrated function within one of the other 14 categories, and Foundational / Systemic Support appears only as a Secondary Core, for Agrimony, Angelica Root, Nettle Leaf, Sarsaparilla, Sea Buckthorn, and Yarrow. Modern network pharmacology offers a genuinely useful research model for plants with multiple constituents and potential biological targets, examining how compounds, molecular targets, and physiological networks interact rather than assuming one isolated mechanism, though these findings are principally hypothesis-generating. Research on herbal synergy similarly shows that constituents within an extract can interact in additive or synergistic ways, a real and active area of study, even though synergy must be demonstrated experimentally rather than assumed from botanical complexity.

## Representative Herbs

Because Category XV contains no Primary-Core herbs, the following are included as Secondary-Core representatives; they should not be interpreted as pharmacologically equivalent to one another.

- Agrimony (*Agrimonia eupatoria*)
- Angelica Root (*Angelica archangelica*)
- Nettle Leaf (*Urtica dioica*)
- Sarsaparilla (*Smilax* species)
- Sea Buckthorn (*Hippophae rhamnoides*)
- Yarrow (*Achillea millefolium*)

## Major Areas of Scientific Investigation

- Multi-component and multi-target botanical pharmacology
- Systems biology and network-based models of herbal action
- Pharmacodynamic and pharmacokinetic synergy among constituents
- Additive, antagonistic, and modifying constituent interactions
- Effects across inflammatory, metabolic, immune, vascular, and digestive pathways
- Whole extracts compared with isolated constituents
- Bioavailability and metabolism of complex botanical preparations
- Quality control, botanical identity, and adulteration
- Limitations of computational target prediction

- Herb–drug interactions and cumulative effects across physiological systems

## Selected Scientific Literature


1. **Li S, Zhang B.** Traditional Chinese medicine network pharmacology: theory, methodology and application. *Chinese Journal of Natural Medicines.* 2013;11(2):110-120. doi:10.1016/S1875-5364(13)60037-0. PMID: 23787177.
2. **Zhang GB, Li QY, Chen QL, Su SB.** Network pharmacology: a new approach for Chinese herbal medicine research. *Evidence-Based Complementary and Alternative Medicine.* 2013;2013:621423. doi:10.1155/2013/621423. PMID: 23762149.
3. **Lee M, Shin H, Park M, Kim A, Cha S, Lee H.** Systems pharmacology approaches in herbal medicine research: a brief review. *BMB Reports.* 2022;55(9):417-428. doi:10.5483/BMBRep.2022.55.9.102. PMID: 35880436.
4. **Noor F, Tahir ul Qamar M, Ashfaq UA, Albutti A, Alwashmi ASS, Aljasir MA.** Network pharmacology approach for medicinal plants: review and assessment. *Pharmaceuticals.* 2022;15(5):572. doi:10.3390/ph15050572. PMID: 35631398.
5. **Yang Y, Zhang Z, Li S, Ye X, Li X, He K.** Synergy effects of herb extracts: pharmacokinetics and pharmacodynamic basis. *Fitoterapia.* 2014;92:133-147. doi:10.1016/j.fitote.2013.10.010. PMID: 24177191.
6. **Spinella M.** The importance of pharmacological synergy in psychoactive herbal medicines. *Alternative Medicine Review.* 2002;7(2):130-137. PMID: 11991792.
7. **European Medicines Agency, Committee on Herbal Medicinal Products.** European Union herbal monograph on *Agrimonia eupatoria L., herba.* EMA/HMPC/680597/2013. Adopted 28 January 2015.
8. **European Medicines Agency, Committee on Herbal Medicinal Products.** European Union herbal monograph on *Achillea millefolium L., herba. Revision 1.* EMA/HMPC/376416/2019. Adopted 2020.
9. **European Medicines Agency, Committee on Herbal Medicinal Products.** European Union herbal monograph on *Urtica dioica L. and Urtica urens L., herba. Revision 1.* EMA/HMPC/261302/2022. Published 14 June 2024.


## Authoritative Scientific Resources

- European Medicines Agency (EMA) herbal monographs and assessment reports
- PubMed, U.S. National Library of Medicine
- Cochrane Library
- National Center for Complementary and Integrative Health (NCCIH)
- World Health Organization (WHO) medicinal-plant monographs
- Systems-pharmacology and network-pharmacology literature

## Clinical Consideration

The term systemic support should not be interpreted as treatment of systemic disease. Fever, unexplained weight loss, persistent fatigue, generalized swelling, widespread pain, jaundice, recurrent infections, abnormal bleeding, neurological changes, or symptoms involving several organ systems require medical evaluation, since these may reflect autoimmune, endocrine, infectious, malignant, cardiovascular, kidney, or liver disease that should not be managed through broad tonic language alone. An herb's presence in several traditional applications does not establish that it can safely or effectively treat multiple diseases simultaneously, and broad-acting plants may also carry broader interaction potential with prescription medicines.

Agrimony's tannin content may affect gastrointestinal tolerance or medicine absorption in concentrated or prolonged use. Angelica Root contains coumarin-related compounds and requires caution during pregnancy, with anticoagulant or antiplatelet medicines, in bleeding disorders, and with photosensitizing preparations. Nettle Leaf's diuretic activity may be unsuitable in significant kidney disease, heart failure, or alongside prescription diuretics without supervision. Sarsaparilla requires careful species identification, since the common name may refer to different Smilax species or unrelated plants, and controlled human evidence for systemic cleansing or hormone enhancement is limited. Sea Buckthorn's composition varies by plant part (fruit, seed, or pulp oil), so findings from one preparation should not be generalized to all products. Yarrow may trigger allergic reactions in people sensitive to the Asteraceae family and requires caution during pregnancy and with medicines affecting bleeding. For all six herbs, computational network-pharmacology findings should be treated as hypothesis-generating rather than as demonstrated clinical efficacy.

### Research Snapshot

Category XV's scientific value lies primarily in explaining a classification principle: the reference book deliberately assigns no herb here as a Primary Core, keeping the category precise rather than becoming a catch-all for plants described as balancing or generally beneficial. Systems and network pharmacology provide a genuinely useful and active framework for investigating how multiple botanical constituents interact with multiple biological pathways, and research on herbal synergy supports real interactions among constituents within an extract. Agrimony, Angelica Root, Nettle Leaf, Sarsaparilla, Sea Buckthorn, and Yarrow each have distinct, well-documented traditional and scientific profiles in their own right, and their authoritative monographs describe specific, preparation-based traditional indications. Foundational / Systemic Support is best understood as an organizational category describing the breadth of these herbs' traditional roles, with each herb's real evidence base evaluated individually according to its specific preparation and measurable actions.

## 📘 Additional Resources & Continuing Study

Thank you for reading *The Herbal Resurrection: A Foundational Framework for Modern Western Herbal Practice*. This volume was created to serve as a clear, structured, and dependable reference for readers seeking a deeper understanding of herbal traditions and their practical relevance in everyday life.

While this book stands fully on its own as a comprehensive reference, readers who wish to move beyond foundational knowledge into **structured understanding and practical application** may continue their study through the companion materials listed below.

These resources are designed to **extend the system presented in this book**, offering a more guided approach to learning through comparison, pattern recognition, and structured study.

---

## 📚 Available Educational Materials:

**• The Herbal Resurrection Student Workbook**
The primary companion to this volume and the core training instrument of the **Ja'hem™ (Jenkins Herbal Educational Method)**. This workbook introduces a structured, category-based learning system that teaches students how to compare herbs, recognize patterns of imbalance, and understand why one herb is chosen over another. Through guided exercises, visual frameworks, and step-by-step modules, it transforms foundational knowledge into practical understanding.

---

**• The Herbal Resurrection Teacher's Manuals**
Two companion instructional volumes, fully aligned with the Student Workbook and built on the Ja'hem™ (Jenkins Herbal Educational Method). The **Practical Guide** (161 pages) provides a complete module-by-module teaching companion for instructors delivering the Ja'hem™ system in a classroom setting. ISBN: 979-8-9953605-3-7. The **Advanced Clinical Edition** (378 pages) includes everything in the Practical Guide, plus clinical frameworks, instructor psychology tools, and practitioner-level resources for professional herbal education. ISBN: 979-8-9953605-4-4. Available exclusively at herbalresurrection.com.

---

**• The Herbal Resurrection Educational Series (Digital Editions)** *(Upcoming)*
An expanding collection of focused digital guides, each addressing major conditions or categories represented in the medical charts found in this book. These materials will offer deeper exploration, targeted explanations, and organized references for continued study.

---

Information regarding the availability of these materials may be found through official Herbal Resurrection channels, including **herbalresurrection.com**, where readers and educators may follow updates or request additional details.

---

Thank you for adding *The Herbal Resurrection* to your personal or professional library. Whether used for personal reference, family learning, or educational settings, this work was created to bring **clarity, structure, and lasting understanding** to the study of herbs.

# THE HERBAL RESURRECTION'S STUDENT WORKBOOK

The Student Workbook, which is the *companion* to *The Herbal Resurrection*, presents a strikingly *new*, structured, and highly effective way to **teach students and beginners how to understand, compare, and apply herbs with clarity and confidence**.

Rather than relying on memorization of individual plants and their uses, this workbook introduces a **new category-based learning system**, where herbs are studied within the **15 Core Herbal Categories** and understood through direct comparison with **other herbs that serve similar roles**.

This approach allows students to see not only what an herb does, but **why one herb should be chosen over another which is similar to it.**

By learning through **pattern recognition, contrast, and functional grouping**, students develop a deeper and more practical understanding of herbal medicine—one that reflects how herbs are actually selected in real-world use.

Each module is designed to guide the student step-by-step, helping them recognize key distinctions such as:

- **Stimulation vs. calming**
- **Acute vs. long-term support**
- **Deficiency vs. excess**
- **Symptom relief vs. structural support**

Through this structured process, confusion is reduced, patterns become clear, and confidence begins to build naturally.

What makes this workbook stand apart is not simply the information that it contains, but **the way that this information is organized and taught**. It literally transforms herbal study from a scattered collection of facts into a truly coherent system of understanding that **practically anyone is able to learn**.

Students who complete this workbook are not just left with isolated knowledge—**they are equipped with a functional framework** that prepares them for **deeper study**, more **advanced material**, and **practical application**.

In addition, the structure of this workbook makes it especially well-suited for **classroom instruction and guided learning**. Its organized 15 modules, clear comparisons, and built-in reinforcement allow instructors to teach herbal concepts in a logical, step-by-step manner without the confusion often associated with traditional approaches. This makes it easier not only for students to learn—but for educators to teach with clarity and consistency.

This method of learning—**based on categories, comparison, and pattern recognition**—represents a meaningful shift in how herbal knowledge can be taught**. It offers a more structured and accessible pathway that may help shape the future of herbal education**.

The Herbal Resurrection's Student Workbook is one of the few herbal study tools built around a complete educational system rather than a collection of facts. For students, it delivers clarity from the very first module building confidence gradually through structure, comparison, and pattern recognition rather than overwhelming them with information all at once.

For instructors, schools, and herbal educators, it provides **a ready-made teaching framework that is logical, step-by-step, and immediately usable in a classroom setting** without requiring students to have any prior herbal knowledge to begin.

If you are serious about herbal study and want to do more than just read about herbs, then this groundbreaking student workbook, **the Ja'hem**, (which is short for **Jenkins Herbal Educational Method**), is the natural next step on that journey.

The Herbal Resurrection Student Workbook, **The Building Blocks of Practical Modern Herbal Study — The Ja'hem**, is currently available at herbalresurrection.com, Amazon, IngramSpark affiliates and other select book outlets.

To arrange '**Bulk'** or '**Custom**' **Orders** please go to the herbalresurrection.com website for further details.

Full Title: **The Herbal Resurrection: The Building Blocks of Practical Modern Herbal Study — The Official Ja'hem™ Student Workbook**. ISBN: 979-8-9953605-2-0 · Available at herbalresurrection.com, Amazon & IngramSpark and other select book outlets.

## 📘 Teacher's Manuals & Classroom Resources

To support formal instruction and organized study, two companion Teacher's Manuals are available for *The Herbal Resurrection*: the **Practical Guide** and the **Advanced Clinical Edition**. Both are designed for educators, facilitators, and learning communities who wish to teach the system presented in this book within a structured learning environment.

At the center of this system is the **Ja'hem™ (Jenkins Herbal Educational Method)**—a structured approach to learning herbs through **category, comparison, and pattern recognition**, as presented in the **Student Workbook**.

The Student Workbook serves as the **core teaching instrument of the Ja'hem™ system**, guiding students step-by-step through structured comparison, pattern recognition, and applied decision-making. Both Teacher's Manuals are built directly on top of this same foundation, covering all 15 modules and the 52 foundational herbs.

---

**The Practical Guide provides:**

- A six-section structure repeated consistently across all 15 modules
- A pre-session instructor briefing before every module
- Scripted session openings built around real-world scenarios, not definitions
- Quick-reference instructor tables covering all 52 foundational herbs
- Scripted redirects for the four most common student errors per module
- Complete quiz answer keys with wrong-answer guidance
- A three-question readiness check before advancing to the next module
- A reinforcement drill to close and anchor every session

---

**The Advanced Clinical Edition includes everything in the Practical Guide, plus:**

- A full instructor psychology and classroom dynamics section
- Herb-by-herb clinical teaching notes with drug interactions and cautions
- Four scenario exercises per module with complete answer keys
- Clinical decision maps for herb selection under pressure
- Observable module mastery benchmarks
- Three teaching format pacing guides: 15-week, condensed, and self-directed
- A master competency rubric and cross-category bridge for all 15 modules

---

Together, ***The Herbal Resurrection***, the **Student Workbook**, and the **Teacher's Manuals** form a unified and structured educational system.

Rather than relying on memorization or unsupervised application, the Ja'hem™ system trains students to:

- Understand herbs through functional categories
- Recognize patterns of imbalance within the body
- Distinguish between herbs that serve similar roles
- Apply herbal knowledge with clarity, structure, and responsibility

---

This approach supports the development of **health literacy, critical thinking, and disciplined decision-making**, making it suitable for a wide range of learning environments, including:

- Classrooms and academic settings
- Apprenticeship and mentorship programs
- Community herbal education groups
- Structured independent study

---

In addition, the system serves as a **preparatory foundation** for those considering deeper study within the field of herbal medicine. By introducing a clear framework, core categories, and structured learning habits, it allows both students and instructors to assess readiness for more advanced and intensive training.

---

The Practical Guide is built for new instructors, herbal schools, and classroom delivery. The Advanced Clinical Edition is built for experienced educators, clinical programs, and naturopathic training. Both are designed to be practical, instructor-friendly, and fully aligned with the Student Workbook, allowing educators to focus on **guiding students through the learning process rather than constructing curriculum from the ground up**.

Both Teacher's Manuals are available exclusively through official Herbal Resurrection channels, including **herbalresurrection.com**, and are not sold through general retail channels. For institutional licensing or bulk orders, contact the author directly at contact@herbalresurrection.com.

**Ja'hem™ Teacher's Manual — Practical Guide.** ISBN: 979-8-9953605-3-7.

**Ja'hem™ Teacher's Manual — Advanced Clinical Edition.** ISBN: 979-8-9953605-4-4.

# 🌿 Selected Sources & Supporting Context

*The Herbal Resurrection* draws upon a wide landscape of herbal knowledge shaped by long-standing traditions, educational institutions, and publicly available scientific research. While this work is organized and presented through its own independent framework, it exists within a broader continuum of herbal study developed over generations.

**Historical Foundations**

Traditional Western herbalism, Appalachian folk practices, Traditional Chinese Medicine, and Ayurvedic systems have all contributed time-tested observations regarding plant actions, energetics, and practical applications. These historical foundations continue to inform modern herbal understanding and study.

**Modern Botanical & Scientific Context**

General scientific findings related to phytochemistry, active plant constituents, antioxidant activity, immune support, digestive function, circulatory health, and other botanical properties are derived from decades of published research across disciplines including botany, ethnobotany, phytochemistry, and integrative health sciences. This body of publicly accessible research provides contextual support for many commonly discussed herbal concepts.

**Contemporary Herbal Authors & Educators**

The modern herbal landscape has also been shaped by respected educators and authors whose published works are widely used in herbal study and instruction. Among these contributors are:

- **Rosemary Gladstar** — Western herbal educator known for accessible herbal learning
- **David Hoffmann** — Clinical herbalist; author of *Medical Herbalism*
- **Matthew Wood** — Contributor to Western herbal energetics and traditional profiling
- **James Green** — Author of practical herbal preparation guides
- **Michael Tierra** — Founder of Planetary Herbology; integrative TCM and Western perspectives
- **Dr. James A. Duke** — USDA botanist and phytochemical researcher

- **Dr. Vasant Lad** — Ayurvedic educator and author
- **Mark Plotkin, PhD** — Ethnobotanist documenting Amazonian medicinal plant traditions
- **Susun Weed** — Educator associated with the Wise Woman tradition

These individuals represent a cross-section of widely recognized voices within the broader field of herbal education and literature.

**Important Clarification**

The inclusion of the above names is intended solely to acknowledge the broader educational and historical environment surrounding the study of medicinal plants. Their mention does **not** imply endorsement, formal affiliation, editorial contribution, or agreement with the specific interpretations, structure, or educational framework presented in this book.

## The Architecture Behind the 15 Core Herbal Categories

A Unifying Framework for Understanding Herbs

The vast world of herbal medicine can appear overwhelming at first glance. Across cultures, continents, and centuries, thousands of plants have been used to support human health—each described through different languages, traditions, and philosophies. Yet when this global body of knowledge is examined carefully, a remarkable pattern emerges.

Herbs, regardless of where they originate, tend to organize themselves into a limited number of **functional roles** within the human body.

The **15 Core Herbal Categories** presented in *The Herbal Resurrection* arose from the careful observation of these recurring patterns. Rather than being invented arbitrarily, these categories reflect how herbs have consistently been understood, grouped, and applied across the world's major healing traditions.

### A Pattern Seen Across Traditions

Traditional systems such as Western Herbalism, Traditional Chinese Medicine, Ayurveda, Indigenous folk practices, and regional ethnobotanical traditions may differ in terminology and cultural expression, but they repeatedly describe similar herbal actions.

For example:

- Herbs that calm the nerves, ease tension, and support sleep appear in every tradition.
- Herbs that strengthen digestion, improve assimilation, and balance appetite are universally recognized.
- Herbs that support circulation, respiration, immune response, detoxification, hormonal balance, and nourishment appear again and again—regardless of geography.

Though the names change, the **roles remain consistent**.

These repeated groupings reveal that herbs naturally cluster according to how they interact with human physiology—particularly with systems such as the nervous, digestive, immune, cardiovascular, endocrine, respiratory, and eliminative pathways.

### From Observation to Organization

The 15 Core Herbal Categories were formed by comparing shared herbal action patterns across multiple traditions and organizing them into a clear, accessible structure. Each category represents a primary functional role that herbs reliably play within the body.

Rather than focusing on isolated symptoms, this framework emphasizes:
- how herbs behave,
- where they act,
- and what systems they primarily influence.

This approach simplifies learning without oversimplifying the herbs themselves, allowing students and practitioners to understand herbal function more clearly and apply that knowledge with greater confidence.

### A Bridge Between Tradition and Modern Understanding

Modern botanical science, phytochemistry, and physiology have further reinforced what traditional systems observed long ago: herbs contain complex compounds that tend to influence specific biological pathways. While the language of science differs from that of tradition, the underlying patterns often align.

When traditional herbal groupings are viewed alongside modern understandings of bodily systems, the same functional clusters continue to appear—affirming that these categories are not cultural inventions, but reflections of how plants consistently interact with the human body.

### Why the 15 Core Categories Matter

By organizing herbs into these 15 Core Categories, the study of herbal medicine becomes clearer and more approachable. Instead of memorizing hundreds of disconnected plant profiles, learners can begin by understanding **herbal roles**, then see how individual herbs fit within those roles.

**This framework:**

- reduces confusion for beginners,
- creates a shared language for instructors and students,
- and provides a logical foundation for deeper study.

It also explains why a relatively small group of well-chosen herbs can address a wide range of common human imbalances—an idea further explored through the Foundational '52'.

**A Framework for Learning, Not a Shortcut**

The 15 Core Herbal Categories are not meant to replace traditional apprenticeship, clinical training, or guided instruction. Rather, they support it as they provide a **conceptual map**—a way to understand the herbal landscape before navigating it in depth.

This book introduces the architecture of that system. Learning how to apply it skillfully requires structured teaching, guided study, and thoughtful instruction—elements best delivered within educational settings.

What you hold here is the **philosophy and foundation** behind the system. It offers clarity, coherence, and perspective—preparing you to explore the herbs themselves with greater understanding and confidence.

## *Author Biography*

**Fred Vincent Jenkins**, born in Harlem, New York, is the author and principal architect of The Herbal Resurrection series. His work reflects a disciplined commitment to organizing herbal knowledge in a manner that is clear, dependable, and suitable for long-term reference. Guided by years of independent study and a deep respect for both traditional and contemporary herbal traditions, Fred has developed a systematic approach to presenting herbs that prioritizes clarity, safety, simplicity, and practical usefulness.

He is responsible for the organizational framework that defines The Herbal Resurrection, including its core category systems, structured layout, and educational format. His guiding intention has always been to make herbal information accessible to everyday readers and students by presenting it in a clean, consistent, and thoughtfully organized manner.

*His guiding philosophy is simple:*

"Just make sense of it, and they will retain it." — Hizzok and the monkey, 2025

The Herbal Resurrection: A Foundational Framework for Modern Western Herbal Practice brings together historical insight, practical reference, and carefully arranged material into one single comprehensive volume. The work is designed not as an interpretation of herbalism, but as a reliable, structured resource for those seeking to learn from time-tested plant traditions without confusion or fragmentation.

Fred will continue to expand this series through additional reference works and educational projects built upon the same principles of accuracy, clarity, and responsible presentation.

A man of peaceful resolve, he prefers to maintain a low public profile and remain outside of public debate; his contribution, however, to the herbal world lies in the deliberate construction of this comprehensive herbal reference book, which was intended to support readers, teachers, and learning communities for generations to come.

The knowledge of healing must always endure. It must be carried forward—generation after generation—by those willing to keep its light alive.

*The Herbal Resurrection— A Foundational Framework for Modern Western Herbal Practice— together with the many other admirable herbal works that exist today, 'accepts' this responsibility of helping carry that torch forward into the future.*

*The author thanks you for purchasing this book and hopes you find his forthcoming works equally useful and rewarding.*

*See you then.*

For updates, additional materials, and educational resources related to this work, visit: **www.herbalresurrection.com** or contact me directly at contact@herbalresurrection.com

## A special Note to Readers

Thank you for reading *The Herbal Resurrection: A Foundational Framework for Modern Western Herbal Practice.*

If this book has been helpful to you, please consider leaving a brief review on **Amazon, Goodreads, or wherever you purchased this book**— even a few words about your experience can help other people discover the book and decide whether it may benefit them on their own journey toward natural healing and wellness.

Your feedback helps support this work and helps keep the tradition of herbal knowledge alive for generations to come.

With gratitude,
**Fred V. Jenkins**
Author, *The Herbal Resurrection*

## 🌿 For Those Who Wish to Study Herbalism Further — Around the World

Herbal wisdom belongs to no single culture or land. It is one of humanity's oldest systems of observation and one of the Earth's most enduring languages of healing. Across every continent, dedicated teachers, schools, and traditions continue to preserve, teach, and refine the study of medicinal plants.

For readers who wish to pursue formal or guided study beyond this volume, the following examples represent a small cross-section of respected herbal learning paths and educational centers from around the world.

### 🌎 North America

- **The Herbal Academy** (Online, USA) — Modern herbal education from foundational through advanced levels
- **Chestnut School of Herbal Medicine** (Asheville, North Carolina, USA) — Garden-based study and traditional medicine-making
- **East West School of Planetary Herbology** (California, USA) — Integrative Western, Ayurvedic, and Chinese herbal traditions
- **Dominion Herbal College** (British Columbia, Canada) — Canada's oldest herbal school offering diploma and distance programs

### 🌍 Europe

- **College of Naturopathic Medicine (CNM)** (UK, Ireland, Germany) — Herbal medicine and natural health diplomas
- **Heartwood — School of Herbal Medicine** (England) — Traditional clinical herbal practice and materia medica
- **Université Européenne des Savoirs Botaniques** (France) — Botanical tradition and phytotherapy studies
- **European Herbal & Traditional Medicine Practitioners Association (EHTPA)** — Professional association supporting herbal practitioners

🌏 **Asia**

- **Ayurveda Colleges and Gurukuls** (India) — Classical training in Ayurvedic herbal medicine
- **Traditional Chinese Medicine Universities** (China & Taiwan) — Comprehensive study of herbal pharmacology and theory
- **Kampo Medicine Schools** (Japan) — Japanese refinement of classical Chinese herbal formulas
- **Thai Traditional Medicine Programs** (Thailand) — Study of Thai herbal systems and traditional healing arts

🌍 **Africa**

- **African Natural Medicine Programs** (Ghana, Nigeria, South Africa) — Indigenous plant medicine and ethnobotany
- **University of the Western Cape — Department of Pharmacy** (South Africa) — Research in African medicinal plants
- **Traditional Healers Organizations** (South Africa) — Preservation of ethical and culturally rooted healing traditions

🌎 **Latin America & the Caribbean**

- **Instituto Latinoamericano de Plantas Medicinales** (Peru) — Amazonian and Andean herbal traditions
- **Centro de Plantas Medicinales y Etnobotánica** (Costa Rica) — Rainforest ethnobotany and sustainable harvesting
- **The Healing Forest School** (Belize) — Immersive study honoring Maya herbal medicine

🌏 **Oceania**

- **Australasian College of Natural Therapies (ACNT)** (Australia) — Herbal and naturopathic sciences

- **New Zealand School of Herbal Medicine (NZSHM)** — Herbal diploma programs rooted in Pacific and European traditions

**Important Note:**
This list is provided for general informational purposes only. Inclusion does not imply endorsement, affiliation, or recommendation. Herbal traditions, schools, and teaching methods vary widely, and prospective students are encouraged to research programs carefully and choose study paths that align with their values, goals, and local regulations.

---

## 🏵 A Final Word

No matter where you study, remember that every herbal tradition — African, Asian, European, Pacific, or American — is a thread within one great tapestry of healing.

Honor your teachers —

Honor the land —

Honor the plants that make this study possible.

"The more you learn, the more this green world of ours will teach you."

---

**Closing Reflection & Disclaimer**

This book is intended for educational and informational purposes only. It is not designed to diagnose, treat, cure, or prevent disease, nor is it a substitute for professional medical advice. Always consult a qualified healthcare provider before beginning any new health regimen, especially if you are pregnant, nursing, taking medications, or managing chronic conditions. With that understanding, may this book serve as a reminder of the enduring wisdom carried forward through the plants of the earth. Herbs have accompanied humanity since ancient times, offering balance, resilience, and renewal. As you close these pages, may you carry with you not only a deeper appreciation for traditional plant knowledge, but also a renewed sense of connection to the natural world from which it all arose.

***Excelsior***

***For additional information, educational use, or inquiries:***
***www.herbalresurrection.com***
***or contact me directly at fred@herbalresurrection.com***

*FVJ — 2025 [Hizzok]*

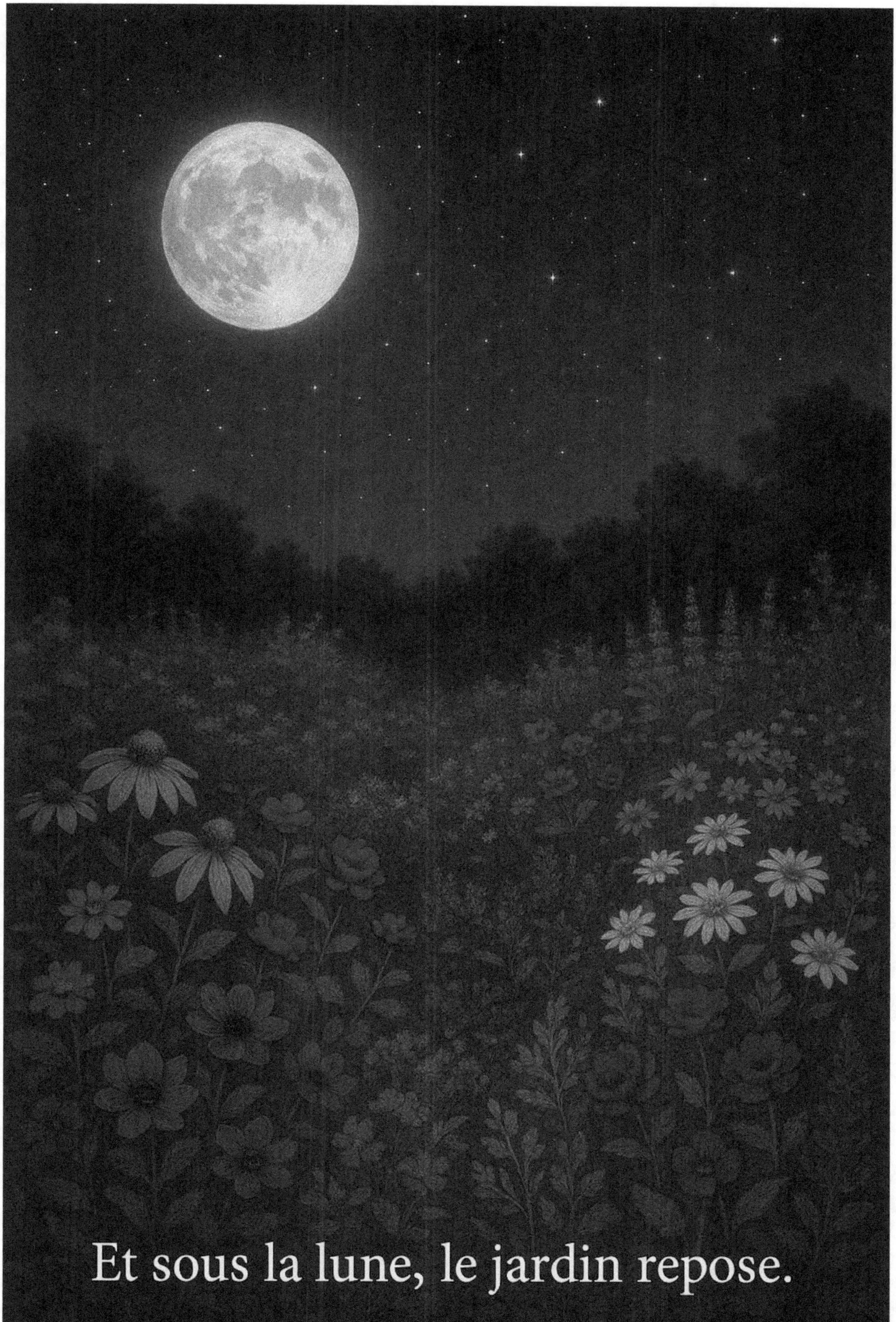
Et sous la lune, le jardin repose.

## YOUR NOTES

www.ingramcontent.com/pod-product-compliance
Lightning Source LLC
LaVergne TN
LVHW060006210926
848481LV00013B/3660
* 9 7 9 8 9 9 5 3 6 0 5 0 6 *